WILLIAM DE MONTIBUS (c. 1140-1213)

The Schools and the Literature of Pastoral Care

by Joseph Goering

The most famous teacher in England during the late twelfth and early thirteenth centuries was William de Montibus. He taught "sacred doctrine" (Bible, theology, morals) at Paris and then, for some thirty years, in the cathedral school at Lincoln. A contemporary described him as "almost the equal of Gregory the Great and Augustine," an exaggerated yet credible assertion in an age that valued encyclopedic learning.

Part One of this study assesses William's life and works and uses the evidence of his teaching at Paris and Lincoln to explore the transition from schools to universities that took place during his lifetime. It also examines William's place in the creation of a new type of didactic literature: "pastoralia," or the popular literature of pastoral care.

Among the primary sources used for this study, William's voluminous writings have a prominent place. Some fifteen treatises in verse and prose together with 149 sermons have been identified and are discussed in Part Two. Six of the shorter texts are printed in working editions based on one or more manuscripts. The remaining texts are represented here in extensive transcriptions and with systematic descriptions of their contents and context. It is hoped that this detailed study of William's writings will stimulate further research into his work and that of his contemporaries, and that it will foster an appreciation of the scholastic and popular culture of the time.

STUDIES AND TEXTS 108

WILLIAM DE MONTIBUS
(c. 1140-1213)
The Schools and the Literature of Pastoral Care

BY

JOSEPH GOERING

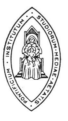

PONTIFICAL INSTITUTE OF MEDIAEVAL STUDIES

Acknowledgment

This book has been published with the help of a grant
from the Canadian Federation for the Humanities, using
funds provided by the Social Sciences and Humanities
Research Council of Canada

CANADIAN CATALOGUING IN PUBLICATION DATA

William, de Montibus, ca. 1140-1213
  William de Montibus (c. 1140-1213) : the schools and the literature
of pastoral care

(Studies and texts, ISSN 0082-5328 ; 108)
Includes extracts in Latin.
Includes bibliographical references and index.
ISBN 0-88844-108-8

1. Pastoral theology — Early works to 1900.
2. William, de Montibus, ca. 1140-1213.   I. Goering, Joseph Ward,
1947- .   II. Pontifical Institute of Mediaeval Studies.   III. Title.
IV. Series: Studies and texts (Pontifical Institute of Mediaeval Studies) ;
108.

BV4009.W55 1992   253   C91-095454-2

© 1992 by
Pontifical Institute of Mediaeval Studies
59 Queen's Park Crescent East
Toronto, Ontario, Canada M5S 2C4

PRINTED BY UNIVERSA, WETTEREN, BELGIUM

For

Fr. Hugh MacKinnon († 1982)
Richard W. Hunt († 1979)
Leonard E. Boyle O.P.

Contents

Preface

Modern histories of medieval scholasticism and of popular religion have distinct origins. The one began with research into developments of doctrine and the writings of the great schoolmen. The other began at the bottom, with collections of the remnants of "folk religion," pious (and not-so-pious) superstitions, and popular customs. Benefitting from the successes and failures of earlier scholarship, both types of history are flourishing today. A tacit assumption underlying much of the current research is that the one has little to do with the other. It would seem that two different worlds and two different types of experience, "learned" and "popular" respectively, are under investigation, and that the student of one need scarcely be concerned with understanding the other.

The present study attempts to identify and explore some of the middle ground. It grew out of the question: "What, if anything, does scholastic theology have to do with popular religion?" At Toronto's Pontifical Institute of Mediaeval Studies and Centre for Medieval Studies I was introduced to the popular theology of medieval Europe and wrote a dissertation whose unwieldy title began: "The Popularization of Scholastic Ideas in Thirteenth-Century England." A figure who loomed in the background of that research was William de Montibus, a master of theology in twelfth-century Paris and chancellor of Lincoln Cathedral until his death in 1213. William's credentials as a schoolman are impeccable. He taught in the Paris schools when Paris was becoming the most important centre for scholastic theology in Europe, and he established at Lincoln the most famous theological school of the time in England. If he is relatively unknown among historians of scholasticism, it is probably because, as Richard Hunt shrewdly observed, "his speculative bent can hardly have been great." Like his contemporaries at Paris, Peter Comestor and Peter the Chanter, William seems to have been little interested in solving speculative problems or in contributing to the definition and development of theological doctrine. Indeed, very few schoolmen in any period were famous or highly respected for such contributions. William's reputation was, instead, that of an outstanding teacher of theology. With his contemporaries in the proto-universities and the diocesan schools, William helped to create new standards of theological education, and to make scholastic theology accessible to a wider audience.

But does this "popular" scholastic theology have anything to do with "popular religion" — with the day-to-day religious experiences of medieval villagers and townspeople? This is a complex question that admits no easy answers. Certainly we cannot presume to find in the writings of the schoolmen direct evidence for the thoughts, beliefs, and values of the common people. Studying even the popular teachings and sermons of the clergy can be no substitute for sensitive investigations of the traditional rites, rituals, and folklore of the towns and villages. Yet it is equally absurd for the student of popular culture to ignore the vast and largely untapped sources of pastoral and practical writings emanating from the schools. Many of the clerics who wrote and studied this literature were, themselves, only little removed from their local communities and traditional religious practices. Nor can we assume that simple peasants and villagers lacked interest in "learned" theology, or that they were isolated from the teachings of the schools. The available evidence suggests that attendance at sermons and at confession, places where scholastic teachings were disseminated, was a form of popular recreation in the thirteenth century rather than a duty imposed by religious authorities. Even popular heresies, so seductive on the Continent if not in England during William's time, imply an alertness among the unschooled to the intellectual and moral questions that were current among the learned. Perhaps we can imagine "learned" and "popular" religion not as two separate and distinct categories but as the two ends of a spectrum. In studying the life and writings of William de Montibus we will find ourselves in the learned portion of the spectrum, but shading perceptibly toward the colours of popular religion.

In the spring of 1982 I approached Father Hugh MacKinnon with a proposal to update his Oxford D.Phil. dissertation on William de Montibus (1957) and to prepare it for publication. We met once in the fall to discuss plans for the project, but his untimely death that winter ended our collaboration. During the succeeding years the work has taken on a new shape and new emphases, but I trust Father Hugh would be pleased with the result.

Part One of this monograph consists of three chapters. The first describes William's life: his early training, his sojourn in Paris and return to Lincoln c. 1185, and his activities as chancellor of the cathedral until his death in 1213.

Chapter Two presents the evidence for William's teaching activities, first on Mont Ste. Geneviève outside Paris and then on the "mountain" of Lincoln. The rich evidence for William's teaching in the Lincoln schools is particularly valuable, and adds significantly to our appreciation of the educational enterprise in diocesan schools before the rise of the universities.

Chapter Three examines William's role in the invention and dissemination of a practical literature of pastoral care. Like Peter the Chanter, Alan of Lille, Gerald of Wales, and others, William was at the beginning of a movement that sought to popularize scholastic teachings and make them accessible to students who wished to learn the "art of arts," the pastoral care of souls. By analyzing the audiences, techniques, and content of pastoral literature as it developed in the late twelfth and thirteenth centuries, I have sought to specify the ways in which William and his contemporaries contributed to this literature, and the limitations of their contributions.

Part Two of this study makes William's fifteen works and 149 of his sermons accessible to scholars for the first time. Six of his treatises are edited here in their entirety : *Peniteas cito* (and gloss), *Errorum eliminatio*, *Tractatus metricus de sacramentis*, *Speculum penitentis*, *De penitentia religiosorum*, and *Epistola ad moniales*. The remaining works are represented by extensive transcriptions designed to convey a full and accurate impression of the contents of each.

Of the many debts incurred in writing this book, the first is owed to Hugh MacKinnon. Father MacKinnon was professor and chairman of the Department of History at the University of Waterloo in Ontario, Canada. A popular teacher and a vibrant presence on the campus, he was also an assistant pastor at St. Teresa's Church in Elmira and, during summer holidays, served as pastor of St. Mary's parish in Huntsville, Ontario. He died in Mexico City at the age of 62, on 28 December 1982. The only editorial decision that we had made together before his death was, at his suggestion, that our book be dedicated to our respective teachers, Richard W. Hunt at Oxford University and Father Leonard E. Boyle at the Pontifical Institute in Toronto.

Colleagues (both students and staff) in many different disciplines have contributed significantly to the final shape of this book. I can acknowledge here only the greater debts : the thoughtful comments and criticisms from John W. Baldwin, Peter Binkley, Jean Hoff, Osmund Lewry, George Rigg, Giulio Silano, and Robert Sweetman. Leonard Boyle has been on leave of absence from Toronto during the writing of this book, but his influence can be found on every page. To Jennifer Rigg, whose nickname for William de Montibus, "Hill-

Billy," has lightened the load of scholarship, goes a special vote of thanks. Finally, I wish to thank the Social Sciences and Humanities Research Council of Canada for their generous financial support, and the libraries and librarians of Europe and North America who have welcomed me into their facilities, provided microfilms of manuscripts in their care, and cheerfully answered my queries. In partial repayment of all these debts I offer this book on the life and writings of William de Montibus.

William was thought to have imitated the bees in drawing raw materials from diverse fields and transforming these into delightful nourishment stored in the honeycombs of his treatises (see pp. 26-27). The bees that found their way into this book were provided by my colleague Heather Phillips.

Toronto

Part One

The Life and Work of
William de Montibus

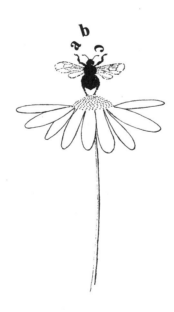

Chapter One

The Life

Early Years

William de Montibus studied and taught in Paris during the twelfth century; he died in Scotland in 1213; but his career began and ended in the English city of Lincoln. There he was probably born, there he lived the last three decades of his life, and there he was buried. The city of Lincoln, on the western fringe of England's fenlands, was a thriving commercial and ecclesiastical centre in the twelfth century.[1] It boasted busy markets and wharves, and numerous wealthy citizens, many of them involved in the lucrative wool trade. The Cathedral Church of St. Mary, crowning the steep hill above the river Witham, was the administrative and spiritual headquarters of England's largest diocese. Sharing the walled enclosure of an old Roman fortress with the royal castle, the cathedral dominated the city both geographically and culturally. In its service William de Montibus spent the most productive years of his life, teaching theology in the schools and sharing in the pastoral and administrative life of the community.

The town itself extended south, down the hill from Lincoln Cathedral and castle, as far as the river Witham. Across the river began the suburb of Wigford, on either side of the main road leading south to London.[2] Many of Lincoln's most important citizens lived or owned land in this

---

[1] See Francis Hill, *Medieval Lincoln* (Cambridge: Cambridge University Press, 1948); Dorothy M. Owen, *Church and Society in Medieval Lincolnshire*, History of Lincolnshire, 5 (Lincoln: History of Lincolnshire Committee, 1971); Graham Platts, *Land and People of Lincolnshire*, History of Lincolnshire, 4 (Lincoln: History of Lincolnshire Committee, 1985).

[2] The best description of this suburb is in B.J.J. Gilmour and D.A. Stocker, *St. Mark's Church and Cemetery*, The Archaeology of Lincoln, vol. 13-1 (Council for British Archaeology: London, 1986), pp. 1-4.

suburb.[3] One of these families bore the surname "de Montibus," thus raising the possibility that William was born within sight of the cathedral where he would spend the latter part of his life.

A thirteenth-century charter in the cartulary of Thurgarton Priory naming "Master William de Montibus" suggests that his family held land in St. Edward's parish, Wigford, and was connected with the rich and powerful in Lincoln. It records a grant of land to the church of St. Peter, Thurgarton, subject to a rent payable to Agnes, the niece of Master William de Montibus. This Agnes was the widow of one important citizen of Lincoln, William of Tattershall, and the daughter of another, James Brand.[4]

The next charter in the cartulary concerns this same property in Wigford, and specifies that it is situated next to the land of a William, son of Richard.[5] This William is not "Magister Willelmus," but he was probably of the de Montibus family, as appears from two other references in the contemporary records. The Final Concords of the County of Lincoln for 1256-1257 record the suit of William, son of Richard de Montibus, and his wife Agnes concerning land in Wigford.[6]

---

[3] Hill, *Medieval Lincoln*, pp. 385-396.

[4] "Omnibus sancte matris etc., Thomas Sampson de Epirston' miles salutem in Domino. Noverit universitas vestra me caritatis intuitu assensu et voluntate Marie uxoris mee pro salute anime mee et antecessorum meorum et pro salute anime Marie uxoris mee concessisse dedisse et hac presenti carta mea confirmasse Deo et ecclesie beati Petri de Thurg' et precipue ad inveniendum lumen in celebracione divinorum ad altare beate et gloriose virginis et ad suum officium cotidianum deputatum inperpetuum terram quam habui in civitate Lincoln' in vico de Wykesford' in parochia sancti Edwardi, illam quam emi pecunia mea munerata de Philipo filio Reinphari le tanur, reddendo inde annuatim unam marcam argenti Agneti nepoti Magistri Willelmi de Montibus et filie Jacobi Brand' quondam uxori Willelmi de Tatershale ..."; Southwell Minster (Notts.) Library MS 3, fol. 155v. I am indebted to Dr. Trevor Foulds for information concerning this cartulary, which he has edited in his unpublished PhD thesis: "Thurgarton Priory and Its Benefactors with an Edition of the Cartulary," 3 vols., University of Nottingham, 1984.

[5] "Universis sancte matris etc., Maria quondam uxor Thome Sampson' salutem eternam in Domino. Noverit universitas vestra me in libera et propria potestate et viduitate mea concessisse dedisse et hac carta mea confirmasse pro salute anime mee et pro anima viri mei et omnium antecessorum et successorum meorum ... terram quam habui in civitate Lincoln' in parochia sancti Edwardi, illam scilicet que aliquando fuit Philipi filii Romphari, que quidem jacet inter Reginaldum Faldecake et Willelmum filium Ricardi. Tenendam et habendam eisdem canonicis in liberam et perpetuam elemosinam faciendo servicium quod ad predictam terram pertinet ..."; ibid, fol. 155v.

[6] *Final Concords of the County of Lincoln*, ed. C.W. Foster (Horncastle: Lincoln Record Society, 1920), 2: 148-149, no. 64: "Between William son of Richard de Montibus, and Agnes his wife, plaintiffs, and Walter abbot of Revesby, tenant, of 2 parts of 1 messuage in the suburb of Lincoln ... . Plea. William and Agnes have acknowledged the whole messuage to be the right of the abbot and his church, and

This same, or another, William de Montibus, son of Richard of Wigford, is mentioned as also holding land in the "Bail" of the city. A quitclaim in the register of Barlings Abbey records the gift of William de Montibus, son of Richard of Wigford, of the return from some houses rented there by a Master Simon.[7] A later Thurgarton charter records the heirs of one Thomas de Monte still holding land and buildings in St. Edward's parish, Wigford, circa 1280.[8]

These documents bear witness to a family, known in the thirteenth century by the surname "de Montibus," that owned property in Lincoln and in the suburban parish of St. Edward, Wigford, and to Master William de Montibus as one of the members of that family. The origins of the family's surname "de Montibus" or "de Monte," however, are obscure. Was William born with this name, or was it a sobriquet that he earned during his teaching career and that was subsequently extended to the rest of his family?[9]

---

have quitclaimed it from themselves and the heirs of Agnes to the abbot and his successors and his church for ever. And for this the abbot has given them 6 marks of silver."

[7] "Omnibus Christi fidelibus ad quos presens scriptum peruenerit, Willelmus de Montibus, filius Ricardi de Wykeford, salutem. Nouerit uniuersitas uestra me remisisse et omnino in perpetuum de me et heredibus meis siue assignatis quietum clamasse Deo et ecclesie beate Marie de Barlinges, idest abbati et canonicis ibidem Deo seruientibus annuum redditum xii den. et quicquid mihi uel heredibus meis quocumque casu inde in posterum accidere poterit, quos iidem abbas et conuentus mihi annuatim soluere tenebantur, de quibusdam domibus in ballio Linc' quas magister Symon de Tresk cementario tenet de eisdem ...''; London, British Library Cotton MS Faustina B.i, fol. 57v. I thank Dr. A.J. Prescott of the British Library for providing the correct reference to this document and a photostatic copy of the original.

[8] "Frater Robertus prior de Thurg' ... . Noverit universitas vestra nos unanimi consensu capituli nostri dedisse et concessisse et hac carta nostra confirmasse Willelmo de Berithby et Agneti uxori sue et Willelmo de Broketon' et Isabelle uxori sue unum mesuagium in villa Lincoln' cum edificiis suis jacentem in vico qui vocatur Wykefford' in parochia sancti Edwardi juxta toftum quod Johannes carpentarius tenet de eisdem Willelmo et Willelmo et eorum uxoribus, quod quidem mesuagium se extendit a regali via usque ad aquam. Tenendum et habendum de nobis et successoribus nostris ... reddendo sacristarie nostre dimidiam marcam ad duos anni terminos, scilicet ad festum sancti Michaelis iij solidos et iiij denarios ad Pascha iij solidos et heredibus Thome de Monte de Lincoln' unam marcam annuatim ad eosdem terminos pro omnibus serviciis exaccionibus et demandis saluo quocumque tallagio si debeatur ...''; Southwell Minster Library MS 3, fol. 155v.

[9] The surname "de Leicester," applied to William by, for example, W.E. Rhodes in his entry "William de Leicester, or William du Mont" in the *Dictionary of National Bibliography* (London: Smith, Elder and Co., 1909), 21: 363-364, has no basis in medieval documents. The error seems to have arisen with John Bale, whose *Scriptorum illustrium maioris Brytannie ... Catalogus* (Basel, 1557-1559), p. 258, refers to "Guilhelmus Leycestrius, a montibus alii cognominant." Bale altered his *Index Britanniae scriptorum*, ed. Reginald L. Poole and M. Bateson (Oxford, 1902), p. 130

Gerald of Wales asserts that Master William was known as William de Monte because he had lectured on Mont Ste. Geneviève in Paris.[10] It was not uncommon for twelfth-century scholastics to draw a surname from the place in which they taught.[11] Alberic de Monte, one of John of Salisbury's teachers, seems to have received his name from the same mountain — Ste. Geneviève.[12] Alexander Neckam plays on the names "de Monte" and "de Montibus" in his eulogy of William in the *Laus sapientie divine* by describing him as a "montanist" (i.e. one who taught on Mont Ste. Geneviève) who left that mount to teach on the "mountain" of Lincoln (i.e. the cathedral close overlooking the city): "Transiit ad montem Montanus, monte relicto."[13] It might be inferred from this text that William was first known in Paris by the surname "de Monte," and that sometime after his return to Lincoln the name was modified to "de Montibus" in acknowledgment of his fame as a teacher of theology on both "mountains." Extant documents refer to William both as "de Monte" and "de Montibus," and although the latter form comes to predominate during the thirteenth century, no

accordingly, adding the words "Leycestre de montibus dictus" over the entry "Guilhelmus Lincolniensis ecclesie cancellarius." Bale did not derive his information from John Leland, who wrote in his *Commentarii de scriptoribus Britannicis* (Oxford, 1709), p. 273: "De Gulielmo Montano. Gulielmus Montanus, theologiae cognitionis professor, inter canonicis supremae Lindiorum urbis celeberrimus vixit; et cancellarii in eadem ecclesia dignitate functus est." The error was doubtless fostered in Bale's mind by a confusion in medieval copies of the very popular *Summa Qui bene presunt*, written by Richard of Leicester, a student of William's, and sometimes ascribed to William.

[10] "Ubi [Lincolniam] sanius atque salubrius in Anglia theologicam scientiam vigere cognovit, sub doctore peroptimo magistro Willelmo de Monte dicto, quoniam in monte S. Genovefae Parisiis legerat, quem etiam ibi archidiaconus tunc noverat, studii causa Lincolniam adivit," *De rebus a se gestis, libri III*, ed. J.S. Brewer, Rolls Series, 21/1 (London: Longman, 1861), p. 93.

[11] For example, the *parvipontani* were those associated with schools on the Petit Pont in Paris, and the *montani* or "montanists" were those associated with schools on Mont Ste. Geneviève. See R.W. Southern, "The Schools of Paris and the School of Chartres," in *Renaissance and Renewal in the Twelfth Century*, ed. Robert L. Benson, Giles Constable, and Carol Lanham (Cambridge MA: Harvard University Press, 1982), p. 114.

[12] R.B.C. Huygens, "Guillaume de Tyr étudiant," *Latomus* 21 (1962) 822, 826.

[13] "Contulit huic primam cathedram Genovefa, secundam
    Mater virgo, sacrae virginitatis honos.
    Transiit ad montem Montanus, monte relicto ... ."

Alexandri Neckam De naturis rerum libri duo. With the Poem of the Same Author, De laudibus divinae sapientiae, ed. Thomas Wright, Rolls Series, 34 (London: Longman, 1863), p. 460. Alexander's reference to the "Mount" of Lincoln is not entirely fanciful; two Lincoln parish churches, St. Andrew's and St. Michael's, bore the epithet "de Monte," apparently to distinguish them from churches dedicated to the same patrons in the suburb of Wigford below the town; see Hill, *Medieval Lincoln*, pp. 111-113.

clear chronological development from singular to plural (as implied by Alexander's story) can be documented.

Whether the surname originated in this way and was thence extended to other members of his family, or whether Gerald and Alexander are simply indulging in rhetorical play on the name which William inherited from his forebears remains a matter of speculation. It is certain, however, that William had relatives in the Lincoln suburb of Wigford who were known by the surname "de Montibus" in the thirteenth century, and who can be presumed to have been settled there in the twelfth century, at the time of William's birth.

The date of his birth, like that of most individuals of the time, is unknown. Gerald of Wales knew him as a master of theology in Paris sometime between 1176 and 1179.[14] Alexander Neckam also may have known William at Paris during the years 1175-1182.[15] If William was a master of theology in 1176, when both Gerald and Alexander were in Paris, he must have already reached his mid thirties. The statutes of Paris of 1215 decree a minimum age of thirty-five for masters of theology,[16] and although this statute was not binding on the twelfth-century schools, it surely reflects a common consensus that a master of theology should be of mature years. If William was roughly thirty-five years of age in 1175, he would have been born around 1140. According to such an estimate he would have been in his seventies at his death in 1213. This is not unlikely. Two of William's acquaintances are known to have lived considerably longer — St. Gilbert of Sempringham died in 1189 at the age of more than one-hundred, and Robert Grosseteste was aged eighty or more at his death in 1253.

St. Gilbert of Sempringham

William's early formation in Lincolnshire had been only a matter for speculation until Albinia de la Mare published her catalogue of the

---

[14] See above, n. 10; Gerald studied in Paris twice, c. 1165-1172 and 1176-1179, but he describes himself as "archdeacon" when he knew William, a title that he acquired in 1175; see Robert Bartlett, *Gerald of Wales 1146-1223* (Oxford: Clarendon Press, 1982), p. 29.

[15] See above, n. 13. For the dates of Alexander's studies in Paris see Richard W. Hunt, *The Schools and the Cloister: The Life and Writings of Alexander Nequam (1157-1217)*, ed. and rev. Margaret Gibson (Oxford: Clarendon Press, 1984), pp. 2-5.

[16] "Circa statum theologorum statuimus, quod nullus Parisius legat citra tricesimum quintum etatis sue annum," *Chartularium Universitatis Parisiensis, Tomus I: Ab anno MCC usque ad annum MCCLXXXVI*, ed. Heinrich Denifle and E.L.M. Chatelain (Paris, 1889), p. 79.

Lyell manuscripts in Oxford's Bodleian Library. In her detailed summary of the contents of Lyell MS 8, she noted a "sermon" by William de Montibus directed to nuns of the Gilbertine Order.[17] In this sermon or pastoral letter William tells the nuns that he, too, owes a great debt to St. Gilbert of Sempringham, "that venerable master and father Gilbert." William had himself been a young boy (*puer*) in Gilbert's household: "Ego itaque patrisfamilias predicti puer."[18] Gilbert, like other important ecclesiastics of the period, had an extended household in which boys were educated and trained for service to the Church. Indeed, an extant charter of the Gilbertine House at Ormsby was witnessed by one William, *puer* of Master Gilbert.[19] This William, of course, need not be William de Montibus, but the document confirms the existence and the importance of *pueri* in Gilbert's household, and gives substance to William's claim of having been a member of that *familia*.

William was to work closely with several saints during his career, but his experience in Gilbert of Sempringham's household was particularly important and was to have a lasting influence on his life and thought. In many ways William's *curriculum vitae* paralleled St. Gilbert's. We are told, for example, that Gilbert left England as a youth to study the liberal arts and theology (*liberalibus et spiritualibus studiis*) in France, where he became a master. He then returned to his native Lincolnshire and began to teach the boys and girls of his province, instructing them in the rudiments of the schools and in moral and monastic discipline.[20]

In a general way, these same words describe William's life. Like Gilbert, he chose to pursue a career as a teacher, and, travelling to France for his training, became a Master there. Upon his return to England, William also devoted himself to teaching that conveyed the rudiments of the liberal arts and scholastic theology while emphasizing practical instruction in a moral and quasi-monastic way of life. He

---

[17] Albinia de la Mare, *Catalogue of the Collection of Medieval Manuscripts Bequeathed to the Bodleian Library Oxford by James P.R. Lyell* (Oxford: Clarendon Press, 1971), pp. 17-18.

[18] Printed below, *Epistola ad moniales*, II.6.

[19] "Hiis testibus magistro Giliberto de Sempyngham ... Willelmo et Herveio et Waltero atque Roberto pueris magistri Gilberti," *Transcripts of Charters relating to the Gilbertine Houses of Sixle, Ormsby, Catley, Bullington and Alvingham*, ed. Frank M. Stenton, Lincoln Record Society, 18 (Horncastle: Morton and Sons, 1922), p. 62. The charter can be dated 1155 x 1189.

[20] *The Book of St Gilbert*, ed. Raymonde Foreville and Gillian Keir (Oxford: Clarendon Press, 1987), pp. 12-16.

was imbued by his paterfamilias with a respect not only for those who chose a cloistered life, like the nuns of the Gilbertine Order, but also for those who led an active life in the world according to the principles of monastic or "religious" discipline.

As a *puer* in Gilbert's household William would have received a grounding in the liberal arts and classical literature as well as an introduction to theological studies. In particular he would have encountered the writings of the twelfth-century English Cistercians with whom Gilbert was closely associated.[21] One work, the *Centum sententiae* of the Cistercian Walter Daniel, may have served William later as a model for his most popular publication, the *Numerale*.[22] No doubt in these years he also learned the art of versification. The ability to transpose doctrine (whether the Bible, or the wisdom and teachings of philosophers, poets, and common people) into verse was widely cultivated in this period, and William became quite proficient. Later, as a master of theology, he used such verses as the basis of much of his teaching, and he left among his writings a number of important collections of didactic poetry.[23]

After his early education in England, William decided, like Gilbert before him, to pursue an academic career in France. He might have studied at any number of schools that flourished on the Continent in the middle of the twelfth century; Paris was not yet the mecca of scholastic theology that it would become in succeeding decades. Nevertheless, we can be fairly certain that he studied in Paris under several masters, including Peter Comestor.[24]

THEOLOGIAN IN PARIS

It is in the suburbs of Paris, as a master of theology, that we first encounter William in the published sources. Gerald of Wales met William during his stay in Paris between 1176 and 1179, and reports

[21] See ibid., pp. xv-xx, 40-47. On the English Cistercians see C.J. Holdsworth, "John of Ford and English Cistercian Writing 1167-1214," *Transactions of the Royal Historical Society*, 5th series, 11 (1961) 117-136.

[22] C.H. Talbot, "The *Centum Sententiae* of Walter Daniel," *Sacris erudiri* 11 (1960) 266-383. See below, *Numerale*, II.7.

[23] See below, the *Peniteas cito*, *Tractatus metricus*, *Versarius*, *Collecta*, II.1, 3, 12, 15.

[24] In his early writings, William sometimes refers to his own masters. One such reference, in sermon no. 3, (p. 527), implies that Peter Comestor was one of William's teachers. William's name is also associated with Comestor's in a collection of disputed questions from Paris, see below, Chapter Two, at note 29.

that William was teaching on Mont Ste. Geneviève just outside of the city.[25] Alexander Neckam, who also knew William in Paris, reports unambiguously that the school on the "Mount" of Paris was William's first. After praising William as "a stable mountain, a pillar of the faith," whose life was devoted to the study of theology (*coelestis pagina*) and to teaching both faith and morals, he tells us that Ste. Geneviève gave to William his first teaching chair and the Blessed Virgin (the Cathedral Church of St. Mary, Lincoln) his second.[26]

No records survive of William's continental education before he began to teach on Mont Ste. Geneviève. Gilbert of Sempringham may have financed his studies, or perhaps William relied on family money for support. Nothing suggests that he enjoyed the income of a clerical benefice during his stay on the Continent.

William's appearance on Mont Ste. Geneviève has led some to conclude that he became a canon of the monastery there, and to identify him with a William, prior of the abbey of Ste. Geneviève, who flourished at the same time.[27] Prior William, however, is known to have died on September 30 of an unspecified year, whereas William de Montibus's death in the spring of 1213 is well attested.[28] Rather, we can presume that William de Montibus was one of the growing number of independent scholars and students converging on Paris at this time, and that he opened a private, theological school on the "Mount" in the 1170's.

---

[25] "... in monte s. Genovefae Parisiis legerat, quem etiam ibi archidiaconus tunc noverat," see above, note 10.

[26] "Lindisiae columen Lincolnia siue columna,
    Munifica, felix gente, repleta bonis,
    Par tibi nulla foret, si te tuus ille magister
    Informaret adhuc moribus atque fide.
    Montanus, sed mons stabilis fideique columna,
    Cui se coelestis pagina tota dedit.
    Montanus, meritis, pius, et servator honesti,
    Veraque simplicitas digna favore fuit.
    Contulit huic primam cathedram Genovefa, secundam
    Mater virgo, sacrae virginitatis honos.
    Transiit ad montem Montanus, monte relicto;
    En montana Syon et loca celsa tenet.
    Haec digressio sit signum seu testis amoris;
    Condigna fateor laus erit ista minor."
    Alexandri Neckam De naturis rerum, p. 460.

[27] Gerald M. Paré, A. Brunet, and P. Tremblay, *La renaissance du XIIe siècle: Les écoles et l'enseignement* (Ottawa: Institut d'Etudes Médiévales, 1933), p. 36, n. 2.

[28] The death of Prior William is recorded in the obituary of the abbey of Ste. Geneviève: *Obituaires de la province de Sens*, Recueil des historiens de la France, 1, ed. Auguste Molinier (Paris: Imprimerie nationale, 1902), p. 511.

While in Paris, William would have been in contact with Peter Comestor, the most famous theologian of the period, and Peter's chosen successor, Peter of Poitiers, as well as many other masters about whom we still know very little.[29]

William was a contemporary of another Parisian theologian whose fame was to be widespread by the end of the century, Peter the Chanter. The respective careers of these two masters deserve comparison. Both began teaching theology at Paris in the 1170's, Peter perhaps as early as 1173 and William by around 1176.[30] Both composed alphabetically arranged *distinctiones* on biblical and moral topics, and both wrote *summae* on the sacraments.[31] Moreover, they shared an interest in adapting for the use of theological students the teachings of the Parisian grammarians and logicians. Toward this end they composed works that circulated under remarkably similar titles: Peter's *De tropis loquendi* and William's *Tropi*.[32]

---

[29] On Peter Comestor see David Luscombe, "Peter Comestor," in *The Bible in the Medieval World: Essays in Memory of Beryl Smalley*, ed. Katherine Walsh and Diana Wood (Oxford: Blackwell, 1985), pp. 109-129; Ignatius Brady, "Peter Manducator and the Oral Teachings of Peter Lombard," *Antonianum* 41 (1966) 454-490. Peter of Poitiers's life and works are described by Philip S. Moore, *The Works of Peter of Poitiers, Master in Theology and Chancellor of Paris (1193-1205)* (Notre Dame IN: University of Notre Dame Press, 1936). Beryl Smalley provides a nice introduction to the Parisian masters of this period in Chapter Five ("Masters of the Sacred Page") of her *Study of the Bible in the Middle Ages*, 2nd ed. (Notre Dame IN: University of Notre Dame Press, 1964), pp. 196-263. Two recent studies of the 12th-century Parisian schools fall on either side of this important period. R.W. Southern, "Schools of Paris," discusses evidence up to 1165, and John W. Baldwin, "Masters at Paris from 1179 to 1215: A Social Perspective," covers the later period; these essays are published in *Renaissance and Renewal*, pp. 113-137 and 138-172.

[30] Neither date is secure. That William was teaching by c. 1176 is inferred from Gerald of Wales's testimony (1176 x 1179), which does not specify when William began to teach in Paris. The date 1173 for Peter the Chanter's mastership is based on a casual remark by Caesarius of Heisterbach in the 1220's; it is accepted by John W. Baldwin, *Masters, Princes and Merchants: The Social Views of Peter the Chanter and His Circle*, 2 vols. (Princeton: Princeton University Press, 1970), 1: 5-6, but elsewhere he has defended, with some cogency, the possibility of a later date for the beginning of Peter's teaching: "A Debate at Paris over Thomas Becket between Master Roger and Master Peter the Chanter," *Studia Gratiana* 11 (1967), pp. 121-132; see also below at note 35.

[31] Peter's *Distinctiones* have not been dated, but their alphabetization is more rigorous and sophisticated than William's (see below, II.8). William's *De septem sacramentis* almost certainly antedates Peter's *Summa De sacramentis*, see Joseph Goering, "The *Diffinicio eucaristie* Formerly Attributed to Robert Grosseteste," *Journal of Theological Studies*, ns 37 (1986) 91-104, at 92-93, and below, II.13, pp. 472-475.

[32] See below, II.11. Peter's *De tropis loquendi* has been discussed on several occasions by Gillian R. Evans. See her "Peter the Chanter's *De Tropis Loquendi*: The Problem

It has been asserted that William was the Chanter's student, but this conclusion seems untenable.[33] Neither author mentions the other by name, and their writings, although similar in form, purpose, and content, provide no evidence of direct borrowing, one from the other. The common elements in their respective works point as easily to a common scholastic milieu as to a direct master/student relationship. The fact that both taught simultaneously in Paris during the 1170's would also argue against one being the other's student. Where their respective teachings can be compared, William's doctrines and methods appear to antedate the Chanter's.[34] Together, William de Montibus and Peter the Chanter provide a valuable picture of the moral and pastoral interests of Parisian theologians in the later twelfth century. Neither, however, had reached the height of his abilities and influence before William left Paris and returned to his native England as a teacher of theology.[35]

St. Hugh of Lincoln

The date and circumstances of William's return to Lincoln are unknown. Gerald of Wales reports that St. Hugh, bishop of Lincoln

---

of the Text," *New Scholasticism* 55 (1981) 95-103; "A Work of 'Terminist Theology'? Peter the Chanter's *De Tropis Loquendi* and Some *Fallacie*," *Vivarium* 20 (1982) 40-58; "The Place of Peter the Chanter's *De Tropis Loquendi*" in *Analecta Cisterciensia* 39 (1983) 231-253; and Appendix 2, "Peter the Chanter's *De Tropis Loquendi*" in Evans's *Alan of Lille: The Frontiers of Theology in the Later Twelfth Century* (Cambridge: Cambridge University Press, 1983), pp. ix, 188-197.

[33] Hugh MacKinnon first proposed that Peter was William's master. His argument, based on similarities between William's and Peter's works on tropes, and on Peter's greater notoriety, are presented in his essay, "William de Montibus: A Medieval Teacher," in *Essays in Medieval History Presented to Bertie Wilkinson*, ed. Thayron A. Sandquist and M.R. Powicke (Toronto: University of Toronto Press, 1969), p. 33. The evidence concerning the *Tropi* is re-examined below (ii.11, p. 350), and found to be inconclusive. MacKinnon's assertion has been repeated by Gillian Evans (see previous note), and by Beryl Smalley *The Gospels in the Schools, 1100-1250* (London: Hambledon Press, 1985), p. 107, but not by Baldwin, *Masters*, who found no evidence that William was a member of Peter's circle.

[34] See above, note 31.

[35] Peter's "circle" in Paris, as described by Baldwin, *Masters*, 1: 17-46, consisted primarily of students who were active in the last decade of the 12th century — none are supposed to have studied with him in the 1170's or early 1180's. The writings of the Chanter that have been dated are from the period after 1186: lectures on the Gospels, 1187 x 1197; *Verbum abbreviatum*, c. 1191 x 1192; *De sacramentis*, 1191/2 x 1197; see Smalley, "The Gospels in the Paris Schools in the Late 12th and Early 13th Centuries: Peter the Chanter, Hugh of St. Cher, Alexander Hales, John of la Rochelle," *Franciscan Studies* 39 (1979) 232-238.

from 1186-1200, instituted William as a canon in the chapter and then as chancellor of the cathedral.[36] The former position William held by 1188, and the latter by 1194.[37] Bishop Hugh may himself have been responsible for bringing William de Montibus back to Lincoln. Hugh, a native of Burgundy, was a popular figure in Paris, familiar with the schools and scholars there, and interested in strengthening the intellectual fabric of his diocese.[38] But schools flourished at Lincoln even before Hugh's episcopate, and William's family ties in that city may have led him back even without Hugh's encouragement. The most that can be said is that William returned to Lincoln sometime during the 1180's, and began a long and notable association with the schools of theology there.

During William's first years at Lincoln, Bishop Hugh's activities helped to set a pattern for pastoral reform that would be taken up and elaborated by many English bishops in the wake of the Fourth Lateran Council of 1215.[39] Hugh issued the earliest surviving *decreta* or synodal statutes for an English diocese;[40] they are recorded by Benedict, abbot of Peterborough, in his *Gesta Henrici*:

> In the meantime, Bishop Hugh, while residing in his diocese, gave edification to the people committed to him, both by his way of life (*conversatione*) and by the word of paternal exhortation, and in his synods he enjoined in virtue of their obedience both his clergy and people to keep without fail the following decrees:
>
> 1. That nothing should be given or received for administering or hastening the administration of justice.
> 2. That nothing should be given or exacted of vicars for their chantries.

---

[36] "Testatus est autem magister Willelmus, quem prefatus pontifex in ecclesia sua Lincolniensi canonicum instituit et cancellarium, quod ..."; *The Life of St. Hugh of Avalon, Bishop of Lincoln 1186-1200*, ed. and trans. Richard M. Loomis, Garland Library of Medieval Literature, 31 (New York: Garland Press, 1985), p. 30.

[37] *Fasti ecclesiae Anglicanae 1066-1300: III, Lincoln*, ed. Diana E. Greenway (London: Institute of Historical Research, University of London, 1977), p. 118 and p. 16.

[38] *Magna Vita Sancti Hugonis: The Life of St. Hugh of Lincoln*, ed. Decima L. Douie and David Hugh Farmer, 2 vols. (rept. with corrections, Oxford: Clarendon Press, 1985), 1: xxviii-xxxv. See also David Hugh Farmer, *Saint Hugh of Lincoln* (Kalamazoo: Cistercian Publications, 1985).

[39] See Marion Gibbs and Jane Lang, *Bishops and Reform, 1215-1272: With Special Reference to the Lateran Council of 1215* (London: Oxford University Press, 1934); Christopher R. Cheney, *English Synodalia of the Thirteenth Century* (1941; rept. with new introd., London: Oxford University Press, 1968).

[40] Christopher R. Cheney, *From Becket to Langton: English Church Government 1170-1213* (Manchester: Manchester University Press, 1956), p. 143.

3. That the archdeacons and their officials should not presume without regular trial to suspend or excommunicate any church or clerk or any one else.

4. That no layman or other person not a priest should have it enjoined upon him as a penance to get Masses said.

5. That no Anniversary Masses or trentals or other fixed Masses should be celebrated for temporal gain.

6. That no one be admitted to the performance of priestly functions unless it be proved that he was ordained canonically by the Archbishop of Canterbury or one of his suffragans.

7. That all who hold ecclesiastical preferment should keep their hair cut short and wear the tonsure.

8. That no cleric should sue another cleric in a temporal court in matters ecclesiastical.[41]

One of Hugh's most important contributions to reforming the diocese of Lincoln was the seeking out of qualified individuals, both in England and in the schools overseas, to fill positions in his cathedral church. Adam of Eynsham, one of St. Hugh's biographers, describes the bishop's conviction that, without the assistance of highly trained *adiutores*, he would be of little use to the clergy and people under him, and unable to do justice to any litigants in the ecclesiastical courts.[42] One of Hugh's first acts as bishop was to appeal to Baldwin, archbishop of Canterbury, for help in securing such individuals. Adam of Eynsham gives this account of his request:

> You are too wise, my reverend Father, not to understand how important it is for my own soul, for the Church over which I rule, and also for yourself, that I should not be a useless pastor. Thanks be to God, I have the will to do what is right; and it is for you to show me the means. I have a special need to surround myself with wise counsellors who will supply for my deficiencies. How can I discover and choose such counsellors, I, who am a stranger in this country? Your long experience must come to my assistance, since you have not feared to lay upon me the burden of the episcopate. Let me beg you then to give me, as my fellow-workers, some of those whom you have trained yourself by word and example.[43]

---

[41] *Gesta Regis Henrici Secundi Benedicti Abbatis*, ed. William Stubbs, 2 vols., Rolls Series, 49 (London: Longman, 1867), 1: 357; quoted here in the translation of Herbert Thurston, *Life of St. Hugh of Lincoln* (London: Burns and Oates, 1898), pp. 326-327.

[42] *Magna Vita*, 1: 110.

[43] Ibid., 1: 111; quoted from Thurston's translation, *Life*, pp. 148-149.

In response the archbishop sent two clerics from his own household, Master Robert of Bedford and Master Roger of Rolleston, who were "conspicuous among all the English clergy" for their learning and virtue, and who came to hold important offices in the diocese of Lincoln.[44]

Hugh's efforts to recruit learned and respected clergy to aid in providing pastoral care in his diocese soon attracted attention, even overseas. Adam of Eynsham tells how one of the most renowned regent masters of theology, a canon of the cathedral of Paris and, apparently, the rector of the schools (*preerat enim scholis Parisiensibus*), praised Hugh for having made his church "more famous than any other church in the world owing to its innumerable distinguished canons." This theologian confided, perhaps facetiously, that he wished to be numbered among Hugh's canons, however modest might be the prebend. Hugh replied at once that he would have him, but on two conditions. First, that he be willing to reside there, and second, that his virtue should equal his learning. The famous theologian blushed at this comment; he was, we are told, more famous for his scholarship than for his good conduct, though it is averred that he reformed somewhat following Hugh's visit.[45] This famous master is unnamed in the story, but the circumstances suggest Peter of Poitiers, the famous, and somewhat scurrilous, master of theology at Paris from c. 1167, who was a canon of the cathedral and its chancellor (and thus *preerat scholis Parisiensibus*) from 1193.[46]

Few of Hugh's appointments worked more credit to Lincoln diocese than his choice of William de Montibus, first as a canon of the cathedral and then as chancellor. In William, Bishop Hugh found not only a kindred spirit, but also an energetic coadjutor in providing pastoral care, and a teacher who established Lincoln as one of the foremost places in England to study theology. William clearly met the criteria

[44] *Magna Vita*, 1: 112-113. Robert became precentor of the cathedral, and Roger first an archdeacon and then dean; see John le Neve, *Fasti*, pp. 9, 13, 33.

[45] "Meminimus autem quendam eo temporis summi fere inter theologos canonicosque Parisienses nominis, dixisse quadam uice Hugoni: 'Gloriosam, domine episcope, pre cunctis totius orbis ecclesiis uestram exhibuistis ecclesiam insignium multitudine clericorum; essetque michi, nec enim id celandum uobis duxi, satis optabile eorum numero quolibet uel perexili titulo sociari.' Cui statim episcopus: 'Et nos', ait, 'eorum uos numero libenti animo iungeremus si etiam inter eos residere uelletis, si quoque ad scientiam mores uobis equis passibus responderent.' Preerat enim scholis Parisiensibus, regens et ipse scholas, celebrior tamen eo tempore scientia quam disciplina. Qui, responso tali accepto, erubuit se nimis libere protulisse quod minus sincere uoluebat in pectore ... . Recedens autem ab eo, castigatioribus de cetero moribus fertur institisse," *Magna Vita*, 1: 120-121.

[46] On Peter's life, see Moore, *Works of Peter of Poitiers*, pp. 1-24.

that Hugh had laid down for the Parisian theologian. He kept residence in Lincoln throughout his tenure, resisting the inclination, common among contemporary scholars, to move frequently from one professional or academic milieu to another. Moreover, William's virtuous behavior won as much respect from contemporaries as did his wide learning.

On a more personal level, Hugh and William appear together in only one story, but it is one that reveals something of the relationship they enjoyed. Both Gerald of Wales and Roger of Wendover tell of a visit made by Bishop Hugh to one of the leper houses in his diocese. Following the visit, William de Montibus observed playfully that St. Martin had healed lepers with his kisses. Hugh responded in kind: "Martin's kiss healed the lepers' flesh, the kiss of these lepers heals my soul."[47]

One final note will serve to introduce the only surviving shred of evidence about William's physical appearance. It is said that St. Hugh, although himself an ascetic of restricted diet and simple habits, kept a sumptuous table for visitors and for his household. He was fond of saying to those about him: "Eat well and drink well and serve God well."[48] If, as one medieval scribe tells us, William de Montibus was nicknamed by his students *mons coagulatus, mons pinguis*,[49] we might surmise that he was of one accord with the bishop concerning the merits of a good table, and had taken full advantage of Hugh's hospitality.

CHANCELLOR OF LINCOLN CATHEDRAL

William's writings tell us little of his career as master, canon, and chancellor at Lincoln, but other evidence helps to shed light on his

---

[47] *Rogeri de Wendover Liber qui dicitur Flores historiarum*, ed. Henry G. Hewlett, 3 vols., Rolls Series, 84, (London, 1886-1889), 1: 304. Gerald of Wales brings out the playfulness in William's comment: "Testatus est autem magister Willelmus, quem prefatus pontifex in ecclesia sua Lincolniensi canonicum instituit et cancellarium, quod in villa Newerc quemdam leprosum osculatus est episcopus sanctus Hugo, et ne magnum quid se in hoc egisse reputaret episcopus, immo pocius defectum suum in hoc attenderet, quod leprosum deosculando non curaret, dixit ei predictus Willelmus, familiaris eius admodum et dilectus, 'Martinus osculo leprosum mundavit'. Et respondit episcopus, dicti causam intelligens, 'Martinus osculando leprosum curavit eum in corpore. Leprosus autem osculo sanavit me in anima.'" Loomis, ed., *Life of St. Hugh*, p. 30 (1:8).

[48] Ibid.

[49] Cf. Ps 67:16; the scribe of MS 34 in Jesus College, Cambridge, comments: "Expliciunt tropi in theologica facultate edita a magistro Willelmo de montibus cancellario lincolniensis ecclesie. Mons iste dicitur a multis mons coagulatus, mons pinguis," fol. 43va.

activities there. It was as a master of theology that he was especially
honoured by his contemporaries, and his role as teacher will be
discussed in Chapter Two. As a pastor and administrator, however,
his influence extended far beyond the classroom.

As chancellor, he held with the dean, subdean, and treasurer, one
of the four great offices of the cathedral.[50] The earliest statement of
the chancellor's duties to have survived at Lincoln is contained in the
fourteenth-century "Black Book," so called from the colour of its
binding. The first document therein is the *Consuetudines et officia
ecclesie Lincolniensis*, copied soon after 1300 from an earlier collection
of customs, now lost.[51] Other documents preserved outside Lincoln,
however, allow us to reconstruct with some accuracy the customary
duties of the chancellor as they were understood early in the thirteenth
century. The most important of these comes from the register of the
diocese of Moray in Northern Scotland. Bishop Brice (1203-1222) was
apparently so impressed by the fame of the Lincoln Chapter under
St. Hugh, that he adopted the Lincoln customs for his own cathedral
church.[52] During the ensuing years a number of written statements
of the Lincoln customs were entered in the Moray registers. Among
these is one entitled *Statuta vicariorum*, which Bradshaw dated c.
1236.[53] It contains the earliest detailed description of the Lincoln
chancellor's duties, and may, indeed, reflect customs that were developed
during St. Hugh's time with the specific interests and abilities of William
de Montibus in mind.

First among the chancellor's duties was to conduct (*regere*) the
cathedral's theological schools, a duty which William performed
assiduously and in person for some twenty-five years.[54] His success
at the task is recorded by Gerald of Wales, who, when unable to return
to Paris to study theology in the 1190's, explained his decision to go
to Lincoln because: "the science of theology flourishes there most

---

[50] For a general description of the chancellor's office, see Kathleen Edwards, *The
English Secular Cathedrals in the Middle Ages: A Constitutional Study with Special
Reference to the Fourteenth Century*, 2nd ed. (Manchester: Manchester University
Press, 1967), pp. 176-216; for a more detailed study, see Christopher Robert Cheney,
English Bishops' Chanceries, 1100-1250 (Manchester: Manchester University Press,
1950).

[51] *Statutes of Lincoln Cathedral*, ed. Henry Bradshaw and Christopher Wordsworth,
2 parts (Cambridge, Cambridge University Press, 1892-1897), 1: 98-99.

[52] Ibid., 1: 40-59; 2: 136-142.

[53] Ibid., 1: 50-59; 2: 143-160.

[54] "Officium Cancelarij est scholas theologie regere," ibid., 2: 158. See Edwards,
English Secular Cathedrals, pp. 196-199.

soundly in all of England, under the best of teachers, Master William de Monte."[55]

Along with the chancellor's duty of teaching in the cathedral's theological schools come two privileges constituting his *dignitas* in relation to the other schools of the city and county of Lincoln. First, no one was to be permitted to teach in the city except by license of the chancellor. Second, the chancellor had the right of appointing masters to all the schools in the county of Lincoln, excepting those situated on the prebendal estates of his fellow canons.[56]

With respect to the exercise of these privileges little can be said. There were almost certainly other schools in Lincoln, and other masters teaching theology, law, medicine, science, or the arts.[57] These masters may have applied to William, as chancellor, for the license to teach, but no records of such applications or licenses survive. It is noteworthy that the chancellor's authority in licensing teachers extended only to the city itself, and not to the other centres of scholastic activity within the diocese such as the schools at Northampton, Stamford, and Oxford.

The second privilege, that of appointment to the schools of Lincolnshire, suggests that the chancellor's right to appoint masters for the schools was similar to the right of a religious or secular patron to present clerics to parochial benefices. In fact the chancellor's power was probably more limited. The early-fourteenth-century Lincoln customs add two clarifications. They specify that his privilege pertains to the county's grammar schools only, and not to "song schools" and other schools maintained by priests for the education of their own parishioners.[58] This privilege would thus seem to encompass appoint-

[55] Quoted above, note 10.

[56] "Dignitas ipsius est, quod nullus potest legere in ciuitate Lyncolniensi nisi de licencia ipsius, et quod omnes scholas in comitatu Lyncolniensi pro suo confert arbitrio exceptis hijs que sunt in prebendis," *Statutes of Lincoln Cathedral*, 2: 160.

[57] The study of 12th- and 13th-century schools in towns that did not become university centres is still in its infancy; see, for example, Nicholas Orme, *English Schools in the Middle Ages* (London: Methuen, 1973); H.G. Richardson, "The Schools of Northampton in the Twelfth Century," *English Historical Review* 56 (1941) 595-605; Edwards, *English Secular Cathedrals*, pp. 185-205; R.W. Hunt, "English Learning in the Late Twelfth Century," *Transactions of the Royal Historical Society*, 4th series, 19 (1936) 19-35; Richard W. Southern, *Robert Grosseteste: The Growth of an English Mind in Medieval Europe* (Oxford: Clarendon Press, 1986), pp. 53-62.

[58] "Idem eciam Cancellarius scolas [gramatice] omnes in ciuitate et commitatu Lincoln pro suo libero conferat arbitrio; scolis cantus, et illis que sunt in prebendis, ac alijs quas tenent ecclesiarum rectores, vel ceteri curati, aut eorum parochiales clerici, in suis parochijs pro suis parochianis in fide et lectura erudiendis, duntaxat exceptis," *Statutes of Lincoln Cathedral*, 2: 300. On song schools offering elementary training in the correct performance (singing) of prayers and liturgy, see Orme, *English Schools*, pp. 59-68.

ments to privately or publicly endowed institutions, and, perhaps even to external schools established by monasteries but taught by secular masters. Such a custom, if rigorously enforced, might have fostered a degree of centralized control and oversight over the schools. But the main purpose was probably less grandiose, seeking simply to ensure that the chancellor could provide a living for some of the students whom he trained in the cathedral schools.

The second duty of the Lincoln chancellor was to preach. The Lincoln statutes of 1236 are quite specific on this point. The chancellor was responsible for preaching in the cathedral when the choir was present. In addition he was bound to preach to the clerics in chapter each Sunday, and to the people on the first three days of Christmas, on the feast of Epiphany, on the first three days of Easter, on the feasts of the Assumption and the Nativity of the Virgin, on All Saints, on Holy Trinity Sunday, and on Ash Wednesday. Finally, on five occasions when there were solemn processions outside the cathedral — Palm Sunday, the Greater Litanies, and the three Rogation Days — he was to preach at a station along the route (*apud locum stacionis*).[59]

William's sermons preserve some indication of these various settings and of the preaching appropriate to each. For example, in an Easter Sunday sermon he describes the people present:

> It is the custom of Holy Church that boys, girls, shepherds, and servants whose work keeps them from church on other days, come together early on the morning of this day. You should know the reason. Know, therefore, that you come to church on this feast, which is greater and holier than all the others, in order to receive light and sustenance ... .[60]

On a Pentecost Sunday William addressed his lay audience as follows:

> "He who has my commandments and keeps them, he it is who loves me" [John 14:1] My beloved brothers, you who are laymen, listen carefully

---

[59] "Officium Cancellarij est ... predicare vel per se vel per alium quem de ecclesia elegerit, dum ex consensu decani et capituli illud extraneo deputet officium. Et hoc intelligendum est quando choro presente predicandum est; alias poterit cui voluerit officium iniungere memoratum. Est autem predicandum hijs diebus populo: singulis dominicis diebus clericis in capitulo, per tres primas dies Natalis Domini, die Epiphanie, item per tres primas dies Pasche, die Assumpcionis, die natiuitatis beate Marie, die Omnium Sanctorum, die Sancte Trinitatis (et hoc fiat vel per canonicos vel per alios viros autenticos si inueniantur qui velint et sciant), item die Cinerum. Per quinque dies apud locum stacionis, scilicet die Palmarum et maiores Letanie, et tribus diebus Rogationis, quando solempnes extra ecclesiam fiunt processiones." *Statutes of Lincoln Cathedral*, 2: 158-159.

[60] See below, II.16, Sermon no. 124.

to these words by which our Saviour declares what is necessary for having true charity and what are the rewards of that charity ... . Go to church gladly, listen attentively to the words of preaching (*uerba predicacionis*), and learn diligently God's commands.

After a brief exposition, appropriate to Pentecost, of the procession of the Holy Spirit from the Father and the Son, he speaks familiarly to the audience:

If you are unable, my brothers, to be with monks (*uiris religiosis*) in mind and body, be with them in mind, be with them in doing favours, or at least in good will.[61]

Several sermons preached to the clerics in chapter constitute small treatises in their own right. William used a sermon for the feast of Holy Trinity, for example, to expound the Apostles' Creed:

On this feast of Holy Trinity I take as the material of my sermon the Apostles' Creed, which contains in brief compass the trinitarian, indeed the catholic, faith. This creed was given to us that we all, clerics as well as lay people, might confess our faith each day. It is thus fitting that everyone understand its content, and especially the clergy, who not only must hold the faith contained therein, but also guard it, and "be always prepared to satisfy any who calls them to account for the faith and hope that is in them" [cf. 1 Peter 3:15].[62]

The sermon for the feast of the Greater Litanies (25 April) was to be preached at a station along the processional route. William was fond of including a brief explication of the origins of the feast:

Behold my brothers, in the holy season of Lent just past, your conscience was cleansed through true penance and good works. With your heart's house swept clean, you worthily received our Lord [i.e. in the eucharist] on Easter Sunday ... . Persevere, therefore, in this cleanliness ... lest you pollute the Lord's dwelling place as once did the Romans. They were gravely punished for this by a plague (*peste inguinaria*), and they instituted today's litanies to ward it off.[63]

In addition to the duties of teaching and preaching, the early Lincoln customs mention some of the chancellor's other responsibilities. He was to care for the cathedral's books, supervise the lectors and ministers at the divine service, take charge of the chapter's seal, compose the

[61] See below, II.16, Sermon no. 127.
[62] See below, II.16, Sermon no. 129.
[63] See below, II.16, Sermon no. 82; cf. Sermon no. 83.

chapter's charters and letters, and read aloud in chapter such documents as were to be read.[64]

The *Registrum antiquissimum* of Lincoln Cathedral records dozens of documents issued or attested by William.[65] In the earliest (c. 1189) he is not yet chancellor and is described simply as "magister."[66] One of the latest documents (c. 1212) describes a transfer of land that took place in the "chancellor's court," which William held in the chapter house.[67] The documents also reveal that William had a clerk named Richard and a seneschal named Gilbert to assist him in his duties.[68]

In addition to his duties as chancellor, William was called upon to act as a papal judge-delegate in cases that had been appealed to the papacy from the ecclesiastical courts.[69] The earliest surviving notice of his appointment as a judge-delegate is found in the Thurgarton cartulary, where he was one of three judges in a case involving Thurgarton Priory and the Gilbertine priory of St. Katherine in Lincoln during the pontificate of Celestine III (1191-1198).[70] Six documents from the pontificate of Innocent III (1198-1216) also show William acting in a judicial capacity in cases brought by St. Peter's (later known as St. Leonard's) hospital at York and Bardney Abbey in Lincolnshire.[71]

While his formal duties as chancellor and judge-delegate provided William ample scope to make his mark in the English ecclesiastical world, his informal and unofficial activities must have been equally important. Only scattered traces of such activities have survived, but

[64] *Statutes of Lincoln Cathedral*, 2: 159-160.
[65] *The Registrum Antiquissimum of the Cathedral Church of Lincoln*, ed. C.W. Foster and Kathleen Major, 10 vols, Publications of the Lincoln Record Society, 27-29, 32, 34, 41, 42, 46, 51, 62, 67, 68 (Hereford: Lincoln Record Society, 1931-1973).
[66] *Registrum Antiquissimum*, 9: 105-106.
[67] "... coram W. cancellario et curia eius quam tunc in predicto capitulo tenuit ..."; ibid., 10: 20.
[68] "Hiis testibus ... Ricardo clerico cancellarii," ibid., 9: 106; "Willelmus Linc' ecclesie cancellarius salutem ... . Hiis testibus ... Gilberto tunc senescallo meo," ibid., 9: 107. This Gilbert is probably the same person who witnessed a grant of c. 1200, noting that he had himself written the document: "hiis testibus ... Gilberto clerico huius carte scriptore," ibid., 10: 178.
[69] For a study of the office of the judge-delegate see Jane E. Sayers, *Papal Judges Delegate in the Province of Canterbury 1198-1254: A Study in Ecclesiastical Jurisdiction and Administration* (Oxford: Oxford University Press, 1971); for reference to William's activities, see pp. 130-131.
[70] Thurgarton cartulary (Southwell Minster Library MS 3), fol. 51r; I owe this reference to Trevor Foulds, see above at note 4.
[71] *The Letters of Pope Innocent III (1198-1216) concerning England and Wales: A Calendar with an Appendix of Texts*, ed. Christopher R. Cheney and Mary G. Cheney (Oxford: Clarendon Press, 1967), pp. 105-106, 119, 124, 145.

one can infer from these something of his extracurricular contributions to life in and around Lincoln Cathedral. For example, when a canon of the Order of Sempringham set out to compile materials for the canonization of Gilbert, the order's founder, he turned to William for advice and assistance. The canon explains in his dedicatory letter (1202 x 1205) addressed to Hubert, archbishop of Canterbury, that his documents have been corrected by, among others, "the very learned theologian, Master William, chancellor of the church of Lincoln."[72]

William also took an active role in the pastoral care of Gilbertine nuns. The medieval catalogue of the books at Peterborough Abbey attributes to William a series of letters or sermons addressed to nuns.[73] With Albinia de la Mare's discovery of one such "sermon" in a Lyell manuscript at the Bodleian Library, we can recover at least a small bit of William's thoughtful and personal style as he addresses the pastoral needs of the women of the Gilbertine Order.[74]

Another description of William's extracurricular activities comes from the caustic pen of Gerald of Wales. As noted above, Gerald had a high regard for William de Montibus and the Lincoln schools of theology that flourished under his tutelage. When Gerald travelled to Lincoln rather than to Paris in the last years of the twelfth century it was not only for the sake of his own studies but also for those of his nephew, whose education and promotion he had undertaken.[75] Apparently, however, this nephew took advantage of his uncle's frequent absences from Lincoln to neglect his studies. When Gerald left England in 1204 for a two-year visit to Ireland he appointed a tutor for his nephew, but upon his return Gerald found the situation worse. He appointed a new tutor, Master William de Capella, who was even less satisfactory. William de Capella apparently colluded with the nephew in defrauding and defaming Gerald.

This situation prompted Gerald to write his *Speculum duorum* or "Mirror of Two Men" (1208 x 1212) exposing the depravities of nephew and tutor alike. He accuses them, among other things, of having

---

[72] "Sane ... uestreque deuotioni quam erga ipsum sanctum satis intensam probaueram, prout a uiro in theologia eruditissimo magistro Willelmo, Lincolniensi ecclesie cancellario, et multis aliis peritis emendata sunt et commendata, sicut iussistis, transmitto." *Book of St. Gilbert*, pp. lxxxiv, 8-9.

[73] See below, *Epistola ad moniales*, ii.6, p. 222.

[74] The sermon (perhaps originally a letter, turned into sermon-form by the scribe of the manuscript) is printed below, ii.6.

[75] The details of this story are set out in *Speculum duorum: or, A Mirror of Two Men*, ed. Yves Lefevre and R.B.C. Huygens, trans. Brian Dawson (Cardiff: University of Wales, 1974), pp. xxx-xxxix.

excerpted passages from his writings and of circulating the excerpts among people who might take offense. Gerald mentions particularly their attempts to slander him with the bishop of Lincoln and with the "elders" of the clergy and chapter of Lincoln.[76]

As one of the senior and respected members of the chapter, William de Montibus may well have been approached by these two for an opinion on the propriety of Gerald's books on Ireland, *The Topography* and *The Prophetic History of the Conquest*. At any rate, Gerald appended to his *Speculum duorum* a letter addressed to William de Montibus in which he defends his Irish histories against William's reported criticisms:

> Our amazement could not have been greater that a man, whom public opinion proclaims to be good and kind, should now, so we hear, dare to condemn our books on Ireland ... on account of the subject matter — books which we gave in one volume to the church of Lincoln, and which he used to praise highly — just because somewhere in them the vice of these people (the vice of coupling with beasts and of beasts' coming to women) is dealt with strict historical accuracy ... .
>
> Besides, you have said that we ought to write theological works and that this would be more becoming to our maturity ... .
>
> It is also our desire that you should know that the above historical works of ours, which you now consider so trivial, in time to come ... will be more valued than very many works. For there is already a superabundance, as it were, of theological books, and even more are being added to the overflowing pile ... .[77]

We are told neither the occasion for William's criticisms of Gerald's writings, nor how Gerald came to hear of them, but the entire episode as recited in Gerald's inimitable prose serves as a reminder of the day-to-day activities and intrigues into which even a respected chancellor might be drawn.

ENGLAND UNDER INTERDICT

During the last five years of William's life, England was under papal interdict.[78] The implementation of this interdict, first published in

---

[76] Ibid., pp. 114, 142.

[77] Ibid., pp. 170-173.

[78] The best general discussion of this interdict is found in Christopher R. Cheney, *Pope Innocent III and England* (Stuttgart: Anton Hiersemann, 1976), pp. 294-356, and idem, "King John and the Papal Interdict," *Bulletin of the John Rylands Library* 31 (1948) 295-317, rept. in *The Papacy and England 12th-14th Centuries* (London: Variorum Reprints, 1982).

England on Sunday, 23 March 1208, varied from place to place, but the general intent was to permit no ecclesiastical services except baptism and confession of the dying. The annals of the Augustinian priory of Dunstable in Bedfordshire offers a nuanced account of the effects of this interdict on Lincoln diocese. The dead were being buried outside the cemeteries, with no priest present; betrothals and ritual purifications of new mothers took place outside the churches; Sunday sermons also were preached outside the churches, where blest bread and water were distributed to the faithful. Inside the churches, priests conducted baptisms with chrism that had been augmented, with papal approval, by the addition of (unconsecrated) oil. The laity were permitted access to the altar to make offerings, if they so desired.[79]

More specific information concerning the practical implementation of the interdict has survived in copies of Pope Innocent's letter to the English executors dated 14 June 1208.[80] This letter forbids all public church services. Pilgrims were to be admitted inside a church only through inconspicuous entrances. Doors of the churches were to remain closed except on major feasts, when parishioners could enter to pray. Baptisms were to be celebrated inside the churches, but with the doors closed and only the parents and sponsors present. The sacrament of penance and penitential discipline were to be administered as before the interdict. Priests were permitted to say their prayers and devotions privately, and on Sundays they were allowed to preach and distribute blest bread and water in the cemetery. They were also to visit the sick, hear their confessions, and celebrate the *commendatio animarum* as usual, but not to offer last communion, or to follow the bodies of the dead to their burial place. Finally, on Good Friday priests were permitted to place the cross outside the churches so that parishioners could exercise their customary devotions in that place, but without any accompanying liturgical ceremony.

---

[79] "Eodem anno, Dominica qua cantatur *Isti sunt dies*, interdictae sunt tota Anglia et Wallia, ita quod omnes privilegiati cessaverunt ... . Tunc corpora defunctorum extra coemiterium absque praesentia sacerdotum sepeliebantur. Sponsalia et purificationes ad ostium ecclesiae fiebant, quibus evangelium legebatur; diebus Dominicis fiebat sermo ad populum extra ecclesiam, et ibi panis benedictus et aqua benedicta dabatur eisdem; sacerdotes in ecclesiis baptizabant; et ne chrisma deficeret, oleum de licentia papae admiscebant; et offerre volentibus accessum ad altaria concedebant." *Annales Monastici, III*, ed. Henry Richards Luard, Rolls Series, 36 (London: Longman, 1866), p. 30; cf. Cheney, "King John," p. 298.

[80] See *Selected Letters of Pope Innocent III concerning England (1198-1216)*, ed. Christopher R. Cheney and W. H. Semple (London: Thomas Nelson and Sons, 1953), pp. 107-109.

Inside the cathedrals ecclesiastical services may have continued much as before the interdict, but with certain modifications. In 1208 Innocent III expressed his willingness to permit the regular clergy (*viri religiosi*) to celebrate "the divine offices with doors shut, no ringing of church bells, and in quiet tones, all excommunicated persons and those under interdict being excluded."[81] This dispensation for regular clergy would have included the chapters of the English monastic cathedrals, and might well have been extended in practice to the communities of canons in secular cathedrals and collegiate churches.

William de Montibus makes almost no reference to the interdict or its effects on the English Church and people. A single, enigmatic couplet in his *Versarius*, entitled "Complaint of the suspended church-men," may be an expression of his consternation at the damage done by the withdrawing of ecclesiastical justice in England during the interdict:

> Nobis suspensis, Christi suspenditur ensis;
> Quando reuertetur Domini uindicta sequetur.[82]

Most of William's activities would have continued even under the new and strained circumstances. The schools, for example, seem to have remained open throughout this period.[83] Sermons, as noted above, were still preached, although in the cemetery or churchyard rather than inside the church. Pastoral care and ecclesiastical business continued much as before,[84] and William himself is recorded as holding court and carrying on routine business in the cathedral's chapter house in 1212.[85] The see of Lincoln was vacant in 1208, the previous incumbent, William of Blois, having died in May 1206. The election of Hugh of Wells proceeded unhindered in 1209, although the new bishop soon joined his episcopal colleagues in exile, to return only after the interdict was lifted.[86] Even in the bishop's absence, however, ecclesiastical administration continued, as can be seen in the *Rotuli* of Lincoln diocese for these years.[87]

[81] Ibid., p. 109.

[82] See below, II.12, no. 228.

[83] See Richard W. Southern, "From Schools to University," in *The History of the University of Oxford*, I, *The Early Oxford Schools*, ed. Jeremy I. Catto (Oxford: Clarendon Press, 1984), pp. 1-36, at pp. 26-27.

[84] Cheney, *Pope Innocent III and England*, pp. 310-317; "King John," pp. 307-311.

[85] See above, at note 67.

[86] Cheney, "King John," pp. 309-311.

[87] *Rotuli Hugonis de Welles, Episcopi Lincolniensis, A.D. MCCIX-MCCXXXV*, ed. W.P.W. Phillimore, 3 vols. (London: Canterbury and York Society, 1907-1909);

The interdict ended with the reconciliation of King John in May of 1213, and with his penitential restitutions during the following year.[88] William, however, did not live to see these events. Shortly after Easter (14 April) of 1213 he died in Scotland. His death is noted in two Scottish works, the chronicles of Melrose and of Lanercost.[89] They tell us only that "William of blessed memory, the chancellor of Lincoln, died after Easter. When the interdict on England was lifted, his body was translated to Lincoln Cathedral and buried there with due reverence."[90] William's death in Scotland is unexplained. Neither the cause of death nor the reasons for his presence in Scotland occasioned comment by the chroniclers. Perhaps he had travelled to Scotland to celebrate the Easter holy days free from the restraints imposed by the interdict on England. At least two English bishops were in exile there,[91] and the Lincoln chapter had established close relations with several Scottish churches.[92]

After William's death, Matthew of Rievaulx composed four sets of commemorative verses in his honour.[93] The first seems to have been intended for inscription in a copy of one of William's treatises. It describes him as a soldier of Christ, and avers that his writings are redolent of balsam and incense, and are filled with honey:

> Filius in matris utero merito sepelitur,
> Vas electum quod condidit istud opus.

---

cf. David Smith, "The Rolls of Hugh of Wells, Bishop of Lincoln 1209-35," *Bulletin of the Institute of Historical Research* 45 (1972) 155-195.

[88] Cheney, *Pope Innocent III and England*, pp. 331-356.

[89] *Chronica de Mailros* (Edinburgh, 1835); *Chronicon de Lanercost* (Edinburgh, 1839); both edited by Joseph Stevenson. The Lanercost chronicle is dependent on Melrose here.

[90] "Obiit pie memorie magister Willelmus de Montibus, cancellarius ecclesie Lincolnensis, post pascha [Apr. 14], cujus corpus anno sequenti, reddita Christianitate per Angliam, in ecclesiam Lincolnensem est translatum, ibidemque cum debita reverentia est tumulatum." *Chronica de Mailros*, p. 114. Cf. *Chronicon de Lanercost*: "Circa, vel paulo ante, haec tempora videtur sanctus Hugo, episcopus Lincolniae, claruisse; nam piae memoriae magister Willelmus de Montibus, doctor sacrae thelogiae, in supramemorati sancti diebus officio cancellarii functus est ejusdem Lincolnensis ecclesiae, ac post Deo placitam vitam et doctrinam, ex hac luce subtractus est post finem paschae, qui tamen supervixisse probatur beato Hugoni diebus multis ... . Corpus vero venerandi magistri Willelmi anno sequenti, Christianitate Angliae reddita, in ecclesiam Lincolniae est translatum, et ibidem cum debita reverentia tumulatum," p. 10.

[91] Cheney, *Pope Innocent III and England*, p. 314, n. 52

[92] See *Statutes of Lincoln Cathedral*, 1: 40-44.

[93] These verses have been edited by André Wilmart, "Les mélanges de Mathieu Préchantre de Rievaulx au début du XIIIe siècle," *Revue bénédictine* 52 (1940) 60.

Christi miles in ecclesia Christi requiescit:
 Coccus bis tinctus, coctus amore Dei.
Dulcia mella uide; loquor: eius opuscula fragrant
 Balsama; thus redolet littera, plena fauis.

The second calls him a "leader and teacher of Lincoln," and makes him almost the equal of Gregory the Great and Augustine:

Dux tuus et doctor fuit, urbs Lincolnia; flere
Debes; orba sedes, tanto uiduata paterno.
Dulcis aroma mely condiuit eum, quia pene
Par est Gregorio mellito gutture; pene
Dico nec ex toto: minor est paulominus illo.
Augustine, tibi soli uix cedere nouit.

In the third poem Matthew praises one of William's most popular writings, his *Numerale*, and prays for William's happiness in heaven:

In libro uite numeretur, qui Numerale
Fecit; in hoc numero fidei lux magna relucet.
Da, bone Messya, de uirgine nate Maria,
Willelmo te posse frui, sine fine beari.

The last set of verses, an epitaph for William's tomb, concludes with the familiar yet appropriate sentiment, "flower of the English without a thorn":

Dormit in hoc tumulo mundissima gleba; sed eius
Spiritus ante deum respirat nunc et in euum.
Ille deo carus et plenus aromate morum
Diues erat meritis, Anglorum flos sine spina.

Alexander Neckam also remembered William fondly, and his praise of William as a teacher and theologian, if less extravagant than Matthew's, is none the less telling. In Distinction Five of his *Laus sapientie divine* Alexander describes important cities of the world. When he comes to Lincoln ("Bountiful Lincoln, the pillar of Lindsey; fortunate in its people and filled with good things"), he pauses to commemorate William de Montibus: "None would be your equal if that master were still instructing you in faith and morals." Playing on William's surname, he calls him a "steadfast mountain and a pillar of the faith, who gave himself wholly to the study of theology." This is a pertinent comment for Alexander, who was something of a polymath and had devoted his life not only to theology but also to the mundane sciences and the literary arts. He goes on to describe the three *cathedrae* or seats that had been conferred on William: the first by Ste. Geneviève on her mountain at Paris, the second by the Virgin Mother in the church of St. Mary on the Mount of Lincoln, and finally, having left one mountain for another, he now can be found in Heaven, enthroned on Mount Zion. Alexander concludes with two lines suggesting that he and William may have been personal friends as well as professional colleagues: "Let this digression be a sign or witness of love; as praise it will be less than he deserves."[94]

Fame, of course, is fleeting. William's reputation as the learned chancellor under whom the theological schools of Lincoln became famous was quickly overtaken by circumstances. By the middle of the century Robert Grosseteste, bishop of Lincoln from 1235 to 1253, had begun to supplant William in popular memory and to earn for himself the honorific title *Lincolniensis*. The Lincoln schools were soon to be eclipsed by the nascent universities at Oxford and Cambridge. William's writings, widely copied during the first half of the thirteenth century, were superseded, on the one hand, by the more systematic and theoretical works of the scholastic theologians,[95] and on the other by a flood of practical treatises designed to educate students in the art of arts, the *cura animarum*.[96]

Nevertheless, it was such schools as those at Lincoln, and teachers such as William de Montibus, that made these very developments possible. The following chapters will explore William's scholastic career and his writings in order to delineate the contributions made by this "flower of the English without a thorn."

[94] Quoted above, note 26.
[95] See below, Chapter Two.
[96] See below, Chapter Three.

Chapter Two

The Schools

THE SCHOOLS OF PARIS:
Contulit huic primam cathedram Genovefa

William began his teaching career on Mont Ste. Geneviève, outside of Paris. During the 1170's Paris, with its suburbs, was becoming one of the most notable centres of scholastic activity in Western Europe. The Parisian schools began not only to overshadow the other important monastic and cathedral schools of Gaul, but also to attract scholars from throughout Christendom to teach and study there.[1] William was one of many Englishmen who taught in the twelfth-century Parisian schools. Astrik Gabriel discusses such illustrious English (and Welsh and Scots) scholars at Paris as Robert of Melun, Robert Pullen, Roger the bishop of Worcester, John of Salisbury, Richard and Andrew of St. Victor, Adelard of Bath, Alexander Neckam, Gerald of Wales, and Adam of Eynsham — the biographer of St. Hugh of Lincoln.[2] John Baldwin has identified sixteen English masters teaching at Paris between 1179 and 1215.[3] The schools of Paris were one of the marvels of the day, and their attraction for William de Montibus need occasion no surprise.

The scholastic geography of Paris in the twelfth century can be inscribed roughly within a triangle extending from the cathedral, on

---

[1] Recent scholarship on the schools of Paris is summarized by R.W. Southern, "Schools of Paris"; John W. Baldwin, "Masters at Paris" in *Renaissance and Renewal in the Twelfth Century*, pp. 113-137, 138-172; and by Jacques Verger, "Des Ecoles à l'université: La mutation institutionelle," in *La France de Philippe Auguste: Le temps des mutations*, ed. Robert-Henri Bautier (Paris: C.N.R.S, 1982), pp. 817-845.

[2] See "English Masters and Students in Paris during the Twelfth Century," chapter one of *Garlandia: Studies in the History of the Mediaeval University* (Notre Dame IN: Mediaeval Institute, 1969), pp. 1-37.

[3] "Masters at Paris," pp. 165-172; these include five masters of arts, five canonists, one master of medicine, and five theologians.

the island of the city, south and east to the abbey of St. Victor on
the left bank of the Seine, then west to the abbey of Ste. Geneviève
on the "mountain" south of the cathedral, and back to the Petit Pont
connecting the left bank with the city.[4] At the corners of this triangle
stood three institutions that played important roles in the growth of
the Parisian schools: the Cathedral of Notre Dame, the monastery of
St. Victor, and the abbey of Ste. Geneviève. Schools seem to have
flourished first in the cathedral cloister, a collection of houses for the
canons and cathedral dignitaries situated to the north and east of the
church. These schools were under the loose jurisdiction of the *écolaitre*
or chancellor of the cathedral. By the 1120's the bishop had agreed
to build a covered building adjacent to the episcopal palace to house
the schools.[5]

At the beginning of the century William of Champeaux, an archdeacon of the cathedral and a famous master in its schools, "converted"
to the monastic life. Crossing to the left bank of the Seine, he entered
the monastery of St. Victor and continued his teaching there. This
may mark the beginning of the schools of St. Victor that would become
famous under masters Hugh, Richard, and Andrew. Under the
guidance of its learned penitentiaries such as Robert Flamborough and
Peter of Poitiers (of St. Victor), it also became an important centre
of pastoral care and penitential discipline for the transient student
population.[6] While William of Champeaux was holding classes in the
monastery of St. Victor early in the twelfth century and one of his
students was teaching in William's former school in the cathedral
cloister, the young Abelard came on the scene hoping to establish
himself as an important master in Paris.[7] Around 1108 he opened a
school on Mont Ste. Geneviève, whence he intended to besiege and
capture the cathedral school on the island of the city. Abelard's choice
of Mont Ste. Geneviève as a base for his assault was, perhaps,

---

[4] See Gerard M. Paré, et al., "Foyers scolaires et centres intellectuels," in *La
renaissance du XIIe siècle*; John W. Baldwin, *The Scholastic Culture of the Middle
Ages 1000-1300* (Lexington MA: Heath, 1971), pp. 26-30; idem, *Masters*, 1: 63-87.

[5] Astrik L. Gabriel, "The Cathedral Schools of Notre-Dame and the Beginning
of the University of Paris," in idem, *Garlandia*, pp. 39-64; Southern, "Schools of Paris,"
pp. 119-121.

[6] Carolus Egger, "De praxi paenitentiali Victorinorum," *Angelicum* 17 (1940) 156-
179; and Jean Longère's introduction to his edition of Peter of Poitiers, *Petrus
Pictaviensis <Summa de confessione> Compilatio praesens*, CCL 51 (Turnhout:
Brepols, 1980), pp. lxxv-lxxxvii.

[7] This story is told, in all its military rhetoric, in Abelard's *Historia calamitatum*,
ed. Jacques Monfrin (Paris: Vrin, 1959), pp. 64-70; cf. Southern, "Schools of Paris,"
pp. 122-123.

influenced by the immunity from episcopal jurisdiction enjoyed by the abbey of Ste. Geneviève and its territory since at least 1107.[8] Abelard's attack on the cathedral school failed, but his school on the Mount flourished, and during the next decades other masters also began to teach there. John of Salisbury, describing his own studies between 1136 and 1148, names three masters certainly teaching on Mont Ste. Geneviève: Abelard, Alberic de Monte, and Robert of Melun. He names three others who were teaching either on the Mount or in Paris — Gilbert of Poitiers, Robert Pullen, and Simon of Poissy.[9] As private schools flourished in the territory of Ste. Geneviève, so too did the abbey itself gain an academic reputation under the guidance of its most illustrious abbot, Stephen of Tournai (1176-1191), who had studied at Orleans, Chartres, and Bologna.[10]

The cathedral precincts, the priory of St. Victor, and the abbey of Ste. Geneviève defined the geographical and institutional framework of scholastic culture in Paris before the emergence of a university or corporation of masters early in the thirteenth century. Similar configurations of cathedral, monastic, and private schools could be found in many parts of Europe during the twelfth century, but Paris was distinguished by the great number of private schools that sprang up within this triangle, among them the school of William de Montibus (or de Monte) on the Mount of Ste. Geneviève.[11]

William's choice of this site for his school may best be explained by practical considerations. The lack of space and the difficulty of acquiring suitable facilities in the city or near the Petit Pont are reason enough for him to have sought the suburbs. William also may have wished to align himself with the pastoral and "monastic" atmosphere of education at Ste. Geneviève, against the more raucous elements of scholastic culture nearer to the city. It is probable that the abbot of

---

[8] *Cartulaire général de Paris, 528-1180*, ed. R.C. de Lasteyrie du Saillart (Paris, 1887), p. 160, n. 142; Hastings Rashdall, *The Universities of Europe in the Middle Ages* (Oxford, 1895), new ed. by F.M. Powicke and A.B. Emden, 3 vols. (Oxford: Clarendon Press, 1936), 1: 341-342.

[9] Southern, "Schools of Paris," p. 129; Nikolaus Häring, "Chartres and Paris Revisited," in *Essays in Honour of Anton Charles Pegis*, ed. J. Reginald O'Donnell (Toronto: Pontifical Institute of Mediaeval Studies, 1974), pp. 268-329, at 317-329.

[10] See Joseph Warichez, *Etienne de Tournai et son temps, 1128-1203* (Tournai: Casterman, 1936).

[11] Southern, "Schools of Paris," pp. 114-121, 128-133. A bibliographical summary of recent research on the local schools of the 12th century is found in Stephen C. Ferruolo, *The Origins of the University: The Schools of Paris and their Critics 1100-1215* (Stanford: Stanford University Press, 1985), pp. 320-324.

Ste. Geneviève had jurisdiction over the schools on the Mount,[12] and William would have found in Abbot Stephen a sympathetic soul.[13] But we know too little about the politics of school-founding in this period to do more than raise the possibility.

The physical aspect of William's school is likewise unknown. The only indispensable element was a hall or room large enough to accommodate the students wishing to hear the master teach. Evidence from the early twelfth century suggests that class sizes could vary from three or four to 300 or more students.[14] A class of the latter size could only be accommodated in such places as the bishop's hall, but most schools were held in private houses leased to a master for this purpose.[15]

As an unbeneficed teacher of theology at Paris, William must have depended on student fees or donations to support his profession.[16] Some flexible method of remuneration must have been customary at Paris in the twelfth century to provide the economic basis for one of the most salient characteristics of scholastic culture there — the frequent movement of students from one master and one classroom to another. The surviving accounts of Parisian academic careers from

[12] Insofar as any jurisdiction was exercised over them; see Southern, "Schools of Paris," p. 120. The right of the abbey of Ste. Geneviève to license masters of theology, canon law, and arts within their jurisdictional boundaries was recognized by Pope Gregory ix in 1227: "Gregorius episcopus ... cancellario Parisiensi salutem ... . Dilecti filii ... abbas et conventus Sancte Genovefe Parisiensis nobis insinuare curarunt, quod cum ad jus eorum pertineat, ut doctores theologie, decretorum ac liberalium artium de ipsorum licentia libere regere valeant in parrochia et terra eorum infra Parisiensium murorum ambitum constituta, tu theologie decretorumque doctores ad regendum inter duos pontes astringis vinculo juramenti. Propter quod et si doctores artium de licentia ipsorum regant in predicta parrochia, theologie tamen et decretorum doctores non audent regere in eadem, unde non solum honori, sed etiam utilitati monasterii sui plurimum derogatur. Volentes igitur ejusdem monasterii honores et jura illibata servari, discretioni tue per apostolica scripta mandamus, quatinus si premissis veritas suffragatur, illos qui predictas scientias in parrochia et terra ipsa docere voluerint ... id facere sine contradictione permittas ... "; *Chartularium Universitatis Parisiensis*, 1: 111 (no. 55). No evidence of the exercise of jurisdiction by the abbot and canons of Ste. Geneviève over 12th-century schools within their territories has survived, but the restriction of the Paris chancellor's authority to the territory "between the two bridges" is tacitly acknowledged by all sides in the document above. On the chancellor of Ste. Geneviève in the 13th century see Rashdall, *Universities of Europe*, 1: 341-342.

[13] See below, pp. 38-39.

[14] Southern, "Schools of Paris," p. 124.

[15] Ibid., pp. 120-121; cf. Häring, "Chartres and Paris Revisited," pp. 327-329; William A. Pantin, "The Halls and Schools of Medieval Oxford: An Attempt at Reconstruction," in *Oxford Studies Presented to Daniel Callus* (Oxford: Clarendon Press, 1964), pp. 31-100.

[16] See Baldwin, *Masters*, 1: 117-130.

the mid twelfth century are striking in this regard.[17] John of Salisbury describes his nearly twelve years of study (1136-1148) under twelve different masters at Paris and at Chartres. William of Tyre mentions sixteen masters under whom he studied from 1145-1165 in Bologna and Paris; ten of these masters taught liberal arts and theology, four taught law, and two instructed him in classical literature and mathematics.

Alexander Neckam's seven-year sojourn in Paris, during William de Montibus's tenure there, is typical of many (perhaps most) students' experience. During those years (c. 1175-1182) he studied and taught arts, and attended lectures on theology, civil and canon law, and medicine.[18] At roughly the same time Gerald of Wales demonstrated a similar interest in attending the schools of many different masters. He claims to have studied theology, law, and arts during his two sojourns in Paris (c. 1165, and from 1176-1179).[19]

Few examples can be found of twelfth-century students who attached themselves to a single master and followed his courses exclusively for an extended period. Student *reportationes* reflect a master's lecture course for a single year or term; the numerous collections of disputed questions report the disputations not of a single master, but of several teachers on important issues of the day.[20] It was, indeed, the abundance of opportunities for attending the lectures and disputations of several masters that made Paris an attractive place to study.

Given such a fluid academic environment, one often looks in vain for the specific students of a given master. Most students could refer to a number of individuals as *magistri mei*. Neither Neckam nor Gerald of Wales says explicitly that they studied under William de Montibus, but they, like other Englishmen at Paris in the 1170's and 1180's, may be presumed to have attended William's school at least occasionally during their stay. Nor should we limit William's audience to Englishmen in Paris. Several copies of William's Parisian treatise *De septem sacramentis* are found in German libraries; indeed, these are the only extant copies that ascribe the work to William.[21] This may be explained as an accident of manuscript transmission, but it may just as plausibly

---

[17] These are conveniently summarized by Häring, "Chartres and Paris Revisited," pp. 317-329, and Southern, "Schools of Paris," pp. 128-132.

[18] Richard W. Hunt, *The Schools and the Cloister*, pp. 5-6.

[19] Baldwin, "Masters at Paris," pp. 143, 146.

[20] Such collections need further study. See Ignatius Brady, "Peter Manducator and the Oral Teachings of Peter Lombard," pp. 455-465; Franco Giusberti, *Materials for a Study on Twelfth Century Scholasticism* (Naples: Bibliopolis, 1982), pp. 113-154.

[21] See below, II.13, p. 473.

suggest that someone with connections in southern Germany heard
William lecture at Paris and returned to his homeland with a copy
of William's work.

As a master of theology in the Parisian schools, William can be
expected to have preached, lectured, and disputed questions.[22] Of these
activities, preaching is the most problematic. The actual context of
preaching in the twelfth-century schools is yet to be elucidated.[23] Did
masters "preach" in their own classrooms, or in the local churches?
Was preaching a formal part of the masters' instruction or a separate
and independent exercise? These are some of the outstanding questions
concerning scholastic preaching in the twelfth and early thirteenth
centuries. William's career sheds no new light on these issues. His extant
sermons seem to date from the period of his Lincoln regency and his
tenure as chancellor of the cathedral there. He composed his *Similitudinarium, Distinctiones, Proverbia*, and other writings with the
preacher as well as the student and teacher in mind, but these, too,
he compiled after leaving the Parisian schools. Although he certainly
began collecting materials for his sermons and treatises during his
Parisian sojourn, these works reflect only in a general way the preaching
activities of the Parisian masters. If William preached at all in the
Paris schools, and we presume that he did, no certain evidence of his
activities in this regard has been identified.

Direct evidence for William's Parisian lectures is also lacking. He
almost certainly lectured on the Bible, as is testified by his familiarity
with both text and glosses of the Scriptures in his subsequent writings.
Specific information on the formal curriculum of lectures in the twelfth-
century schools, however, is very meagre; customs of the thirteenth-
century universities, specifying how and when masters would lecture
and the texts they would expound, are inapplicable to the earlier
period.[24] The most that can be said is that the curriculum in William's

---

[22] See Smalley, *Study of the Bible*, pp. 196-213; Baldwin, *Masters*, 1: 90-116.

[23] Like most scholarship on the subject, the recent study by Jean Longère, *La
prédication médiévale* (Paris: Etudes Augustiniennes, 1983), tells us much about the
preachers and their sermons but very little about the physical and institutional context(s)
in which they preached. The issue of context is raised in the questionnaire on sermon
studies, circulated by the French School in Rome for the volume entitled *Faire croire:
Modalités de la diffusion et de la réception des messages religieux du XIIe au XVe
siècle* (Rome: Ecole Française de Rome, 1981).

[24] The best description of the 13th-century theology curriculum remains Palémon
Glorieux, "L'enseignement au moyen âge: Techniques et méthodes en usage à la Faculté
de Théologie de Paris, au XIIIe siècle," *Archives d'histoire doctrinale et littéraire du
moyen âge* 43 (1968) 65-186. Beryl Smalley has greatly expanded our knowledge of
12th-century lectures on the Bible; see *Study of the Bible*, and *Gospels in the Schools*,

day was characterized by a good deal of flexibility. William may have lectured, for example, on a collection or "harmony" of the gospels rather than on each book individually,[25] or he may have lectured on the Bible "histories" of one of his own teachers, Peter Comestor.[26]

The clearest positive evidence for William's Parisian teaching is the collection of his lectures and questions on the Church's sacraments. It has been recognized that the two activities of lecturing and disputing, clearly distinguished in the thirteenth-century universities, grew originally from the lecture techniques of the twelfth-century masters. William's *De septem sacramentis* illustrates the original conflation of these two activities. He begins the treatment of each sacrament with a brief exposition or lecture, which is followed by a longer series of *quaestiones* and *responsiones*. The work itself is probably not a *viva voce* report, but it conveys accurately the general tenor of discussions concerning the sacraments in the late-twelfth-century Parisian classrooms.[27]

One further document may preserve a record of William's teachings in the Parisian schools. An interesting collection of questions in the British Library (MS Royal 10.B.vii, fols. 205ra-211va) records the disputations of an unidentified master concerning theological, moral, and sacramental topics.[28] The manuscript was in the possession of the monks of Bardney Abbey during the thirteenth century, but the questions themselves seem to stem from the late-twelfth-century Parisian schools. Two masters only are cited by name. One is Peter Comestor, and the other William de Montibus (*de Monte*).[29] William

---

but much work remains to be done on the lectures and disputations of the 12th-century schools.

[25] Beryl Smalley makes the suggestion in her "Gospels in the Paris Schools," pp. 238-239, and note 14; and *Gospels in the Schools*, p. 107, n. 14; I have been unable to attribute to William any of the anonymous commentaries mentioned by Smalley.

[26] As late as 1253 the statutes of Oxford University, influenced by early customs in Paris, still envision the possibility of lectures on Comestor's *Histories* in the theology curriculum: "(De theologis licenciandis ad incipiendum). Statuit vniversitas Oxonie, et, si statutum fuerit, iterato consensu corroborat quod nullus in eadem vniuersitate incipiat in theologia nisi ... legerit aliquem librum de canone Biblie uel librum senten-ciarum uel historiarum, et predicauerit publice vniuersitati ... "; *Statuta Antiqua Vniuersitatis Oxoniensis*, ed. Strickland Gibson (Oxford: Clarendon Press, 1931), p. 49. The surviving copies of scholastic commentaries on Comestor, many from the late 12th and early 13th centuries, have received insufficient attention.

[27] See Goering, "*Diffinicio eucaristie*," pp. 91-104.

[28] Artur Landgraf seems to have been the first and the last scholar to utilize these questions; see his *Dogmengeschichte der Frühscholastik*, 4 vols. (Regensburg: F. Pustet, 1952-1956); see 2/1: 258, n. 201 for a reference to "William de Monte."

[29] Peter Comestor is cited on fol. 209rb: "Comestor dixit quod ex solis uirginibus suplebitur ruina angelorum in uno pariete et corrupti in alio pariete erunt."

is reported as having stressed the ordinary human character of the flesh that Christ assumed in the incarnation by arguing that, before the passion, his physical death was as inevitable as anyone else's, unless God should intervene supernaturally.[30] The anonymous author of these questions added that, although Jesus was subject to the general necessity of physical death, his specific and historical death on the cross was not inevitable, but was freely chosen. The careful study of the question-literature of the twelfth-century schools is still in its infancy, and further references to the oral teachings of William de Montibus at Paris may yet be discovered.[31]

Given the relatively free commerce of ideas and the circulation of students among the various disciplines and between one master's classroom and another's, we should be wary of insisting on the existence of distinct "schools" of thought in twelfth-century Paris.[32] Nevertheless it is possible to situate William and his teachings broadly within what Martin Grabmann has called "the biblical-moral orientation" (*die biblisch-moralische Richtung*), and "the practical orientation" (*die praktische Richtung*) of theology in the Parisian schools.[33] Each of these terms — "biblical," "moral," and "practical" — deserves consideration.

A peculiarly biblical approach to theology in the late-twelfth-century schools is difficult to identify, and is the least precise characteristic of Grabmann's description. The Bible had been, and was to remain, the standard theological textbook in the schools.[34] Nevertheless, neither

---

[30] "Si queritur qualem carnem assumpserit Christus, dicendum quod talem qualem habuit uirgo scilicet carnem addictam necessitati moriendi. Vnde dicit magister W. de monte quod ante passionem Christus necessitatem moriendi haberet nisi potencia diuine maiestatis occurreret," ibid., fol. 208vb.

[31] See above, n. 20. For a general orientation see Bernardo C. Bazan, Gérard Fransen, John W. Wippel, and Danielle Jacquart, *Les questions disputées et les questions quodlibétiques dans les facultés de théologie, de droit et de médecine*, Typologie des sources du moyen âge occidental, 44-45 (Turnhout: Brepols, 1985).

[32] See the perceptive comments in William J. Courtenay, *Schools & Scholars in Fourteenth-Century England* (Princeton: Princeton University Press, 1987), pp. 171-192.

[33] Martin Grabmann, *Die Geschichte der scholastischen Methode*, 2 vols. (1909-1911; rpt. Darmstadt: Wissenschaftliche Buchgesellschaft, 1957), 2: 476-501. Grabmann discusses William de Montibus in the chapter entitled "Die von Petrus Cantor ausgehende biblisch-moralische Richtung der Theologie." It might be more accurate to substitute Peter Comestor's name for that of Peter the Chanter; Grabmann mentions Comestor only in passing, p. 477.

[34] The two classic, and complementary, studies are: Smalley, *Study of the Bible*, and Ceslaus Spicq, *Esquisse d'une histoire de l'exégèse latine au moyen âge* (Paris: Vrin, 1944). The impression that some theologians were more interested in speculative than biblical theology has arisen, in part, from the lack of interest among scholars in the biblical and exegetical writings of the early scholastics.

William de Montibus nor his contemporaries in the "biblical-moral school" (e.g. Peter Comestor, Peter the Chanter, and Stephen Langton) limited their teachings to the exposition or interpretation of Holy Scripture.[35] A perusal of William's extant works reveals the range of his interests extending far beyond the simple exposition of the biblical text. Unlike Langton and the Chanter, William seems not to have published a gloss or running commentary on all the books of the Bible, although his thorough familiarity with the Bible and its glosses is evident in all his writings. Nor is William's interest in sacred scripture confined to the Bible itself. He treats the liturgy, the Lives of the Saints, and even the natural world, as authoritative documents, and uses them in his theological teaching just as he does the biblical texts.[36]

If William is to be seen as part of a biblical or biblicist direction in late-twelfth-century theology, this should be understood in the sense that the "sacred page," in its widest connotation, dominated all of his work. When Alexander Neckam singles out for particular praise William's exclusive study of the "sacred page" (*cui se coelestis pagina tota dedit*), he is not implying that William studied and taught only the Bible; rather he is contrasting William to other masters who, like Alexander himself, devoted much of their time and energies to studying the liberal arts and secular sciences.[37] William's devotion to the "sacred page," that is to the teaching and writing of theology, was a predilection that he shared with Comestor, Langton, Peter the Chanter, and others. It was worthy of note in the twelfth-century schools, and perhaps justifies us in characterizing him as having a *biblische Richtung* in theology.

More discriminating than the epithet "biblical," which can be applied in some sense to every Parisian theologian, is the term "moral," which describes accurately an important current of theological activities in the schools. But here again distinctions should be made. What we call

[35] Peter Comestor, for example, wrote one of the first commentaries on Lombard's *Sentences*; see Luscombe, "Peter Comestor," p. 116. Comestor, de Montibus, Langton, and Peter the Chanter all disputed questions on non-biblical topics, and all wrote extensively concerning the Church's sacraments. William and Peter the Chanter both composed works that brought to bear on theological language the teachings of the arts faculties in Paris, see below, *Tropi* ii.11.

[36] In this he followed one of his masters, Peter Comestor; see Beryl Smalley, "Peter Comestor on the Gospels and His Sources," *Recherches de théologie ancienne et médiévale* 46 (1979) 84-129, at 115-123.

[37] *Alexandri Neckam De naturis rerum*, p. 460; quoted above, Chapter One, at note 26.

"moral theology," as distinct from sacramental, dogmatic, and speculative theology, had no independent existence in the twelfth-century schools.[38] The surviving evidence of William de Montibus's Parisian teaching shows his concern with sacramental and dogmatic theology.[39] Peter the Chanter and Stephen Langton, two of Grabmann's premier representatives of a "biblical-moral direction" in theology, also made important contributions to speculative and sacramental theology.[40] On the other hand, such speculative theologians as Abelard, Gilbert of Poitiers, and Peter of Poitiers were also skilled in moral analysis and moral exhortation. Nevertheless a distinctive moral approach to the study of theology was to be found in the twelfth-century Parisian schools, and William de Montibus was one of its noteworthy proponents.

Many of William's contemporaries equated moral theology with the moral discipline of the cloister. Stephen of Tournai, abbot of Ste. Geneviève from 1176-1191, sings the praises of education in his abbey in the Parisian suburbs, where the student of theology (sacre pagine) can study truth in the lecture hall and moral virtue in the cloister.[41] When asked by the archbishop of Lund whether his nephew should study on "the Mount" or in the secular schools of Paris, Stephen replied that it is in the cloister where one finds schools both of truth and of virtue. He adds that, if the archbishop should desire his nephew to attend the secular schools, he should choose some city other than

---

[38] Perhaps the earliest reference to moral theology as a distinct discipline is Alan of Lille's comment: "Theologie due sunt species: una rationalis ... alia moralis, que circa mores sive informationes hominum vertitur," quoted by Georg Wieland, *Ethica — Scientia practica: Die Anfänge der philosophischen Ethik im 13. Jahrhundert* (Münster: Aschendorff, 1981), p. 80, n. 119. But note that Alan emphasizes the practical end of moral theology, not its existence as an independent scientific discipline.

[39] See especially the discussion of his *Numerale* and *De septem sacramentis*, II.7 and 13, below.

[40] For an appreciation of Peter and Stephen's contributions to speculative theology see Edouard Dumoutet, "La théologie de l'eucharistie à la fin du XIIe siècle: Le témoignage de Pierre le Chantre d'après la 'Summa de sacramentis,'" *Archives d'histoire doctrinale et littéraire du moyen âge* 14 (1943-1945) 181-262; F.M. Powicke, *Stephen Langton* (Oxford: Clarendon Press, 1928).

[41] "Sacre pagine studens scolas veritatis in auditorio, scolas virtutis frequentat in claustro: cum neque hic sine veritate virtutem, neque ibi sine virtute combibat veritatem. Duo suggens ubera cito poterit impinguari," letter of Stephen to Absalon, archbishop of Lund, *Chartularium Universitatis Parisiensis*, 1: 42 (no. 41). For a general appreciation of this educational sensibility among the regular canons in the 12th century see Carolyn Walker Bynum, *Jesus as Mother: Studies in the Spirituality of the High Middle Ages* (Berkeley: University of California Press, 1982), esp. pp. 22-80.

Paris, where the nephew will learn to be disputatious but not to be good.[42]

In other letters Stephen admitted the possibility of moral theology being learned outside the cloister, illuminating, incidentally, a "moral direction" in the Parisian schools. He wrote, for example, to the archbishop of Reims that Peter the Chanter, who was "famous throughout the whole church," was a good choice for bishop of Tournai because "in him the twofold knowledge, of doctrine and moral discipline, shines so clearly."[43] This twofold knowledge distinguishes the moral direction in theology from a predominantly intellectual one. Just such an understanding of moral theology was obviously in the mind of St. Hugh of Lincoln when he chided another famous Parisian theologian (Peter of Poitiers?) for not having virtue to equal his learning.[44]

William de Montibus's interests and his early training led him into the biblical-moral current of Parisian theology. He had learned from Gilbert of Sempringham the importance of pursuing knowledge and virtue hand-in-hand.[45] Although himself a secular teacher, William never lost his appreciation for the discipline of the cloister. His choice of Mont Ste. Geneviève as the site of his school may reflect a tacit sympathy with the educational ideals set out so forcefully by Abbot Stephen, and it is not impossible that some of William's students came from the abbey to hear his lectures. In later years William continued to address monastic as well as secular audiences, urging both to study theology as a moral and an intellectual discipline. It is in this twofold approach to theology, uniting the intellectual curiosity of the secular schools with the moral discipline of the cloister, that the moral orientation of twelfth-century scholasticism can be recognized most clearly.

---

[42] "Quod autem de ipso nobis per litteras vestras intimastis, vel in monte, vel ad Parisienses secularium scolas et venditores verborum mittendo, salva gratia vestra non admittimus ... . Habet in claustris sapientia regulas suas, habet et regulares suos, erigens sibi scolas inde veritatis, hinc virtutis. Quod si forte consilium vestrum in hoc declinaverit, ut de regulari secularem facere credatis, aliam quam Parisium civitatem in qua studeat eligite, ne in oculis nostris pro matutino et vespertino sacrificio quod nobiscum offerre debuerat Domino, verborum strepitus et disputationum anfractus offerat ... "; *Chartularium Universitatis Parisiensis*, 1: 43 (no. 42).

[43] "Vir est cujus per omnes ecclesias fame suavis diffunditur opinio, qui gemina scientia efficacissime clarens et doctrinam monitis ornat et moribus disciplinam," ibid., 1: 46 (no. 46).

[44] See above, Chapter One, at notes 45 and 46.

[45] See above, Chapter One, at note 20.

One further characteristic of the biblical-moral school identified by
Grabmann is its practical approach to theology. If "practical" be taken
here in simple contradistinction to "theoretical" or "speculative theology"
we might well hesitate to place any of the twelfth-century theologians
exclusively in one camp or the other. More appropriate is to distinguish
between those theologians whose primary interest was investigating and
elucidating theological questions (the speculative theologians), and
those, like William, who were primarily interested in teaching theology
and elucidating its implications for everyday life (the practical theologians). The former have been studied copiously for their original
contributions to the development of doctrine; the latter, less interested
in making definitive contributions to doctrine than in making the fruits
of scholastic discussions available to students in the schools, have
received less attention. It is this practical aspect of scholasticism that
is now beginning to receive its due.

Like Peter Comestor and Peter the Chanter, William's fame among
his contemporaries lay in his abilities as a teacher of theology. For
the modern historian wishing to study the developments in this practical
aspect of scholastic theology, the most valuable sources extant are the
handbooks and *summae* that these masters composed as aids to
students in the schools, and the sermons that they preached as a part
of their teaching there. Peter Comestor's *Historia scholastica* and Peter
the Chanter's *Verbum abbreviatum* are two of the most famous
examples of the practical writings from this period, and the latter has
been used as the basis for a thoughtful reconstruction of Peter the
Chanter's influence and activities.[46] Stephen Langton's preaching and
the complicated manuscript traditions that preserve it have also been
studied.[47] These works, however, represent only a fraction of the
practical writings that poured out of the Parisian schools at the end
of the twelfth century.

The originality and popularity of such practical writings can be
inferred from the works themselves and from the large number of extant
manuscripts containing them. Eloquent testimony to their ubiquity and
to their novelty can also be found in contemporary criticisms of this
practical approach. For example, the same Stephen of Tournai who
had praised the "biblical-moral" approach to scholastic theology was

---

[46] Baldwin, *Masters*. The practical teachings of Peter Comestor are awaiting study;
see the suggestive comments in Luscombe, "Peter Comestor," pp. 109-121.

[47] Stephen Langton, *Stephanus de Lingua-tonante: Studies in the Sermons of
Stephen Langton*, ed. Phyllis Barzillay Roberts, Studies and Texts, 16 (Toronto:
Pontifical Institute of Mediaeval Studies, 1968).

quite troubled by the flood of practical writings engulfing the schools. After leaving the abbey of Ste. Geneviève to become bishop of Tournai in 1192, he complained to the Pope (either Celestine III or Innocent III) about the ruinous state of theology, canon law, and arts as taught at Paris. He singled out for particular comment "the recent and novel *summulae* and commentaries on theology that are everywhere being written ... as if the works of the holy Fathers no longer sufficed" for the study of sacred letters.[48]

In a letter addressed to William de Montibus, Gerald of Wales also disparages these novelties of practical theology:

> There is already a superabundance, as it were, of theological books, and even more are being added to the overflowing pile. These are concoctions of all sorts of different books and are taken from the outstanding works of great writers, then presented as though they are something new, but with some artificial rearrangement and a change of title. In fact these modern booklets are not truly genuine, for they are patched together from the earlier original works of others; they are attempts to snatch the reputation from the deserving and attach it to the undeserving.[49]

William, however, makes no apologies for his own impressive contribution to this practical literature of theological education; he freely acknowledges the derivative nature of his writings. In his *Similitudinarium*, William claims to have collected examples "whencesoever God gives them," for use in all kinds of theological discourse.[50] In his *Proverbia*, he proffered useful things, excerpted from wheresoever: flowers for the readers' enjoyment, pearls for their adornment, honey-

---

[48] "Id tantum, quod dolet, significare volumus sancte paternitati vestre, cui Deus contulit et potestatem corripiendi errores, et scientiam corrigendi. Lapsa sunt apud nos in confusionis officinam sacrarum studia litterarum, dum et discipuli solis novitatibus applaudunt, et magistri glorie potius invigilant quam doctrine, novas recentesque summulas et commentaria firmantia super theologia passim conscribunt, quibus auditores suos demulceant, detineant, decipiant, quasi nondum suffecerint sanctorum opuscula patrum, quos eodem spiritu sacram scripturam legimus exposuisse, quo eam composuisse credimus apostolos et prophetas." *Chartularium Universitatis Parisiensis*, 1: 47 (no. 47).

[49] "Scire vos etiam volumus quod predicta scripta nostra hystorica ... longeviora ... in posterum erunt quam scripta plurima, que theologica et theologice facultati tanquam ex superhabundanti et superflue superaddita, ex aliorum scriptis undique corrogata et transpositionibus quibusdam artificiosis et titulorum mutationibus ex magnorum virorum laboribus egregiis excerpta et quasi de novo nunc fabricata, sed verius quidem artificialiter innovata, quatinus ex aliorum operibus antiquis et autenticis consuta sic nuper opuscula et dignis laudem adimere et indignis adquirere queant." *Speculum duorum*, pp. 172-173.

[50] See below, II.9.

combs for nourishment, and health-giving candies (*electuaria*) for their strengthening.[51]

No doubt William began this work of collecting and excerpting in the Parisian schools, but it was during his nearly three decades of teaching in Lincoln that he brought it to fruition in the classroom, in the pulpit, and in his scholastic compositions. There one can see most clearly the practical problems that confronted a teacher, and the various techniques that William developed to make accessible to students the fruits of twelfth-century scholastic theology.

THE SCHOOLS OF LINCOLN:
Transiit ad montem Montanus, monte relicto

The scholastic geography of England at the end of the twelfth century was much like that of France in the middle of the century. Schools flourished in the monasteries and in the cathedrals, and independent masters could be found teaching students in many locales.[52] None of these centres of learning had attained the density of academic population that characterized the schools of Paris. English students who had the interest and the financial means travelled to Paris to study, and often to teach, throughout the second half of the twelfth century.[53] This free concourse of Englishmen to the French capital must have been encouraged by the proximity of the English duchy of Normandy, only a short distance down the Seine from Paris. In the latter part of the century, however, relations between the French and English became increasingly strained, and travel to and from the Continent became more hazardous. Gerald of Wales, who had studied twice in the Parisian schools, c. 1165, and c. 1176-1179, found himself prevented from a third journey in the 1190's because of the outbreak of hostilities. Forced to remain in England, he sought out the schools of Lincoln because "the science of theology flourishes there most soundly in all of England, under the best of teachers, Master William de Monte."[54] Others had similar experiences, and contributed to the growing concentration of students and masters in the indigenous English schools. By the third decade of the thirteenth century, Englishmen would no longer have felt the necessity of travelling to the Continent for a quality education.

[51] See below, II.10.
[52] See above, Chapter One, note 57.
[53] See above, at notes 2 and 3.
[54] Quoted above, Chapter One, note 10.

During the formative years of the English educational establishment (c. 1180-1220), however, it was far from certain that a single locale would come to dominate in the way that Paris had in France. The growth of Oxford and Cambridge as incorporated universities at the expense of monastic, cathedral, and proto-university centres throughout England happened only slowly, and was not a foregone conclusion.[55] The history of the schools that failed to become famous university centres in the thirteenth century and their contributions to the scholastic culture of Europe still await investigation. Of all the English schools flourishing before 1230, the theological school of William de Montibus at Lincoln is one of the best suited to study. Elsewhere only scattered documents and casual references survive. From Lincoln, thanks to the popularity of William as a teacher, and to his unusual *stabilitas loci* as canon and then chancellor of the cathedral, from c. 1186 to 1213, an unusually full picture of scholastic life in this period has been preserved.

William's *translatio studii* from the mount of Paris to the mount of Lincoln took place sometime during the 1180's. He was surely teaching in Lincoln by 1189, when he first appears in a Lincoln document designated simply as "magister,"[56] and his reputation was established by the 1190's, when Gerald of Wales sought out the Lincoln schools on account of William's presence there.

We might infer from Gerald's comment that other masters were also teaching at Lincoln, and that the concourse of masters and students presented a suitable alternative to the Parisian schools wherein Gerald could exercise his own skills. He makes no mention of studying under William, but rather of the "flourishing studies" in Lincoln — a milieu in which he could study, write, and participate in the academic life of lectures and disputations as he had done at Paris and Oxford on other occasions.[57]

Evidence concerning other schools at Lincoln in this period is sparse, but this is not unusual, as our knowledge of the schools and teaching masters in the period is quite imperfect. A cursory review of the Lincoln Cathedral canons and officials alone, however, reveals the names of

---

[55] See M.B. Hackett, *The Original Statutes of Cambridge University: The Text and Its History* (Cambridge: Cambridge University Press, 1970); Southern, "From Schools to University," pp. 1-36.

[56] See above, Chapter One, n. 66.

[57] Quoted above, Chapter One, note 10. Gerald composed several theological works while at Lincoln; see Bartlett, *Gerald of Wales*, App. I, pp. 213-221.

some seventy masters (*magistri*) holding Lincoln prebends during the twenty-five years from 1188 to 1213.[58] These and others, whose names, reputations, and writings are lost to us, may well be said to have comprised an academic milieu in which schools and study might flourish.

As at Paris, the fame of the Lincoln schools depended on the numbers and quality of the students as well as the masters. The most easily identifiable group of students at Lincoln is the cathedral clergy.[59] The canons, canon-vicars, officials, and their respective *adiutores* were well situated, physically and financially, to take advantage of academic pursuits in the city. William's sermons illustrate the kind of instruction that they might have received on an informal basis.[60] It is likely that some of them also took advantage of the classroom instruction, whether to better themselves and improve their chances for promotion in ecclesiastical service, or simply out of an interest in the things being taught.

Monks and regular canons in and around the diocese of Lincoln also were attracted to the cathedral schools. Many of the surviving manuscripts of William's writings were preserved in monastic houses, and William often refers, in these writings, to the monastic life.[61] The example of the Gilbertine canon who sought William's advice when composing his life of St. Gilbert illustrates the kinds of ties established between the regular clergy and the master of a cathedral school.[62] The Gilbertine canons served as chaplains, teachers, and preachers to the nuns and lay-brothers of the order. They were expected to provide learned pastoral care in the Order of Sempringham, and would have received excellent training for this service in William's school. Matthew, the Cistercian precentor of Rievaulx who composed several sets of memorial verses in William's honour, seems to have known him

---

[58] Le Neve, *Fasti ecclesiae Anglicanae 1066-1300*: III *Lincoln*. The term "magister" in documents of this period does not necessarily indicate either that the bearer is a "graduate" of some school or that he is actually teaching at the time the document was issued. The title does indicate, however, that the person has had some formal education and is perceived as capable of teaching in a school should the opportunity arise. Bishop Hugh's insistence on the residence of his canons would suggest that many of the "magistri" were not absentees.

[59] See Edwards, *English Secular Cathedrals*, pp. 33-96, 251-317.

[60] See especially sermons 1-73, in II.16, below.

[61] See, for example, the entry "Monachus," in William's *Similitudinarium* (II.9) and *Versarius* (II.12). The provenance of manuscripts containing William's writings is recorded in Appendix A, below.

[62] See above, Chapter One, at note 72

personally, and may also have been among his students.[63] So, too, the unidentified recipient of two sermon-collections composed by William, probably an Augustinian canon, may be presumed to have studied under William at Lincoln.[64]

A third group of students to be found frequenting William's school included those with private means of support who attended the schools as a road to advancement in the Church or in secular government. We have no way of estimating the numbers of such students, and their names are almost all lost to us. A few, however, are known through their writings. One of these was Richard of Wetheringsett, who tells us explicitly in his *Summa Qui bene presunt* that William was one of his masters.[65] Richard subsequently became a master in his own right, and was perhaps one of the first chancellors of Cambridge University.[66]

Another of William's students known to us through his writings is Samuel Priest (*Presbyter*).[67] The surname "Priest" is probably a family name rather than an indication of occupation or office. The name is known in the Jewish community of Lincoln, and appears often as a translation of the surname "Cohen."[68] Samuel may have been a christian convert from Judaism, or have belonged to a family of such converts.

Gerald of Wales describes another "private" student at Lincoln. In his *Speculum duorum* ("A Mirror of Two Men"), Gerald tells in great detail how he established his nephew along with a tutor in the Lincoln schools during William's chancellorship, and how these two managed to squander the educational opportunities there. Although this nephew was presumably studying introductory subjects rather than theology, he may be taken as a representative of one type of student, usually lost to history, who frequented the schools in William's day.

---

[63] See above, Chapter One, at note 93; cf. Wilmart, "Les mélanges de Mathieu," p. 50.

[64] See sermons 74-113 in ɪɪ.16, below.

[65] This work is discussed below, Chapter Three, pp. 86-91.

[66] The most recent discussion of Richard's career is by Fritz Kemmler, *"Exempla" in Context: A Historical and Critical Study of Robert Mannyng of Brunne's "Handlyng Synne"* (Tübingen: Gunter Narr, 1984), pp. 46-48. A study of the *Qui bene presunt* and its author is being prepared by J. Goering.

[67] See Josiah Cox Russell, *Dictionary of Writers of Thirteenth Century England* (1936; rpt. New York: Burt Franklin, 1971), p. 147; cf. below, *Super Psalmos* (ɪɪ.14) and *Collecta* (ɪɪ.15).

[68] See John Paul Bischoff, "Economic Change in Thirteenth Century Lincoln: Decline of an Urban Cloth Industry" (PhD diss.: Yale University, 1975), pp. 103-104.

This group of "secular" students would also include clerics in minor orders who enjoyed some of the fruits of an ecclesiastical benefice while they attended the schools. The number of beneficed clerics in the schools would grow during the later Middle Ages, when official sanction was given to the practice of financing one's education through the possession of a benefice. Pope Boniface VIII's bull *Cum ex eo* (1298) formalized the process by which licenses for study could be given to beneficed clergy.[69] The numbers of such clerics in William's school should not, however, be overestimated. The earliest episcopal ordination records for Lincoln diocese are found in the registers of Bishop Hugh of Wells (1209-1235). These note thousands of presentations to benefices, and include some references to appointments made conditional on the appointee attending the schools. The editor of the *Rotuli* has presumed that such clerics would attend universities or schools of theology like William's,[70] but in fact the expectations seem much more limited. The ordinands are almost certainly being referred to the local song or grammar schools that they might "learn letters," or "learn chant and song," or simply "learn something." Only a few of the entries mention clerics leaving their parishes to pursue higher studies.[71]

Once committed to the Lincoln schools, students may have had a choice of masters and of academic curricula. Our sources, however, are limited to the teachings of the most famous Lincoln master, William de Montibus. William's own writings are extensive, and provide valuable information about the academic milieu of the Lincoln schools. Many of them take the form of aids-to-study, and constitute what might be called the "informal" curriculum of William's school, that is, works that students could study at their leisure as supplements to the formal course of lectures and disputations. These writings will be discussed below.

Evidence concerning William's actual classroom teaching, and thus for the formal curriculum of his school, survives in three collections made by his students. Two were made by Samuel Presbyter, of whom little is known except that he was a student in William's school and an inveterate "collector" of religious verses and theological materials.[72]

---

[69] Leonard E. Boyle, "The Constitution 'Cum ex eo' of Boniface VIII: Education of Parochial Clergy," *Mediaeval Studies* 24 (1962) 263-302; rept. in his *Pastoral Care, Clerical Education and Canon Law, 1200-1400* (London: Variorum Reprints, 1981).

[70] See W.P.W. Phillimore's comments in his introduction to *Rotuli Hugonis de Welles*, 1: xvii.

[71] Ibid., 1: xii-xviii; cf. Orme, *English Schools*, pp. 12-21.

[72] See above, note 67.

Samuel is meticulous in recording the origins of his collections. At the head of one he writes: "Hec collecta sunt ex auditis super Psalmos in scola magistri Willelmi de Montibus."[73] As the title suggests, this is not a commentary on the Psalms officially published by William, but rather a student's collection of classroom notes.

These lectures conform to the general pattern of classroom teaching in late-twelfth-century Paris. The Bible was the standard theological text, and the master of theology was expected to lecture on it. William's choice of the Psalms as the subject of his lectures is also typical. The expectation that a master would lecture on all the books of the Bible, if it ever existed in practice, was hardly current in William's day.[74] If a choice of books was to be made, the Psalter, with its deep roots in the familiar liturgy and devotion of the Church, was a clear favourite.[75]

The content of William's lectures on the Psalms is also typical of the classroom use of the Bible in this period. He provided no systematic or definitive commentary on the text and accumulated glosses. Rather William and most of his contemporaries used the biblical text as a means of introducing students to the entire scope of theological knowledge. Like the Psalter commentaries of Peter Comestor and Peter the Chanter, William's lectures were quite discursive. His favourite technique was to use a single word from a Psalm as the basis for distinguishing the many uses of that word, not only in the sacred scriptures, but in all theological and moral discourse. William's commentary constitutes a *summa theologiae* — a summary of sacred doctrine rooted in the biblical text but extending to all aspects of theology. This method of commenting on the Psalms as an introductory exercise in theology was popular in Paris during the last decade of the twelfth century, and was used not only by the so-called "biblical-moral" theologians but also by such "speculative" writers as Peter of Poitiers and Praepositinus.[76]

Another of Samuel's school collections fits less easily into what we have come to view as the standard pattern of scholastic lecturing. His *Collecta ex diuersis auditis in schola* consists entirely of glossed verses

[73] See the *Super Psalmos*, below, II.14.

[74] Peter the Chanter is said to have been the first to comment on the whole Bible, as did Stephen Langton; see Smalley, *Study of the Bible*, p. 197.

[75] See C. Spicq, *Esquisse d'une histoire de l'exégèse*, pp. 62, 396.

[76] On Peter of Poitiers's Psalm-commentary, see Moore, *Peter of Poitiers*, pp. 78-96; on Praepositinus's, see Georges Lacombe, *La vie et les oeuvres de Prévostin* (Kain: Le Saulchoir), pp. 104-130.

on various theological topics.[77] The verses appear to be compositions of William de Montibus; many are found in his *Versarius*, and the glosses repeat materials from William's other lectures and writings. If Samuel's collection does indeed represent materials heard in William's school, it would seem that William not only lectured on existing texts such as the Bible, but also provided his own texts in the form of didactic verse, and commented on them in the same way that later masters would comment on the text of Peter Lombard's *Sentences*. In the context of late-twelfth- and early-thirteenth-century scholasticism, such a procedure is understandable. The establishment of a standard curriculum with set lecture-texts (the Bible and Lombard's *Sentences*) was an accomplishment of the thirteenth century. Earlier masters had a good deal of freedom in choosing their texts, and apparently experimented with a number of options.[78]

The use of versified materials for teaching in such advanced disciplines as law and theology can be inferred from the number of scholastic textbooks translated into verse. The Bible, Lombard's *Sentences*, Comestor's *Scholastic histories*, Gratian's *Decretum*, and Raymund of Peñafort's *Summa de casibus* all received verse renditions and summaries.[79] The purpose of these texts and the audiences for which they were intended need investigation, but that they were used in the schools can hardly be questioned.

In William's case we have the explicit testimony of Samuel Presbyter that he heard expositions of verse-texts in William's school. Samuel's testimony is confirmed in the writings of another of William's students, Richard of Leicester, *alias* Wetheringsett.[80] Shortly after William's death in 1213, Richard composed a *summa* of pastoral theology that became extremely popular in the thirteenth and succeeding centuries. It is known by its incipit, *Qui bene presunt presbyteri*.[81] This pastoral *summa* is an avowed collection of William's teachings (*dicta*). Some of these "sayings" can be traced to William de Montibus's writings rather than to his classroom teaching, but many of the explicit references to William's *dicta* seem to derive from his oral teachings.

[77] See the *Collecta*, below, II.15.

[78] See above, at notes 24-26. The scholastic context of the many expositions of the *Ave Maria*, the creeds, the *Pater noster*, the canon of the Mass, etc., produced in the late 12th and early 13th century still awaits investigation.

[79] See Joseph de Ghellinck, "Medieval Theology in Verse," *Irish Quarterly Review* 9 (1914) 336-354. Further bibliographical information is found below in the discussion of William's versified texts (II.1, 3, 12, and 15).

[80] See above, at note 66.

[81] Kemmler, *"Exempla" in Context*, pp. 46-59; see below, Chapter Three, pp. 86-91.

Often these references are to brief verses and the master's exposition. For example, Richard quotes lines 15 to 30 of William's *Peniteas cito peccator*, and then reports William's exposition: "modo exponit magister tres primos uersus."[82] This example is particularly enlightening because the gloss reported by Richard differs somewhat from the written gloss that circulated with the poem. Such a variance is understandable if we presume that William recited pieces of didactic verse and then expounded them extemporaneously for his students.

Further evidence of the curriculum in William's school can be garnered from his own extant writings. Although these works are literary creations, at least one stage removed from his actual teaching, they elucidate his pedagogical style, and illustrate the range of topics and materials that he employed in teaching theology. One of his briefest, but most influential, works is the just mentioned *Peniteas cito peccator*. A version of this poem with a standard gloss circulated widely during the thirteenth century, and became a mainstay in the grammar schools of the later Middle Ages. In origin, however, this didactic poem may have been part of a larger undertaking in William's school, an exposition of the seven sacraments of the Church. The verses of the *Peniteas cito* are all included in a "Metrical treatise on the Church's seven sacraments."[83] Each of the sacraments is there represented by a selection of didactic verse illustrating the main elements of doctrine and practice concerning the sacrament. The unique manuscript copy of the treatise is unglossed and therefore cannot be connected directly with classroom activities, but the evidence from William's students, Samuel Presbyter and Richard Wetheringsett, suggests that such verses were a mainstay of William's school. In twelfth-century Paris the academic context for expositions of the sacraments was the *quaestio*. By the mid thirteenth century the sacraments were discussed primarily in lectures on Book Four of Lombard's *Sentences*. William apparently created another context for teaching sacramental doctrine by collecting or composing a text of his own from easily memorized verses, and using these as the basis for scholastic exercises.

Another of William's compositions, one of his most popular to judge by the number of extant manuscripts and contemporary references, he named the *Numerale*. In a brief preface to the work, William describes it as a compendium of introductory materials that will prepare

---

[82] London, British Library MS Royal 9.A.xiv, fol. 115va; see below, II.1, at notes 14 and 15.

[83] See *Tractatus metricus*, below, II.3.

the student to progress more competently in the study of theology.[84] The *Numerale* is a literary work rather than a record of classroom lectures and disputations. It was meant to be read outside the classroom, and to be used, in conjunction with other writings, as a resource for theological students.[85] In it one finds brief summaries of the elements of christian doctrine as they were being taught in William's school. The contents of the doctrine thus imparted are the commonplaces of theology and morals that should be known by all theologians. They form, as William tells us, the basis for any further progress in theological study. His teachings are neither innovative nor controversial. Similar doctrines could be garnered by an ambitious student from the writings of the Fathers and from the works of contemporary teachers and preachers. But William presents them systematically, in brief compass, and in a memorable way, so that the beginning student will have before him a useful introduction to theological studies.

The *Numerale* not only introduces the beginning theology student to the content of christian doctrine but also to the scholastic techniques by which this doctrine is taught and learned. In chapters dealing with such topics as the unity of God, the Trinity, the Incarnation, and the power of the sacerdotal keys, William presents the opinions current in the schools, and offers his own resolutions of the various disputes.[86] In other chapters he demonstrates how the theologian uses examples from the natural world to understand and expound doctrine. He also demonstrates the importance of *distinctiones* in clarifying points of doctrine, and the usefulness of a knowledge of figures of speech (*tropi*) for interpreting sacred texts. The techniques illustrated in this introductory guide formed the bases for William's theological lectures and for his preaching. Although the *Numerale* is a literary exercise, removed from the classroom, it illustrates clearly the types of instruction that one would encounter in his Lincoln school.

Another work that permits some indirect insight into William's approach to theological education is his *Tropi*.[87] Of all the interpretive techniques that a student of theology must master, the most subtle

---

[84] "Ad introducendam facultatem theologicam quedam conpendiose prelibanda sunt ut conpetentius ad altiora fiat progressus," see below, ii.7, p. 236.

[85] See William's colophon: "Et hic gratias agendo huius summe finem facimus cui nomen Numerale imponimus. Plura quidem hic omissa in aliis opusculis nostris copiosius sunt exarata," ibid.

[86] See, for example, William's comment, ibid., at the end of section 1.1: "Queritur an in disputatione sancti dicendi sint dii. Respondeo non. Alia est enim ratio scripture que tropis utitur, alia disputationis que nudam querit ueritatem."

[87] See below, ii.11.

pertain to the interpretation of Scripture and sacred writings. Among the skills judged necessary for this undertaking in the twelfth- and thirteenth-century schools, perhaps the most important were those learned through constant exercise in the principles of grammar, rhetoric, and logic.[88] These skills were taught in the arts curriculum of the medieval schools, and William assumed in his students at least a rudimentary familiarity with the vocabulary and the techniques of these disciplines. Building on this foundation, he provided them with a guide, his *Tropi*, that applied the principles of the arts curriculum to the interpretation of the sacred scriptures. Like the *Numerale*, this work was intended for private, extracurricular study, but it, too, illuminates the informal curriculum of William's school and the teaching of theology in this diocesan school at the end of the twelfth century.

In addition to these introductory guides for the student of theology, William produced four substantial reference works as practical aids for the preachers and teachers that he was training in his school.

His *Versarius*[89] is an unusual work that fits uneasily into any of the recognized genres of medieval literature. It comprises some 4,400 lines of verse, many accompanied by extensive glosses. These verses are grouped under some 900 alphabetically arranged subject headings. The user, wishing to write, preach, teach, or learn about God's love, for example, can turn to the title "Caritas" or "Largitas Dei," and find there several lines of verse summarizing William's teachings and a gloss explicating the doctrine memorialized therein. Should he wish to learn about the priestly office, the entries under "Confessio," "Penitentia," "Predicatio," "Prelatus," "Sacerdos," and "Sacrificium" would be particularly helpful. William himself refers the auditors or readers of his sermons to the *Versarius* for further information.[90] The *Versarius* is neither a long poem, nor a dictionary of poetic quotations; it lacks the unity and coherence of a poem, and many of its verses are incomprehensible without the accompanying gloss, making them unsuitable for use by a writer seeking an appropriate poetic tag to summarize or adorn his own work. Rather, the verses collected there are to serve as the basis for study and learning. Most of William's writings are littered with such verses; many of the verses quoted by

[88] See Gillian Evans, *The Language and Logic of the Bible: The Earlier Middle Ages* (Cambridge: Cambridge University Press, 1984); idem, *Alan of Lille*.
[89] See below, II.12.
[90] See below, II.16, Sermon nos. 132 and 139.

Samuel Presbyter and Richard Wetheringsett, and almost all of those
comprising William's *Peniteas cito* and *Tractatus metricus* are collected
under various titles in the *Versarius*. William composed this work rather
late in his career, and it should perhaps be seen as a *summa* or
compendium of verse texts suitable for school lectures and scholastic
teaching. Just as the Bible, the *Decretum*, and Lombard's *Sentences*
brought together various prose texts to serve as the basis for classroom
teaching in the universities, so William's *Versarius* collected a variety
of verse texts that evidently formed an important part of his theological
instruction in the Lincoln schools.

Three other substantial collections of alphabetically arranged aids
for theologians are William's *Distinctiones*, *Proverbia*, and *Similitudinarium*. These he conceived as repositories of three distinct kinds
of theological resources. The first contains explications of the diverse
significations of words and things in theological discourse. The second
is a florilegium of proverbs and authoritative *dicta*. The third collects
similitudes or *exempla* from the natural world and applies them to
a wide range of theological and moral topics. William's choice of these
three types of materials was a considered one, as he explains in the
prologue to the *Similitudinarium*: "⟨Theological⟩ arguments are
proven or elucidated by authorities and reasons, by examples and
similitudes adduced therein."[91] The student wishing to write or speak
cogently would find the materials for rational arguments conveniently
organized in the *Distinctiones*, authorities in the *Proverbia*, and
similitudes and examples in the *Similitudinarium*. These three works,
like the *Versarius*, are organized alphabetically, and together they
constitute the most ambitious and sustained attempt by any author
in this period to make information easily accessible by means of the
new techniques of alphabetization.[92]

William's *Distinctiones*[93] fit into a loosely defined genre of scholastic
literature that developed during the twelfth century. Masters used
distinctiones to collect and expound diverse materials in a systematic

[91] "Propositiones in medium prolatas probant seu dilucidant auctoritates et rationes,
exempla et similitudines," see below, ii.9, p. 313; cf. *Tropi*: "*Iudicium*: Iudicandum
est et probandum est secundum auctoritates, rationes, exempla, similitudines," ii.11,
p. 387.
[92] See Richard H. Rouse and Mary A. Rouse, "*Statim invenire*: Schools, Preachers,
and New Attitudes to the Page," in *Renaissance and Renewal in the Twelfth Century*,
pp. 201-225; idem, *Preachers, Florilegia and Sermons: Studies on the "Manipulus
florum" of Thomas of Ireland*, Studies and Texts, 47 (Toronto: Pontifical Institute
of Mediaeval Studies, 1979), pp. 3-42.
[93] See below, Chapter Three, pp. 70-71, and ii.8.

way. Students were taught to "distinguish" the various significations of a word or thing as a means of interpreting authoritative texts and resolving apparent contradictions among several authorities. A highly technical type of *Distinctio* was already in use among the Bolognese lawyers by the mid twelfth century,[94] but the genre reached its zenith at Paris, toward the end of the century, where it was exploited as a practical tool by theologians and lawyers alike. Recent scholarship has begun to appreciate the importance of biblical *distinctiones* as a method of commenting systematically on the text of Scripture.[95] As a pedagogical method, however, the *distinctio* had much broader applications. Richard de Mores (Ricardus Anglicus) used the new "Parisian" *distinctio* to expound Gratian's *Decretum*,[96] and William de Montibus devoted the first part of his *Tropi* to the use of distinctions in theological discourse. The so-called *Distinctiones monastice* utilize this method for the liberal education of monastic readers.[97] William de Montibus's and Alan of Lille's *Distinctiones*, and Peter the Chanter's *Summa Abel* were among the earliest works to adopt the new technique of alphabetical organization that enabled these authors to summarize a wide range of theological and philosophical topics.[98] All proved to be very popular collections among theologians at the turn of the century.

Distinctiones and distinction collections served a valuable purpose as resources for preachers throughout the thirteenth and fourteenth centuries, but they had other applications beyond the construction of popular sermons.[99] The early scholastics found in the *distinctio* a

[94] Stephan Kuttner, *Repertorium der Kanonistik (1140-1234): Prodromus Corporis Glossarum, I* (Vatican City: Biblioteca Apostolica Vaticana, 1937), pp. 208-227.

[95] See especially, Richard H. Rouse and Mary A. Rouse, "Biblical *Distinctiones* in the Thirteenth Century," *Archives d'histoire doctrinale et littéraire du moyen âge* 41 (1974) 27-37. The most ambitious collection of biblical distinctions is the *Pantheologus* of Peter of Cornwall, a massive work in four parts, completed by 1189. See Hunt, "English Learning," pp. 33-34, 38-42; Peter Hull and Richard Sharpe, "Peter of Cornwall and Launceston," *Cornish Studies* 13 (1986) 5-53.

[96] Giulio Silano, "The 'Distinctiones Decretorum' of Ricardus Anglicus: An edition," 2 vols. (PhD diss.: University of Toronto, 1981).

[97] See André Wilmart, "Un répertoire d'exégèse composé en Angleterre vers le début du XIIIe siècle," *Mémorial Lagrange* (Paris, 1940), pp. 307-346.

[98] See Gillian Evans, "Alan of Lille's *Distinctiones* and the Problem of Theological Language," *Sacris erudiri* 24 (1980) 67-86.

[99] For *distinctiones* as preaching aids, see Rouse and Rouse, *Preachers*, pp. 3-42; "*Statim invenire*," pp. 212-218. See also David L. d'Avray, *The Preaching of the Friars: Sermons Diffused from Paris before 1300* (Oxford: Clarendon Press, 1985), under "distinctions" in his index. Their wider applicability, however, should not be ignored. A 15th-century writer makes explicit the broad usefulness of such *distinctiones*: "One

powerful tool for systematizing instruction and for clarifying doctrine.
The habit of "distinguishing" was inculcated not only in sermons but
also in lectures, disputations, and occasional writings. William uses
the *distinctio* technique in nearly all of his writings; he teaches it as
an important skill for those who wish to construct clear, accurate, and
persuasive arguments in the schools.

   Another ambitious collection of theological materials for the schools
is William's *Proverbia*, or, as it is named in two of the manuscripts,
"Proverbs and other edifying sayings."[100] Like the *Distinctiones*, it is
organized around numerous alphabetically arranged topics of interest
to the teacher and preacher. A scholar wishing to construct persuasive
arguments, to adorn them with telling aphorisms, or simply to meditate
on the topics listed, could find collected here apposite quotations from
the classical authors, Church Fathers, canonical authorities, and from
the popular wisdom of the time. The value of such a collection to
the work of the schools should not be underestimated. Then, as now,
a student was expected to have read widely in the classical and
ecclesiastical authors, and to have learned the wisdom of the ages from
the original documents.[101] The problem confronting students and
teachers was that of making this wisdom more easily accessible for
use in various kinds of written and spoken communication.

   Early medieval florilegia represent an initial response to this problem.[102] More sophisticated solutions were pursued by the Dominican
friars of St. Jacques, Paris, who perfected the first topical concordance
of the Bible in the 1230's;[103] by Robert Grosseteste, who invented an
ingenious table of authorities and a system of reference symbols to
keep track of his readings;[104] and by many other writers in the thirteenth
century. William's *Proverbia* is a precocious example of this scholastic

---

finds listed here in alphabetical order, like a concordance, the more important and
commonest topics that arise *in both lectures and sermons*, and, indeed, those topics
which might be *helpful to a man in all things*" (emphasis added); quoted by Richard
H. Rouse, "Backgrounds to Print: Aspects of the Manuscript Book in Northern Europe
of the Fifteenth Century," *Proceedings of the PMR Conference*: Annual Publication
of the Patristic, Mediaeval, and Renaissance Conference, 6 (Villanova: Augustinian
Historical Institute, 1981), p. 42.

   [100] See below, ii.10.
   [101] See Joseph de Ghellinck, "'Originale' et 'Originalia,'" *Archivum latinitatis medii
aevi* 14 (1939) 95-105; Rouse and Rouse, "*Statim invenire*," pp. 222-223.
   [102] See the discussion of William's *Prouerbia*, below, ii.10, pp. 334-336.
   [103] Richard H. Rouse and Mary A. Rouse, "The Verbal Concordance to the
Scriptures," *Archivum Fratrum Praedicatorum* 44 (1974) 5-30.
   [104] Southern, *Robert Grosseteste*, pp. 186-193, and the bibliography there.

activity. His organization of the authorities (among whom he included
the authority of popular wisdom as represented by the proverbial
sayings of his countrymen) under several hundred alphabetically
arranged topics helped to invent the format, and to stimulate the
development, of such modern reference tools as the dictionary of
quotations.

These efforts to encapsulate received wisdom in brief scope and
usable form were neither idle exercises nor contemnible substitutes for
real scholarship. We know that Gerald of Wales, who professed scorn
for those who produced collections of other people's writings, himself
used florilegia in constructing his theological treatises.[105] Robert
Grosseteste apparently consulted his own *Tabula* or concordance of
authorities when he wrote and taught in the schools, and even when
he composed his letters.[106] It will come as no surprise that collections
of quotable authorities were indispensable for preachers, but the
importance of such collections in the lecture hall and in the private
study may prove to have been equally great.[107] The energy that went
into compiling William's *Proverbia et aliis verbis edificatoria* testifies
clearly to the importance of such works in the scholastic milieu of
the thirteenth century.

A final alphabetically arranged compilation, the *Similitudinarium*,[108]
completes this list of William de Montibus's extracurricular aids for
theologians. Similitudes are comparisons or analogies drawn between
phenomena of the natural world and human or divine behavior.
William conceived of them as essential elements in theological discourse,
and ranked them with "reasons," "authorities," and "*exempla*" as the
chief ways in which arguments are proven or elucidated.[109] Modern
scholarship has tended to link similitudes and *exempla* primarily with
the preaching office, and to describe these as devices for adorning
sermons;[110] William's collection reminds us of their value for the

[105] A.A. Goddu and Richard H. Rouse, "Gerald of Wales and the *Florilegium
Angelicum*," *Speculum* 52 (1977) 488-521.

[106] Southern, *Robert Grosseteste*, pp. 211, 213.

[107] See, for example, the index of "authorities" adduced in the *Summa fratris
Alexandri, Alexandri de Hales ... Summa Theologica: Indices in Tom. I-IV* (Grottaferrata: Collegii S. Bonaventurae, 1979), pp. 167-242; the place of concordances and
florilegia in transmitting these authorities deserves careful investigation.

[108] See below, II.9.

[109] See above, note 91. For William's differentiation between similitudes and
exempla, see II.9, pp. 304-305.

[110] Claude Bremond, Jacques Le Goff, Jean-Claude Schmitt, *L'"exemplum*,"
Typologie des sources du moyen âge occidental, 40 (Turnhout: Brepols, 1982); J.-Th.
Welter, *L'exemplum dans la littérature religieuse et didactique du moyen âge* (Paris:

scholastic theologian as well. The theologian could draw equally on evidence from the natural world, as created by God, as on human reason and the wisdom of sages, to construct his arguments. He would learn about the world of nature from his own thoughtful observation, from bestiaries and lapidaries, and from the teachings of natural scientists whose experiments and observations were finding increasing favour in the schools. In the *Similitudinarium*, William tells us, he has collected a number of these examples from nature, taking pains to organize them in alphabetical order so that he and others might be able to find pertinent similes quickly and easily. William used similitudes in all of his teaching and writing. His *Similitudinarium* made these resources available both to students and teachers in the schools and to writers and preachers who wished to apply this aspect of "scholastic method" in wider arenas.

A discussion of the formal and informal curriculum of studies in William's school at Lincoln would be incomplete without a discussion of his sermons. As a master of theology, William would have been expected to preach as well as lecture and hold disputations. Failing any direct evidence that William preached to his students in the classroom, we might presume that the sermons he preached in the cathedral and in the chapter house served simultaneously to fulfill his pastoral duties as cathedral chancellor and his academic responsibilities to teach by preaching. Because preaching, like lecturing, is an ephemeral act, our knowledge of these academic exercises in the schools is limited to the chance survival of written reports, quotations, and summaries. No student reports of William's scholastic sermons survive to illuminate this aspect of his day-to-day teaching. William, however, conceived of his sermons not only as *viva voce* instructional discourses but also as written tools for research and learning. He made collections of his own sermons, and intended that they should serve as extracurricular aids to the student of theology. In his introductory textbook, the *Numerale*, William often refers his reader to one of his sermons for further information on a particular topic.[111] Clearly, his sermons

---

Guitard, 1927); Louis-Jacques Bataillon, "*Similitudines* et *Exempla* dans les sermons du XIIIe siècle," in *The Bible in the Medieval World*, pp. 191-205. Fritz Kemmler, in his "*Exempla*" in *Context*, places *exempla* in the broader context of pastoral instruction.

[111] For example: "Huiusmodi bestie et reptile uersantur in nemore quod plantauit Abraham in Bersabee ... de quo in sermonibus nostris si quesieris inuenire poteris"; London, British Library MS Cotton Vespasian E.x, fol. 167v.

continued to play an important educational rôle long after their immediate occasion in the school and the cathedral had been forgotten.

This study of William's writings reveals something of the scope and substance of theological education at Lincoln, where, according to Gerald of Wales, "the science of theology flourishes most soundly in all of England, under the best of teachers, Master William de Monte."[112]

Although the schools and scholars of Paris dominated the theological landscape during William's lifetime, most students obtained an advanced education not at Paris but at local monastic and cathedral schools. If Paris was at the headwaters of scholastic theology, then schools like William's at Lincoln were the channels through which this theology flowed. William's writings, and those of his students, offer a unique opportunity to explore the permutations of one stream as it moved away from its source.

For more than twenty-five years William ruled the school of theology at Lincoln. He left a large body of writings that can be associated with his teaching there. His students preserved further records and reminiscences. From these we can catch a glimpse of the workings of one cathedral school and its rôle in the development and dissemination of scholastic theology. When the full history of the thirteenth-century "faculties" of theology is written, the pioneering efforts of teachers like William de Montibus and his contemporaries in local schools throughout Europe will form an important chapter.

But the predominance of theology as an academic discipline, indeed as the "queen of the sciences," is only one aspect of the history of scholasticism. Of equal, if not greater, historical importance is the process by which scholastic ideas became part and parcel of the everyday experience of medieval men and women. The popularization of learned theology, and the extension of this learning to those who lacked the interest or the opportunity to pursue a long and arduous course of study in the schools, deserves careful investigation. William de Montibus's contribution to the popularization of theology is the subject of the following chapter.

---

[112] Quoted above, Chapter One, note 10.

Chapter Three

The Literature of Pastoral Care

Two years after the death of William de Montibus in 1213, the Fourth Lateran Council turned its attention to the pastoral reform of the Church and the education of the clergy. The Council asserted that the most important of all the arts was the pastoral care of souls (*Cum sit ars artium regimen animarum* ...),[1] thus giving its authoritative solution to a *quaestio* that had been disputed in the contemporary schools.[2] By implying that pastoral care could be taught and learned just like grammar, logic, medicine, and theology, the Council gave voice to a growing consensus that pastors could and should receive special education for their task. During the course of the thirteenth century a vast literature of pastoral care grew up as an adjunct to the more formal instruction in theology, law, and the arts. This literature sought

---

[1] *Conciliorum oecumenicorum decreta*, ed. Joseph Alberigo, J.A. Dossetti, P. Joannou, C. Leonardi, and P. Prodi, 3rd ed. (Bologna: Istituto per le Scienze Religiose, 1973), p. 248. The canons of the Council are also edited, along with medieval commentaries, in *Constitutiones Concilii quarti Lateranensis una cum Commentariis glossatorum*, ed. Antonius Garcia y Garcia, Monumenta iuris canonici, Series A, Corpus glossatorum 2 (Vatican City: Biblioteca Apostolica Vaticana, 1981). A thoughtful summary of the pastoral provisions of the Council is found in Michele Maccarrone, "'Cura animarum' e 'parochialis sacerdos' nelle costituzioni del IV concilio lateranense (1215). Applicazioni in Italia nel sec. XIII," in *Pievi e parrocchie in Italia nel basso medioevo (sec. XIII-XV)* (Rome: Herder, 1984), 1: 81-195.

[2] Although the ultimate source of this quotation is Gregory Nazianzen and Gregory the Great (see Maccarrone, "Cura animarum," p. 134, note 163), its immediate context was the 12th-and 13th-century schools. See, for example, the text quoted from a late-12th-century logical tract by Lambertus Marie de Rijk, in his *Logica modernorum: A Contribution to the History of Early Terminist Logic*, 2 vols. (Assen: Van Gorcum, 1962-1967), 2: 418: "Quid est dyaletica. Dyaletica est ars artium, scientia scientiarum, quia sola facit scire et nescientem posse manifestare. Contra. Theologia est ars artium, scientia scientiarum; non ergo dyaletica. Dicendum quod dyaletica est ars artium, scientia scientiarum, quia sine illa nulla ars perfecte potest scire." Innocent III's "determination" of this question is that neither logic nor theology is the "art of arts"; the title belongs to the pastoral care of souls.

to present in simple terms and accessible forms the practical knowledge required of the pastor of souls. Leonard E. Boyle, who has taken the lead in identifying and studying this genre of literature, coined the term *pastoralia* to encompass the many and diverse works produced in the thirteenth and subsequent centuries to educate clerics (and, gradually, the laity) in those things pertaining to the care of souls.[3]

No discussion of William de Montibus's career would be complete without a study of his rôle in the development of this practical literature of pastoral care. Although the great florescence of pastoral manuals came in the years after his death, *pastoralia* had their roots in the scholastic milieu of the late twelfth and early thirteenth centuries.[4] By the end of the thirteenth century a new audience for pastoral literature had been identified, techniques for popularizing scholastic doctrines had been developed, and an appropriate content for pastoral instruction had been identified. In this chapter we will seek to specify the ways in which William and his contemporaries contributed to these developments, and the limitations of their contributions.

THE AUDIENCE FOR PASTORALIA: STUDENTS IN THE SCHOOLS

Implicit in the growth of a new literature of pastoral care in the thirteenth century is the emergence of a demand for such popularizing texts and the cultivation of a new audience of readers. It is tempting to assume that this audience was comprised of actual pastors — the simple priests in their parishes. With hindsight we can say that the parish priest was an obvious and appropriate recipient of the new pastoral education, and he was already beginning to be treated as such

---

[3] Leonard E. Boyle's unpublished Oxford D.Phil dissertation, "A Study of the Works Attributed to William of Pagula with Special Reference to the *Oculus sacerdotis* and *Summa summarum*," 2 vols. (1956), is still indispensable; parts of this research are published in various essays conveniently assembled in Boyle's *Pastoral Care, Clerical Education and Canon Law, 1200-1400* (Variorum Reprints: London, 1981). His most recent thoughts on the genre are contained in three articles: "*Summae confessorum*," in *Les Genres littéraires dans les sources théologiques et philosophiques médiévales: Définition, critique, et exploitation*, Actes du Colloque international de Louvain-la-Neuve, 25-27 mai 1981 (Louvain: Institut d'études médiévales, 1982), pp. 227-237; "The Fourth Lateran Council and Manuals of Popular Theology," in *The Popular Literature of Medieval England*, ed. Thomas J. Heffernan (Knoxville: University of Tennessee Press, 1985), pp. 30-43; "The Inter-conciliar Period 1179-1215 and the Beginnings of Pastoral Manuals," *Miscellanea Rolando Bandinelli Papa Alessandro III*, ed. Filippo Liotta (Siena: Accademia Senese degli Intronati, 1986), pp. 45-56.

[4] See Boyle, "Inter-conciliar Period"; Baldwin, *Masters*, passim.

by the Fourth Lateran Council.[5] The Council may be seen as giving the first official recognition to the parish priest as one of the primary elements in a renewal of the Church's pastoral care. During the following centuries the parish priest gradually would be expected to exercise at the local level all of the pastoral duties previously expected only of bishops and learned monks; he would become a preacher and a learned teacher, a judge, and a doctor of souls.

But did the demand for didactic literature in the early thirteenth century emanate from the parishes? Did parish priests actively seek out educational texts? Did their pastoral vocation require them to become learned, or did the communities they served expect much book learning of them? Were they, indeed, literate (in the modern sense), and capable of reading with understanding the pastoral *summae* and handbooks produced in ever-greater numbers during the course of the century? The answers to these questions are elusive, but some clarifications are possible.

The modern expectation that priests be educated in the schools and readers of learned books is the product of many centuries of development; even today such learning is less than universally espoused. In the thirteenth century such an expectation could scarcely have been more than a gleam in some reformers' eyes. Throughout most of the Middle Ages the parish priest was, first and foremost, a member of the local community. His primary loyalties were to the local church and to the patron who appointed him. His activities were shaped by local traditions and responded to local needs. He might or might not be married, he might or might not have paid for his office or inherited it from his father, and he might or might not be educated, depending on the prevailing customs and expectations of the local community. Seldom a holy-man (in the technical sense that Max Weber has called a *virtuoso*), he was the administrator of the local cultus, dispenser of blessings for flocks, crops, wells, swords, salt, fish, eggs, and for all important occasions, the spiritual, and sometimes (as leader of the local militia) the physical protector of the local community, and the intercessor for the souls of the dead. His education was more often that of a traditional apprenticeship under the incumbent priest than formal training in the schools of arts, canon law, or theology.[6]

---

[5] See Boyle, "Inter-conciliar Period," and "Manuals of Popular Theology"; Maccarrone, "Cura animarum," pp. 81-195.

[6] See Joseph Goering, "The Changing Face of the Village Parish: The Thirteenth Century," in *Pathways to Medieval Peasants*, ed. J.A. Raftis (Toronto: Pontifical Institute of Mediaeval Studies, 1981), pp. 323-333.

Both local communities and higher ecclesiastical authorities shared this traditional understanding of the priest's rôle. William of Pagula's advice, early in the fourteenth century, summarizes well the prevailing expectations of a parish priest's educational attainment:

> Ordinands should not be examined too rigidly, but rather in a summary fashion and leniently. Too great a degree of perfection is not required as long as a reasonable literacy, a legitimate age and a good character are not wanting in the candidate. The good opinion in which a candidate publicly is held can be the equivalent of an examination; indeed it is clear from the *Decretum* that local candidates for the priesthood are to be spared examination.[7]

The emphasis here on good behaviour and local reputation rather than on academic proficiency and book-learning is an under-appreciated aspect of the medieval expectations of parish priests. Pagula's instruction is not a counsel of despair. Most priests had little need for formal or advanced education. They were expected to be the custodians of the Church's rites and rituals, to bless the community's activities, to pray for the souls of the departed, and to make God present in the Mass. For none of these traditional activities was it necessary that the priest have spent time at the schools or universities.

He would need to be "reasonably literate," as Pagula says, but such literacy implied primarily the ability to pronounce correctly the Latin texts of the liturgy and sacramentaries — not the ability to read, write, and construe grammar and syntax that was taught in the schools of liberal arts.[8] Such passive literacy was still being taught to clerics in Chaucer's day,[9] and, if the story is true, it was just such literacy that

---

[7] Quoted by Leonard E. Boyle, in "Aspects of Clerical Education in Fourteenth-Century England," *The Fourteenth Century*, ACTA, 4, Proceedings of the State University of New York Conferences in Medieval Studies, ed. Paul E. Szarmach and Bernard S. Levy (Binghamton NY: Center for Medieval and Early Renaissance Studies, 1977), pp. 19-20; rpt. *Pastoral Care*.

[8] John Balbi of Genoa defines "literatus" in his *Catholicon* (c. 1286): "Literator uel literatus non dicitur ille qui habet multos libros et inspicit et reuoluit ut monachus qui proprie potest dici antiquarius, quia antiquas historias habet ad manum. Sed ille dicitur literator uel literatus qui ex arte de rudi uoce scit formare literas in dictionibus, et dictiones in oracionibus, et oraciones scit congrue proferre et accentuare. Vnde Ieronimus super Math' literator inquit erat qui grammatos grece dicitur. Literatus componitur cum in- et dicitur illiteratus -ta -tum, idest sine literis, non literatus, idiota" (Mainz, 1460). For examples of priests who are illiterate even in this limited sense and still considered worthy of their office, see Caesarius of Heisterbach's "De simplicitate," in *Caesarii Heisterbacensis monachi Ordinis Cisterciensis Dialogus Miraculorum*, ed. Josephus Strange, 2 vols. (Cologne, 1851), pp. 340-390.

[9] See Geoffrey Chaucer, "The Prioress's Tale," in *The Riverside Chaucer*, ed. Larry D. Benson, 3rd ed. (Boston: Houghton Mifflin Company, 1987), p. 210, lines 502-536.

permitted John Milton's daughters to read the texts of the classics to their blind father, mellifluently but without comprehension.

When Robert Grosseteste, the zealous reforming bishop of the mid thirteenth century, wished to encourage the parish priests in his diocese to preach regularly (i.e. to expound the "simple history" of the gospel pericope to their people each Sunday), he recognized that some of them would be unable to understand the Latin text. He urged these to seek out a neighbouring priest who understood Latin and who would charitably expound the Scriptures to them.[10]

Some parish priests, of course, had a formal education and had gained an active command of Latin by reading, writing, and speaking it in the schools. Encouragement was given for such studies by both the Third Lateran (1179) and Fourth Lateran Councils. By the end of the thirteenth century a formal mechanism was instituted whereby rectors or vicars holding benefices with the care of souls could be excused from residence for up to five years in order to study at a school or university.[11] These persons were, indeed, part of the audience for which *pastoralia* were written. We should be wary, however, of overestimating the size of this audience, and of idealizing the perceived benefits of a scholastic education for all parish priests. The numbers of episcopal licenses for study in the schools increased gradually during the thirteenth century, but so did the complaints that persons with no zeal for souls were using their pastoral benefices as an excuse for getting an education.

Most parish priests, vicars, and chaplains, however, would seem to have had little interest in books (other than those necessary for the liturgy), great difficulty in obtaining and copying them, and small skill

[10] "Potest ... quilibet persona uel sacerdos repetere in septimana nudum textum Euangelij diei dominice, ut tunc sciat saltem historiam grossam subditis suis referre; et hoc dico si Latinum intelligat ... . Si uero non intelligit Latinum, saltem potest adire vicinum aliquem intelligentem qui caritatiue ei exponet. Et sic vlterius gregem suum doceat, et in vno anno potest repetere sic epistolas festorum, et in secundo vitas sanctorum, et deinde subditis referre." From the sermon *Scriptum est de Levitis*, quoted in Joseph Goering and F.A.C. Mantello, "The *Meditaciones* of Robert Grosseteste," *Journal of Theological Studies*, n.s. 36 (1985) 122, n. 16. This advice from the great bishop of Lincoln was still being repeated in Lollard circles at the end of the 14th century; see Southern, *Robert Grosseteste*, p. 308.

[11] See above, Chapter Two, at notes 69-71. Boyle, "Constitution 'Cum ex eo,'" stresses, rightly, that the students who availed themselves of *Cum ex eo* licenses in the 14th century "were not 'parish' priests, or priests in any capacity, at the time of the granting of a license"; rather they were promising young men who were being given financial incentive to study in the schools before undertaking the *cura animarum* (pp. 275-277).

in understanding them. Nor should they be disdained for this lack of interest. The traditional expectations of parish priests stressed values other than the ability to read, write, and converse in Latin. If they were competent custodians of the local cultus, of good character, and of good reputation in the local community, then they were living up to both the official and the unofficial requirements of their calling. When the need arose for these priests to be instructed in some of the new developments in theology and law emanating from the schools, more efficient ways of instructing them could be found — in the archidiaconal or decanal synods and visitations, in the confessional, or from the pulpit — than in the new-fangled literature of pastoral care.[12]

If the robust demand for this pastoral literature did not arise (originally) from the practising parish priest, whom might the authors have had in mind as readers of their works? The intended audience must have been able to read and understand Latin with some facility, individuals interested in learning new approaches to the pastoral care, who were familiar with the techniques of learning from books and written documents, and with the ways of acquiring or copying these written materials for their own use. Such an audience could most easily be found in the secular and religious schools of medieval Europe where Latin was taught and spoken as a "living" language, where people with a patent interest (and investment) in learning congregated, and where the techniques of book-learning were cultivated.

The enormous success of scholastic institutions by the middle of the twelfth century is one of the surprises of medieval history. By the end of the twelfth century book-learning and higher education had become respectable occupations, not just for "philosophers" and gentlemen of leisure but for a significant cross-section of the European population. As the numbers of students frequenting the schools grew, education came to be seen less as a way of life open to only a few, and more as a desirable preparation for many practical careers.

A term that emerges during the twelfth century to designate this body of students in the schools is *clericus*.[13] The history of this term

---

[12] See Robert Grosseteste, *Templum Dei*, ed. Joseph Goering and F.A.C. Mantello, Toronto Medieval Latin Texts, 14 (Toronto: Pontifical Institute of Mediaeval Studies, 1984), pp. 6-7; Goering, "Village Parish"; Roy M. Haines, "Education in English Ecclesiastical Legislation of the Later Middle Ages," in *Councils and Assemblies*, ed. G.J. Cuming and Derek Baker, Studies in Church History, 7 (Cambridge: Cambridge University Press, 1971), pp. 161-175.

[13] See M.T. Clanchy, *From Memory to Written Record: England, 1066-1307* (Cambridge MA: Harvard University Press, 1979), pp. 177-181; Alexander Murray,

still awaits careful investigation.[14] It has different connotations in different contexts. In one sense it can be translated as "clergy," and used to distinguish those in Holy Orders from the "laity" who are not.[15] In another sense it is used to describe ordained persons who are still in minor orders, and who will be designated *subdiaconus*, *diaconus*, *presbyter*, etc. if and when they proceed to major orders.[16]

A third usage of the term, the one that concerns us here, is as a designation for students in the schools. It seems to connote no ecclesiastical or pastoral vocation. Peter the Chanter expresses this clearly: "There are two kinds of clerics ... namely those who are ecclesiastics and those who are scholastics."[17] Richard Rufus of Cornwall, in the 1250's, equates *clerici* with arts students in this striking description of a city:

> For example, there are many types of persons in a city; there are laymen, and among them there are many different sub-groups; there are also clerics, and many types of these as well, such as grammarians, logicians, and naturalists.[18]

Reason and Society in the Middle Ages (Oxford: Clarendon Press, 1978), pp. 263-265. The term *clericus* is already a synonym for "student" in Petrus Alfonsi's *Disciplina clericalis*, from the beginning of 12th century; see *The Scholar's Guide: A Translation of the Twelfth-Century "Disciplina clericalis" of Pedro Alfonso*, trans. Joseph Ramon Jones and John Esteen Keller, Medieval Sources in Translation, 8 (Toronto: Pontifical Institute of Mediaeval Studies, 1969), pp. 17-20. The reference to classes of "sixty or a hundred clerics" that Theobald of Etampes is said to have taught at Oxford early in the 12th century also stresses the academic, rather than the ecclesiastical, status of these schoolboys; see Richard W. Southern, "Master Vacarius and the Beginning of an English Academic Tradition," in *Medieval Learning and Literature: Essays Presented to Richard William Hunt*, ed. J.J.G. Alexander and M.T. Gibson (Oxford: Clarendon Press, 1976), pp. 257-286, at pp. 267-268.

[14] See *Dictionary of Medieval Latin from British Sources*, Fasc. II C (London: Oxford University Press, 1981), pp. 359-360, *clericus*.

[15] See Aldo Luigi Prosdocimi, "Chierici e laici nella societa occidentale del secolo XII: a proposito di Decr. Grat. C. 12 q. 1 c. 7: Duo sunt genera," *Proceedings of the Second International Congress of Medieval Canon Law* (Vatican City: S. Congregatio de Seminariis et Studiorum Universitatibus, 1965), pp. 105-122.

[16] See H.S. Bennett, "Medieval Ordination Lists in the English Episcopal Registers," in *Studies Presented to Sir Hilary Jenkinson*, ed. J. Conway Davies (London: Oxford University Press, 1957), pp. 20-34.

[17] "Clericorum duo sunt genera et in utroque boni et mali: quidam ecclesiastici, quidam scholastici." Quoted by Baldwin, *Masters*, 2: 51, n. 57, from the Chanter's *Summa Abel*.

[18] "Verbi gratia, multi modi hominum sunt in civitate, ut laici, et inter alios multi modi laicorum; et etiam clerici et inter istos multi modi clericorum, ut grammatici, logici et naturales." Quoted by Timothy B. Noone, "An Edition and Study of the *Scriptum super Metaphysicam*, bk. 12, dist. 2: A Work Attributed to Richard Rufus of Cornwall" (PhD diss.: University of Toronto, 1988), p. 325.

It is these *clerici*, students in the schools, who become the earliest audience for the practical literature of pastoral care. When the Fourth Lateran Council referred to the care of souls as the art of arts (*ars artium*) it was as a suggestion to students of various disciplines — liberal arts, philosophy, medicine, law, even theology — that the noblest study of all was the simple *regimen animarum*. All students, not just theologians, gradually came to be seen as potential recipients of pastoral education. All students, even those engaged in the study of arts, law, and medicine, eventually were regarded as a fitting audience for the literature of pastoral care.[19] But such an audience was only slowly identified and cultivated, as can be seen in an examination of the writings of William de Montibus and his contemporaries.

William saw himself first and foremost as a theologian and a teacher of other theologians. His major literary efforts were directed to a rather specialized audience — students who wished to learn the scholastic discipline of theology. His *Numerale* was to serve as a basic introduction to the discipline, his *Tropi* as a sophisticated guide to the grammatical and logical intricacies of sacred scriptures, and his *Distinctiones*, *Proverbia*, and *Similitudinarium* as source books for the practising theologian. Even his metrical works, the *Versarius*, *Tractatus metricus de sacramentis*, and the *Peniteas cito*, were designed for the student of theology. They were composed with neither simple priests nor the general population of the schools in mind. Their terse phrases and laconic glosses demanded of the reader a certain familiarity with the sacred scriptures and their glosses, and with the classics of theology. In a later day William's *Peniteas cito* would be used as a set text in the grammar schools, but William himself seems not to have envisioned it as functioning in this way.[20]

William took cognizance of the wider student audience in the schools, but he wrote no pastoral treatises for their instruction. His *Speculum penitentis* and *Errorum eliminatio* are both directed to theologians, and his *Quomodo uiri religiosi* to learned monks. Under the rubric "De clericis" in his *Proverbia*, William includes ninety-seven examples of proverbial wisdom appropriate for students; this is one of the longest

---

[19] The importance for prospective pastors of training in philosophy, the liberal arts, law, and medicine was stressed by Archbishop John Pecham at the Council of Reading (1279); see Boyle, "Constitution 'Cum ex eo,'" pp. 269-270.

[20] The *Peniteas cito* may have originally been composed as a part of the *Tractatus metricus*, and only later separated and circulated as an independent treatise on penance; see above, p. 49. Its success as a scholastic summary of penance seems eventually to have recommended it for popular use.

sections in the work. But the sayings collected there are for use by theologians who wish to edify students in the schools; they make no effort to train the *clerici* themselves for the pastoral care of souls.[21]

As a pastor and "prelate" in the cathedral William also adverts to the wider clerical audience. His *viva voce* sermons in the cathedral no doubt constituted a kind of "clerical" instruction aimed at more than just the theologians, but William addressed no *pastoralia* or written sermon collections to such students, nor did he take pains in the sermons themselves to instruct this audience in the art of preaching or of pastoral care. The one sermon collection that William manifestly intended as a pastoral aid was directed neither to students nor to simple parish priests. Its recipient was someone who was already quite learned, but who, out of laziness or incompetence, had neglected to undertake the preaching office that was required of him.[22] William seems never to have envisaged his works as practical guides to pastoral care that would be of use to non-theologians.

William inherited his conception of theological education from the twelfth-century scholastics. He viewed theology, like philosophy, as a moral and intellectual discipline that required a full commitment of one's time and energies. The audience for which he wrote consisted of theologians-in-training who would learn from him the intricacies of textual interpretation, the wisdom of the Scriptures, and the techniques of arguing correctly and persuasively with reasons, authorities, examples, and similitudes. They would master these skills by hearing lectures on the Bible and its glosses, disputing questions, listening to learned sermons, and practising the art of versification as an aid to understanding and remembering the lessons learned in the schools.

Theologians trained in this way in William's school might go on to teach others — the laity as well as clerics (students and churchmen).[23]

[21] The "proverbs" concerning *clerici* contain a good deal of advice about the liberal arts, and often urge students to proceed to higher studies, i.e. to become theologians: "Studia liberalia meritoria artificia sunt, hactenus utilia si preparent, ingenium non detinent. Tamdiu enim istis immorandum est quamdiu nihil agere animus maius potest. Rudimenta sunt nostra non opera," Oxford, New College MS 98, fol. 70ra. Many entries consist of simple exhortation or admonition concerning the academic life: "Bernardus: sunt clerici quidam qui habitu milites, questu clericos, actu neutrum exhibent," ibid., fol. 70rb; "Pars sciencie est scire quod nescias, iuxta illud socraticum: scio quod nescio," ibid., fol. 70va; "Magistrum te pocius audire quam ut magistrum delectet audiri," ibid., fol. 70vb.

[22] See below, II.16, Sermon nos. 74-115.

[23] Such instruction would often take the form of preaching. See Michel Zink, *La prédication en langue romane avant 1300* (Paris: Champion, 1976); C.A. Robson, *Maurice of Sully and the Medieval Vernacular Homily* (Oxford: Blackwell, 1952).

But these non-theologians comprised a secondary audience, for which William wrote no pastoral *summae*, treatises, or handbooks. No one doubted that they should receive christian instruction; but few could have imagined that the laity and simple clerics would be introduced to the subtleties of scholastic theology by means of written texts. *Pastoralia*, the written literature of pastoral care, began to flourish in the decades after William's death, when all students, not just theologians,[24] came to be recognized as appropriate audiences for the theological teachings of the schools.

Hand in hand with the recognition of this new and important audience, however, went the task of identifying an appropriate body of knowledge to be taught, and the necessity of discovering pedagogical methods that would permit the transmission of the teachings of the schools to those who lacked time, interest, or ability to follow a course of study such as William expected of his "theologians." It is to the techniques of popularization and to the content of the pastoral literature that we now turn.

THE TECHNIQUES OF POPULARIZATION

The process by which difficult or complex doctrines are made accessible to a broader audience the French call *vulgarisation*; we will refer to it as "popularization." It was practised on a large scale in the schools of the late twelfth and early thirteenth centuries, where the burgeoning of knowledge and the availability of authoritative texts in all disciplines — arts, philosophy, medicine, law, and theology — far outstripped the abilities of all but a few individuals to master thoroughly even one discipline. As more and more students flocked to the schools, demanding to learn something of one or more of these disciplines, teachers developed a number of techniques to meet the demand. A full discussion of these techniques is beyond the scope of this essay. Here we will draw attention only to those that came to be crucial for the writing of *pastoralia* in the thirteenth and subsequent centuries.

---

[24] The same gradual recognition of a wider audience for scholastic ideas, described here with respect to the theological schools, took place in the schools of law. The contemporaneous process needs investigation; see Paul Anciaux, *La théologie du sacrement de pénitence au XIIe siècle* (Louvain: Nauwelaerts, 1949); Pierre Michaud-Quantin, *Sommes de casuistique et manuels de confession au moyen âge (XII-XVI siècles)* (Louvain: Analecta mediaevalia Namurcensia, 1962).

Language

First among the requirements of a popular literature was that it be easily read and comprehended. The learned Latin of the twelfth-century "humanists," based in part on classical models and cultivated as a mark of sophistication, was ill suited to the purpose.[25] An alternative, however, was to be found in the spoken language of the schools. Latin was the language of instruction and of everyday communication among students in many schools. Without this common language, the diverse native languages and dialects of students and masters would have made education impossible. Although taken for granted as a means of oral discourse, this common or "low" Latin was employed only hesitantly in written texts.[26] Writers were loath to give up the rhetorical refinements that were the mark of twelfth-century learning. Those who composed works in the simple style felt compelled to apologize for doing so. Gerald of Wales's intricately composed introduction to his *Gemma ecclesiastica* is typical: "I know that to learned readers and delicate ears ... I will appear in this work either wearisome or superfluous. But let them know that these things are written exclusively for our own country of Wales, and are set forth in plain and common language without ornamentation ... so that they might be understood."[27] Only when this common Latin, with its simple and straightforward style, became an acceptable vehicle for written communication could a popular literature flourish.[28]

[25] For a description of the humanist style in 12th-century literature and a bibliography on the subject, see Janet Martin, "Classicism and Style in Latin Literature," in *Renaissance and Renewal*, pp. 537-568.

[26] See Joseph de Ghellinck, *L'essor de la littérature latine au XIIe siècle*, 2nd ed. (Brussels: Desclée de Brouwer, 1954); Erich Auerbach, *Literatursprache und Publikum in der lateinischen Spätantike und im Mittelalter* (Bern: Francke, 1958), especially pages 206-208, where he distinguishes two streams of high medieval Latin literature — a rhetorical-humanistic style and the "dialektisch-wissenschaftliche Latein der Scholastik." We would propose a third category — the low Latin of the schools.

[27] "Scio tamen quod eruditis auribus delicatisque quibus trita sunt ista lectoribus, vel taediosus esse videbor in hoc opusculo vel superfluus. Sed sciant illi quod Walliae nostrae soli scripta sunt ista, publicis admodum et planis absque ornatu tam verbis quam sententiis rudibus solum ad intelligendum exposita," *Gemma ecclesiastica*, ed. J.S. Brewer, Rolls Series 21/2 (London: Longman, 1862), p. 6.

[28] The use of vernacular languages for pastoral instruction also became widespread during the 13th century. Robert Grosseteste played an important part in introducing Anglo-Norman as a language for written instruction, but this development is beyond the scope of this study. For recent bibliographical surveys, see Siegfried Wenzel, "Vices, Virtues, and Popular Preaching," *Medieval and Renaissance Studies* 6 (1976) 28-54; Fritz Kemmler, *"Exempla" in Context*.

William de Montibus, however, makes few concessions to the linguistic abilities of his readers. He expects his theologians to have learned the classical authors and to be at home with the rhetorical nuances of twelfth-century Latin literature. His introduction to theology, the *Numerale*, is written in a less complex Latin than many of his other works. But this simpler Latin is only a propaedeutic vehicle serving to introduce the readers to the higher reaches of theology and to the learned language of that discipline.

William's expectations of his students are illustrated clearly in the two sets of sermons that he composed for an acquaintance who was neglecting his preaching duties.[29] The sermons themselves, designed to be preached to a non-academic audience, are composed in a plain and unadorned style. They are introduced to their recipient, however, by two masterful examples of the scholastic *ars dictaminis*. The forceful rhetoric of these introductions, replete with ornate sentences and obscure words, would have failed to move anyone who was ill at ease with the learned literary conventions of the schools. The sermons indicate that William could write a simple Latin that echoed the common vocabulary and speech patterns of daily life. The prefaces to these sermons, however, reveal an author who expected of his readers a sophisticated fluency in the rhetorical Latin of the schools.

Pedagogical methods

If William was in the rear guard with respect to the language of popular literature, he was in the van of those developing new literary techniques of popularization. The twelfth century is remarkable for the production of new genres of scholastic literature. The law schools witnessed the emergence of *Quaestiones*, *Distinctiones*, *Summae*, *Notabilia*, and *Brocarda*,[30] while the schools of theology produced their own *Sententiae*, *Glossae*, *Postillae*, *Quaestiones*, *Lecturae*, and *Summae*.[31] Less well known are other types of literature that sought to popularize scholastic teachings and make the fruits of learned discussions accessible to a wider audience. These emerged at the end of the twelfth century, primarily in England and northern France. William de Montibus's *Distinctiones*, *Proverbia*, *Similitudinarium*, and *Versarius* are four excellent and early examples of this popularizing literature.

---

[29] See below, II.16, Sermon nos. 74-115.

[30] See Kuttner, *Repertorium*.

[31] In general see Nikolaus M. Häring, "Commentary and Hermeneutics," in *Renaissance and Renewal*, pp. 173-200.

Learned legal commentaries known as *Distinctiones* first emerged from the famous law schools of Bologna during the twelfth century.[32] It was in Paris and the north of Europe, however, where these were transformed into a genre of popular literature.[33] By the end of the twelfth century, *distinctiones* were one of the most important pedagogical implements of the schools.[34]

In their simplest form, *distinctiones* served to organize and present the various meanings of a word or thing in different contexts. Thus, in theology one might "distinguish" the literal, moral, tropological, and anagogical significance of the holy city, Jerusalem. William's distinctions concerning the word *arcus* (meaning both the archer's bow and the rainbow) are more complex, but exemplify the same technique.[35] He begins by stating that the "bow" can signify Christ, God's graciousness, Holy Scripture, judgement, strength, purpose, treachery, and grief. The rainbow, placed in the clouds of heaven as a sign of the covenant between God and humankind following the flood (Gen 9:12-17), represents Christ, who was found amidst the doctors in the temple as if in the clouds of heaven. Like the rainbow, Christ appears to us regularly "in the clouds," that is, in the sermons of preachers, who are likened to "clouds" in a subsequent distinction. The rainbow's verdant colour represents Christ's divinity; its reddish colour, the blood of his humanity. The rainbow-like visions seen by Ezekiel (1:26-28) and by John (Apoc 4:3) represent Christ in the flesh, his ascension, and his coming again on the day of judgement, as well as God's graciousness in encircling and protecting us.

William explicates the Psalmist's reference to God as an archer bending his bow (Ps 7:13) as a representation of sacred scripture. The bow is composed of two different elements — the bow itself, which is rigid, and the bowstring, which is soft and flexible. The Old Testament provides the strength and rigidity of Scripture's bow, while the bowstring of the New Testament bends and controls this rigidity.

The archer's bow also represents God's fearsome judgements. The solid wood of the unstrung bow represents God's power and strength.

---

[32] Kuttner, *Repertorium*, pp. 208-227.

[33] Ibid. Giulio Silano, "'Distinctiones Decretorum'," illustrates how Ricardus Anglicus (de Mores) utilized the distinction-style of the Parisian theologians rather than the more cumbersome and technical style of the Bolognese jurists.

[34] Although *distinctiones* have received considerable attention in recent years, we still have no comprehensive study of the texts or history of the genre. See above, Chapter Two, at notes 95-99, and below, Part ii.8, pp. 261-264.

[35] Printed below, ii.8.

At the day of judgement, the bow will be strung, and God will shoot the sharp arrows of his hard verdicts.

Two further interpretations of the word *arcus* in sacred scripture are explicated briefly — the bow is a metaphor for "strength" in Hosea 1:5: "I will break Israel's bow in the valley of Jezreel"; and a metaphor for "purpose" or "intention" in 1 Samuel 2:4: "The bow of the strong is overcome." Both steadfast strength and firm purpose to do good are implied in the Psalmist's exclamation: "You have made my arms like a bronze bow" (Ps 17:35).

Finally, William presents several texts wherein the bow represents deceit and evil intent. The evildoers in Psalm 10:3 and Psalm 36:14 are bent on sin and deceit as much as on physical warfare. The enigmatic reference to an evil bow (*arcum prauum*) in Psalm 77:57, "they are bent like an evil bow," might refer either to a weak and overly pliable bow, or to one that is turned in perverse fashion against the shooter himself.

The practical nature of these *distinctiones* is remarkable. The genre has small pretensions to literary elegance; its primary goal is the summation and organization of doctrine in a simple and accessible format. This format could be further simplified by presenting the elements of each distinction in a schema or diagram. Texts like Robert Grosseteste's *Templum Dei*, composed in large part of *schemata* summarizing the doctrine of theologians and canonists, illustrate the usefulness of the *distinctio* in the popular literature of pastoral care.

Distinctio collections sought to digest complex doctrines, and to represent them in easily accessible form. Medieval florilegia sought to collect the "flowers" or apt sayings of ancient and medieval authorities as an aid to the student, the scholar, and the pastor of souls. Such collections were not new in the twelfth century, but they were brought to a new level of practical organization and usefulness by William de Montibus and his contemporaries. William's *Proverbia* is a notable example of the florilegial literature of this period.[36] Much more comprehensive than its precursors, William's collection brings together aphorisms and quotations drawn from many sources — from ancient and modern writers, from prose works and poetry, from secular and religious writings, and from humble as well as exalted authorities. All of these quotations are organized under topical headings, and arranged alphabetically, which enabled the reader to find apposite materials quickly and easily. By the end of the thirteenth century such collections

---

[36] See below, ii.10.

were in common use among preachers and pastors. Their usefulness
was the result of the techniques of popularization developed by William
de Montibus and his contemporaries.

As the *Proverbia* constitutes a handy thesaurus of learned and
popular quotations, so William's *Similitudinarium* makes accessible to
theologians the fruits of scholastic research and pious meditation
concerning the natural world.[37] Although not the first to make use
of similitudes and metaphors in teaching, William was one of the first
to conceive of a vast encyclopedia of such metaphors. His *Similitudinarium*, like the aforementioned collections, was divided into alphabetically arranged topics, "so that we might find more quickly and
easily some simile pertaining to a proposed topic of discourse." Judging
from the large number of extant manuscript copies of this work, it
was an immediate success. This technique of collecting and presenting
similitudes for practical use by the preacher and teacher was quickly
adopted by others. Most important are the collections of *exempla*,
closely related to *similitudines*, that flourished during the thirteenth
and fourteenth centuries.[38]

William's *Versarius* represents yet another experiment in the field
of popular didactic literature.[39] Poetry had long been considered an
appropriate medium for teaching and study. Verse summaries of almost
every field of human knowledge appeared in the eleventh and twelfth
centuries; even texts of scholastic theology and law were turned into
verse. In addition to formal didactic poems and the verse translations
and epitomes of major works, one encounters in manuscripts of the
thirteenth and subsequent centuries a plethora of brief poetic tags
intended to convey in a memorable fashion the essential elements of
some doctrine. Scribes and readers copied these verses on the flyleaves
and in the margins of manuscripts, and authors frequently inserted
them into prose treatises as an integral part of the composition.[40]
Although scholastic theologians and lawyers were not above including

[37] See below, ii.9.
[38] See above, Chapter Two, note 110.
[39] See below, ii.12.
[40] See de Ghellinck, "Medieval Theology in Verse," pp. 336-354; Siegfried Wenzel,
Verses in Sermons: "Fasciculus Morum" and Its Middle English Poems (Cambridge
MA: Mediaeval Academy of America, 1978), pp. 61-65; Lynn Thorndike, "Unde versus,"
Traditio 11 (1955) 163-193; C.M. Joris Vansteenkiste, "'Versus' dans les oeuvres de
Saint Thomas," in *St. Thomas Aquinas 1274-1974: Commemorative Studies*, ed.
Armand A. Maurer, 2 vols. (Toronto: Pontifical Institute of Mediaeval Studies, 1974),
1: 77-85.

such verses in their writings, authors of practical, pastoral treatises were their most assiduous users.[41]

William's *Versarius* is a unique attempt to provide a systematic encyclopedia of Latin poetry useful to the theologian. He composed and collected some 1,300 verses, couplets, and short poems, and organized them under alphabetical topics like those in his *Distinctiones*, *Proverbia*, and *Similitudinarium*. With this opus in hand, the writer of a pastoral treatise, a sermon, a letter, or any such work, could easily and quickly find apposite verses to serve as the basis for his exposition.

Books

Underlying all of these experiments in popularization was a new attitude toward books and book-learning that would have tremendous impact on the western world in succeeding centuries.[42] Our modern facility with the written word and our presumption that one can learn almost anything by reading books is an important legacy from this period of the Middle Ages. William and his contemporaries devoted a great deal of effort to the invention of techniques that would transform books into didactic tools and make book-learning an easier process.

William's writings illustrate the early and inchoate attempts to transform "literature" into an educational tool. His large collections of distinctions, similitudes, proverbs, and verses are artless and repetitive — they correspond to no classical model or standard of literary presentation. He chose an alphabetical format for these works not for its beauty but for its practical effectiveness. As one of the first authors to use alphabetization on this grand a scale, William helped to make the technique acceptable as a legitimate form of literary expression.[43]

---

[41] Perhaps the most conspicuous example is one of William de Montibus's students, Richard of Wetheringsett, whose *Summa Qui bene presunt* is discussed below. Wenzel, *Verses in Sermons*, pp. 63-100, gives many other examples, to which should be added Aag of Denmark; see, Angelus Walz, "Des Aage von Dänemark, *Rotulus pugillaris* im Lichte der alten dominikanischen Konventstheologie," *Classica et mediaevalia* 15 (1954) 198-252, and 16 (1955) 136-194.

[42] An excellent description of this new attitude and its various manifestations in the 13th century is in Rouse and Rouse, "*Statim invenire*," pp. 201-225; idem, *Preachers*, pp. 3-42.

[43] Rouse and Rouse, *Preachers*, pp. 28-29, distinguish between the invention of techniques (such as alphabetization) and their consistent application. William was not the inventor but one of the first and most persistent users of alphabetical order as the organizing principle of his writings.

The artificial structure of William's *Numerale* is yet another expression of his search for effective (if artless) means of literary presentation. Under the numbers One to Twelve, William assembles the basic theological concepts he wishes to teach, from One God, One Faith, and One Baptism, to the Twelve Articles of Faith, the Twelve Hours of the Day, and the Twelve Prerogatives of the Blessed Virgin. The immediate popularity of this work indicates that it met a need in the early-thirteenth-century schools; the absence of imitators later in the century only shows that other, more effective, modes of presentation had been created to meet the same need.

William and his contemporaries played tirelessly with this new idea that books should be practical tools rather than works of art. Their various experiments helped to create new attitudes toward books, and toward learning from books, that had important consequences in all fields of human endeavor. Literacy and book-learning became, for the first time, a practical virtue and not simply an adornment for the chosen few. One of the first to formulate clearly this new attitude was Robert Grosseteste, a cleric in Bishop Hugh of Lincoln's household in the 1190's and subsequently the bishop of Lincoln from 1235 to 1253.[44] During the 1220's Grosseteste wrote a pastoral handbook for the education of priests. In it he presents the human body as the temple of God (*templum Dei*) and the cardinal virtues of temperance, fortitude, and prudence as the foundation, walls, and roof of that temple. The virtue of prudence, he tells us, has several elements. One is docility (*docilitas*), which he defines as "the ability to teach the unskilled, first oneself and then others, *through the written word*."[45] These last words — *per res scriptas* — are harbingers of the modern world. The suggestion, that everyone, not just schoolmen, should learn by reading, marks a turning point in the history of popular literature and practical education.

By elevating book-learning to the status of a general virtue, thirteenth-century scholastics set the stage for the outpouring of *pastoralia* that characterized the subsequent centuries. They recognized in the growing student population a suitable audience for written instruction concerning the exercise of pastoral care. By refining the educational experiments of William de Montibus and his contemporaries, they developed techniques for popularizing scholastic doctrine

---

[44] Although Grosseteste was at Lincoln during the 1190's, there is no evidence that he studied theology there under William de Montibus.

[45] "Docilitas: per res scriptas sciencia erudiendi imperitos, primo se et deinde alios," *Templum Dei*, p. 31.

and educating non-specialist readers through the written word. One last ingredient was necessary, however, for the creation of a recognizable genre of pastoral literature; some consensus had to be reached about the proper content of instruction for the *cura animarum*. Such a consensus emerged, it seems, only in the years after William's death. But two English writers, one a student of Peter the Chanter of Paris and the other a student of William de Montibus, played crucial rôles in this development.

THE CONTENT OF PASTORALIA

When the Fourth Lateran Council defined pastoral care as the art of arts, it was expressing a growing consensus that soul-care, like theology, law, medicine, and the arts, was a distinct discipline that could be taught and learned in the schools.[46] When it came to defining the content of this discipline, however, the Council was understandably vague. Canon 11, *De magistris scholasticis*, required that theologians be appointed in each metropolitan cathedral to teach priests and others "those things which are known to pertain to the care of souls."[47]

But what are those things? Might they include, for example, the art of preaching and of hearing confessions? Canon 10 of the Council, *De praedicatoribus instituendis*, addressed the need for the appointment of fit and holy men to assist busy bishops in their pastoral task of preaching to the people. These episcopal assistants (*coadiutores et cooperatores*) were also to help in hearing confessions, assigning penances, and in other activities "which pertain to the care of souls."[48] Such skills, then, are among the things "that are known to pertain

---

[46] See above, at note 2.

[47] "Sane metropolitana ecclesia theologum nihilominus habeat, qui sacerdotes et alios in sacra pagina doceat et in his praesertim informet, quae ad curam animarum spectare noscuntur." *Concilium oecumenicorum decreta*, p. 240.

[48] "Inter caetera quae ad salutem spectant populi christiani, pabulum verbi Dei permaxime sibi noscitur esse necessarium. ... Unde cum saepe contingat, quod episcopi propter occupationes multiplices vel invaletudines corporales aut hostiles incursus seu occasiones alias — ne dicamus defectum scientiae, quod in eis est reprobandum omnino nec de caetero tolerandum — per se ipsos non sufficiunt ministrare populo verbum Dei, maxime per amplas dioeceses et diffusas, generali constitutione sancimus, ut episcopi viros idoneos ad sanctae praedicationis officium salubriter exequendum assumant, potentes in opere et sermone, qui plebes sibi commissas vice ipsorum, cum per se nequiverint, sollicite visitantes, eas verbo aedificent et exemplo ... . Unde praecipimus tam in cathedralibus quam in aliis conventualibus ecclesiis viros idoneos ordinari, quos episcopi possint coadiutores et cooperatores habere, non solum in praedicationis officio verum etiam in audiendis confessionibus et poenitentiis iniungendis ac caeteris, quae ad salutem pertinent animarum," ibid., pp. 239-240.

to the care of souls," but can they be taught in the schools? And if so, how? The Council offered no guidance in this regard. Certainly there was cause for optimism. Peter the Chanter in his school at Paris, William de Montibus in his at Lincoln, and many others had been successful in teaching and inspiring students to undertake these and other pastoral tasks. Perhaps the Council, encouraged by these examples, saw no need for more specificity. If the *ad hoc* teachings of the contemporary masters were producing the type of persons who would be suitable episcopal assistants, then simply making this instruction more easily and widely available would suffice to meet the needs of the reforming Church of the thirteenth century. Vagueness about the proper and specific content of pastoral instruction in the schools is understandable in 1215. The teachers themselves, as we shall see, were only feeling their way toward a consensus about those things that pertain to the pastoral care of souls.

It is one thing to train and appoint a few good men to aid bishops in their pastoral duties, and quite another to educate all of the parochial clergy concerning the care of souls. Canon 11 of the Council had provided for learned assistants to help the bishop in hearing confessions and assigning penances, but Canon 21 of the same Council required that every parishioner confess at least once a year to his or her own priest (*proprio sacerdoti*).[49] Should not these simple priests, too, be instructed in the things pertaining to pastoral care?

The Council addressed this question in Canon 27, *De instructione ordinandorum*. It required that the bishop or his representative should take care to instruct and inform prospective ordinands to the priesthood about the correct celebration of the Church's rites and sacraments.[50] We note that the bishop is not ordered to send clerics to the schools,

[49] "Omnis utriusque sexus fidelis ... omnia sua solus peccata confiteatur fideliter, saltem semel in anno proprio sacerdoti, et iniunctam sibi poenitentiam studeat pro viribus adimplere ..."; ibid., p. 245. The Council's use of the phrase *proprius sacerdos* would seem to be intentionally vague so as to cover all of the various jurisdictional possibilities. For most people, this would refer to their parish priest. For monks, canons, inmates of some hospitals, etc. it would designate their abbot, prior, or someone delegated by the superior to hear confessions. Parish priests themselves would confess to the official designated as their confessor by the bishop. For those studying in the schools special penitentiaries (from the abbey of St. Victor at Paris, or St. Frideswide in Oxford, for example) could serve as the students' *proprii sacerdotes* for the hearing of confessions.

[50] "Cum sit ars artium regimen animarum, districte praecipimus, ut episcopi promovendos in sacerdotes diligenter instruant et informent vel per se ipsos vel per alios viros idoneos super divinis officiis et ecclesiasticis sacramentis, qualiter ea rite valeant celebrare ... "; ibid., p. 248.

nor to ensure that they had attended a school where the "art of arts" was taught.[51] Neither is it implied that the bishop should instruct prospective priests in all the details of conducting the liturgy and performing the sacraments of the Church. Ordinands would have had to learn these basics in their progress through the clerical ranks by aiding and observing a practising priest. Rather the canon envisages a more careful episcopal oversight over the ordination of candidates to ensure that they had, indeed, learned the basics. "The ordination of ignorant and untrained candidates," the Council asserts, "can easily be discovered, and both the ordinands and the ordainers will be severely punished."[52]

But what positive "instruction" and "information" concerning the liturgy and sacraments does the Council envisage in this canon? The answer would seem to lie in the words *rite ... celebrare*: bishops should teach ordinands *to celebrate* the rituals *correctly*. If bishops would be unable to teach ordinands everything about how these are to be celebrated, they could at least correct obvious errors and misunderstandings. The content of such instruction is adumbrated elsewhere in the legislation of Lateran IV. It is elaborated further in synodal constitutions of individual dioceses throughout Europe.[53] And it gradually finds its way into the pastoral literature of the thirteenth century.

---

[51] Canon 30, *De idoneitate instituendorum in ecclesiis*, insists that ordinands be virtuous (*morum honestas*) and have a knowledge of letters (*scientia litterarum*), but not that they have studied in the schools. Canon 32, *Ut patroni competentem portionem dimittant clericis*, acknowledges that in certain regions scarcely any parish priest can be found who is even slightly skilled in letters, but the Council finds both the cause of this abuse and its remedy to lie in the economic rather than the educational sphere: "Nam ut pro certo didicimus, in quibusdam regionibus parochiales presbyteri pro sua sustentatione non obtinent nisi quartam quartae, id est sextamdecimam decimarum. Unde fit ut in his regionibus pene nullus inveniatur sacerdos parochialis, qui vel modicam habeat peritiam literarum," ibid., pp. 249-250.

[52] "Quoniam si ignaros et rudes de caetero ordinare praesumpserint, quod quidem facile poterit deprehendi, et ordinatores et ordinatos gravi decrevimus subiacere ultioni," ibid., p. 248. Examinations of candidates became an integral part of the ordination ceremony during the 13th century; see Bennett, "Medieval Ordination Lists," pp. 20-34.

[53] See Bishop Richard Poore's statutes for the diocese of Salisbury (1217 x 1219), in *Councils & Synods*, 1: 57-96. Poore wanted his archdeacons and rural deans to distribute the decrees rapidly, "ut sacerdotes, ipsas frequenter habentes pre oculis, in ministeriis et dispensationibus sacramentorum sint instructiores et in fide catholica bene vivendo firmiores" (p. 96). Cf. Haines, "Education in English Ecclesiastical Legislation," pp. 161-175; Vincent Gillespie, "*Doctrina* and *Predicacio*: The Design and Function of Some Pastoral Manuals," *Leeds Studies in English*, ns, 11 (1980) 36-50.

Although the wording of Canon 27 is vague, other canons of the Council speak eloquently and at length about various errors and abuses in the celebration of divine offices and sacraments. Canons 14 to 17 discuss aspects of the behaviour and dress of clerics that interfere with the proper exercise of their duties. Canon 18 forbids clerical participation in judicial ordeals — a popular liturgico-sacramental activity. Canon 19 concerns abuses of liturgical ornaments and utensils. Canons 20 to 22 discuss details of the correct celebration of the eucharist, penance, and the last rites, respectively. Canons 47 to 49 concern the correct forms of excommunication. Canons 50 to 52, concerning the sacrament of marriage, draw particular attention to the rôle of the parish priest (*parochialis sacerdos*) in prohibiting clandestine marriages. Canons 53 to 56 describe abuses of ecclesiastical tithes, and again the parish priest (*presbyter parochialis*) is invoked, this time to warn him against assigning tithes to laymen. Finally, Canon 66 discusses the "frequent reports" that clergymen extort payments for the performance of such pastoral services as funerals, weddings, and the celebration of other sacraments.

All of these canons contain examples of the kind of "instruction" that ordinands should receive about the correct celebration of the divine offices and sacraments. Similar instructions were already being recorded in the synodal statutes for individual dioceses before 1215, and would become commonplace during the thirteenth century.[54] The actual teaching of parochial clergy envisaged by the councils and synods was, no doubt, to be *viva voce*. The bishop or one of his officials was expected to examine and instruct his clergy personally, either at the time of ordination or during pastoral visitations and convocations. Written directives for such examinations and teachings began to appear in the thirteenth century.[55] These, along with the statutes themselves, form a part of the new literature of pastoral care, and illustrate an important element of this literature's proper content.

[54] For a bibliographical orientation to the growing literature on councils and synods, see Odette Pontal, *Les statuts synodaux*, Typologie des sources du moyen âge occidental, 11 (Turnhout: Brepols, 1975).

[55] See, for example, the questionnaire appended to Robert Grosseteste's synodal statutes (1239?), *Councils & Synods*, 1: 276-278. An extremely detailed and informative set of instructions is found in the *Libellus pastoralis de cura et officio archidiaconi*, from the mid 13th century, edited by F. Ravaisson from Laon, MS 157, in an appendix to his *Catalogue général des manuscrits des bibliothèques publiques des départements de France, I* (Paris, 1849), pp. 592-649. Ravaisson's ascription of this work to Raymund of Peñafort is erroneous; see Stephan Kuttner, "The Barcelona Edition of St. Raymond's First Treatise on Canon Law," *Seminar* 8 (1950) 52-67, at p. 53, note 5.

The Fourth Lateran Council of 1215 is significant, not for defining the content of pastoral education, but for giving support to many of the inchoate and unsystematic experiments in education that were current at the time. We have identified in the conciliar documents two main thrusts of these experiments. First was the interest in training scholars in "those things that are known to pertain to pastoral care" — especially the arts of preaching and of hearing confessions and assigning penances. Second was the insistence that the parochial clergy should be informed concerning the correct performance of their duties as ministers of the divine offices and administrators of the Church's sacraments. The Council's vagueness concerning the specific content of instruction that would achieve these ends is perhaps best understood as caution and circumspection. The Fathers of the Council could scarcely do better than to encourage experiments and wait patiently for some consensus to emerge.

The decades immediately following the Council witnessed a tremendous outpouring of *pastoralia* in the form of instructional *summae*, handbooks, and treatises, many seeking to combine the pastoral teachings of the schools with the practical instruction of simple priests. This unique synthesis of the two (separate) interests expressed by the Council came to define the proper content of pastoral literature. But before describing the emergence of this consensus, it would be well to look back to the pre-conciliar period, and especially to the works of William de Montibus, to examine the materials out of which it was formed.

The schools of the later twelfth century produced a plethora of idiosyncratic works concerning preaching, penance, and the sacraments, as well as expositions of the various creeds, the *Pater noster*, the rituals of the Mass, the vices and virtues, and, of course, the Bible.[56] Each dealt, in its own way, with "those things that are known to pertain to the care of souls." Nevertheless the diversity of these writings testifies to their experimental nature and to the lack of consensus at the time about the proper content (not to mention "audience" and "style") of a pastoral literature. Perhaps the finest example to emerge from the

---

[56] See Häring, "Commentary and Hermeneutics," p. 189, nn. 147-151. The failure of many works to fall under clearly defined categories of "scholastic" literature (i.e. lectures, disputations, and sermons) has resulted in their being ignored or misunderstood. Studies of individual authors reveal the extent of their interest in extracurricular subjects. See d'Alverny, *Alain de Lille*, where not only the "oeuvres de théologie pratique" but all the other genres identified there contain works of potential pastoral significance.

Parisian schools was Peter the Chanter's *Verbum abbreviatum*.[57] It is a pastiche of information on preaching, confession, virtues and vices, and many other topics, garnered from Peter's own teachings and from those current in the twelfth-century schools. The subject matter made it appealing to many readers, and it enjoyed a tremendous popularity. But the absence of a clear or coherent plan of organization, and the heterogeneity of its contents, made it less than ideal as a teaching instrument for the *cura animarum*.

William de Montibus's scholastic writings share with Peter's many of the same limitations. His *Distinctiones* and *Numerale*, for example, are filled with insights and casual asides concerning the care of souls, but the reader must devote a good deal of time and energy to ferreting them out. Neither William nor Peter attempted to distinguish the content of professional, theological education from the content appropriate for pastors involved in the day-to-day exercise of the *cura animarum*.

William was not unaware of the needs of the wider clerical audience at the Lincoln schools and in the surrounding communities. But the content of his practical instruction has an incidental and *ad hoc* quality. This becomes clear if we examine William's writings in terms of the pastoral categories adumbrated in the Fourth Lateran Council and elaborated during the following century, i.e. (1) preaching, (2) penance, and (3) instruction about the correct celebration of the Church's rites, rituals, and sacraments.

Gems of instruction concerning the importance of preaching and the qualities of good preachers are scattered throughout William's writings.[58] He took the preaching office seriously and inspired others to do so as well. But nowhere does he set out systematically the principles by which preachers should be trained, nor does he define (as did one of his students) the content of doctrine and instruction that pastors should convey in their sermons. William's students and other auditors could learn some of these things by hearing and reading the chancellor's sermons, but they would search in vain for a concise and easily accessible summary of the preaching office. William did compose a collection of sermons to aid a specific pastor in fulfilling his preaching duties, but these sermons were tailored for the needs

---

[57] The "shorter" version of this work is printed in PL 205: 1-554; cf. Baldwin, *Masters*, 2: 246-265.

[58] In addition to the rubrics "Predicator," etc. in his *Distinctiones* (II.8), *Similitudinarium* (II.9), and *Proverbia* (II.10), see the *Numerale*, "De altari aureo," p. 247, and the *Super Psalmos*, p. 497.

and interests of that particular individual.[59] They were not "model" or "generic" sermons such as became popular later in the thirteenth century, nor do they represent a conscious attempt on William's part to compose an integral guide to the pastoral art of preaching.[60]

William's contributions to defining the content of pastoral instruction concerning penance were similarly *ad hoc* and incidental. He writes eloquently and often about aspects of penance and confession in all of his longer works, but his comments are scattered and disjointed. He composed a brief treatise to help confessors learn how to elicit confessions of the more subtle and dangerous sins,[61] and another to advise monastic confessors in the art of enjoining penances appropriate for their cloistered brothers and sisters.[62] But nowhere does he define clearly and comprehensively those things that should be taught in the schools concerning the art of hearing confessions and enjoining salutary penances. Even his famous *Peniteas cito peccator*, which was later to be treated as an epitome of all that a priest needed to know in exercising his penitential office, seems not to have been conceived as such by William.[63] The *Peniteas cito* is not a systematic poem, but rather a medley of didactic verses, chosen from among many others, to illustrate specific aspects of penitential discipline. He surely would have been pleased to see the success that his "poem" enjoyed in later years. But he can scarcely have imagined that this *ad hoc* scholastic exercise would come to be so useful and so highly esteemed as a popular summary of the content of penitential education.

The Church's liturgy and sacraments also receive extensive but unsystematic treatment in William's writings. Like his contemporaries, William included the prayers and rites of the Church among the sacred scriptures, adducing them along with biblical citations to argue and illustrate various points of doctrine. He also collected a number of *quaestiones* on the sacraments, and composed a metrical treatise *de sacramentis*.[64] Both include useful information about the interpretation

[59] See below, *Sermones* (II.16), nos. 74-115.

[60] On "model sermons" see the excellent study by d'Avray, *The Preaching of the Friars*. Maurice of Sully, Alan of Lille, and Alexander of Ashby were some of William's predecessors and contemporaries who also experimented with methods of teaching the art of preaching. All were pioneers in a movement that would bear fruit in many types of *pastoralia* during the subsequent centuries. These authors produced model sermons and *artes praedicandi*, but no systematic discussions of the proper *content* of pastoral preaching as it should be taught in the schools.

[61] Printed below, *Speculum penitentis* (II.4).

[62] Printed below, *De penitentia religiosorum* (II.5).

[63] See below, *Peniteas cito* (II.1).

[64] See below, *De septem sacramentis* (II.13), and *Tractatus metricus* (II.3).

and the celebration of the sacramental offices. His *Errorum eliminatio* might seem particularly relevant to the Lateran's decree that priests should be taught the correct performance of the Church's rites and sacraments.[65] The bulk of sections 2 to 8 and section 10 of this treatise pertains directly to aspects of the cathedral prayers and readings, and only by extension to the liturgy in parishes and monasteries. Section 1, *De hiis que fiunt in ecclesia*, however, discusses errors that must have been common in the parishes, and section 9, *De erroribus laicorum*, is given over entirely to errors common among parishioners that it was the duty of the clergy to extirpate. Such instructions may well have been necessary and useful for ordinands, but they have an incidental quality here. However interesting this miscellany of instructions may be, it neither attempts comprehensiveness nor does it reflect a consensus concerning the appropriate content of pastoral education for ministers of the Church's rites and sacraments.

All of these scattered examples testify to William's abiding interest in penance, preaching, and the Church's rites and sacraments, but they also reveal an absence of any clear and systematic programme for teaching pastoral care in the schools.

Within a few years of William's death in 1213, however, two pastoral *summae* appeared that helped to define for future generations the proper content of instruction concerning the *cura animarum*. One of these emanated from Peter the Chanter's school at Paris and took as its starting point the art of penance. The other emerged from William de Montibus's school at Lincoln, and was couched in terms of the art of preaching. The first is Thomas Chobham's *Summa Cum miserationes Domini*,[66] the second Richard Wetheringsett's *Summa Qui bene presunt presbyteri*.[67] Both were very popular in the thirteenth

---

[65] Printed below, *Errorum eliminatio* (II.2).

[66] *Thomae de Chobham Summa confessorum*, ed. F. Broomfield, Analecta mediaevalis Namurcensia, 25 (Louvain and Paris: Nauwelaerts, 1968). Robert Courson's *Summa Tota celestis philosophia* (1208 x 1213) is sometimes seen as rendering a similar service for the Chanter's teachings, but Robert's *summa* is aimed at a sophisticated academic audience; it is not a "popularizing" *summa*. For a work that attempts to popularize the Chanter's and Courson's teachings, see Vincent L. Kennedy, "The Handbook of Master Peter Chancellor of Chartres," *Mediaeval Studies* 5 (1943) 1-38; this handbook, however, had no imitators, and did little to establish a proper "content" for the literature of pastoral care. Finally, I have ignored Robert of Flamborough's *Liber poenitentialis*, edited by J.J. Francis Firth, Studies and Texts, 18 (Toronto: Pontifical Institute of Mediaeval Studies, 1971), and the tradition of *summae de penitentia* that follow it. The development of this genre of pastoral literature deserves separate treatment (see above, n. 24).

[67] No edition; for the manuscripts see Morton W. Bloomfield, B.-G. Guyot,

century and continued to be copied and read until the end of the Middle Ages. But these works are even more significant in that they marked a new departure in the literature of pastoral care. Each reflected, and in its own way helped to establish, a common and enduring consensus about "those things that are known to pertain to the care of souls."

Thomas Chobham's Summa Cum miserationes Domini

Thomas Chobham's *summa* is one of the most accessible works of practical theology produced in the Middle Ages.[68] Here the theological teachings of Peter the Chanter and others, the doctrines of the canonists, and the legislation of Church and State, come to life in pithy summaries and reflections on everyday life. Chobham sets out to describe, without abstruse and theoretical digressions, the actions and practical considerations necessary for the priest who will hear confessions and enjoin penances.[69] In doing so, he placed himself in a tradition that stretched back into the twelfth century and beyond — to the "Penitentials" of the earlier Middle Ages.[70] But Chobham's achievement embraces far more than was envisioned in the earlier penitential literature. His is one of the first *summae* of pastoral care and clerical education. Known to medieval writers as the *Summa Cum miserationes*, its manuscript copies also bore such descriptive titles as *Liber ad instructionem sacerdotum, Manuale sacerdotum, Summa de sacramentis, Summa de casibus, Summa iuris,* and *Speculum ecclesie.*[71] Chobham's work illustrated how, under the guise of a penitential *summa*, one could teach almost everything that a priest needed to know in exercising the care of souls.

Chobham begins with a definition of penance and of various types of penitential activities, from solemn, public, and private penance to the paying of tithes, giving of alms, daily recitation of the *Credo* and

---

D.R. Howard, and T.B. Kabealo, *Incipits of Latin Works on the Virtues and Vices, 1100-1500 A.D.* (Cambridge MA: Mediaeval Academy of America, 1979), no. 4583.

[68] On Chobham's *Summa* see Broomfield's introduction to his edition, pp. xi-lxxv; cf. Baldwin, *Masters,* 1: 34-36; Kemmler, *"Exempla" in Context,* pp. 35-39.

[69] "De penitentia igitur dicturi subtilitates et inquisitiones theoricas pretermittemus et operationes et considerationes practicas que ad audiendas confessiones et ad iniungendas penitentias sacerdotibus necessarie sunt diligentius prosequemur," *Summa confessorum,* p. 3.

[70] See Cyrille Vogel, *Les "Libri paenitentiales,"* Typologie des sources du moyen âge occidental, 27 (Turnhout: Brepols, 1985).

[71] See Leonard E. Boyle's review of Broomfield's edition in the *Catholic Historical Review* 57 (1971) 487-488.

Pater noster, and prayers for the dead.[72] He then describes in detail the types of sins for which penance should be enjoined.[73] He helps the reader to distinguish between venial (*venialia*) and deadly sins (*mortalia peccata*), and discusses briefly the standard division of the latter into seven criminal sins (criminalibus peccatis). He introduces Moses's Decalogue or Ten Commandments as another tool for recognizing what vices should be shunned and what virtues cultivated. Likewise the ten plagues of Egypt, each parallel to one of the commandments, "are useful for priests to know in many cases of conscience (*casibus confessionum*)."[74] Chobham completes this discussion of sins by introducing priests to the seven petitions of the *Pater noster*, the seven beatitudes, the seven gifts of the Holy Spirit, and the seven theological and cardinal virtues. Each of these, he says, is important in the pastoral care of souls. For example: "The priest must also know the four cardinal virtues — prudence, justice, fortitude, and temperance — so that he will know how to teach the penitent to distinguish good from evil through prudence, how to avoid evil and do the good through justice, how to uproot vices and plant virtues through courage, and, through temperance, how to avoid gluttony and lust."[75]

Next Chobham explains the importance of considering the circumstances of sins (time, place, intention, etc.) so one can know how serious each sin is, and thus know what penance to enjoin for each.[76] Finally, just as sins are mitigated or exacerbated by the circumstances in which they are committed, so are individuals affected by their personal circumstances. Some of these, such as illegitimate birth or natural deformities, are beyond an individual's control; others like bigamy and infamy result from the person's own actions. The priest must be aware of all such circumstances because some render the individual incompetent (*irregularis*), and prevent him or her from marrying or being admitted to holy orders, and from exercising such legal acts as testifying or accusing someone in a court. Chobham illustrates each type of "irregularity" and explains its implications.[77]

Having summarized what the priest needs to know about penance, sins, and sinners, Chobham then turns his attention to the priest himself:

[72] *Summa confessorum*, pp. 5-14
[73] Ibid., pp. 14-44.
[74] Ibid., p. 33.
[75] Ibid., p. 44.
[76] Ibid., pp. 45-61.
[77] Ibid., pp. 61-79.

"Who and what sort of person should he be who ought to enjoin penances" (*Quis et qualis debeat esse ille qui penitentias iniungere debeat*).[78] He begins by comparing priests to monks: "Just as a monk ought to know his Order's Rule by which he regulates his life, so the priest should know his 'rule,' in accordance with which he ought to be ordained and to minister in his priestly orders."[79] This "rule" Chobham finds in the scriptural letters to Timothy (3:2-7) and to Titus (1:6-8). It begins: "Oportet episcopum esse irreprehensibilem, sine crimine, unius uxoris virum ... ." Although these words were addressed to bishops, Chobham assures his readers that, of old, even simple priests (*minores sacerdotes*) were called bishops, and that this "rule" pertains to all clergy with the care of souls.[80]

Next Chobham discusses the specific knowledge required of priests. He begins with a lucid exposition of the ancient prescription requiring all priests to know the books of the liturgy: the Sacramentary, the Lectionary, the Calendar, the penitential canons, a book of homilies, etc.[81] Then, because "the priest must know what a sacrament is, how many sacraments there are, and how these ought to be administered,"[82] Chobham undertakes to provide a comprehensive, practical guide to six of the Church's seven sacraments: baptism, eucharist, orders, marriage, confirmation, and extreme unction. (He reserves detailed treatment of the sacrament of penance for later chapters of his *summa*). This discussion represents an elegant summary of what one must know in order to instruct ordinands concerning the Church's sacraments, "qualiter ea rite valeant celebrare."

The remainder of Chobham's *summa* treats in fascinating detail practical aspects of administering the sacrament of penance. Nowhere else in medieval literature are we brought so near to the practice of penance as it was conceived by learned scholars and recommended to the simple clergy. Much of Chobham's advice to the confessor and

[78] Ibid., p. 79.

[79] Ibid.

[80] See ibid., pp. 80-81, where Chobham discusses briefly the legal and theological issues involved in identifying priests with bishops. For a recent review of this question see Roger E. Reynolds, "Patristic 'Presbyterianism' in the Early Medieval Theology of Sacred Orders," *Mediaeval Studies* 45 (1983) 311-342. By considering all priests as "bishops" Chobham is not so much entering the scholastic fray on this vexed question as expressing a growing consensus that the discipline and education that once was expected primarily of high ecclesiastical officials should now be required of even simple priests as well.

[81] *Summa confessorum*, pp. 86-88.

[82] Ibid., p. 88.

many of his practical observations were, no doubt, commonplace among churchmen of the time. But never before had they been given such extensive literary treatment.

Much more than a *summa de penitentia*, Chobham's *summa* is an innovative synthesis of practical theology, canon law, local and regional legislation, and what we might call "popular spirituality," as these pertain to the pastoral care of souls. This brief summary of his work gives an inadequate picture of the wealth of learned detail and common observations on the needs and interests of practising pastors. Although the materials themselves were not new, they had been available previously only in scattered references or in oral teachings. Chobham's contribution was to bring these together in a work that ignored the boundaries of scholastic disciplines (law, theology, arts, etc.), and that helped to establish a standard programme or curriculum for pastoral education in the centuries to come.

The very length and detail of his *summa* made it less accessible to the simple clergy with little desire or ability to read long books (or any books at all); nevertheless it marks a turning point in pastoral literature. Educated priests and teachers, comfortable with the techniques of book-learning, could and did read Chobham's *summa*. Some, no doubt, handed on the fruits of their reading to less learned priests, whether in casual conversation, in the pulpit, in the confessional, in local, diocesan, and provincial synods, or on other occasions. Other scholars, perhaps inspired directly or indirectly by Chobham's work, or simply responding to similar intellectual and literary currents in the early thirteenth century, composed their own pastoral handbooks and *summae*. In doing so they built, wittingly or not, on the emerging consensus that Chobham helped to create concerning the proper content of "those things that are known to pertain to the care of souls."

Richard of Wetheringsett's Summa Qui bene presunt

Thomas Chobham shaped his pastoral *summa* from the odds and ends of theological and pastoral instruction current in the circle of Peter the Chanter. The framework he chose for conveying these teachings was the *summa de penitentia*, a pre-existing type of literature that he transformed to suit his own purposes. What Chobham did for the Chanter's teachings, Richard of Wetheringsett did, at roughly the same time, for the teachings of William de Montibus. Richard, however, chose a different framework for his pastoral *Summa Qui bene presunt*. He presents a summary of the things that are necessary for the care of souls under the guise of a guide for preaching. Taken together, these two innovative *summae* bid fair to establish a programme by which suitable candidates (*viros idoneos*) could be trained in the schools, "not only in the office of preaching but also in that of hearing confessions and enjoining penances, and of other things that pertain to the health of souls."[83]

The only certain fact known about Richard of Wetheringsett is that he was a student in William de Montibus's school.[84] We can infer from ascriptions in various manuscript copies of his *summa* that he was rector of the parish of Wetheringsett in Suffolk, that he was associated with Leicester, and that he may have become one of the first chancellors of the University of Cambridge.[85] But of his contribution to the early development of a literature of pastoral care there can be no doubt. His *summa* brought order and discipline to William de Montibus's teachings, and, like Chobham's *summa*, helped to establish a canon of instruction for those engaged in the *cura animarum*.

Richard acknowledges his debt to William de Montibus in the first chapter of the *Qui bene presunt*. "The aforesaid topics," Richard explains, "can be elucidated by means of scriptural authorities and the doctrines of <modern> teachers, and especially the sayings (*dicta*) of Master William de Montibus, the former chancellor of Lincoln Cathedral."[86] Scarcely a page of Richard's text fails to witness to one or another of William's teachings. He refers readers explicitly to William's *Numerale* and *Distinctiones*, he attributes to William many of the didactic verses that are found throughout the *summa*, and he uses the simple appellative "magister" to introduce William's teachings.[87] The entire eleventh section of the *Qui bene presunt* (see below) is

[83] See above, note 47.

[84] On Richard see A.B. Emden, *A Biographical Register of the University of Cambridge to 1500* (Cambridge: Cambridge University Press, 1963), p. 367 ("Leycestria alias Wetheringsette"), p. 632 ("Wetherset"), p. 679 ("Leycestria ... Richard de"); Wenzel, "Vices, Virtues, and Popular Preaching," pp. 28-54; Kemmler, *"Exempla" in Context*, passim; d'Avray, *Preaching of the Friars*, pp. 82-86.

[85] See above, Chapter Two, note 66.

[86] "Et ad manifestationem singulorum predictorum per ordinem possunt auctoritates induci scripturarum, et sententie magistrorum, et specialiter dicta magistri Willelmi de montibus quondam Lincoln' cancellar'"; London, British Library MS Royal 9.A.xiv, fol. 18vb.

[87] "Hos articulos <fidei> et eorum auctoritates et similitudines quibus facilius possunt mentibus rudibus persuaderi predictus magister Willelmus de montibus in fine libelli sui quem Numerale appellauit sic composuit," ibid., fol. 19vb. "Et est inuenire auctoritates premisse similitudinis et de effectu peccati in Distinctionibus cancellarii Lincolniensis," ibid., fol. 108vb. "Hic ponit magister [i.e. William de Montibus] exempla de deitate et humanitate Christi: est Deitas in carne sicut lux in sole ... "; ibid., fol. 20vb.

inspired by William's *Errorum eliminatio*. Most of Richard's borrowings from his master, however, are unacknowledged. He combed William's writings and collected from his diverse teachings those doctrines, similitudes, authorities, poems, and expositions that are relevant to the life and duties of a priest charged with the care of souls. These Richard reassembled, along with his own materials and those of other people, into a unique pastoral *summa* without precedent in the earlier literature.

The *Qui bene presunt* begins with a scriptural similitude comparing the priest and the elder. "'Priests who rule well are considered worthy of a twofold honour' [1 Tim 5:17]: especially those whose labour is in word and doctrine. For *presbyter* in Greek means *senex* in Latin, and the two things that pertain to an old person by nature, namely continence and wisdom, pertain by grace to the priest."[88] "Through wisdom the priest should teach the ignorant by his words, and through continence he should impart morals by his example."[89] "Incontinent priests are like the elders who lusted after Susannah in the book of Daniel [Dan 13:1-64]. Those who lack wisdom are like the sons of Eli, knowing neither God nor their priestly duties, they ministered to the people [1 Sam 2:12-13]; the many unskilled priests of today are like these."[90]

Richard continues his exposition of the priestly office and of the twofold honour due to it, and then draws attention to the gloss that he appended to the text of 1 Timothy: "especially those whose labour is in word and doctrine." This he expounds: "In word, that is in exhorting the learned; in doctrine, that is in instructing those who are not. In word with respect to morals, and in doctrine with respect to faith (for the word 'doctrina' implies the nature or 'dogma' of the 'Trinity,' and thus pertains to the faith). The goal (*summa*) is that those who are themselves instructed should instruct the people in faith and morals, for the substance (*summa*) of the christian religion is in faith and morals."[91]

[88] "Qui bene presunt presbiteri duplici honore habeantur, maxime qui laborant in uerbo et doctrina. Presbiter uero Grece senex dicitur Latine, et debent presbitero duo conuenire per gratiam que senibus conueniunt per naturam, scilicet continentia et sapientia," ibid., fol. 18ra.

[89] "Ut <presbiter> per sapientiam instruat uerbo nescientes, per continentiam exemplo informet ad mores," ibid.

[90] "In continentia defecerunt presbiteri qui exarserunt in Susannam, ut legitur in ultimis Danielis, unde eis assimulantur omnes incontinentes. In sapientia defecerunt filii Ely, filii Belial, nescientes Dominum neque officium sacerdotum ad populum ministrabant quibus hodie multi assimulantur imperiti," ibid.

[91] "Et notandum est quod sequitur: 'maxime qui laborant in uerbo et doctrina';

Richard concludes his preface with a list of those things that are most pertinent to instruction in faith and morals, and which the priest should frequently preach to his people. This list is a detailed table of contents for the *Summa Qui bene presunt*, and amounts to a kind of syllabus for pastoral education:

The things that belong most especially to faith and morals and must be preached very frequently are:

[1] The creed of faith. It contains twelve articles, as is explained below.

[2] The Lord's Prayer, which has seven petitions.

[3] The general and particular gifts of God; the latter are the seven gifts of the Holy Spirit as enumerated in Isaiah 11: Wisdom, Understanding, Counsel, Fortitude, Knowledge, Piety, and Fear.

[4] The four cardinal virtues, which are Justice, Prudence, Fortitude, and Temperance.

[5] The three theological virtues, those conferred by grace, which are Faith, Hope, and Charity.

[6] One should preach especially about the seven deadly vices, which are Pride, Anger, Envy, Avarice, Sloth, Gluttony, and Lust.

[7] So too should one make known the seven sacraments, which are Baptism, Confirmation, Eucharist, Penance, Holy Orders, Marriage, and Extreme Unction.

[8] Also, the two commandments of love, namely loving God and one's neighbour.

[9] The ten moral teachings of the law which are God's Commandments, namely, on worshipping one God, on not taking God's name in vain, on observing the Sabbath (i.e. feast days), on honouring one's parents, not killing, not committing adultery, not stealing, not bearing false witness, not coveting your neighbour's wife or maidservant, or anything of his.

[10] The rewards in body and soul of the just in heaven, and the punishments in body and soul of the evil in hell.

[11] Also the priest should teach his flock about those things in which many are misled.

[12] And about what they should avoid (*uitare debeant*), namely sin and tacit assent to sin, and those things forbidden <by God or> by their superiors; and what they should do (*agere debeant*), namely what pertains to the office or status of each individual, and especially those things that are commanded by God or by their superiors.

---

in uerbo idest in exhortatione scientium, in doctrina idest in instructione nescientium; in uerbo quoad mores, in doctrina quoad fidem (dicitur enim doctrina quasi Trinitatis forma uel dogma, quod ad fidem pertinet). Et est summa ut ipsi instructi populum instruant in fide et moribus. In fide enim et moribus consistit summa Christiane religionis," ibid., fol. 18va.

These things can be remembered by means of the following verses:

> Hec sunt precipue sermonibus insinuanda,
> Bis sex articuli fidei septemque petenda,
> Virtutes, uitia, presertim crimina septem,
> Septem sacra, duo Domini mandata decemque [precepta]
> Legis, iustorum merces peneque malorum,
> In quibus erratur, quid uitandum, quid agendum.[92]

Richard's *summa* achieved immediate popularity, and remained useful for several centuries. As late as the fifteenth century students were keeping an eye out to buy it in the Oxford book market.[93] But irrespective of its actual use and influence, the *Summa Qui bene presunt* marks an important stage in the development of the literature of pastoral care. Richard no more created this literature than did his master, William de Montibus, or the Parisian masters and their students. But he wrote what can be seen in retrospect as one of the first true pastoral *summae*. Drawing on the various pedagogical experiments current in the late-twelfth- and early-thirteenth-century schools, Richard created a coherent *summa* that identified clearly the

---

[92] "Maxime uero ad fidem et mores pertinentia predicanda sunt frequentius: Simbolum fidei duodecim continet articulos sicut inferius dicetur in hac summa Qui bene presunt. Item oratio dominica; septem habet petitiones. Dona Dei generalia et specialia; specialia sunt septem dona Spiritus sancti que enumerat Ys. xi, que sunt sapientia, intellectus, consilium, fortitudo, scientia, pietas et timor. Item uirtutes cardinales sunt quatuor, que sunt iustitia, prudentia, fortitudo, temperantia. Item tres sunt uirtutes gratuite uel theologice, que sunt fides, spes, caritas. Item predicanda sunt precipue septem mortalia uitia, que sunt superbia, ira, inuidia, auaritia, accidia, gula, luxuria. Item innotescenda sunt septem sacramenta, que sunt baptismus, confirmatio, eucharistia, penitentia, ordo, coniugium, extrema unctio. Item predicanda sunt duo mandata caritatis, scilicet de diligendo Deo et proximo. Item predicanda sunt decem moralia legis que sunt mandata Dei scilicet de uno Deo colendo, nomen Dei non in uanum assumendo, de sabbatis idest festis obseruandis, de parentibus honorandis, non occidendo, non mechando, non furtum faciendo, non falsum testimonium perhibendo, non concupiscendo uxorem proximi tui, uel ancillam, uel aliquam rem proximi. Item predicandum est que sit merces iustorum in celo tam in corpore quam in anima, et que sit pena malorum tam in corpore quam in anima in inferno. Item instruendi sunt subditi in quibus a multis erratur, quid uitare debeant scilicet peccatum et consensum peccati et quod a superioribus est prohibitum. Item quid agere debeant scilicet quod pertinet ad officium uniuscuiusque uel statum, et maxime quod a Deo uel a superioribus est preceptum. Et possunt premissa sic retineri per hos uersus sequentes: Hec sunt precipue sermonibus insinuanda ... "; ibid., fol. 18va-vb.

[93] See the note on fol. iiiᵛ of MS 328/715 in Gonville and Caius College Library, Cambridge: "Fiat scrutamen in foro nuncupato Jaudewyn market de libris subscriptis si poterint ibi venales reperiri, videlicet: Qui bene presunt; Legenda sanctorum; Speculum ecclesie; Abstinentia [i.e. John Balbi's *Catholicon*?]; Gemma sacerdotalis." Cf. Montague Rhodes James, *A Descriptive Catalogue of the Manuscripts in the Library of Gonville and Caius College*, 2 vols. (Cambridge: Cambridge University Press, 1907), 1: 371.

audience for *pastoralia*. He used the pedagogical techniques of William de Montibus to write a work that was accessible and useful to that audience. And he expressed clearly and succinctly the growing consensus of his contemporaries about the proper content of instruction for those engaged in the pastoral care of souls.

The audience to which Richard directed this *summa* was neither monastic nor scholastic, but one that cut across both of these traditional categories. He wrote the *Qui bene presunt* for priests (actual and potential) who wished to learn about the *cura animarum*. In the penultimate paragraph of the work Richard addresses this audience directly. It comprises both those who teach the "art of arts" (*magistri*) and those who exercise this art in fulfilling the sacerdotal office (*presbiteri*): "so you <are> teachers and priests, on whom depends the soul of the people (Iudith 8:21). Now, 'the priests who rule well are worthy of (or are considered worthy of) a twofold honour.' ... Do your work, then, so that you might receive that reward."[94]

The techniques of popularization favoured by Richard are those of his master, William de Montibus. He weaves together distinctions, similitudes, *exempla*, and mnemonic verses. Writing a clear and simple Latin prose, he glosses obscure words or expressions and sometimes offers an equivalent in the vernacular (usually English, occasionally Anglo-Norman).

The contents of his *summa* express neatly and succinctly the consensus about the proper content of pastoral education. The twelve topics encompassed here became, in one form or another, the basis for instruction of parish priests from the thirteenth century to the end of the Middle Ages. Wetheringsett's programme for training priests by teaching them about those things that they should preach frequently in their parishes struck a particularly sympathetic chord among English readers.[95]

Alexander of Stavensby, the first teacher of St. Dominic's friars, in Toulouse, added to his synodal statutes for the diocese of Coventry

---

[94] "Igitur uos magistri et presbiteri, ex quibus pendet anima populi, ut legitur Iudith viii [8:21]. Nam qui bene presunt presbiteri dupplici honore digni sunt (uel digni habeantur), ut premissum est in principio huius summe. Operemini igitur sic opus ut uobis reddatur merces, quia 'labores manuum tuarum manducabis' etc. [Ps 127:2]. Hiis igitur circa ministerium sacerdotum tractatis, finem libet facere sermonis. Et si quidem bene ut honori Dei competit, hoc et ipse uelim. Si quid autem residuum fuerit, filiis Aaron relinquimus; faciendi quidem libros nullus est finis. Hic erit ergo consummatio uel consummatus," BL MS Royal 9.A.xiv, fol. 112rb-va.

[95] See Wenzel, "Vices, Virtues, and Popular Preaching," pp. 28-31; and d'Avray, *Preaching of the Friars*, pp. 82-90.

and Lichfield (1224 x 1237) two pastoral treatises, one on confession and one on the seven deadly sins. He begins the latter with the injunction: "Let all parishioners on all Sundays or other feasts be told by their priests: 'There are seven criminal sins which you must flee ... .'"[96]

Robert Grosseteste, bishop of Lincoln from 1235 to 1253, began his own synodal statutes thus: "Since there is no salvation of souls without keeping the Commandments, we exhort in the Lord and firmly enjoin that each shepherd of souls and each parish priest know the Decalogue, that is, the Ten Commandments of the Mosaic Law, and preach and expound them frequently to the people in his care. Let him also know which are the seven criminal sins and preach them likewise to the people as something to be fled. Let him, moreover, know the seven sacraments of the Church, at least in a simplified way; and let those who are priests know especially what is necessary for the true sacrament of confession and penance, and teach the laity frequently the form of baptizing in the common tongue. Let in addition each of them have understanding of the faith, at least in a simplified form, as it is contained in the Creed, the major as well as the minor, and in the form beginning 'Quicumque vult,' which is daily recited in the Church at Prime."[97]

Walter of Cantilupe, bishop of Worcester from 1236/7 to 1266, composed a pastoral treatise beginning *Omnis etas hominum*, apparently to supplement his own synodal statutes of 1240.[98] The tract begins with a discussion of the Ten Commandments, the seven deadly sins, and other matters pertaining to confession and penance. It concludes with a chapter on the articles of faith, and an injunction that "the priest should teach the layperson to believe and know the Creed, at least in his mother-tongue, and know the *Pater noster*, and the *Ave Maria*."[99]

Roger Weseham, Grosseteste's successor as lector to the Oxford Franciscans, dean of Lincoln Cathedral, and bishop of Coventry and

---

[96] *Councils & Synods*, 1: 214.

[97] Ibid., 1: 268.

[98] See Boyle, "William of Pagula," 2: no. A.17; Cheney, *English Synodalia*, pp. 42-43; the manuscripts are listed in Bloomfield, *Incipits*, no. 3663. Except for the introduction and conclusion, this treatise is identical with the *Summula* of Peter Quinel or Quivel, bishop of Exeter 1280-1291, edited by Powicke and Cheney in *Councils & Synods*, 2: 1059-1077. Peter seems to have borrowed his predecessor's work entire, substituting only a new prologue and conclusion (pp. 1060-1062, 1077). A study of the *Omnis etas* is in preparation.

[99] *Councils & Synods*, 2: 1076.

Lichfield (1245-1256), composed a treatise for the clergy of his diocese that includes many of the topics set out in the *Qui bene presunt*.[100] He introduces the reader to the seven sacraments, the seven gifts of the Holy Spirit, the seven virtues, the seven petitions of the Lord's Prayer, the eight beatitudes, the Ten Commandments, and the seven deadly sins. He continues: "We wish also that the faith and its articles be mentioned often in the churches and sometimes preached simply and without discussion, instructing rather by examples than by subtle reasonings or questionings or discussions." The twelve articles of faith are then expounded in just such a way. Roger concludes with a brief discussion of the things that are to be avoided.

The most influential injunction of this type in England was that promulgated by the archbishop of Canterbury, John Pecham, in 1281. The ninth canon of his provincial constitutions, beginning with the words *Ignorantia sacerdotum*, requires: "that each priest who has the cure of souls, four times a year, that is during each quarter of the year, on one or several feast days, himself or through a substitute, must expound to his people in their vernacular language, without any subtle and fanciful embellishment: the fourteen articles of faith, the ten commandments of the Decalogue, the two precepts of the gospel, that is, the twin commandments of love, further the seven works of mercy, the seven capital sins with their offspring, the seven chief virtues, and the seven sacraments of grace."[101]

The striking element of these decrees is their provision for simple "catechetical" preaching by the parish priest. The particular lists of *predicanda*, if not the requirement of such preaching in the parishes, is new in the thirteenth century. By the seventeenth century such elementary pastoral preaching had become a commonplace part of the homiletic tradition, at least in France.[102] If it was so in the thirteenth century, little written evidence of it has survived. But the absence of actual thirteenth-century sermons on these matters in the surviving manuscripts tells little against the growing consensus, witnessed in numerous pastoral handbooks and *summae*, that priests should and could be taught both the art of simple preaching and the simple content to be conveyed thereby.[103]

---

[100] The text is printed by Cheney, *English Synodalia*, pp. 149-152, from MS Bodley 57 of the Bodleian Library Oxford. Another copy is in Lambeth Palace MS 499, fols. 72v-73r.

[101] *Councils & Synods*, 2: 900-905.

[102] See d'Avray, *Preaching of the Friars*, p. 82 and n. 1.

[103] See ibid., pp. 82-90.

Thomas Chobham and Richard of Wetheringsett in their pastoral *summae* gave tangible form to the vague provisions of the Fourth Lateran Council, provisions that were, themselves, but reflections of a widely felt and inchoate desire to apply the fruits of contemporary scholarship to the pastoral care of souls. The Council had called for the training of special adjutants to the bishop who could help him in preaching and in administering penance. It had also admonished bishops to instruct all candidates for the priesthood in the proper administration of the sacraments and celebration of the rites of the Church. Chobham, basing his *summa* on the teachings of Peter the Chanter and his school, suggested a way to accomplish the Council's goals by focusing on the sacrament of penance. Wetheringsett chose the preacher's art as his subject and, drawing especially on the teachings of William de Montibus, invented another way to achieve the desired end of educating preachers, confessors, and candidates for the priesthood.

These two *summae* were the vanguard of a vast literature of pastoral care that appeared in the thirteenth and subsequent centuries.[104] Some works, like Robert Grosseteste's very popular *Templum Dei*, followed Chobham in using penance as the organizing principle for pastoral education. Others related their diverse materials to the preaching office.[105] Some authors invented new and unusual frameworks for their treatises, but in doing so they strayed very little from the consensus about the content of *pastoralia* established early in the thirteenth century.

Perhaps the most ambitious pastoral *summa* of the thirteenth century was the anonymous *Speculum iuniorum*, written in England c. 1250, perhaps by a Dominican friar.[106] Writing for "juniors," i.e. young clerics, he organized his work around the topics Evil (Book One), and Good (Book Two).[107] In Book One the author discusses sin and

---

[104] The best survey of pastoral writings in England during the 13th and 14th centuries is still Leonard E. Boyle's unpublished dissertation, "William of Pagula"; see also Boyle's annotated schema of *pastoralia* in "Manuals of Popular Theology," pp. 30-43. No comparable research has been undertaken concerning works produced on the Continent. Some idea of the vast numbers of pastoral texts produced in these centuries can be gleaned from Bloomfield, *Incipits*.

[105] See, for example, Roger Weseham's treatise, above, at note 100.

[106] See Leonard E. Boyle, "Three English Pastoral Summae and a 'Magister Galienus,'" *Studia Gratiana* 11 (1967), pp. 135-144; Joseph Goering, "The Popularization of Scholastic Ideas in Thirteenth-Century England and an Anonymous *Speculum iuniorum*" (PhD diss.: University of Toronto, 1977).

[107] Three further books were apparently planned, one treating the virtues, the gifts of the Holy Spirit, and the beatitudes; one on the soul and its powers; and one on

punishment. In Book Two he describes the goods of nature and grace, and then treats each of the Church's seven sacraments. In each section of the *Speculum* the author begins with the teachings of the scholastic masters. He quotes long passages from Alexander of Hales, Philip the Chancellor, William of Auxerre, Albert the Great, Robert Grosseteste, and the English Dominican masters Robert Bacon and Richard Fishacre. He then proceeds to draw on the pastoral writers. Quoting extensively from Chobham and Wetheringsett, as well as from Raymund of Peñafort's *Summa de penitentia*, Peraldus's *Summa vitiorum* and *Summa virtutum*, and Grosseteste's *Templum*, he produces a striking tapestry of practical, pastoral instruction. Although idiosyncratic in his approach, the author of the *Speculum iuniorum* shared with the other pastoral writers an implicit consensus about the proper content of education concerning "those things that are known to pertain to the care of souls."

William of Pagula

In many ways the culmination of these thirteenth-century experiments in defining the content of *pastoralia* is found in the still unedited *summae* of William of Pagula.[108] William was born in the Yorkshire village of Poul (Pagula). In 1314 he was appointed perpetual vicar of the parish church at Winkfield, near Windsor Forest. He was a master of arts and a deacon upon his appointment, and was ordained to the priesthood just over a year later, in June of 1315. He then went to Oxford, where he studied canon law for six or seven years. After completing his Oxford regency, William returned to residence in his parish church. In 1321 he was given added duties by the bishop of Salisbury, who appointed him *penitentiarius* for the deanery of Reading, and later for the entire archdeaconry of Berkshire. "Penitentiaries" are episcopal officials charged with overseeing penitential

---

the angels and God. These seem never to have been written; see Goering, "*Speculum iuniorum*," pp. 203-205.

[108] See William A. Pantin, *The English Church in the Fourteenth Century* (Cambridge: Cambridge University Press, 1955), pp. 189-218. The following summary is derived from several of Leonard Boyle's publications, especially, "The *Oculus sacerdotis* and Some Other Works of William of Pagula," *Transactions of the Royal Historical Society*, 5th series, 5 (1955) 81-110; "The '*Summa summarum*' and Some Other English Works of Canon Law," in *Proceedings of the Second International Congress of Medieval Canon Law*, ed. Stephan Kuttner and J.J. Ryan (Vatican City: Biblioteca Apostolica Vaticana, 1965), pp. 415-456; "Constitution '*Cum ex eo*,'" and "Aspects of Clerical Education". All are reprinted in his *Pastoral Care*.

discipline in the local parishes. William took the job seriously and even produced a handbook on the subject for parish priests, other penitentiaries, and bishops.[109]

William of Pagula composed four major works during the years 1319 to 1332. Most ambitious was his *Speculum praelatorum*,[110] a vast compilation in three books that combined devotional, pastoral, and homiletic materials of William's own invention with extracts from such influential continental *summae* as Hugh of Strassburg's *Summa theologicae veritatis*, John of Freiburg's *Summa confessorum*, and James of Milan's *Stimulus amoris*. Although it survives in a single manuscript copy, it was perhaps William's most important and most characteristic work. It reveals "a rigorous attention to detail, a remarkable ability to manipulate the sources of canon law, a strong sense of the place of the legislation of the Church in England, and that balance of law and theology which is due to Pagula's discerning use of the *Summa confessorum* of John of Freiburg."[111] Books One and Two of this *Speculum* cover much the same material as William's *Oculus sacerdotis* and *Summa summarum*. Book Three, however, is unique. It treats the preaching duties of priests, and is one of the finest summaries of the homiletic art to be produced in medieval England. For each Sunday and for almost every other liturgical occasion Pagula gives three or four sermon outlines, following these with as many as seven or eight sermon *themata*. He then adds an extensive dictionary of patristic quotations (complete with cross-references to Book Two of the *Speculum*) that could be used by preachers to elaborate the *themata* and fill out the outlines *ad libitum*. This remarkable treatise deserves further study.

A shorter and more accessible work, the *Speculum religiosorum*, was derived from the *Speculum praelatorum*.[112] This "Mirror" for non-mendicant religious is an important compendium of law, theology, and ecclesiastical legislation as these pertained to the care of souls in monasteries. The pastoral instruction of monks has been largely neglected in modern scholarship. William of Pagula's treatise, like William de Montibus's *De penitentia religiosorum*, reminds us of the

[109] See remarks on the *Pars oculi*, below.

[110] See Boyle, "*Oculus sacerdotis*," pp. 102-103; "*Summa summarum*," pp. 432-434.

[111] Boyle, "*Summa summarum*," pp. 433-434; cf. L.E. Boyle, "The *Summa confessorum* of John of Freiburg and the Popularization of the Moral Teaching of St. Thomas and Some of his Contemporaries," in *St. Thomas Aquinas, 1274-1974*, 2: 245-268; rpt. in *Pastoral Care*.

[112] See Boyle, "*Oculus sacerdotis*," p. 102; "*Summa summarum*," pp. 434-438.

importance of such instruction. It would serve as an excellent starting point for further investigations.

More popular still was Pagula's *Summa summarum*.[113] Its subtitle, *Repertorium iuris canonici*, might give a misleading impression of this fascinating amalgam of theology, canon law, ecclesiastical legislation, and local discipline. William composed this *summa* while he was studying and teaching law at Oxford, but it is anything but a scholastic summary of canon law. He tells us that he wrote the work, not for legal scholars and students, but for the unlearned and those wholly ignorant of canon law, and especially "for prelates and priests, since their ignorance of canon law is especially dangerous."[114] It is, in other words, a detailed, comprehensive, and extremely useful reference work for those involved in the *cura animarum*.

But far-and-away the most popular and most influential work produced by William of Pagula was his *Oculus sacerdotis*. The *Oculus* is divided into three parts, each representing an aspect of pastoral education adumbrated in the Fourth Lateran Council of 1215. The *Dextera Pars* (or Right Eye) concerns those things that the priest should preach and expound regularly to the people. These include such practical matters as the proper forms of baptism in case of necessity, the importance of annual confession and of the Mass, the meaning of confirmation, details concerning the sacrament of marriage and the collection of tithes, and warnings about subtle forms of usury. General parochial misbehaviour, especially such as might be serious enough to result in excommunication, receives particular attention. This discussion is followed by an elaboration of Archbishop Pecham's *Ignorantia sacerdotum*, which, as noted earlier, obliged parish priests to instruct the laity in the fourteen articles of faith, the seven sacraments, the Ten Commandments, the seven deadly sins, the seven works of mercy, and the seven virtues.[115]

The *Sinistra Pars* (or Left Eye) provides instruction necessary for the correct administration of the Church's rites and sacraments. Pagula teaches what the priest needs to know about each of the Church's seven sacraments, and includes, for example, a chapter in which each of the ritual actions of the Mass is examined and explained. Excerpts from this and other chapters found their way into the missals, *rituales*,

---

[113] Boyle, "*Summa summarum*," pp. 415-456.
[114] Ibid., p. 442.
[115] Boyle, "*Oculus sacerdotis*," pp. 88-90.

and *manuales* (liturgical handbooks for the parish priest) of the later medieval Church.[116]

These two parts of the *Oculus* were written between 1319 and 1322, while Pagula was finishing his Oxford course and exercising the care of souls in Winkfield parish. Some five years later (1327-1328), after considerable experience as pastor and as penitentiary for the bishop, he added another book to his *Oculus*. He entitled it the *Pars Oculi* (or A Part of the Eye). This book completes the priest's "eye" by instructing him in the art of hearing confessions and assigning penances.[117]

William of Pagula's *Oculus sacerdotis* became a classic text of the pastoral care during the fourteenth and fifteenth centuries. It survives in more than fifty manuscript copies. Within a decade of its publication an anonymous author had added an eyelid (*Cilium oculi*) to Pagula's "eye." John de Burgh, the chancellor of Cambridge University, synthesized William's teachings in his own, very popular, *Pupilla oculi* (1384). Countless other writers of both Latin and vernacular treatises borrowed, directly or indirectly, from William's *Oculus*.[118]

For us, it expresses clearly a mature consensus about the proper content of pastoral education. A century earlier the Fourth Lateran Council had suggested, vaguely, that promising students be trained in the art of preaching and hearing confessions, and that all priests be instructed in the proper performance of the Church's rites. With the benefit of one-hundred years of experience and experiments behind him, William of Pagula was able to specify the content of such instruction, and to make it accessible in written form to all priests charged with the *cura animarum*.

CONCLUSIONS

What can we say, then, about William de Montibus's rôle in the creation of a practical literature of pastoral care? It is surely doing William no injustice to say that he and his contemporaries could scarcely have imagined the tremendous vitality of such a popular literature in the later Middle Ages. William wrote for a select audience of monks and clerics who wished to become learned theologians and pastors. He made no particular attempt to address the "simple" priest

[116] Ibid., pp. 91-92.
[117] Ibid., pp. 85-87.
[118] Ibid., pp. 94-96.

or the wider audience of young students who were thronging to the schools in search of a liberal education. His pedagogical techniques were those of the twelfth-century schools. He required of his students a thorough grounding in the classical and ecclesiastical authors. He expected them to read and write Latin fluently, and to apply the techniques of the grammarian, rhetorician, dialectician, and exegete to the interpretation of sacred scriptures. The content of his teaching was the academic discipline of theology, not the practical art of pastoral care. The learned theologian should, of course, be able (and willing) to preach, to hear confessions, and to administer the Church's sacraments and rites correctly; but he would learn these skills, not for their own sake, but as part of his general education in the scholastic discipline of theology.

The next step in creating a popular literature of pastoral care was taken by the generation of students trained by William de Montibus, Peter the Chanter, and other teachers of the "inter-conciliar period" (1179 to 1215). Although individual works on preaching, confession, practical law, and theology were composed before 1215,[119] the concerted and conscious effort to address a nonprofessional audience, to write practical works that were accessible to the casual reader, and to distinguish clearly the proper content of pastoral instruction from the broader training in a scholastic discipline, came into its own in the years after the Fourth Lateran Council.

William de Montibus stands at the beginning of this movement, not as its originator, but as theologian and teacher who prepared the ground for its growth. A consideration of his writings, edited and described below, will reveal the reasons for his high esteem among contemporaries, and illustrate the wealth of materials that he made available to subsequent teachers of the practical art of pastoral care.

[119] See Boyle, "Inter-conciliar Period."

Part Two

The Writings of William de Montibus

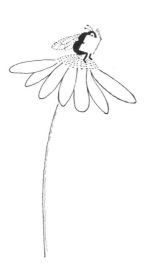

Introduction

Only one of William de Montibus's writings, the brief *Peniteas cito peccator*, has appeared previously in print. Other works have been noted on occasion, but the complex manuscript traditions of the texts, and the unfamiliar literary genres in which William wrote, have helped prevent a proper understanding of his oeuvre. The following catalogue of William's writings, based on an examination of nearly all of the known manuscript copies, describes the content of each work and the context in which it was composed and in which it circulated.

The groundwork for this study was laid in Father Hugh MacKinnon's Oxford D.Phil dissertation (1959), "The Life and Works of William de Montibus," written under the supervision of Richard Hunt. Other scholars have made important contributions to recovering William's authentic writings and identifying the manuscripts containing them.[1] Further discoveries will, no doubt, be made, but this catalogue represents the state of our current knowledge. It includes a discussion of the contents and historical context, authenticity and date, sources, and manuscripts of the following fifteen works and 149 sermons attributed to William de Montibus. Six of the works (nos. 1-6) are printed in their entirety from selected manuscript witnesses. The others are represented by extensive transcriptions that seek to convey an accurate and substantial guide to the materials found therein.

1. *Peniteas cito peccator* (a collection of glossed didactic verses on penance and confession)
2. *Errorum eliminatio* (a treatise on common "errors" in the liturgy and on various malpractices and superstitions in the churches)

---

[1] Especially Leonard E. Boyle in his D.Phil dissertation (1956), "A Study of the Works Attributed to William of Pagula with Special Reference to the *Oculus sacerdotis* and *Summa summarum*." Boyle drew attention to the *De septem sacramentis* (below, no. 13), which MacKinnon left out of his study. Boyle also attributes to William de Montibus a *summa*, beginning: "Scire debent sacerdotes quod non habent potestatem absolvendi penitentes ab enormibus peccatis nisi in articulo necessitatis." This *summa* is, in fact, an excerpt from the *Summa Qui bene presunt* written by William's student, Richard of Wetheringsett.

3. *Tractatus metricus de septem sacramentis ecclesie* (a collection of verses on the sacraments and on other "catechetical" themes)

4. *Speculum penitentis* (a penitential treatise for theologians and confessors)

5. *De penitentia religiosorum* (a guide for the administration of penance in monasteries)

6. *Epistola ad moniales* (pastoral letter[s] to nuns of the Gilbertine Order at Sempringham)

7. *Numerale* (an introductory *summa* of theology)

8. *Distinctiones theologice* (an alphabetical source book of theological doctrine)

9. *Similitudinarium* (an alphabetical source book of similes and *exempla* for the theologian)

10. *Prouerbia* (an alphabetical source book of proverbs and other edifying sayings)

11. *Tropi* (an hermeneutical *summa* for the theologian)

12. *Versarius* (an alphabetical compendium of didactic verse, with glosses)

13. *De septem sacramentis* (a treatise, in question form, on the sacraments)

14. *Super Psalmos* (a student *reportatio* of lectures on the Psalms)

15. *Collecta* (a student *reportatio* of didactic verses and their exposition in William's school)

16. *Sermones* (four collections of sermons, for diverse audiences and occasions)

Each work is discussed according to a common format. Introductory comments give a brief description of the work and a sketch of its historical and literary context. These are followed by a section entitled AUTHENTICITY AND DATE, in which arguments for William de Montibus's authorship of each work are presented, along with a discussion of the date of composition. Although the writings can seldom be dated precisely, the following chronological arrangement represents the tentative conclusions achieved in the individual studies below.

> *De septem sacramentis* (before 1186?)
> *De penitentia religiosorum*
> *Errorum eliminatio* (before 1200?)
> *Distinctiones theologice*
> *Prouerbia*
> *Similitudinarium*
> *Tropi* (cites the *Distinctiones*; after 1200?)

Numerale (cites the *Distinctiones*)

Epistola ad moniales (after 1202)

Super Psalmos

Collecta

Sancti estote (printed below as a part of the *Speculum penitentis*; written before that work.)

Speculum penitentis (cites the *Numerale*)

Tractatus metricus de septem sacramentis ecclesie (before the *Peniteas cito*?)

Peniteas cito peccator (before the *Versarius*?)

Versarius (cites the *Distinctiones*, the *Similitudinarium*, the *Speculum penitentis*, and the *Errorum eliminatio*; after 1208?)

Sermons (preached at various dates from the 1190's, or before, until the end of William's life)

The section on SOURCES notes both explicit sources (those authorities cited by William) and implicit sources (those from which he seems to have drawn his materials without acknowledgement). Finally, under MANUSCRIPTS, all of the known manuscript copies of each work are listed and, where possible, described. The dates assigned are for the writing of each individual work in the manuscript. In most cases dates are based on paleographical evidence alone, and make no pretence to precise accuracy; a work described as "early 13th century" might, in fact, have been written in the late twelfth century, etc. One peculiarity of English scribal practice (most of the manuscripts were written in England) helps to specify the date of writing somewhat. Before the middle of the thirteenth century, English scribes were in the habit of writing above the top line of ruling on each page; after c. 1250 they began to write below the top line.[2] The phrase "above top line" in the manuscript descriptions draws attention to this peculiarity of the English manuscripts.

The Title (if given in the manuscript), the Incipit and Explicit of the text, and the Colophon (if any) are noted. Round brackets ( ) enclosing Latin words in this section indicate that the words are written in red ink. Peculiarities of the codex or of the manuscript copy are noted in a separate paragraph.[3]

---

[2] Neil R. Ker, "From 'Above Top Line' to 'Below Top Line': A Change in Scribal Practice," *Celtica* 5 (1960) 13-16.

[3] Modern catalogue descriptions of the manuscripts are cited only in exceptional instances. References to catalogues printed before 1960 can be found in Paul Oskar Kristeller, *Latin Manuscript Books Before 1600: A List of the Printed Catalogues and Unpublished Inventories of Extant Collections*, 3rd ed. (New York: Fordham

This introductory material is followed by either an edition of the text (nos. 1-6) or by a transcription of selected parts (nos. 7-16). Unless otherwise noted, the orthography of the base manuscript is retained in the printed text, except that assibilated ci/ti is printed as "ti," and u/v is printed as "u" in lowercase and "V" in uppercase. Punctuation, capitalization, and paragraph divisions conform to modern practice. Rubrics in the manuscripts are indicated by small capitals in the transcriptions.

Three appendices complete Part Two of this study. The first provides a geographical listing of all of the manuscripts containing William's writings. The second lists alphabetically the 1,379 first lines of verse found in William's *Versarius*. Appendix Three lists alphabetically the *themata* of William's sermons.

University Press, 1960). See also R.A.B. Mynors, *Catalogue of the Manuscripts of Balliol College Oxford* (Oxford: Clarendon Press, 1963); other recent catalogues are cited in the text and footnotes.

II.1

Peniteas cito peccator

This brief poem, seldom longer than 150 lines in any of its versions, became one of the most popular vehicles for conveying the essentials of penance to medieval European confessors. Its influence can be measured only partially by the large number of extant copies. Well over 150 manuscript copies have been identified. The poem was printed at least fifty-one times between 1485 and 1520, introducing thousands of copies into circulation throughout Europe at the end of the Middle Ages and testifying to its continued popularity and usefulness.[1] More important than the physical remains, however, is the evidence that this poem was one of the mainstays of European primary education. As an introductory text, memorized by students during their formative years in grammar and theological schools, it circulated much more widely, if less tangibly, than the extant copies alone can indicate.[2]

Neither the fame of its author nor the poetic beauty of the text itself can account for its extraordinary popularity. The identity of its author was forgotten by the middle of the thirteenth century. A few copyists ascribed the work to other famous writers, but the majority of copies and all the early printed texts are anonymous. As poetry, the *Peniteas cito* is undistinguished. Barthélmy Hauréau describes it as "un très méchant poème."[3] In fact it is not a poem at all but a collection of discrete units of didactic verse assembled *ad hoc* to form a kind of textbook of penitential doctrine.

---

[1] See T.N. Tentler, *Sin and Confession on the Eve of the Reformation* (Princeton: Princeton University Press, 1977), pp. 47-48, and *passim*.

[2] Br. Bonaventure [John N. Miner], "The Teaching of Latin in Later Medieval England," *Mediaeval Studies* 23 (1961) 1-20; J. de Ghellinck, "Mediaeval Theology in Verse," pp. 336-354; Vansteenkiste, "'Versus' dans les œuvres de Saint Thomas," pp. 77-85; Orme, *English Schools in the Middle Ages*, p. 104.

[3] *Notices et extraits de quelques manuscrits latins de la Bibliothèque Nationale* (Paris, 1891), 2: 65. Elsewhere, however, he comments on its surprising humanity, ibid., 3: 226-227.

The popularity of the *Peniteas cito* arose precisely from its success in conveying, in brief compass and in memorable terms, the essentials of the doctrine of penance as they were understood from the late twelfth century until the end of the Middle Ages. In a few lines of verse the author has summarized the orthodox consensus concerning penance that emerged from the twelfth-century schools. His summary, both balanced and humane, was presented in a form that was easily accessible to generations of students as they began their academic studies. Few penitential texts or *summae confessorum* can be said to have exercised such a widespread and continuous influence throughout the later Middle Ages.

In addition to the early modern printings, the *Peniteas cito* was published twice among the works of Peter of Blois, once in the seventeenth century and again in the nineteenth century. The last edition, with all its faults, was reprinted in Migne's *Patrologiae*, and has formed the basis for most scholarly discussions of the poem.[4] The modern editions treat it as a single poem, suppressing the rubrics that divide the work in most early copies and giving a false impression of its poetic unity. Medieval scribes also took liberties with the topical rubrics, feeling free to add, ignore, and modify them to fit their own conceptions of the work. Nevertheless the rubrics are important for understanding both the genesis and the use of the poem. As we know from William's *Versarius* and from the *dicta* preserved by his students, his didactic poetry consists of brief verse-units, only a few lines long, that served as the basis for a scholastic exposition. A reading of the *Peniteas cito* reveals that it, too, comprises numerous smaller units that are separable in theory and were often separated in fact.[5] The work as it circulated in the schools had a didactic rather than a poetic unity, but this scarcely deterred countless teachers and students from using it as a useful introduction to the doctrine and practice of penance.

---

[4] The seventeenth-century printing is in Pierre de Goussainville's edition of Peter of Blois, *Petri Blesensis ... Opera omnia* (Paris, 1667); the nineteenth-century edition is by J.A. Giles, *Petri Blesensis ... Opera omnia* (London, 1847), 4: 369-373. Giles used MS 36 of Lambeth Palace, London, as a base text, silently emending this on the basis of readings in MS 1968 of the Bibliothèque Royale in Brussels. His edition was reprinted by J.P. Migne, PL 207: 1153-1156, where a number of misprints were introduced into the text.

[5] See Hans Walther, *Initia carminum ac versuum medii aevi posterioris latinorum* (Göttingen: Vandenhoech and Ruprecht, 1959), whose index of first lines includes not only line 1, "Peniteas cito" (no. 13564), but also lines 7, 10, 22, 23, 40, 46, 53, 57, 63, 69, 78, 86, 117, 124, and 136.

Another measure of the usefulness of the *Peniteas cito* is the energy that went into glossing the text. The gloss printed below is the earliest, and was probably composed by William himself. During the subsequent centuries, however, the text was endowed with numerous, often lengthy glosses, each designed to develop the theological, canonical, and/or practical teachings implicit in the verses.[6] More than a dozen distinct commentaries are noted by Bloomfield in medieval manuscripts,[7] and Tentler has drawn attention to the glosses accompanying the early printed editions.[8]

Innumerable guides, handbooks, and penitential *summae* were composed in Latin and in all the vernacular languages during the thirteenth and subsequent centuries, but the *Peniteas cito*, composed at the beginning of this period, continued to serve as a useful introduction to the doctrine and practice of penance well into the sixteenth century. It circulated throughout Europe, and exerted an influence far out of proportion to its unprepossessing appearance.

AUTHENTICITY AND DATE

Manuscript copies ascribe this work to Peter of Blois, John Garland, Thomas Chobham, Robert Grosseteste, St. Bonaventure, Bernard Sylvester, and even Pope Sylvester and St. John Chrysostom,[9] but the majority of copies are anonymous. As recently as 1962, Pierre Michaud-Quantin, in his authoritative survey of penitential *summae*, could claim that none of the suggestions concerning the authorship of the *Peniteas cito* was persuasive.[10] In 1969, however, Hugh Mac-Kinnon argued that "it seems highly likely that William de Montibus himself made the initial compilation of the *Peniteas cito*."[11] MacKinnon drew attention to two early manuscript copies of the poem independently

---

[6] See Pierre Michaud-Quantin, *Sommes de casuistique*, p. 19.

[7] Bloomfield, et al., *Incipits*, nos. 3804-3811, 3813-3821.

[8] *Sin and Confession*, pp. 47-48, and *passim*.

[9] See Hauréau, *Notices et extraits*, 2: 65; *Thomae de Chobham Summa confessorum*, p. 598; Samuel Harrison Thomson, *The Writings of Robert Grosseteste, Bishop of Lincoln, 1235-1253* (New York, 1971), pp. 257-258; Balduinus Distelbrink, *Bonaventurae scripta: Authentica, dubia, vel spuria critice recensita* (Rome: Istituto Storico Cappuccini, 1975), p. 199.

[10] *Sommes de casuistique*, p. 19.

[11] "William de Montibus: A Medieval Teacher," pp. 40-44; his argument was accepted by Richard W. Hunt, "A Manuscript Containing Extracts from the *Distinctiones monasticae*," *Medium aevum* 44 (1975) 241.

ascribing it to William,[12] and also to the inclusion of the entire poem in another of William's writings, his *Versarius*, where the verses are found dispersed under such alphabetical headings as *Confessio, Penitens, Qualis debeat esse prelatus, Que sunt necessaria penitenti*, and *Satisfactio penitentialis*.

Many of the verses and glosses of the *Peniteas cito* are also quoted in an early-thirteenth-century pastoral *summa*, the *Qui bene presunt*, composed by William's student Richard of Wetheringsett (of Leicester).[13] Although Richard mentions William as the principal source of the materials included in his *summa*, he quotes numerous verses, usually without citing any author or source, and only a thorough study or an edition of the *Qui bene presunt* will reveal the full extent to which he has utilized the writings and oral teachings of his master. Occasionally, however, he cites William's teachings explicitly. In the description of a good confession, Richard quotes lines 21 to 38 of the *Peniteas cito* as edited below, and then reports his master's exposition of the first three verses: *modo exponit magister tres primos uersus*.[14] The exposition is apparently a *reportatio* of William's own lectures or *dicta* concerning these verses, and it bears a close resemblance to the formal gloss on the poem.[15]

Further evidence of William's authorship of the *Peniteas cito* is found in the other glosses. Many were drawn from such standard resources of the late-twelfth- and early-thirteenth century theologian as the Bible, Lombard's *Sentences*, and Gratian's *Decretum*. Several of the more idiosyncratic glosses, however, bear close comparison with passages in other works written by William de Montibus. One of these is the

[12] See MSS *C* and *V*, below. A third early manuscript copy ascribing the work to William has been identified in the Huntington Library, San Marino, California, MS HM 19914. This codex was written in England before 1250. The *Peniteas cito* begins on fol. 227r with the rubric: *Penitentiarius magistri Willelmi de montibus*, and ends, incomplete on fol. 228v, in the gloss on *contraria* in line 107 of the poem as edited below: ... *Quod gula peccaverit ieiunium*. A final rubric on fol. 229r comments: *Explicit penitentiarius magistri Willelmi de montibus set incompletus*. Because this copy is incomplete its readings are not reported in the edition below.

[13] Concerning Richard's *summa*, see Chapter Three. Two manuscript copies of this *summa* have been used in preparing the present arguments; they are London, British Library MS Royal 9.A.xiv, fols. 18ra-112va, and San Marino, Huntington Library MS HM 19914, fols. 115ra-158rb.

[14] MS Royal 9.A.xiv, fol. 75ra-b.

[15] Compare the following: "VERA ... ne quis causa humilitatis dicat se fecisse quod non fecit. Vnde Augustinus ... . (S)CITA ... Ne tardes conuerti ad Dominum etc ... . FIRMA ... ne sint treuge set firma pax inter Deum et hominem ... . DISCRETA, id est discrete facta, ut sit sal in omni sacrificio ..."; ibid., fols. 75rb-va, with the glosses to ll. 21-23, a, d, e, and k below.

gloss on the word *discreta* in line 23. The manuscripts of the *Peniteas cito* preserve only the terse quotation from Leviticus, "Sal in omni sacrificio." In his *Numerale*, however, William elaborates: "... Et reddam Tibi uota mea que distinxerunt labia mea, id est discrete protulerunt, ut sit sal in sacrificio."[16] William seems to have been fond of applying this scriptural phrase to the notion of "discretion." He adduces it elsewhere in the *Numerale*,[17] and his student, Richard of Wetheringsett, noted it in his *Qui bene presunt* as one of his master's sayings.[18]

The gloss on *preces*, in line 61 of the *Peniteas cito*, also reflects something of William's own teachings. It consists of a quotation from "Gregory" describing how the souls of the dead, who are beyond the help of penance, can be set free by the works of living friends and relatives, through fasting, offerings, prayers, and almsgiving. The quotation was not a commonplace in the twelfth- and thirteenth-century literature, but William cites it explicitly in another of his works, the *Proverbia*: "Gregorius: Anime defunctorum quatuor modis soluuntur, aut oblationibus, aut precibus sanctorum, aut carorum elemosinis, aut ieiunio cognatorum."[19]

A third example, in line 154 of the *Peniteas cito*, is the interpretation of Psalm 103:26, "Draco iste quem formasti ad illudendum ei," as implying the overthrow of the devil through penance (glosses on s and t). The same interpretation is found, in almost the same words, in William's *Numerale*: "Hic est draco formatus ad illudendum ei. Ei autem illuditur cum eius temptationem resistitur, uel labor eius per penitentiam cassatur."[20]

William's role in composing and glossing these verses is fairly certain, but a date of composition is difficult to assign. The gloss, in its present form, can perhaps be dated to the later years of William's career by the parallels with his *Numerale* and *Versarius*. The verses may have been composed earlier, and may also have circulated originally as part of a quite different work such as the *Tractatus metricus* on the seven sacraments.[21]

---

[16] In section 10.3 of the *Numerale* (see below, II.7).

[17] Ibid., sect. II.3: "Ita in opere quinque sunt attendenda, scilicet ... discrecio: sal in sacrificio, et plectrum in cithara ... ."

[18] See above, n. 15.

[19] See below (II.10); the quotation is included under the topical heading *De morte*.

[20] *Numerale*, section 3.16.

[21] See discussion of the manuscripts below.

MacKinnon argued that the verses constituting the *Peniteas cito* were excerpted from William's *Versarius*,[22] but the opposite relationship is equally plausible. The *Versarius* was compiled late in William's career as a kind of alphabetical repository for the verses he used in his classroom teaching. It contains numerous verses and verse-units on confession in addition to those found in the *Peniteas cito*. If we assume that the *Versarius* is the source of the verses that comprise the *Peniteas cito* we must then explain how these particular verses were chosen from the mass of available materials, and how they circulated as a discrete penitential "poem" from at least the early years of the thirteenth century. A consideration of the glosses in both texts suggest that those in the *Versarius* are abbreviated forms of the glosses in the *Peniteas cito*, and some are omitted entirely in the longer work. On balance it seems more likely that the *Peniteas cito* had an independent existence and use in William's classroom, and that its verses were later distributed under appropriate rubrics in his alphabetical *Versarius*.

SOURCES

The verses of the *Peniteas cito* seem to be of William's own composition although some may be free adaptations of earlier verse or prose. The first line, for example, may be thought to paraphrase Publilius Syrus: "Ad paenitendum properat cito iudicat."[23] In at least one instance the verses have been shown to be unprecedented. In his study of the circumstances of human acts, Johannes Gründel demonstrated that the list of *circumstantiae* aggravating sins in lines 53-55, was a new formulation, previously unknown in the scholastic literature.[24]

No sources are adduced in the body of the poem, but the glosses include quotations from the Bible and the Church Fathers (Augustine, Bede, Chrysostom, Gregory, Jerome), and includes one sentence each from Seneca (*Philosophus*) and Ovid (*Poeta*). William's debt to

[22] "William de Montibus: A Medieval Teacher," pp. 43-44. Father MacKinnon confided that his thesis director, Dr. Richard Hunt, considered this argument a "suasio" but not a "persuasio."

[23] *Publilii Syri sententiae*, ed. Eduard von Wölfflin (Leipzig: 1869), p. 67, no. 32. This was suggested to me by Professor Pierre Payer.

[24] *Die Lehre von den Umständen der menschlichen Handlung im Mittelalter* (Münster: Aschendorffsche Verlag, 1963): "Wir begegnen hier einem neuen, bisher unbekannten Schulvers, der alle erschwerenden Umstände in folgendem dreizeiligen Hexameter zusammenfassen will," pp. 395-396. Gründel notes the subsequent popularity of this list of circumstances in the thirteenth century, especially among the Franciscans (ibid., pp. 396, 416, 529, 651).

contemporary teachers and writers is less easily specified. Many of the quotations and interpretations proffered in the gloss were commonplaces in the twelfth-century schools. One author, however, who exercised an important, if unacknowledged, influence on William was Bartholomew of Exeter. William drew from Bartholomew's *Penitentiale* a handful of quotations from canonical and theological authorities (ll. 71-72 glosses a and b; l. 100 gloss a, etc.), but he also quoted extensively and verbatim from Bartholomew's own advice to the confessor (l. 7 gloss a; l. 82 gloss a; l. 147 glosses dd and ee, etc.)

MANUSCRIPTS

The most recent census of manuscripts containing the *Peniteas cito* lists more than 150 examples.[25] This enumeration is manifestly incomplete; the variety of titles, glosses, and rubrics with which copies were adorned make the work virtually impossible to identify with certainty from the brief descriptions provided in many manuscript catalogues.[26] The following manuscripts were used in this edition:

1. *C* = Cambridge, University Library MS Ii.1.26E, fols. 1ra-3va. Early 13th century (above top line).
   Inc. Gloss: *Ne tardas conuerti*
   Inc. Txt.: (*Que sunt neccessaria penitenti*) *Peniteas cito peccator*
   Expl. Gloss: *ut fiat restis longa.*
   Expl. Txt.: *consuetudo ruina.*
   Colophon: *Explicit liber penitentialis secundum magistrum W. de montibus Cancellarium Lincolniensem.*

2. *A* = London, British Library Cotton MS Vespasian D.xiii, fols. 114rb-115rb. Early 13th century (above top line).
   Title: *Qualis debet esse confessio hic per uersus notificatur.*
   Inc.: *Peniteas cito peccator*
   Expl.: *consuetudo ruina.*
This copy is unglossed and has no rubrics, but is divided into subsections by paragraph signs in the margins. It is followed by sixteen miscellaneous verses on fol. 115ra-b, and then by a glossed version of the poem, ascribed explicitly to William de Montibus, designated here by the siglum *V.*

---

[25] Bloomfield, et al., *Incipits*, nos. 3804-3821.
[26] See, for example, ibid., no. 3191, the *De emendatione peccatoris* of Richard Rolle, where the authors' comment: "Some of these MSS may contain *Peniteas cito* rather than *De emendatione peccatoris* because of the similarity of incipits."

3. *V* = London, ibid., fols 115rb-118va.

> Title: *Incipit tractatus magistri Willelmi de montibus de confessione.*
> Prol.: *Bernardus dicit super Cantica sermone xvi°: Confessio eo periculosius noxia quo subtilius uana. Cum etiam ipsa inhonestia et turpia de nobis detegere non ueremur, non quia humiles simus set ut esse putemur. Appetere autem de humilitate laudem humilitatis non est uirtus, set subuersio. Verus humilis uilis uult reputari, non humilis predicari; gaudet contemptu sui. Hoc solo sane superbus quod laudes contempnit. Quid peruersius, quid indignius ut humilitatis custos confessio superbie militet, et inde uult uideri melior unde uideris deterior.*
> Inc. Gloss: *Ecclesiastico xiiii.*
> Inc. Txt.: *(Que sunt necessaria penitenti) Peniteat cito*
> Expl. Gloss: *ut fiat longa restis.*
> Expl. Txt.: *consuetudo ruina.*

The unusual "prologue," consisting solely of a quotation from St. Bernard, accompanies other copies of the *Peniteas cito*; see, for example, San Marino, Huntington Library ms hm 19914 and London, bl ms Royal 12.F.xv, fol. 180rb.

4. *B* = London, British Library ms Royal 9.A.xiv, fols. 296ra-298rb. Later 13th century.

> Inc. Gloss: *Non tardes conuerti*
> Inc. Txt.: *(Que sunt necessaria penitenti) Peniteas cito peccator*
> Expl. Gloss: *ab eo scilicet exigatur.*
> Expl. Txt: *Affectus causa, uicium, persona notetur* [line 125].

5. *P* = London, Lambeth Palace ms 36, fols. 95v-97v. Mid 13th century.

> Inc. Txt.: *Peniteas cito peccator*
> Inc. Gloss: *Unde Iob: Etiam si occiderit me.*
> Expl. Txt.: *et consuetudo ruina.*
> Expl. Gloss: *ut sit longa restis.*

Giles used this copy as the base text for his edition of the poem, which was reprinted by Migne in pl 207: 1153-1156. It has no rubrics or paragraph divisions. Several longer quotations from Augustine and other Church Fathers have been intruded among the marginal glosses; these have been ignored in the present edition.

A second and distinct witness to the earliest version(s) of the poem is found in the two manuscripts containing William's *Versarius*. The manuscripts of this work are described below (ii.12), and have been assigned the following *sigla* in the present edition:

6. *K* = Cambridge, Corpus Christi College ms 186.

7. *L* = London, British Library MS Add. 16164. Because the glosses in these manuscripts are sporadic and less detailed than those in MSS *BCP* and *V* of the *Peniteas cito*, variant readings in the glosses of the *Versarius* have been ignored.

A third source for this edition is the copy of the *Peniteas cito* that forms the section on "Penance" in the *Tractatus metricus de septem sacramentis ecclesie*, discussed below (II.3). This copy of the poem is unglossed, but its presence as a discrete and complete unit in a treatise on the sacraments that may have been composed by William de Montibus makes it worthy of consideration. The text of this copy bears striking resemblances to the text of *C*, an early ascribed copy of the *Peniteas cito*. The unique manuscript containing this work is:

8. *O* = Oxford, Bodleian Library MS 419, and the *Peniteas cito* is found on fols. 204ra-vb.

> Inc. Txt.: (*De hiis que necessaria sunt In confessione*) *Peniteas cito peccator.*
> Expl.: *et consuetudo ruina.*

The text has no gloss. It is followed immediately by three lines of verse:

> Fercula, festa, canes et equi, numerusque clientum
> Vestibus et uasis, domibus curaque parentum
> Excelsus superesse negant bona danda potentum

and then by the rubric: *Explicit de penitentia. Incipit de uerbis apostoli Pauli de prelatis ecclesie.*

The text printed here is edited from all eight manuscripts, and variant readings are reported in an *apparatus criticus* keyed to the line numbers of the poem. The gloss is edited from the four witnesses that report it, MSS *BCP* and *V*. Each gloss is keyed to the word or phrase that it elucidates by superscript arabic numerals.

Lines 115 to 134 and 148 to 155 of the text, marked with asterisks (*), are found in MS *C* of the *Peniteas cito* but not in MSS *ABP* or *V*. They appear in the same order in MS *O* — the *Tractatus metricus* — and are also found in MSS *K* and *L* of the *Versarius*; they may have been part of an early redaction of the poem. The edition of the glosses to these lines reports the readings of MSS *KL* and *C*, MS *O* has no gloss. Also within square brackets are references to the sources actually utilized in the gloss, where these can be identified, or to related passages in works that circulated in William's milieu. The following abbreviations are used in identifying the sources:

Barth = Bartholomew of Exeter, *Penitentiale*, ed. Adrian Morey, *Bartholomew of Exeter, Bishop and Canonist ... with the Text of Bartholomew's Penitential from the Cotton Ms. Vitellius A.XII* (Cambridge, 1937).

Decretum = *Decretum magistri Gratiani*, ed. E. Friedberg (Leipzig, 1881).

Cantor = Peter the Chanter, *Verbum abbreviatum*, PL 205: 23-554.

Comestor = Peter Comestor, *De sacramentis*, ed. R. Martin, in H. Weisweiler, *Maitre Simon et son groupe* "De sacramentis" (Louvain, 1937).

Lombard = *Magistri Petri Lombardi ... Sententiae in IV libris distinctae*, 3rd ed., vol. 2 (Grottaferrata, 1981).

Glossa = *Biblia sacra cum glossa ordinaria et glossa interlineari ... et postilla Nicolai Lyrani*, 7 vols. (Lyons, 1545; 1590; Paris, 1590; Venice, 1603).

Peniteas cito peccator

QVE SVNT NECESSARIA PENITENTI

Peniteas cito[a] peccator cum sit miserator
  Iudex.[b] Et sunt hec quinque tenenda tibi:
Spes[c] uenie, cor[d] contritum, confessio[e] culpe,
5   Pena satisfaciens,[f] et fuga[g] nequitie.

1 Que ... penitenti *om. P*: Qualis debet esse confessio hic per uersus notificatur *A*: De hiis que neccessaria sunt in confessione *O*   2 Peniteas] Peniteat *V*

a Ecclesiastico xiiii [5:8]: Non tardes conuerti ad Dominum Deum tuum.
     Ecclesiastico ... tuum *om. P*   Non tardes] Ne tardas *C*   ad ... tuum *om. B*   conuerti] uenire *V*

b Secundo Esdre iv [Neh 9:1-37].
     Secundo ... iv *om. BCP*

c Sperate in eo omnis congregatio populi; effundite coram illo corda uestra etc. [Ps 61:9].
     Vnde Iob [13:15], Etiam si occiderit me sperabo in eum. *add. P*

d Cor contritum et humiliatum Deus non despicies [Ps 50:19].

e In Prouerbis [28:13]: Qui abscondit peccata sua non dirigetur; qui autem confessus fuerit et reliquerit ea, ueniam consequetur. Item [Jac 5:16]: Confitemini alterutrum peccata uestra.

> In Prouerbis *om. BCP*   Item ... uestra *om. BCP*

f Id est penitentia. Vnde [Mt 3:8; cf. Lc 3:8]: Facite dignos fructus penitentie.

> Vt qualitas et quantitas pene, respondeat qualitati et quantitati culpe. *add. P*

g Quasi a facie colubri fuge peccatum [Eccli 21:2]. Conuertere ad Dominum et relinque peccata [Eccli 17:21]. Fugite fornicationem [1 Cor 6:18].

> fuge] fugite *PV*   conuertere ... peccata *om. PV*   Fugite fornicationem *om. BCP*

DE REMISSIONE INIVRIARVM

7 Vt dimittaris,[a] aliis peccata remittas,
   Hiisque satisfacias[b] quos te[c] lesisse fateris.

> 6 De remissione iniuriarum *om. AKLOP*   iniuriarum *om. V*   7 remittas] remitte *AKL*: remittis *C*   8 satisfacias] satisfaciens *BV*

a Dimitte nobis debita nostra sicut et nos dimittimus debitoribus nostris [Mt 6:12]. Oportet etiam penitentem satisfacere hiis in quos ipse delinquit, et ex toto corde dimittere hiis qui in ipsum delinquerunt. Hec enim ad peccatorum remissionem precipue sunt necessaria [*Barth* c.11 p.182]. Dimittite et dimittemini [Lc 6:37]. Conseruis offensas non imputando [cf. Mt 18:21-25].

> in quos] quibus *PV*   peccatorum] delictorum *B*   precipue *om. V*   Dimittite ... imputando *om. P*

b Quocumque modo. Vnde Dominus [Mt 5:23-24]: Si offers munus tuum ad altare, et ibi recordatus fueris quod frater tuus habet aliquid aduersum te, relinque ibi munus tuum ante altare et uade prius reconciliari fratri tuo et tunc ueniens offer munus tuum.

> Quocumque modo *om. BP*   aduersum] aduersus *V*   ante altare *om. V*   reconciliari] te conciliari *C*

c Mattheo iiii [5:23-24]: Vnde si offers etc. Verbo uel facto.

> Matheo ... facto *om. BCP*

DE SATISFACTIONE

10 Sperne uoluptates,[a] lusus,[b] spectacula mundi;[c]
    Desere consortem[d] prauum populique[e] tumultum,
    Secretasque[f] preces et opus[g] pietatis amato.

9 De satisfactione] *om. ABP*: Satisfactio penitencialis *KL*: Que sunt
uitanda in hoc seculo *O*   10 uoluptates] uoluntates *AV*   lusus] luxus
CO   11 Desere] Dissere *V*   consortem prauum] consortes prauos *O*
12 Secretasque ... amato *om. KL*

   a Carnales. Vnde Ieronimus [*Decretum*, De pen. D.1 c.66]: Penitens
   dormiat in sacco ut preteritas delicias per quas Deum offenderat, uite
   austeritate compenset.
      Carnales *om. BCP*   Vnde Ieronimus *om. VP*   dormiat] dormitet
      V   preteritas *om. V*

   b Seculares. Cum ab aliis luditur, tu sancti honestique aliquid tractabis.
   Tobia iii [3:17]; Ieremia lxii [15:17].
      Seculares *om. BCP*   aliquid] aliud *V*   Tobia ... lxii *om. BP*

   c Res uana. Vnde Philosophus [Seneca, *Epistolae morales* 7.2]: Quo
   maior est populus cui miscemur, hoc periculi plus est. Nihil enim tam
   dampnosum bonis moribus quam in aliquo spectaculo residere.
      Res uana *om. BCP*   Philosophus ... est *om. C*   miscemur] misertur
      V   bonis moribus *om. P*   moribus] operibus *V*

   d Qui cum sapientibus graditur sapiens erit; amicus stultorum similis
   efficietur [Prov 13:20].
      similis] singulis *V*

   e Vnde Dominus surdum et mutum curandum seorsum a turba ducit
   [cf. Mc 7:34-37], id est a strepitu mundi. Quotiens, inquit Ieronimus,
   inter homines fui, minus homo me redii [*Cantor*, c.178, col.206].
   Ieremia [15:17]: Interius solus sedebam. Qui tangit picem etc. [Eccli
   13:1].
      fui minus] fuimus *C*   me *om. P*   Ieremia ... etc. *om. BCP*

   f Secundum illud [Mt 6:6]: Clauso ostio ora Patrem tuum in abscondito.

   g Id est elemosinam. Nam ut ait Apostolus [1 Tim 4:8]: Pietas ad omnia
   utilis est, promissionem habens uite que nunc est et future.
      elemosinam] ecclesiam *V*   cum gemitibus et suspiriis. Excercere ad
      pietatem ad thimoth. *add. V*

QVOD PLENARIA DEBET ESSE CONFESSIO

14 Omnia[a] peccata plangat contritio uera,
   Scrutans etates,[b] sensus,[c] loca,[d] tempora, membra.[e]

   13 Quod ... confessio *om. AP*: Qualiter inquirende sunt circumstancie *O*
plenaria] plenaris *V*   14-15 Omnia ... membra *om. KL*   15 Scrutans]
Seruans *P*

   a Ne pars ciuitatis compluatur et ex parte arida remaneat [cf. Amos

4:7]. Hoc est, ne penitens quedam uitia deploret et deserat, et in aliis grauiter perduret. Quid enim prodest si peccata luxurie quis defleat, et adhuc estibus auaricie anhelet? [*Decretum*, De pen. D.3 c.6].

   ne penitens] penitens *C*   anhelet] anelat *P*

b Quid in pueritia, quid in iuuentute commiserit, et sic de ceteris.

c Quomodo per gustum, uel illicita uerba, uel per tactum, uisum, auditum, uel odoratum peccauerit.

d Quid in hoc, quid in illo loco, uno uel alio tempore egerit.
   egerit *om. PV*

e Quomodo uno, quomodo alio membro peccauerit.

DE FLETV

17 Deplores[a] acta, nolens committere flenda.[b]
Plangas amissa[c] cum commissis[d] et omissis,[e]
Offensasque Dei,[f] quod fratres dampnificasti.

   16 De fletu *om. AKLOP*   17 Deplores ... flenda *om. KL*   Deplores] Deplorans *A*   18 Plangas ... omissis *om. C*: Plango quod amisi, quod commisi, quod omisi *L*   amissa] admissa *P*   19 Offensasque ... dampnificasti *om. KL*   fratres] fratrem *ABPV (ante corr.)*

a O penitens.
   om. PV: omnipotentes *C*

b Penitere est enim ante acta peccata deflere, et iterum flenda non committere uel nolle committere [*Comestor*, p.60*; cf. *Lombard*, D.14 c.2, p.317].
   Penitere ... committere *om. P*   iterum flenda non] flenda *B*: iterum non *V*

c Statum et tempus; innocentiam et famam.

d Malis.

e Bonis. Hoc est plangere dampna tua, et peccata et delicta.
   plangere] plange *C*   et peccata *om. B*   et delicta] Delicta *V*

f Plange et quod Deum offendisti et proximum dampnificasti.
   offendisti] ostendisti *P*

QVALIS DEBET ESSE CONFESSIO

21 Vera[a] sit, integra[b] sit, et sit confessio munda.[c]
Sit cita,[d] firma,[e] frequens,[f] humilis,[g] spontanea,[h] nuda,[i]

Propria,[j] discreta,[k] lacrimosa,[l] morosa,[m] fidelis.[n]
Peniteas plene[o] si uere peniteat te,
25 Non per legatum, non per breue, set refer ipse.[p]

20 Qualis ... confessio *om. AP*   21 Vera ... munda] Integra sit culpe
confessio mundaque uera *KL*   22 Sit] Et *KL*   cita] scita *AO*   nuda]
nudus *A*   24 plene] plane *O*

a Nemo humilitatis causa fateatur se reum illius peccati quod se non
   commisisse noscit, quia sic peccatorem se constituet. Vnde Augustinus
   [*Lombard*, D.21 c.8, p.385]: Cum humilitatis causa mentiris, si non
   eras peccator antequam mentireris, mentiendo efficieris quod uitaras.
       illius] alicuius *PV*   se[2] ... constituet] non omisit *P*   noscit] notuit
   C   constituet] constitueret *C*   si] set *B*   eras] erat *C*

b Vt penitens omnia peccata mortalia uni sacerdoti confiteatur cum
   circumstantiis.
       peccata *om. BV*   confiteatur *om. C*

c Vt contritus se mundet interius confitendo spiritualia, exterius pandendo
   carnalia. Vnde Dominus [Mt 23:25-26]: Ve uobis scribe et pharisei
   ypocrite, qui mundatis quod deforis est calicis et parapsidis, intus autem
   pleni estis rapina et immunditia. Pharisee cece, prius munda quod intus
   est calicis et parapsidis, ut fiat et id quod deforis est mundum.
       spiritualia *om. V*   pandendo] puniendo *P*   intus[1] ... parapsidis *om.*
   V   Pharisee ... munda *om. C*   deforis] deterius *P*

d Ne tardes conuerti ad Dominum Deum tuum [Eccli 5:8], exemplo
   Marie Magdalene [Lc 7:37-38] et mulieris Chananee accelerantis et
   orantis pro filia [Mt 15:21-28]. Ne differatur.
       conuerti] uenire *V*   exemplo ... differatur *om. P*   accelerantis et *om.*
   V   Ne differatur *om. V*

e Id est in pace firma. Ne penitens recidiuet; non sint treuge set firma
   pax inter ipsum et Deum. Vnde Apostolus [Hebr 4:14]: Teneamus
   confessionem.
       Id est ... firma *om. BCP*   non ... confessionem *om. P*   Vnde Apostolus
   om. B

f Confitebimur tibi Deus, confitebimur [Ps 74:2]. Item [cf. Rom 10:10]:
   Deo facta frequens confessio uitam parit.
       Confitebimur ... confitebimur *om. P*   parit] panit *C*

g Cor contritum et humilis [cf. Ps 50:19]. Vnde dicitur de Dauid [cf.
   2 Sam 11-12]: Qui humiliter confitetur, mox ueniam meretur.
       Cor ... humilis *om. BCP*   Dauid] deo *B*

h Sicut sponte quis peccauerit. Quia extorta confessio meritum non habet.
   Sicut enim spontanea precessit peccati perpetratio, sic uoluntaria
   sequatur confessio et satisfactio. Vnde Psalmista [Ps 27:7]: Ex uoluntate
   mea confitebor illi.

Sicut ... peccauerit *om. BC*   satisfactio] satisfacit *P*   Psalmista *om.*
BC   illi] ei *V*

i Aperta scilicet non operta, sine excusatione uel simulatione, quia non
   potest sanare medicus nisi prius sit detectum uulnus.
         Aperta *om. PV*   sine] non *B*: sit *P*

j Confitemini alterutrum peccata uestra [Jac 5:16], quasi non aliena.

k Sal in omni sacrificio [cf. Lev 2:13].
         Sal] sit *add. PV*

l Lacrimando. Lacrime lauant delictum quod pudor est confiteri. Vt in
   Maria Magdalena [Lc 7:37-38] et Petro [Mt 26:75].
         Lacrimando *om. BC*: Lacrime lauant *P*   quod pudor ... confiteri *om. BC*

m Morietur penitens coram sacerdote peccata illi confitendo, illum
   diligenter audiendo, et onus satisfactionis deuote suscipiendo. In
   cognoscendo augmentum peccati innuat penitens cuius etatis fuerit,
   cuius sapientie, cuius ordinis; immoretur in singulis istis, et sentiat
   modum criminis, purgans lacrimis omnem qualitatem uitii [cf. *Lombard*,
   D.16 c.2, p.338].
         Morietur] Moretur *PV*   innuat] inuentat *B*: inueniat *C*   qualitatem]
   quantitatem *P*

n iii Numeris [Thren 3:40]: Scrutemur uias nostras, et reuertamur ad
   Dominum. Vt contritus confiteatur sub spe uenie, de indulgentia non
   diffidens, set confidens. Judas [Mt 27:3-5], Cain [Gen 4:13-16] confessi
   sunt set diffisi sunt. Vtriusque confessio infidelis fuit.
         iii ... Dominum *om. BCP*   spe] specie *B*   set[2]] et *BP*

o Sine suppressione et tergiuersatione.
         suppressione] peccati *add. P*   tergiuersatione] teguminis actione *P*:
   transgressione *V*

p Dic tu iniquitates tuas ut iustificeris [cf. Is 43:26].
         tu] ipse *add. P*

CVI DEBEAS CONFITERI

27 Compatienti,[a] plus sapienti, dic meliori.[b]
   Presbiteris multis prodest si confitearis;[c]
   Copia presbiteri si desit pande sodali.[d]

      26 Cui ... confiteri] *om. CP*: Confessio *KL*: Quod penitens debet querere
superiores prelatos in arduis confitendis set cum licencia *O*   27 plus] dic
P   29 Copia ... sodali] Dicere si pudeat semel uni dicito saltem/Quod
si non iteras non iterabis idem *O*

a Qui cum potestate habeat et scientiam. Vnde Augustinus [*Decretum*, De pen. D.6 c.1]: Qui uult confiteri peccata sua ut inueniat gratiam, querat sacerdotem qui sciat ligare et soluere, ne ambo in foueam cadant.

    Qui ... scientiam *om. P*   cum potestate] cum potestatem *C*: potestatem *V*

b Querat penitens licentiam a proprio sacerdote, et si non dederit nihilominus sumat, uel suo inuito adeat superiorem, uel prius confiteatur proprio sacerdoti, deinde alii.

    Querat] Petat *V*   nihilominus *om. B*   adeat] sumat *B*   uel] ut *BP*   deinde] demum *C*

c Augustinus [*Decretum*, De pen., D.1 c.88]: Quia quanto pluribus confitebitur penitens turpitudinem criminis in spe uenie, tanto facilius consequetur ueniam remissionis.

    confitebitur] confitetur *V*   in ... uenie *om. P*   consequetur] consequitur *C*   Peccatorum namque confessio demonum est ingens confusio *add. V*

d In necessitatis articulo. Augustinus [*Decretum*, De pen. D.6 c.1]: Tanta uis est confessionis ut si deest sacerdos, confiteatur proximo. Sepe enim contingit quod penitens non potest uerecundari coram sacerdote, quoniam desideranti nec locus nec tempus offert, et si ille cui confitebitur potestatem non habeat soluendi, tamen fit dignus uenia ex desiderio sacerdotis, qui confitetur socio turpitudinem criminis. Mundati enim sunt leprosi dum irent ostendere se coram sacerdotibus antequam ad eos peruenirent. Vnde patet Deum ad cor respicere dum ex necessitate prohibentur ad sacerdotes peruenire.

    In ... Augustinus *om. PV*   deest] est *V*   contingit] contigit *C*   quoniam] quem *P*   habeat] habet *P*   soluendi *om. C*   amen fit] cum sit *B*   irent] ibant *CP*   coram] ora *B*   prohibentur] prohiberentur *V*

DE CORPORALIBVS ET SPIRITVALIBVS PECCATIS

Corporis ut maculas anime sic crimina pandas.[a]
Carnea sunt periuria, crapula, furta, libido;
Mente latet liuor, odium, tumor, ira, cupido.[b]
Precipue pestes septem memores capitales,[c]
35 Non solum fontes set riuos inde fluentes.[d]
Fonte suo riuus magis est quandoque nociuus;[e]
Vnde Loth incestus peior fuit ebrietate,
Atque Cain grauior cedes fraterna furore.

    30 De ... peccatis] *om. ACP*: Quod sacerdos debet predicare in genere subditis peccata capitalia uitanda *O*: in confessione pandendis *add. L*   31 crimina] crimine *O*   pandas] pande *CV*   33 tumor] timor *K*   cupido] libido *P*   36 riuus] riuis *V*   est *om. P*   37 peior] grauior *A*   38 Atque] At *C*   furore] cruore *O*

a Sic confiteris exteriora et carnalia peccata, ita interiora et spiritualia.

b Hec sunt spiritualia.

c Confitendo septem capitalia uitia.
    om. P

d Id est alia peccata que ex hiis oriuntur.
    peccata] uicia *P*

e Vt homicidium grauius est ira ex qua nascitur.

QVE SVNT VITIA CAPITALIA

40 Culparum fontes sunt fastus,[a] liuor,[b] et ira,[c]
    Accidie[d] neuus et auaritie,[e] gula,[f] luxus.[g]

    39 Que ... capitalia] *om. A P*: Septem uicia capitalia *L*: Septem peccata
capitalia *O*: Que sunt septem capitalia uicia *V*   41 Accidie] Accidieque
A   neuus] uenus *ACO*: genus *V*   Hec mala curantur sua si contraria
dentur *add. V*

a Id est superbia. Superbia est amor proprie excellentie.
    om. BCV

b Inuidia. Inuidia est aliene felicitatis afflictio.
    om. BCV

c Ira est irrationabilis motus animi, que Dei officium non operatur.
    om. BCV

d Tristitia siue accidia est tedium eterni boni.
    om. BCV

e Auaritia est immoderatus amor habendi.
    om. BCV

f Gula est immoderatus appetitus edendi.
    om. BCV

g Luxuria est turpis motus desiderans uenerem.
    om. BCV

QVOD MORTALIA SINT SPECIFICANDA ET CETERA IN GENERE CONFITENDA

    Cum singillatim[a] mortalia dixeris[b] uni,[c]
    Cuncta simul[d] quecumque grauant comitantia[e] culpas,
45 Dic citra factum committere que uoluisti.[f]
    Dic uenialia,[g] dic que sunt a mente relapsa,[h]

Dic tua delicta,[i] generaliter[j] ista reuela.[k]
Nam reus in multis[l] quando peccata fatetur,
Vel queuis[m] dicat,[n] uel nil dixisse uidetur.
50 Postremum crimen si pure quis fateatur,
Ille tacere potest quicquid redit et comitatur.

42 Quod ... confitenda] *om. ABKLP*: Quod penitens debet omnia et
uni dicere *O*   et ... confitenda *om. C*   44 culpas] culpa *B*   45 factum]
facta *O*   46 uenialia] venalia *P*   relapsa] repulsa *P*   47 reuela]
reuera *L*   49 nil] nihil *P*   51 et] aut *K*

    a Manifeste specificando.
       om. V

    b Id est penitens.
       om. V

    c Sacerdoti, uel socio in necessitate.
       in necessitate *om. V*

    d Vt sit integra confessio.
       Vt] Cum *V*

    e Scilicet circumstantias aggrauantes.
       Scilicet ... aggrauantes] Cunctas circumstantias *P*

    f Id est confitere peccata que uoluisti facere et non fecisti.
       fecisti] fecistis *BC*

    g Cotidiana et leuia.
       leuia] uenalia *P*

    h Id est obliuioni tradita.

    i Id est omissiones bonorum.
       omissiones] remissiones *V*

    j In genere.
       om. V

    k Quatuor scilicet predicta genera peccatorum.
       Quatuor *om. P*

    l Id est peccatis.
       om. PV

    m Mortalia que tunc occurrunt memorie.
       memorie] ei in memoria *B*

    n Non tamen oportet ut quotiens confitemur totiens omnia que prius
      confessi sumus confiteamur. Si enim post specialem et generalem
      confessionem rite factam recidiuet penitens, purgato per confessionem
      illo peccato in quo recidiuauit, remittuntur omnia que causa illius
      redierunt.

ut] quod *CP*   totiens] totius *P*   que ... sumus] prius confessa *V*
confiteamur] iterum confitemur *V*   specialem] spiritualem *C*   rite] rete
C   per] post *V*   in quo] quo *P*: in quod *V*

QVE CIRCVMSTANTIE AGGRAVANT PECCATA

Aggrauat ordo,[a] locus,[b] peccata, scientia,[c] tempus,[d]
Etas,[e] conditio,[f] numerus,[g] mora,[h] copia,[i] causa,[j]
55 Et modus[k] in culpa, status[l] altus, lucta[m] pusilla.

52 Que ... peccata] *om. P*: Circumstantie aggrauant peccatum *KL*: In
quibus casibus peccatum aggrauatur *O*   54 numerus] iuuenis *A*   55 Et]
Est *O*   altus] almus *K*

    a Sacer.
       Sacer] Sacerdotum *P*: Sacerdotum uel alius sacer ordo *V*

    b Ecclesia uel cemeterium.

    c Seruus sciens uoluntatem domini sui et non faciens uapulabit multis
      [cf. Luc 12:47].
       uoluntatem domini sui *om. BCP*

    d Sollempne, uel ieiunium.
       Sollempne] festum *add. PV*   ieiunium] ieiunii *B*

    e Plus peccat senex fornicando quam iuuenis.

    f Lex Moysi iussit mulierem liberam pro fornicatione lapidari, ancillam
      uero flagellari [cf. Lev 19:20].
       pro fornicatione] propter fornicacionem *P*   lapidari] liberari *V*

    g Vnde [Ier 2:36]: Quam uilis facta es nimis iterans uias tuas.
       Vnde] Ysa *add. V*   Quam] quasi *P*

    h Peccatum enim quod non statim diluitur per penitentiam, mox pondere
      suo trahit ad aliud [*Cantor*, c.149 col.356]. Sanguis sanguinem tetigit
      [Os 4:2]. Manens quidem in mortali, thesaurizat sibi iram in die iusti
      iudicii Dei secundum cor suum impenitens [cf. Rom 2:5].
       ad aliud] aliquid aliud *B*: ad illud *V*   in die *om. PV*   Dei *om. B*
      secundum ... impenitens *om. PV*   suum] tuum *B*

    i Cui plus committitur, ab eo plus exigitur, et magis ingratus efficitur
      cum Deum offendit [cf. Lc 12:48].
       ab ... et *om. BCP*

    j Cum quis ex odio facit quod tamen alias iustum esset.
       tamen] non *B* Item nota quod grauiter peccat qui contempnit, grauius qui
      impunitatem promittitur, grauissime qui ignorat *add. C*

k Vt si uir dormiens cum muliere utatur membro non concesso ad concubitum.

> ad concubitum *om. P*: uel more canino *add. V*

l Quanto gradus altior tanto lapsus grauior.

> lapsus] casus *V*

m Modica. Plus peccat qui modice temptationi cedit quam qui graui uincitur impugnatione. Sunt enim quidam qui se ultro offerunt peccato, nec expectant tentationem, set preueniunt uoluptatem [*Barth*, c.26, p.195].

> Modica *om. PV*   cedit] cecidit *B*: ceditur *CP*   uincitur impugnatione] impugnacioni *P*   enim quidam *om. V*   offerunt] efferunt *P*   uoluptatem *om. CP*

DE PENITENTIA INFIRMORVM

Eger peniteat et crimina confiteatur.
Non imponetur huic pena, set insinuetur;
Hanc tamen explebit si firma salus sibi detur.
60 Si migret, absoluat contritum presbiter egrum;
Huncque preces[a] releuent, ieiunia, dona[b] suorum.

> 56 De ... infirmorum] *om. P*: Quod laborans in extremis omnia peccata sua debet detegere reiterando, nec tamen imponenda est ei penitencia set insinuanda *O*   infirmorum] infirmi *KL*: egri *V*   57 et] qui *C*   58 imponetur] imponatur *VP*   insinuetur] insinuatur *C*   59 explebit] implebit *AV*   si] set *O*   sibi detur] reparetur *P*   61 Huncque] Hincque *V*

a Gregorius [cf. *Comestor*, pp.84*-85*]: Anime namque defunctorum quatuor modis absoluuntur: aut ieiunio cognatorum, aut oblationibus sacerdotum, aut precibus sanctorum, aut elemosinis carorum.

> carorum *om. C*

b Elemosine carorum, Parabola xxxvii [cf. Tob 12:8-9].

> *om. V*   Parabola xxxvii *om. P*

CVR INSTITVTA SIT CONFESSIO

63 Vt sit pena rubor tibi, uilis ut efficiaris,
Doctior ut fias, iniungitur ut fatearis.

> 62 Cur ... confessio *om. AKO*   63 Vt] Et *V*   tibi] uel *O*   ut] sit ut *P*   64 iniungitur] iunguntur *B*   fatearis] efficiaris *C*

Qvantvs sit effectvs confessionis

66 Iudicio teget extremo confessio culpas,[a]
Ne uideat Deus[b] aut demon[c] uel qui facit[d] illas.

65 Quantus ... confessionis *om. AKOP*: Effectus confessionis *L*
66 extremo] extrema *O*   67 Deus] Dominus *O*

> a Beati quorum remisse sunt iniquitates et quorum tecta sunt peccata
>   [Ps 31:1].
>
> b Ad dampnandum.
>
> c Ad accusandum.
>
> d Ad erubescendum.
>   *om. P*

Qvalis debeat esse confessor

Confessor mitis, affabilis atque benignus,
70 Sit sapiens, iustus, sit dulcis, compatiensque.
Vt crimen proprium celet peccata reorum.[a]
Sit piger[b] ad penas, sit uelox ad miserandum,
Et doleat quotiens facit illum culpa ferocem.
Infundat mulcens oleum uinumque flagellans
75 Nunc uirgam patris, nunc exerat ubera matris.
Sibilet et cantet, stimulet cum cogit oportet.

68 Qualis ... confessor] *om. AP*: Quod omnis prelatus debet esse mitis
et compatiens subditis suis *O*   confessor] prelatus *KL*   69 Confessor]
Prelatus *KL*   70 sit^2] set *O*   71 celet] celat *V*   72 miserandum]
miserendum *BCKL*   73 Et] Sic *P*   culpa] pena *O*   74 mulcens]
miscens *O*   flagellans] flagellis *O*   75 Nunc uirgam] Hunc uirga *P*
nunc exerat] habeat nunc *AV (in ras.)*: non exerat *P*   76 Sibilet] Silibet
C   stimulet] rumilet? *O*   cogit] cogi *L*

> a Gregorius [*Barth*, c.29, p.198]: Sacerdos ante omnia caueat ne illorum
>   qui confitentur ei peccata alicui recitet, non propinquis, non extraneis,
>   nec quod absit pro aliquo scandalo. Nam si hoc fecerit deponatur,
>   et omnibus diebus uite sue ignominiosus peregrinando pergat.
>   qui *om. C*   non ... non] nec ... nec *PV*   deponatur] dampnabitur
>   *P*   et] in *C*
>
> b Iohannes Crisostomus [*Barth*, c.34, p.201]: Si fascem super humeros
>   adolescentis quem non potest baiulare posueris, necesse habet ut fascem
>   reiciat, aut sub pondere confringatur. Sic et homo cui graue honus

penitentie imponis, aut penitentiam reiciet, aut suscipiens dum ferre
non potest, scandalizatus, amplius peccabit. Demum et si erramus
modicam imponentes medicinam, nonne melius erit propter misericordiam rationem dare quam propter crudelitatem? Vbi enim paterfamilias
largus est, dispensator non debet esse tenax. Si Deus benignus, ut quid
sacerdos eius austerus uult apparere?

habet] est *V*   confringatur] constringatur *B*   graue ... penitentie] onus
importabile *B*   suscipiens] suscipiat *C*   Demum] *om. P*: Deinde *C*
medicinam] penitenciam *P*   propter crudelitatem] crudelitatem *P*   Vbi]
Vnde *C*

QVE SVNT INQVIRENDA IN CONFESSIONE

78 In primis querat contritus quomodo credat;
Si credit corde sane fateatur et ore.

77 Que ... confessione] *om. AKLP*: Penitens primo conueniendus est
de fide *B*: Penitens coniu<...> in primo <...> *C*: Qualiter debet inquisicio
fieri in confessione *O*   79 credit] credat *APV*

SACERDOS CAVTE INQVIRAT DE PECCATIS

81 Post hec rimetur peccantis uulnera caute.
Contra naturam[a] culpam non exprimat ullam,
Ne super enormi si simplex conueniatur,
De quo nil sciuit ad agendum sic moneatur.

80 Sacerdos ... peccatis *om. AKLOPV*   81 rimetur] rimentur *P*
uulnera] uiscera *O*   82 exprimat] exprimit *CO*: exprimet *A*   84 agendum sic] noscendum *B*   sic moneatur] si moneatur *O*: commoneatur *K*:
sic moueatur *APV*

a In enumeratione uitiorum, caueat sacerdos ne penitentem conueniat
super aliquo peccato quod sit contra naturam, uel aliter multum
abhominabile, nisi forte ea persona sit quam ex auditu, uel ex aliis
probabilibus coniecturis de tali crimine suspectam habeat. Set sine
alicuius peccati expressione poterit simpliciter dicere: frater recogita
tecum si aliquando aliquod peccatum commisisti quod fuerit contra
naturam, uel aliter multum abhominabile fecisti. Ideo autem peccata
abhominabilia coram hominibus exprimi non consulimus, quoniam
audiuimus tam uiros quam mulieres per expressam nominationem
ignotorum criminum in peccata que prius non nouerant incidisse
[*Barth*, c.38, p.205].

enumeratione] numeracione *P*   aliter ... abhominabile[1]] quia multum abhominabile est *P*: super aliquo multum abhominabili peccato *V* abhominabile[1]] abhominabilem *B*   ea persona] talis persona *V*: ea perita *B*   commisisti] fecisti *P*: *om. V*   fuerit] fuit *B*   aliter multum[2]] aliquod aliud *P*   abhominabile fecisti] abhominabilem *B*: abhominabile *CP* coram hominibus *om. P*   hominibus] omnibus *B*   criminum *om. P* prius *om. P*   nouerant] nouerunt *PV*

De cavtela inivngendi penitentiam

Vxor adulterii rea confessore perito
Sic luat admissum ne sit suspecta marito.
Sepe sibi moneat confessos ne recidiuent,[a]
Siue relabantur confestim confiteantur[b]
90 Et uitent[c] causas ad lapsus allicientes.
Solliciti[d] penam complere satisfacientem,
Os seruent[e] caute, sensus[f] cum pectore,[g] renes:[h]
In prauos casus horum procliuior usus.
Hoc est difficile magis et seruare necesse.

85 De ... penitentiam] *om. APKLV*: Quod caute agunt cum nuptis ne possint comprehendi *O*   penitentiam] penitentia *C*   86 confessore] confessoreque *B*: confessione *C*: prelato *KL*   perito] sapiente *KL* 87 luat] lauet *A*   88 Sepe sibi] Sepius *A*   sibi] tibi *B*   confessos] confessor *APV*   recidiuent] recidiuet *PV*   89 Siue relabantur] Et si labantur *A*: Siue relabuntur *C*   90 Et uitent] Vitenti *P*   lapsus] lapsum *O*: lansusa *L*   allicientes] allicienta *L*   92 Os seruent] Obseruent *BPV* 93-94 In ... necesse *om. P*   94 est] tibi *AV*   magis et] magisque *V*

a Sicut Dominus dixit languido curato [Ioh 5:14]: Ecce sanus factus es; iam amplius noli peccare ne deterius tibi contingat.
　　Ecce ... es] Es sanus *C*   amplius *om. C*

b Ne tardes conuerti ad Dominum Deum tuum.
　　conuerti] uenire *V*

c Vt commessationes et potationes, otia et solitudines et ceteras oportunitates et commoditates que peccatis prestant incitamenta uel fomenta, penitens euitet. Vnde Poeta [Ovid, *Remedia amoris*, ll.139, 579]: Otia si tollas periere cupidinis artus. Quisquis amas loca sola nocent, loca sola caueto.
　　euitet] euiterunt *V*   poeta *om. V*   amas] amans *P*   sola caueto] caueto *B*

d Vnde Dauid [Ps 37:19]: Quoniam iniquitatem meam annuntiabo tibi, et cogitabo pro peccato meo; uel: sollicitus ero pro peccato meo.
　　Vnde Dauid *om. BCV*   cogitabo] cogitacio *V* peccato meo] peccatis meis *BV*

e Vnde Salomon [Prov 21:23]: Qui custodit os suum custodit ab angustiis
animam suam.

   Vnde Salomon] Solucio *V*

f Ne mors ingrediatur per fenestras [cf. Ier 9:21]; quia ut ait Beda: Qui
corporeos non seruat sensus mortis sibi ipse reserat aditus.

   Ne ... ingrediatur] Mors ingreditur *B*   non *om. C*   ipse *om. P*

g Secundum illud Salomon [Prov 4:23]: Omni custodia serua cor tuum,
quia ex ipso uita procedit.

   Salomon *om. BCV*   serua] custodi *PV*

h Sint lumbi uestri precincti et lucerne ardentes in manibus uestris [Lc
12:35].

QVOD SACERDOS NON DEBET ESSE ACCEPTOR PERSONARVM

Vtque fori iudex pro persona prohibetur
Flectere iudicium, medicus uariare medelas,
Sic anime iudex odio caueat uel amore
Confessos penis onerare uel alleuiare;
100 Ecclesie morem uel patrum scripta sequatur,[a]
Sitque modus pene iuxta moderamina culpe,
Et tanto leuior quanto contritio maior.[b]

   95 Quod ... personarum] *om. AKLP*: Exemplum *O*   personarum]
om. V   96 Vtque] Vt *O*   persona] pecunia *O*   97 uariare] narrare
BCK   medelas] medelam *KL*   98 Sic] Dic *C*   caueat] cauet *L*
100 scripta] scriptaque *L*   sequatur] sequantur *O*   101 iuxta] tempus
add. C   Quod contricio est pars maxima satisfaccionis *add. O (rubr.)*
102 quanto] quanta est *P*

   a Scilicet sacerdos iniungendo penitentiam. Ex Concilio Magociensi
[*Barth*, c.33, p.200]: Modus tempusque penitentie peccata sua confi-
tentibus aut per antiquorum canonum institutionem, aut per sacrarum
scriptuarum auctoritatem, aut per ecclesiasticam consuetudinem pro-
batam, imponi debet a sacerdotibus.

      Scilicet ... penitentiam *om. B*   tempusque] Christus quia *B*   sua *om.*
C   sacrarum] sanctarum *B*: *om. P*   consuetudinem] auctoritatem *P*
probatam] approbatam *V*

   b Mensuram temporis in agenda penitentia ideo non satis aperte prefigunt
canones pro unoquoque crimine ut de singulis dicant qualiter unumquodque emendandum sit, set magis in arbitrio sacerdotis intelligentis
relinquendum statuunt, quia apud Deum non tam ualet mensura
temporis quam doloris, nec abstinentia tantum ciborum quantum

mortificatio uitiorum. Ideoque tempora penitentie pro fide et conuersatione penitentium abbreuianda precipiuntur, et pro neglegentia
protelanda [*Lombard*, D.20, c.3, p.376].

prefigunt] prefigurat *C*   unumquodque ... sit] emendenda sunt *V*   in-
telligentis] intelligentes *B*   quia] quod *B*   tam] tantum *V*   quam]
quantum *V*   tantum *om. PV*   quantum] quam *P*   pro²] per *P*

Antidotvm spiritvale

Vt medici curant uario medicamine corpus,
105 Non sanat febrem quod uulnus siue tumorem,
Sic anime uarias egre poscunt medicinas.
Opponas igitur anime contraria[a] morbis:
Propria det cupidus, se castret luxuriosus;
Inuide liuorem depone, superbe tumorem;
110 Sobrietasque gulam, patientia reprimat iram;
Amoueat lesus rancorem, tedia mestus;
Potus aque redimat excessus ebrietatis;
Carnis delicias castiget uirga flagellans.
Vt bene peniteat ablatum predo reponat.

103 Antidotum spirituale] *om. ALP*: De antidoto spirituali *V*   103-
114 Antidotum ... reponat *om. K*   104 Vt] Et *B*   105 Non sanat]
Nunc sanent *A*: Infirmans *C (in ras.)*: Nunc sanat *V*   quod] nunc *AV*
106 poscunt] possunt *C*   Contraria contrariis curantur *add. O (rubr.)*
107 morbis] morbos *O*   108 castret] castet *AC*   110 reprimat] deleat
A: comprimat *O*   112 ebrietatis] ebrietates *A*: ebrietatum *P*   113 cas-
tiget] castigat *P*   flagellans] flagellas *O*   114 Augustinus, non dimittitur
peccatum nisi reddatur ablatum *add. O (rubr.)*

a Super Leuiticum lxxxiii [*Glossa*, ad Lev 25:27]: Secundum ea que
peccauerit homo, oportet pretium reddi: quod gula peccauerit ieiunium
corrigat, quod garrulitas amisit silentium doleat, et similiter contraria
contrariis curantur.

Super] Vt medici super *P*   lxxxiii] lxxx *B*: *om. P*   peccauerit¹] peccant
B   peccauerit²] peccauit *B*   garrulitas] garuli *V*   amisit ... doleat]
admisit ... deleat *B*   et ... curantur *om. P*

115 *Ex uiridi ligno limphas calor exprimit ignis,
*Sic de corde pio lacrimas iacit ardor amoris.

*Nos quia peccati medicina semper egemus,
*Contra peccatum medicinam semper habemus.

*Culpa reo nox est, contrito gratia lux est.
120 *Obtenebrat culpa, dat lucida gratia corda.

*Sunt extrema crucis contriti quatuor ista:
*Spes[a] Dominique timor[b] ac festinatio,[c] finis.[d]

> 115 Confessio *add. KL (rubr.)*   115-122 Ex ... finis *om. ABPV*
> 117 medicina ... egemus *om. C*   118 Contra peccatum *om. C*   122 Spes ...
> finis *om. K*

> a In Dei misericordia et de uenia.

> b Propter imperfectum, ne scilicet nondum perfecte penituerit, uel
> recidauerit.
>> Propter] semper *L*   uel recidauerit] et recidiuum *KL*

> c Propter septem pericula que sunt consuetudo peccandi, ruina de
> peccato in peccatum, mors subitanea, egritudo corporalis, purgatio
> diutina in purgatorio, difficultas uere penitendi, erubescentia confitendi
> [cf. *Cantor*, c.149 cols.355-358].

> d Id est consummatio. Christus et Andreas renuunt in corpore uiui. De
> cruce deponi, tu penas in cruce fini.
>> uiui] ui *C*   deponi] poni *C*

*QVIBUS PVNITVR PECCATVM

*Sit tibi potus aqua, cibus aridus, aspera uestis,
125 *Dorso uirga, breuis somnus durumque cubile.
*Flecte genu, tunde pectus, nuda caput, orans,
*Hereat os terre, mens celo, lingua loquatur,
*Cor dictet. Sit larga manus, ieiunia crebra,
*Mens humilis, simplex oculus, caro munda, pium cor,
130 *Recta fides, spes firma; duplex dilectio semper
*Ferueat; assiduis precibus, iustis tamen, ora.
*Hec age peccator quem uere penitet. A te
*Tu potius penas peccatis exige dignas
*Quam te perpetuis addicat iudicis ira.

> 123 Quibus ... peccatum] *om. C*: Austeritas penitentis *K*: Austeritas uite
> penitentis *L*   123-134 Quibus ... ira *om. ABPV*   128 dictet] ditet *C*
> 132 Hec] Hoc *O*   penitet. A te] peniteat te *C*   133 Tu] Vt *C*

QVE SVNT ATTENDENDA IN SATISFACTIONE

Vestio,[a] poto,[b] cibo,[c] tectum do,[d] uisito,[e] soluo,[f]
Commodo,[g] compatior,[h] conuerto,[i] dono,[j] remitto,[k]
Arguo,[l] consulo, supplico, do quodcumque talentum.[m]
Flecto genu,[n] uigilo,[o] ieiuno,[p] laboro,[q] flagellor,[r]
140 Vestio dura,[s] pedes nudor,[t] tero cor,[u] peregrinor.[v]
Peniteo,[w] lego,[x] ploro,[y] precor,[z] caro sic maceratur.
Hiis que confessis sint iniungenda notabis:
Publica[aa] sit pena, fuerit si publica noxa;[bb]
Si lateat licet enormis, lateat quoque pena.
145 Hoc est, qui peccat occulte, peniteat clam.
Singula confessor prudentius ut moderetur,
Affectus[cc] causa, uitium,[dd] persona[ee] notetur.

135 Que ... satisfactione] *om. AP*: Opera misericordie *K*: Septem opera misericordie *L*: Sex opera caritatis *O*   136 Quo defunctus eget non tua cura neget. *add. KL*   137 Commodo] Hoc modo *P*   138 Arguo ... talentum *om. APV*   consulo supplico] supplico consulo *O*   139-145 Flecto ... clam *om. K*   flagellor] flagello *L*   140 Vestio] Induo *L*   peregrinor *om. P*   141 sic] ne *B*   maceratur] miseratur *C*   142 sint] sunt *AP*: sic *V*   Quod pena debet esse quandoque occulta et quandoque manifesta *add. O*   143 fuerit] fiunt *A*   144 lateat²] latet *B*   146 Singula] Vincula *B*   Singula confessor] Hec igitur cuncta *KL*   147 Affectus] Actus *P*   notetur] uetetur *C*   *explicit B*

a Nudum. Cum uideris nudum operi eum [cf. Mt 25:36].
    Nudum] Nudus *B*

b Sitientem. Si sitit, potum da illi [Rom 12:20].
    Sitientem] Sciciens *B*

c Esurientem. Si esurierit inimicus tuus ciba illum [Rom 12:20].
    Esurientem] Esuriens *B*

d Peregrinum. Egenos uagosque induc in domum tuam, exemplo Abrahe [Gen 18:1-5] et Loth [Gen 19:1-29]; et Iob xxvi [31:32]: Foris non mansit peregrinus, etc.
    Peregrinum] Peregrinus *B*   induc *om. V*   et Iob ... etc. *om. P*   xxvi *om. B*

e Infirmum. Infirmus eram et uisitastis me [Mt 25:36].
    Infirmum] Infirmus *B*: Infirmos *CP*

f Vinctum a carcere. In carcere eram et uenistis ad me [Mt 25:36].
    Vinctum a carcere] Vinctus et in carcere *B*   eram] fui *V*

g Iustus tota die miseretur et commodat [Ps 36:26]. Item [Ps 111:5]:

Iocundus homo qui miseretur et commodat; et Mattheo iiii [5:42]: Qui petit a te da ei.

> *om. P*   Iustus] Intus *C*

h Item Iob xxvi [30:25]: Flebam super eo qui afflictus erat et compatiebatur anima mea pauperi.Apostolus, secunda ad Corinthios [2 Cor 11:29]: Quis infirmatur, etc.; et Ecclesiastico xxvi [7:38]: Non desis plorantibus in consolatione etc.

> *om. P*   Item Iob xxvi] *om. B*: Item Iob *V*   eo] eum *C*   Apostolus
> *om. BC*   secunda ad Corinthios] *om. P*: xxvi *V*   et Ecclesiastico xxvi
> *om. C*

i Iacobus [5:20]: Qui conuerti fecerit peccatorem ab errore uie sue, saluabit animam eius a morte.

> Iacobus *om. BCP*

j Quod superest date elemosinam et ecce omnia munda sunt uobis [Lc 11:41].

k Item [Lc 6:37-8]: Dimittite et dimittemini. Date et dabitur uobis. Ecclesiastico lxxiiii [cf. 28:1-2].

> Dimittite ... dimittemini *om. P*   Ecclesiastico lxxiiii] *om. B*: Ecclesiastico
> lxxxiiii *C*

l   Argue, obsecra, increpa in omni patientia et doctrina [2 Tim 4:2]. Prouerbia xxvii [24:25]: Qui arguunt laudabuntur et super eos ueniet benedictio.

> Argue ...benedictio *om. PV*   Prouerbia xxvii *om. B*   laudabuntur]
> laudabunt *B*

m Ad multiplicandum.

> Ad multiplicandum *om. PV*

n Vnde in Actibus apostolorum [7:59]: Stephanus positis genibus, etc. Luca xix [22:41]; Michea xvi [6:6].

> Vnde ... Stephanus] *om. P*: Dominus *BC*   Luca ... xvi] *om. P*: Mc
> xvi *V*

o Dominus pernoctans erat in oratione [Lc 6:12]. Deus Deus meus, ad te de luce uigilo [Ps 62:2].

p Vt Moyses [Ex 34:28] et Helyas [3 Reg 19:8], Christus [Mt 4:2] et Anna [Lc 2:36-37]. Item [Mt 17:20; Mc 9:28]: Hoc genus demonii in nullo potest eicere nisi in oratione et ieiunio.

> demonii ... eicere] demoniorum non potest eici *P*: non eicitur *V*   eicere]
> euenire *C*

q Laboraui in gemitu meo [Ps 6:7]. Item: Vide humilitatem meam et laborem meum [Ps 24:18], dicat penitens.

> in] cum *C*   Item ... penitens *om. P*   laborem ... penitens] eripe me
> *V*   dicat penitens] dicit penitenti *B*

r Apprehendite disciplinam etc. [Ps 2:12]. Item: Pro mensura peccati
   et plagarum modus, Deut c. xxxi [25:2].

   Apprehendite] Apprehende *PV*   Deut c. xxxi] Deuteronomium *P*: *om. V*

s Vt Iohannes baptista habens uestimentum de pilis camelorum [Mt 3:4].
   Iob xvi [16:16]: Saccum.

   Iob ... saccum *om. P*

t Vt Moyses cui dixit Dominus [Ex 3:5]: Solue calceamentum de pedibus
   tuis. Isaia liiii [20:2].

   Dominus *om. C*   tuis ... liiii *om. V*

u Psalmista [Ps 50:19]: Cor contritum et humiliatum Deus non despiciet.
   Daniele viii [3:39]: Set in anima contrita.

   Psalmista *om. BCP*   Daniel ... contrita *om. PV*   viii] fere m. co.
   add. B   Set] si *C*

v Vt eunuchus qui uenit adorare in Ierusalem [Act 8:27].

   eunuchus] ethnicus *V*   qui uenit] quieuit *V*   qui ... Ierusalem *om. P*

w A penitentia sermonem incohat Iohannes baptista (Mattheo ii) [3:1-2],
   et Iesus (Mattheo iii) [4:17], Apostoli [Act 2:38].

   sermonem incohat] sermones inchoant *B*   Mattheo ii ... Apostoli] Marc
   iii *add. B*: Mt ii, iiii, apostoli, Mt. v, Vnde *C*: *om. P*: Apoc. ii, Marcus v,
   Iohannes iii *V*

x Super Lucam xvi: Nihil tam accepta Deo quam meditatio legis cum
   executione operis.

   Super Lucam xvi *om. P*   Lucam] n *B*: enim *C*   tam] tamen *C*
   accepta] acceptum *PV*

y Beati qui lugent, etc. [Mt 5:5]. Item: Lacrime lauant delictum.

z Sine intermissione orate [1 Thess 5:17].
   ieiunium domatur *add. C*

aa Id est penitentia iniuncta.
   om. P   penitentia *om. B*

bb Super Mattheum ix, Iohanne iiii, [*Glossa* ad Mc 5:43]: Publica noxa
   publico eget remedio; leuis et secreta leuiori, et secreta potest deleri
   penitentia.

   Super ... iiii *om. P*   Iohanne iiii] iiii.iii.f. *B*: et iiii, inferri *C*   leuis
   et secreta] leuis *B*: Peccata leuis *C*: secreta uel priuata *V*

cc Id est intentio.
   om. P

dd Considerandum est an peccatum sit ueniale an mortale, utrum publicum
   uel occultum, si scienter uel nescienter, si sponte uel non sponte
   commissum, si cum deliberatione uel non, si sola cogitatione uel
   locutione uel opere [*Barth*, c.26, p.194].

nescienter] non *PV*   sponte commissum *om. PV*   si sola] *om. B*: si commissum sit sola *V*

ee Attendendum est de penitente utrum liber sit an seruus; si clericus, si laicus, si monachus. Si clericus, cuius ordinis sit et cuius dignitatis. Si laicus, an coniugatus uel sine coniugio. Item si penitens sit diues uel pauper; si puer uel adolescens; si uir uel etate senex; si hebes uel gnarus; si sanus uel infirmus; si uirgo uel corrupta; si continens uel incontinens; si officium gerat quod sine peccato administrari possit uel non. Et ex hiis relique penitentium differentie perpendantur, secundum quas augenda est uel minuenda penitentia, ita scilicet ut cui plus commissum est plus exigatur ab eo [*Barth*, c.25, p.194].

et cuius] aut *V*   uel sine coniugio] uel non *C*   etate senex] etate uel sexu *PV*   gnarus] etate gnarus *C*   Si sanus ... corrupta *om. B* infirmus] eger *P*: Si uir uel mulier *add. C*   gerat] gerens *PV*   differentie] differe *B*   quas] quos *B*: quo *C*   exigatur] exigitur *C*   eo] illo *V* et cui minus minus *add. P*

*Mos,[a] cumulus,[b] mors[c] et morbus,[d] rubor[e] acta fatendi,
*Difficilisque salus,[f] purgatio dura per ignem,[g]
150 *Detenta culpa[h] tardanti[i] sunt metuenda.
*Accelerent nos conuerti,[j] deflere[k] reatus:
*Horror duritie,[l] grauitatis,[m] mortis[n] et ignis,[o]
*Temporis[p] ac operum[q] lucrum cum celicolarum[r]
*Plausu, Tartarei confusio[s] multa ministri,[t]
155 *Et fuga Cocyti[u] felix, et adeptio celi.[v]

148 Attendas cur peniteas et quomodo, quando *precedit in K*   Mos] Mors *C*   148-150 Mos ... metuenda *om. ABLPV*   149 purgatio] purgato *C*   150 Detenta] Detento *KO*   tardanti] tardendi *C*: tardandi *K*   Vt cito peniteat peccanti sunt memoranda *add. K*   151 Accelerent ... reatus] Cur acceleranda sit penitentia *V (rubr.)*   151-155 Accelerant ... celi *om. ABPV*   152 duritie] diuicie *C*   153-154 Temporis ... celicolarum] *ll. 131-132 rev. O*   ac] hac *C*   155 adeptio] adoptio *O*

a Consuetudo insconsa.
   om. C

b Accumulatio peccatorum succedentium.
   om. C

c Incerta uel preoccupans.
   om. C

d Ventrem absorbens.
   om. C

e Erubescentia confitendi.
   om. C

f Sicut curatio uulneris diutina.
    om. C

g Purgatorium.
    om. C

h Mortali.
    om. C

i Penitere.
    om. C

j Ad Deum.

k Hoc est penitere, quia penitere est ante acta deflere, et deflenda non committere.

l Ne tradat Deus hominem in reprobum sensum [cf. Rom 1:28].
    tradat] tardet *C*

m Quia peccatum pondere suo trahit ad aliud.

n Que est fur perfodiens domum [cf. Mt 24:43].
    perfodiens] fodens *C*

o Gehennalis uel purgatorii.

p Conserua tempus [Eccli 4:23].
    tempus] corpus *C*

q Si hec et hec fecero, caritatem autem non habeam, nihil mihi prodest [cf. 1 Cor 13:1-3].
    autem *om. KL*

r Gaudium erit coram angelis super uno penitente [cf. Lc 15:7].
    coram angelis *om. C*   penitente] peccatore penitentiam agente *C*

s Draco iste quem formasti ad illudendum ei [Ps 103:26].

t Cuius diutina machinatio cassatur, rete rumpitur, et ipse superatur.
    cassatur] cessator *C*   rete] rite *C*

u Quis ostendet uobis fugere a uentura ira? Facite ergo fructus dignos penitentie [Mt 3:7-8; cf. Lc 3:8], id est, uitatio gehenne. Dicitur autem Cocytus fluuius inferni, et interpretatur luctus. Iob. xx, in fine.
    Facite] Facito *C*   uitatio] uisitatio *C*

v Vnde [Mt 4:17]: Penitentiam agite, appropinquabit enim regnum celorum.

156 Ad Dominum festinandi[a] sunt hee tibi[b] cause:
  Ignis purificans,[c] mors,[d] egritudo[e] ruborque,[f]
  Et cure grauitas,[g] et consuetudo,[h] ruina.[i]

156 sunt] sint *AKV*   hee] hec *C*   156-158 Ad ... ruina *om. BL*
158 et² *om. C*

a Scilicet per penitentiam et confessionem.
     om. P

b Scilicet peccatori.
     om. P

c Grauis.
     om. P

d Fur.
     om. P

e Turbans.
     om. P

f Nude confitendi.
     Nude confitendi] confitendi *P*

g Satisfactionis. Vt sint condigni fructus penitentie.

h Lapis super Lazarum [cf. Io 11:38-39; *Cantor*, c.149, p.356].
     Lapis] lapsis *V*

i De peccato in peccatum; ut fiat longa restis [cf. *Cantor*, ibid.].
     fiat] sit *P*

II.2

Errorum eliminatio

William's treatise "for eliminating errors in those things that are read and sung in the Church," provides an unusual and fascinating glimpse into popular beliefs and liturgical practices at the end of the twelfth century. He begins the treatise with a discussion of errors arising in the day-to-day celebration of Church rites (section 1), and then solves various grammatical, metrical, and textual problems arising from Psalter readings (section 2). Sections 3 and 4 treat the chants and hymns of the liturgy. Prayers of confession, absolution, and intercession are discussed in section 5, and questions arising from the Epistle and Gospel readings in sections 6 and 7. Section 8, on Prefaces, completes William's discussion of errors "in those things that are read and sung in the Church." He then discusses briefly some of the errors and superstitions to be found among the laity (section 9). The reference in paragraph 14 to lay persons who "adore the elevated host as if it were Christ" is perhaps the earliest reference to the popular "desire to see the host" in the Middle Ages.[1] One of William's students, Richard of Wetheringsett, later developed this ninth section into an extended treatise in his popular *Summa Qui bene presunt*.[2] Apparently as an afterthought, William appended a tenth section that returns to a discussion "concerning those things that are sung in the Church."[3]

---

[1] See E. Dumoutet, *Le désir de voir l'hostie et les origines de la dévotion au saint sacrement* (Paris: Beauchesne, 1926); Vincent L. Kennedy, "The Moment of Consecration and the Elevation of the Host," *Mediaeval Studies* 6 (1944) 122-123 and n. 8.

[2] On the *Qui bene presunt* see Chapter Three. In MS Royal 9.A.xiv of the British Library, London, Richard's treatment of the errors of the laity begins on fol. 104v: "Sequitur de erroribus laycorum a quibus sunt cohibendi, qui sic possunt retineri:
In quibus erratur sunt hostia, gleba, repertum ... ."
It concludes on folio 108r.

[3] This chapter, "De hiis que cantantur in ecclesia," is omitted in MSS 2 and 3, below, but its presence in the independent witnesses of MSS 1 and 4 suggests that it is authentic.

Although commentaries and explications of the Mass abounded in the twelfth and thirteenth centuries, William's *Errorum eliminatio* bears little resemblance to any of these.[4] It is an unusual example of an important scholastic activity — the study of the Church's liturgy and rites as theological documents. Artur Landgraf drew attention to this activity in a brief communication concerning "Scholastische Texte zur Liturgie des 12. Jahrhunderts."[5] Citing a number of occasional arguments concerning the liturgy found in various *summae*, scriptural commentaries, and sentence commentaries, Landgraf argued that such texts, although rare, are important for reconstructing the idiosyncracies of local liturgical practices as well as for investigating the influence of scholastic/dogmatic theology on the liturgy.

Two examples noted by Landgraf concerning the Parisian liturgy are echoed in William's *Errorum eliminatio*. The first is found in a twelfth-century gloss on Lombard's Sentences in MS VII C 14 of the Biblioteca Nazionale in Naples, and should be compared with the first paragraph in section 3 of William's text:

> Sed miror, quare ecclesia Parisiensis ultimum "Sanctus" in eadem distinctione et prolatione iungat cum eo quod sequitur "Dominus Deus Sabaoth." Alie enim ecclesie non ita faciunt, immo una pars chori dicat primum "Sanctus" et altera pars secundum "Sanctus," et iterum illa pars que dicit secundum "Sanctus" dicit "Dominus Deus Sabaoth." Sed in ecclesia Parisiensi illa pars chori, que dicit tertium "Sanctus," dicit etiam "Dominus Deus Sabaoth." Et potest fieri hac ratione, ut ostendatur, quod istud, scilicet "Dominus Deus Sabaoth" eidem precedentia spectat, et preterea ideo, ut sicut ibi Trinitas insinuatur, ita tantummodo trina prolatio fiat.[6]

A second example noted by Landgraf, in MS Vat. lat. 10754 in the Vatican Library written at the end of the twelfth century, concerns the hymn *Nunc sancte nobis Spiritus*, and can be compared with William's discussion of the hymn in paragraph 6 of section 4:

---

[4] Cf. Honorius Augustodunensis, *Gemma animae* (PL 172: 541-738); *Iohannis Beleth Summa de ecclesiasticis officiis*, ed. Heribert Douteil, 2 vols., CCL 41, 41a (Turnhout: Brepols, 1976); Innocent III, *De sacro altaris mysterio* (PL 217: 773-914); Peter of Roissy, *Manuale de mysteriis ecclesiae* (see V.L. Kennedy, "The Handbook of Master Peter Chancellor of Chartres," pp. 1-50); *Praepositini Cremonensis Tractatus de officiis*, ed. James A. Corbett (Notre Dame IN: University of Notre Dame Press, 1969); Guy of Orchelles, *Summa de officiis ecclesiae* (see V.L. Kennedy, "The 'Summa de officiis ecclesiae' of Guy d'Orchelles," *Mediaeval Studies* 1 [1939] 23-62).

[5] *Ephemerides liturgicae* 45 (1931) 211-214.

[6] Ibid., p. 213.

Nos autem dicimus quod hoc nomen unus aliquando exclusive, aliquando distinctive ponitur, aliquando ponitur essentialiter. Distinctive ut dictum est: Pater est unus, Filius est unus. Exclusive, ut Pater et Filius et Spiritus Sanctus sunt unus, id est non sunt plures. Essentialiter duobus modis: primo quando subiective ponitur per subintellectum articuli, ut cum dicitur: Pater et Filius et Spiritus Sanctus sunt omnipotens, iustus et huiusmodi. Unde dicimus, quod bene dicitur: Nunc sancte nobis Spiritus, unus Patri cum Filio. Quidam vero dicunt, ut magister Petrus Lombardus, quod debet dici: unum cum Filio Patri. Unde in quibusdam ecclesiis ita dicitur, scilicet in Parisiensi. Unde quidam sic exponunt: Cum dicitur unus Patri et Filio, id est una spiratione spiratur a Patre et Filio. Vel sic: Unus Patri cum Filio id est equalis Patri et Filio, vel communis Patri et Filio, vel subintelligitur Spiritus.[7]

Both examples illustrate an interest in liturgical texts and practices as matters for scholastic inquiry and theological clarification. The traditional axiom "lex orandi lex credendi" finds its twelfth-century expression in these and other passages of William's treatise. Landgraf notes the rarity of such texts in which liturgical practices are used to solve theological questions on the one hand, and theological principles are invoked to alter the shape of local liturgies on the other.[8] A proper appreciation of William's *Errorum eliminatio* and its historical context must await a systematic study of many other neglected treatises, but William's work is an outstanding example of this genre.

AUTHENTICITY AND DATE

Two of the four extant copies ascribe the work to William de Montibus, and the other copies bear no ascription. Internal evidence confirms the ascription to William. Of particular note is the blessing of infirm eyes (*oculorum infirmorum*) presented in the last paragraph of section 1. The author introduces this ritual blessing in a way to suggest that it is a new liturgical formula rather than an existing one in need of

---

[7] Ibid., pp. 213-214. On the text of the hymn see Guido Maria Dreves, *Hymnographi Latini: Lateinische Hymnengedichter des Mittelalters*, in Analecta hymnica medii aevi, 2nd series (1907) 50: 19-20.

[8] "Unbekannt dürfte aber bis heute geblieben sein, dass man im Mittelalter und zwar bereits in den Zeiten der Frühscholastik aus den Feinheiten der Liturgie scholastische Fragen zu lösen versuchte und dass umgekehrt die einseitige Stellungnahme in einer scholastischen Streitfrage den Anlass bot für Aenderungen in den liturgischen Werken einzelner Provinzen. Texte dieser Art finden sich allerdings selten genug, und aus diesem Grund möchte ich diejenigen, welche mir aufstiessen, hier mitteilen." Landgraf, "Scholastische Texte," pp. 212-213.

correction or emendation. The blessing did, in fact, find its way into
several liturgical handbooks containing sacerdotal blessings, and manuscripts not only in England but also in Germany ascribe it to William
de Montibus.[9]

Several circumstances suggest that the work was composed at Paris,
or shortly after William moved to England in the 1180's. One is the
existence of similar types of scholastic discussions to be found scattered
among twelfth-century writings connected with Paris. A second indication of an early date of composition is the presence, rare among
William's extant writings, of one and possibly two references to his
own teachers. The first is in paragraph five of section seven: "sed hoc
non approbant magistri nostri." The second, in the final paragraph
of the work, refers vaguely to the wiser masters: "ut aiunt magistri
saniores." Neither of the opinions has been identified, but the issues
being debated point toward a date early in the second half of the twelfth
century rather than later. In any case, the fact that William refers to
his own masters at all would suggest that the work was written early
in his career, and before he became a respected authority in his own
right.

SOURCES

The basic source for this work is the Church's liturgy as practised
and understood in William's day. The prayers and hymns mentioned
here can be identified in various editions of pre-Tridentine missals,
manuals, and hymnaries,[10] but the specific liturgical use(s) that William
has in mind remains unidentified.

In addition to the opinions of his own masters noted above, William
refers explicitly to a number of authorities. Most prominent is the
Glossa ordinaria on the Bible. In a few instances William acknowledges

---

[9] *Manuale ad usum percelebris ecclesiae Sarisburiensis*, ed. Arthur J. Collins, HBS
91 (London, 1960), p. 69; Christopher Wordsworth and Henry Littlehales, *The Old
Service-Books of the English Church* (London: Methuen, 1904), p. 235; Adolph Franz,
Die kirchlichen Benediktionen im Mittelalter (1909; rept. Graz: Akademische Druck,
1960), 2: 496.

[10] See *Missale Romanum Mediolani, 1474*, ed. Robert Lippe, 2 vols., HBS 17, 33
(London, 1899, 1907); *The Sarum Missal Edited from Three Early Manuscripts*, ed.
John Wickham Legg (Oxford: Clarendon Press, 1916); *Manuale ... Sarisburiensis*; *The
Gilbertine Rite*, ed. Reginald Maxwell Wooley, 2 vols., HBS 59-60 (London, 1921-
1922); *The Canterbury Hymnal*, ed. Gernot R. Wieland, Toronto Medieval Latin Texts,
12 (Toronto: Pontifical Institute of Mediaeval Studies, 1982). No comparable editions
of the Parisian liturgy and rites in William's day are available for consultation.

other scriptural glosses. He cites both Peter Lombard's and Gilbert of Poitiers's gloss on the Psalms (section 2, paragraph 2), and certain "glossed books" concerning a text of Ecclesiasticus (section 6, paragraph 15).

Most of William's references to the Church Fathers come from the *Glossa ordinaria*, but he quotes accurately from sermons of Gregory the Great and Augustine in section 6, paragraph 16.

Implicit references to debates and opinions in the twelfth-century schools abound, but few can be identified with certainty. The reference in section 1, paragraph 9 to those who believe that the soul of Christ is his divinity can be compared to *sententiae* from the school of Gilbert of Poitiers,[11] as can the opinion, *secundum quosdam*, concerning bad works and good works as causes of damnation and salvation in section 10, paragraph 2.[12]

MANUSCRIPTS

1. Cambridge, Peterhouse MS 255, fols. 133va-137ra. Early 13th century (above top line). Printed below.

2. Oxford, Bodleian Library MS Add. C. 263 (sc 27646), fols. 115rb-118ra. Early 13th century (above top line).
   Inc. Prol.: *Ad eliminandum quorundam errores*
   Inc. Txt.: *Decollatio Iohannis baptiste*
   Expl.: *nisi restituatur ablatum si restitui potest.*
   Colophon: *Explicit errorum quorundam eleminatio* (sic).
The text has neither rubrics nor clear divisions of subject matter. It omits some of the material in the other MSS, and arranges other material idiosyncratically.

3. Oxford, Bodleian Library MS Laud lat. misc. 345 (sc 1273), fols. 15ra-18va. 14th century.
   Title: *De eliminacione errorum.*
   Inc. Prol.: *Ad eliminandum quorundam errores*
   Inc. Txt.: *Decollacio sancti Johannis Baptiste*
   Expl.: *nisi restituatur ablatum si restitui potest.*

---

[11] See Nicholaus Häring, "Die *Sententie magistri Gisleberti Pictavensis Episcopi*," *Archives d'histoire doctrinale et littéraire du moyen âge* 45 (1978) 125 and 126 (nos. 14 and 19).

[12] In his lectures *Super Psalmos* William attributes this "sentence" to Gilbert (Oxford, Bodleian Library MS Bodley 860, fol. 88vb).

Colophon: *Explicit liber magistri Willelmi de Montibus de errorum eliminacione.*

4. Paris, Bibliothèque Mazarine MS 730, fols. 67v-68r. Early 13th century (above top line).

Title: *Incipit errorum elim<in>atio, de hiis que fiunt in ecclesia.*
Inc. Prol.: *Ad eliminandum quorundam errores*
Inc. Txt.: *Decollatio Iohannis baptiste*
Expl. (imperfect in section 10): *Feria sexta in ieiunio quatuor temporum.*
A note on the bottom of fol. 68v, in a slightly later hand, reads: "Dicit beatus Franscicus in vita sua: Qui pauperi maledicit Christo iniuriam facit."

William's *Errorum eliminatio* is printed here from Cambridge, Peterhouse MS 255, the most complete and careful copy. Emendations and expansions, printed within angle brackets, are drawn from the consensus of the other manuscripts and from the text of the liturgy, when, for example, the incipit of a liturgical passage is not given.

Errorum eliminatio

Incipit Errorum eliminatio.
Ad eliminandum quorundam errores de hiis que in ecclesia leguntur et cantantur, quedam in unum breuiter compegimus in hunc modum.

1 DE HIIS QVE FIVNT IN ECCLESIA

5 Decollatio sancti Iohannis baptiste celebratur in ecclesia quando capud eius inuentum est, sed circa pascha decollatus est.

Michael pungnauit cum dracone, id est diabolo, non cum aliquo dracone corporali et uisibili.

Albis indutus sacerdos ad altare dicens "confiteor Deo" etc. credit
10 se mundum esse, cum penitere sit ante acta deflere et flenda non committere.

Credunt crismale proferendum ante tribunal Christi.

Puerpere dant post missam in purificatione panem benedictum et
in die ieiunii, <uel> dant eukaristiam non precurrente confessione.
15 Non iniungunt fidem uel iuramentum uel uotum obseruare, sed
permittunt stultis ista agere: transgredi et penitentiam agere.
Paciscuntur in tricennariis.
Falsas iniungunt penitentias et non competentes.
Credunt animam Christi nihil aliud esse quam eius deitatem, cum
20 anima tristis et a corpore recessit.
Benedictio oblationum post ewangelium ex radice cupiditatis uel ex
uitio adulationis processit, et ideo non est facienda. Neque enim habetur
ex auctoritate, nec ex prelatorum consuetudine, nec uerba ad hoc sunt
instituta; Apostoli [Act 4:35] etiam nec tangere dignati sunt, sed ad
25 pedes proici fecerunt, calcandumque docet quod subdunt gressibus
aurum. Item sic uilificatur benedictio sacerdotalis cum adeo sollempniter
fiat super reprobam monetam sicut super eukaristiam, ita affectuose
super quadrantem sicut super calicem.
Benedictionem uero oculorum infirmorum neccesitas inducit et
30 deuotio postulantium, et potest fieri in hunc modum: Domine Ihesu
Christe qui aperuisti oculos ceci nati, serena (uel sana) oculos huius
famuli tui (uel -le tue, uel -orum, uel -arum), dans in eis uisum
perspicacem, sufficientem, idoneum, et competentem in obsequium
tuum, per uirtutem huius sacramenti, et per hoc signum sancte crucis
35 tue. In nomine Patris et Filii et Spiritus sancti, amen. Hoc autem
signum crucis faciat sacerdos cum corporali, et eodem uentilet in oculis
eius, cum dicit "In nomine Patris et Filii et Spiritus sancti, amen."

2 DE PSALTERIO

"Saturati sunt filiis" [Ps 16:14], ablatiui casus.
40 "Sicut letantium" [86:7], hic debet fieri distinctio secundum magnam
glosaturam, scilicet magistri Petri Lumbardi; secundum uero glosaturam
magistri Giliberti Porretani dicetur coniunctim "sicut letantium omnium," et tunc fiet distinctio quam quidam uocant metrum.
"Prope es tu Domine" [118:151], et non "esto."
45 "Si memor fui tui" [62:7], et non "sic."
"Sicut in exitu super summum" [73:5], et non "sompnum."
"Minuisti eum paulo minus ab angelis" [8:6]. Hic sunt due dictiones,
"paulo" et "minus," ut patet in Glosa; sed cum dicitur "paulominus
consummauerunt me in terra" [118:87], hic est una dictio, et est sensus
50 paulominus fere consumpnauerunt, hoc est pene destruxerunt.
"Et aures eius in preces eorum" [33:16], non "ad." Vnde ibi Glosa

dicit: Nota quod non ait "ad preces" sed "in preces," in quo notatur celeritas audiendi.

"Et edificentur muri Ierusalem" [50:20]; "Et non dominetur mei
55 omnis iniustitia" [118:133], <non> "ut."

"Ne tradas bestiis (id est diabolo et angelis eius) animam confitentem tibi" [73:19]. Glosa: Que penitens confitetur peccata. Potest tamen in exequiis defunctorum licite dici: "Ne tradas, Domine, bestiis animas confitentes tibi" sicut singulariter legitur in Psalmo: "In memoria eterna
60 erit iustus" etc. [111:7], et tamen in exequiis pluraliter dicitur "in memoria eterna erunt iusti."

"Memor ero Raab et Babilonis" [86:4] id est gentium. Memor dico scientibus me, id est Apostolis, qui<bus> de illis recipiendis precipiam, sicut diceret aliquis: Memor esto negotii tui, illi scilicet precipiendo
65 ut curet de eo.

"Et eduxit eos in argento et auro" [104:37], uel "cum argento et auro." Nam ponitur "in" pro "cum," more scripture. Ita habetur in Glosa.

"Sacerdotes tui induantur iustitia" [131:9], non -am, nam Glosa
70 suplet "et aliis uirtutibus."

"Laudate nomen <Domini>; laudate, serui, Dominum" [134:1], non "Deum." Nam Glosa suplet: quia serui estis, laudate Dominum.

"Nolite confidere in principibus (id est in angelis, siue bonis siue malis) neque in filiis hominum (id est in hominibus quibuscumque)
75 in quibus non est salus" (id est a quibus) [145:2-3]. Non enim sunt auctores salutis; homines et angeli ministri sunt, solus Deus auctor est.

"Et super dolorem uulnerum eorum addiderunt" [68:27] (et "meorum"), neutri generis, uel masculini generis.
80 "Et inhabitabunt ibi, et hereditate <uel -tem> adquirent eam" [68:36].

"Ego uero egenus et mendicus et pauper sum; Deus adiuua (uel -uat) me" [69:6].

"Adiutor meus et liberator meus esto (uel es tu) Domine ne moreris" [69:6].

85 "Et exultabit lingua mea iustitiam tuam" [50:16], id est cum exultatione annuntiabit. Anselmus ait: Semicocti gramatici emendauerunt exaltabit.

"Similis factus sum pellicano" [101:7], penultima corripitur. Vnde: Non sunt concordes pellicanus et sua proles.

90 "Illuminans (uel -nas) tu mirabiliter" etc. [75:5].

"Immittet angelus Domini in circuitu timentium eum" [33:8], id est immissionem faciet, cum alia translatio habet: "Circumdat angelus

Domini in giro timentes eum, et eruet eos." Ita dicitur: "Numquid irascetur per singulos dies" [7:12], et tamen alia litera habet: "Numquid
95 adducit iram per singulos dies."

"Et in mandatis eius uolet nimis" [111:1], tamen alia littera habet "cupit nimis," et ita in diuersis translationibus sunt uerba diuersorum temporum.

"Dixit Deus ex Basan, conuertam (uel -tar) in profundum (uel
100 -do, uel -dis) maris" [67:23].

"Viderunt ingressus tui (uel -os) Deus" [67:25].

"Sicut ablactatus super matre (uel -trem suam)" [130:2], utrumque habetur.

"Si non proposuero tui Ierusalem" [136:6], id est de te, uel "si non
105 proposuero te," quodlibet istorum congrue dicitur.

"Deficit in salutare tuum anima mea (id est tendens in Ihesum) et in uerbum tuum (id est in Filium tuum, uel in promissum tuum) supersperaui" [118:81].

"Mirabilia testimonia tua" [118:129], non habetur ibi "Domine."
110 "Mittit cristallum suum" [147:17], uel -am, neutri generis, uel feminini. Dicitur enim "hoc cristallum, huius cristalli" uel "hec cristallus, huius cristalli," sicut "hoc margaritum" et "hec margarita."

"Dixit iniustus ut delinquat" [35:2]. Sapiens enim dicit, id est proponit et promittit, ut non delinquat; stultus autem ut delinquat et
115 peccet.

"Vidi impium superexaltatum et eleuatum sicut cedros Libani" [36:35], uel "super cedrum Libani," utrumque habetur.

"Et numerum dierum meorum quis est" [38:5], uel "qui est," utrumque habetur.
120 "Euellet te de tabernaculo tuo" [51:7], uel "suo," utrumque dicitur.

"Fundatur exultatione uniuerse terre" [47:3]. Hic fiat distinctio quia ciuitas fundatur; deinde sequitur "mons," id est Iudei, et "latera aquilonis," id est gentes, sunt "ciuitas regis magni," id est Dei.

"Veniat illi (uel illis) laqueus quem ignorat (uel -rant), et captio quam
125 abscondit apprehendat eum (uel eos), et in laqueum cadat (uel -dant) in ipsum (uel in ipso)" [34:8]; et nota quod "abscondit" singulariter dicitur cum precedat "illis" pluraliter quia plures sunt unum in malitia.

"Et oratio mea in sinum meum" [34:13], uel "sinu meo."

"Exurge et intende iudicium meum" [34:23], uel "-o meo."
130 "Iudica me secundum iustitiam tuam (uel meam) Domine Deus meus" [34:24].

"Nec dicant deuorauimus" [34:25], non deuorabimus; dicit enim ibi Glosa: Non dicit deuorabimus eum ut non resurgeret.

"Quoniam prospicit quod ueniat (uel ueniet) dies eius" [36:13].

135 "Inimici uero Domini mox ut honorificati fuerint" etc. [36:20], uel sine "ut," et tunc exponatur "mox" id est quam statim, sicut habetur in Glosa.

"Iustus autem miseretur et tribuet" [36:21], id est dabit, non retri-.

"In me sunt Deus uota tua que reddam laudationes (uel -nis) tibi" 140 [55:12].

"Apud Dominum gressus hominis dirigentur" [36:23], uel -getur.

"Cum ceciderit" [36:24], non habetur ibi "iustus," sed supletur homo "non collidetur" et cetera.

"In uoce exultationis et confessionis sonus (uel soni) epulantis" [41:5], 145 utrumque habetur.

"Ad me ipsum (uel me ipso) anima mea conturbatur" [41:7], utrumque dicitur.

"A templo tuo in Ierusalem, tibi offerunt reges munera" [67:30]. R<omanum Psalterium> habet "a templo tuo quod est in celo," et 150 hac litera utimur in cantu.

"Mirra, et gutta, et casia" [44:9], fistula scilicet que est arbor aromatica et parua; casia quidem herba est de qua non agitur hic.

"Rigans (uel -gas) montes de superioribus tuis (uel suis)" [103:13].

"Impleta est terra possessione tua" <uel sua> [103:24].

155 "Emitte (uel -tes) spiritum tuum et creabuntur" [103:30].

Non est dicendum "probatum terre" ut sequatur "repurgatum septuplum" [11:7], sed ut habetur in libro glosato: "probatum terre" id est a terra, scilicet nihil terrenitatis habens; et ponitur genitiuus hic pro ablatiuo, more Grecorum, et est "purgatum septuplum" id est 160 perfecte.

"Quoniam Dominus in generatione iusta est" [13:6], non "iuxta," nomen scilicet non aduerbium.

"Consilium inopis confudistis" [13:6], non -disti, pluraliter scilicet non singulariter.

165 In primo Psalmo "Dixit insipiens" habetur: "Cum auerterit Deus captiuitatem plebis sue" [13:7], in altero [52:7]: "Cum conuerterit."

"Memores erunt (uel memor ero, dicit ecclesia) nominis tui, Deus, in omni generatione et generationem" [44:18]. Ieronimus: Idemptitatem ponit casuum semper, uel ablatiui, uel acusatiui, nos uariamus sic: "in 170 generatione usque in generationem."

"Speciem Iacob quam (uel quem) dilexit" [46:5].

"Exultauit (uel -bit) cor meum in salutari tuo" [12:6].

"Defecerunt oculi mei dum spero in Deum meum" (uel -o meo) [68:4].

175   Pronuntiatio Psalterii partim metrica, partim melica, partim prosayca est, et ita mixta est, et ideo nihil officit secundum diuersas consuetudines in eadem ueritate diuersa pronuntiatio.

3 De cantv

Ab una parte chori dicatur "sanctus" et ab altera "sanctus," et iterum
180 a prima "sanctus." Deinde ab altera parte "Dominus Deus sabaoth," quia "sanctus" ibi ponitur personaliter, "Dominus Deus" essentialiter, et ideo non sunt coniunctim proferenda.

    "Venite exultemus Domino" [Ps 94:1]. Psalmus iste inuitat Iudeos ad fidem. Vnde in passione Domini, scilicet in exequiis Christi, non
185 cantatur quia tunc discipuli eius omnes ab eo recesserunt. In exequiis etiam nostris non cantatur quia defuncti nostri non sunt uocandi ad fidem, sed orandum est pro eis ut spem teneant quod fide crediderunt. Hic enim locus est credendi et merendi; in patria locus est fruendi et recipiendi.

190   "Quorum doctrina fulget ecclesia ut sole et luna." Doctrina quidem apostolica comparatur soli totum mundum illuminanti. Vnde "Deus, qui uniuersum mundum beati Pauli predicatione docuisti," etc.

    "Portantes facem et illuminantes patriam"; fax est uerbum Dei secundum illud in Parabolis [6:23]: "Mandatum lucerna est et lex, lux";
195 et in Ecclesiastico [48:1] dicitur: "Surexit Helyas propheta quasi ignis, et uerbum ipsius quasi facula ardebat."

    "Felicia nimium angelorum rutilant agmina," et non felix stat.

    "A rea uirga (id est peccatrice) stirpe prime matris Eue florens rosa processit Maria." Hoc est alibi dictum: "Sicut spina rosam genuit Iudea
200 Mariam."

    "Genuisti modo miro," non "more," quia non fuit consuetudo uirginem parere.

4 De hymnis

In festis alicuius abbatis sic cantetur: "Ihesu redemptor omnium, salus
205 et spes credentium."

    In translatione alicuius confessoris sic cantatur: "Iste confessor Domini sacratus, sobrius, castus, fuit" et sic deinceps.

    Quod quidam dicunt "Maria mater gratie," etc. alii non approbant dicentes quia sola diuina essentia mater est omnium gratiarum.

210   In festo uirginis non martyris cum cantatur "Virginis proles" subticeatur uersiculus ille: "Vnde nec mortem nec amica mortis seua

penarum genera pauescens, sanguine fuso meruit sacratum scandere celum." In alio quidem ymno de confessoribus: <"Iste confessor Domini sacratus ... .> Hodie letus meruit secreta scandere celi."

215 <"Exultet celum laudibus ... .> Nos sempiterni gaudii (non -is) <faciat esse compotes>," sicut dicitur "compos mentis," non mente.

"Nunc sancte nobis Spiritus unum Patri cum Filio," quia unum id est una res, id est una substantia, unus Deus sunt Pater et Filius et Spiritus sanctus; uel ita: "Nunc sancte nobis Spiritus unus Patris cum

220 Filio," id est una persona procedens a Patre et Filio. Non autem approbamus quod dicitur: "Nunc sancte nobis Spiritus unus Patri cum Filio," ne scilicet sonet in ore Christiani quod sonuit in ore heretici, ut Sabellii qui dixit unam personam esse Patrem et Filium et Spiritum sanctum, nisi unus pro communis accipiatur. Spiritus enim sanctus

225 communiter procedit a Patre et Filio una et eadem processione.

"Vita data per uirginem gentes redempte plaudite." <"Vita data" sunt ablatiui casus ubi subintelligatur> ex uel pro.

<"Iam lucis orto sidere ... .> Vt cum dies abcesserit noctemque sors reduxerit," id est diuina gratia, uel "sol reduxerit," recedens scilicet.

230   5 DE CONFESSIONE ET ORATIONIBVS

"Confiteor Deo et beate Marie et omnibus sanctis Dei et uobis, fratres, peccaui cogitatione, locutione, et opere; mea culpa; precor uos orare pro me."

"Misereatur tui omnipotens Deus, et dimittat tibi omnia peccata tua,

235 liberet te ab omni malo, conseruet et confirmet in omni opere bono, et perducat ad uitam eternam."

"Confiteor Deo et beate Marie et omnibus sanctis Dei et tibi, pater, peccaui cogitatione, locutione, et opere; mea culpa; precor te ora pro me."

240 "Misereatur uestri omnipotens Deus, et dimittat uobis omnia peccata uestra, liberet uos ab omni malo, conseruet et confirmet in omni opere bono, et perducat ad uitam eternam."

"Absolutionem et remissionem omnium peccatorum nostrorum per gratiam sancti Spiritus tribuat nobis omnipotens et misericors Domi-

245 nus." Ita breuiter hec dicantur, secundum morem uirorum peritorum et religiosorum.

Quidam dicunt <"Concede nos famulos tuos ... > perpetua mentis et corporis sanitate gaudere," quibus obiciunt: optatis uobis perpetuam corporis sanitatem, ergo numquam uultis egrotare, ita non mori, sed

250 Deus uult hoc, et ita uoluntas uestra diuine uoluntati aduersatur. Ideo

alii dicunt "perpetua mentis et corporis salute gaudere," salus enim
anime proprie est et hec preoptanda est et preferenda sanitati que
proprie corporis est. Potest tamen intelligi perpetua sanitas que erit
in patria que optatur a nobis semiuiuis relictis et corruptibilis nature
255 in uia. Sequitur in oratione "et futura perfrui letitia." Sed quia crastina
futura est, ideo alii expressius dicunt eterna.

    "Qui uenturus est iudicare uiuos et mortuos et seculum per ignem."
Hoc non est dicendum pro defunctis sed tantum in exorcismis, ad
exterendum demones qui ibi exorzizantur, id est adiurantur ut recedant.
260 Cum autem dicitur "Exorzizo te creatura salis" uel "aque," is est sensus:
adiuro te diabole ne impedias sanctificationem per aspersionem salis
et aque faciendum.

    Minus congrue dicitur "quorum corpora hic et ubique requiescunt,"
cum nulla corpora ubique requiescant; nullum enim corpus est ubique.
265 Sed potius dicendum "quorum corpora hic uel ubique requiescunt,"
uel "quorum corpora hic requiescunt."

    <"Fidelium Deus omnium conditor ... > ut indulgentiam quam
optauerunt piis supplicationibus consequentur," non "semper optauerunt," quia non semper fuerunt. Item dum erant in feruore culpe
270 et in intensa libidine peccandi interim non mouebantur ad optandum
ueniam.

    6 De epistolis et qvibvsdam aliis qve legvntvr in ecclesia

"Centum quadraginta quatuor milia" etc. [Apoc 7:4]. Non est numerus
innocentum, sed in Apocalipsi ponitur propter misterium.
275   In epistola ad Galatas [4:6]: "Quoniam autem estis filii Dei," Haimo
subiungat in Glosa dicens scilicet Dei adoptiui, non naturales.

    "Misit Deus Filium suum factum ex muliere" [Gal 4:4]. Huic etiam
consonat illud in principio epistole ad Romanos [1:2-3]: "In scripturis
sanctis de Filio suo qui factus est ei ex semine Dauid secundum
280 carnem."

    In epistola ad Philipenses, capitulo primo [1:10], "ut sitis scinceres,"
id est sine operibus corruptionis, quasi sine cane id est corruptione.
Vnde media huius dictionis "scinceres" corripitur, sed quandoque
producta reperiatur, tunc "sincere" pro "sincerum" ponitur, poetica
285 licentia uel metri neccesitate.

    "Filie tue de latere surgent" [Is 60:4], uel lac sugent; Glosa super
illum locum dicit: Quidam codices habent "de latere surgent," sed hoc
neque in Ebreo neque in Septuaginta inuenitur, neque Ieronimi sensus
ad hoc inclinatur.

290   "Cum complerentur dies pentecostes" [Act 2:1] ita legitur, sed
cantatur "Dum complerentur."

Secunda ad Thimotheum vi [4:8]: "In reliquo reposita est mihi corona
iustitie." Glosa: "In reliquo," id est in futuro; non habetur ibi de reliquo.

"Cunctus autem populus uidebat uoces et lampades et sonitum
295 buccine" etc. [Ex 20:18]. Huic simile est illud in Apocalipsi [1:12]: "Et
conuersus sum ut uiderem uocem, que loquebatur mecum," et in
Mattheo [27:54]: "Senturio autem et qui cum eo erant custodientes
Ihesum, uiso terre motu et hiis que fiebant, timuerunt ualde." Visus
quippe dicitur quia uiuatior sensus est et uelocior, et pro omni sensu
300 ponitur. Vnde Augustinus super predictum locum Exodi ait: Visus qui
primatum optinet in sensibus omnibus intermiscetur. Sic enim dicimus
audi et uide, palpa et uide.

"Videte fratres quo modo (id est quo moderamine) caute ambuletis"
[Eph 5:15], ita habetur in Glosa. Non est ergo ibi "quo modo" una
305 dictio sed due dictiones.

"Quo modo fiet istud quoniam uirum non congnosco" [Lc 1:34] due
dictiones sunt, quo et modo. Vnde Ambrosius super Lucam: Linquit
quod faciendum credit que quo modo fiat querit. Per quomodo uero
quod est aduerbium querit dubitans simul de re et modo, ut Nichodemus
310 dicens: "Quomodo potest homo nasci cum sit senex?" [Io 3:4].

"Porro si in digito Dei eicio demonia, profecto peruenit in uos
regnum Dei" [Lc 11:20]. "Peruenit" dicendum est media producta. Vnde
interliniaris ibi dicit: preteritum pro futuro.

"Velud etiam hic publicanus" [Lc 18:11], "uelud" una dictio est ibi.
315   "Vidimus enim stellam eius in oriente et uenimus adorare eum" [Mt
2:2]. "Venimus" presentis temporis est, hic media scilicet producta.

"Et congregans omnes principes sacerdotum et scribas populi,
scissitabatur" [Mt 2:4]. Per s c i s scribitur sequentibus aliis litteris.

"Et flores mei fructus odoris et honestatis, ego mater pulcre
320 dilectionis et timoris et agnitionis et sancte spei" [Eccli 24:23-24]. Ibi
habetur in libris glosatis, scilicet "odoris" non "honoris," et "agnitionis"
non "magnitudinis."

Gregorius in omelia dominice tertie post octauam pentecostes, super
illud euuangelium: "Accesserunt ad Ihesum publicani et peccatores, ut
325 audirent illum; et murmurabant" etc. [Lc 15:1], ita dicit: Aliud est quod
agitur tipho superbie, aliud quod zelo discipline. Tiphos grece, inflatio
Latine. Vnde in Actibus Apostolorum [27:14] dicitur: "Ventus tiphonicus" id est inflatiuus; et Augustinus in sermone qui sic incipit:
"Sanctorum martirum" ita dicit de uirtute martyrum: Ipsa est uera
330 et sola dicenda uirtus, que non militat tipho sed Deo.

"Aperi eis thesaurum tuum fontem aque uiue" [Num 20:6], ut satiatis scilicet ipsis cesset murmuratio eorum.

"Aggrauata est uia maris trans Iordanem Galilee gentium" [Is 9:1]. Glosa: Quia multe gentes habitabant ibi; et alia Glosa: Galilee due
335 sunt, una gentium in tribu Neptalim, altera in tribu Zabulon. Sequitur [9:2]: "populus qui ambulabat in tenebris uidit lucem magnam." Super hoc nomen "populus" stat Glosa interliniaris: Israel, uel quarumlibet gentium.

In libro Sapientie [4:3] habetur: "et adulterine plantationes non
340 dabunt radices altas"; sed quoniam Grece "moscos" uitulus dicitur, mosceumata quidam non intellexerunt esse plantationes, et uitulamina interpretati sunt, qui error tam multos codices preocupauit ut uix inueniatur aliter scriptum, ita habetur ibi in Glosa, et dicunt quod uitulamen nichil est.

345 Petrus sub Herode incarceratus est tempore paschali, sicut habetur [Act 12:1-3]: "Misit Herodes rex manus" etc. usque ibi "apposuit apprehendere et Petrum. Erant autem dies azimorum" etc. De hoc autem sollempnizat ecclesia in Kalendis Augusti, propter euentum quendam qui accidit Rome tunc temporis prout habetur in legenda
350 eiusdem solempnitatis.

<"Deus qui ad salutem humani generis ... > ut creatura tua misterii tui (id est inuestigabilis potentie, uel "misteriis," id est secretis efficaciis que scilicet sunt in sacramentis et in sacramentalibus, ut in baptismo et in aqua benedicta) tibi (id est ad honorem tuum) seruiens."

355 Iniquitas sedet non super sed subter talentum plumbi; ita enim legitur in Zacharia [5:8] de angelo et muliere: "Dixit angelus, hec est impietas, et proiecit eam in medio amphore, et misit massam plumbeam in os eius"; uel prius sedit super, deinde subter.

"Ecce ego mittam angelum meum, et preparabit uiam ante faciem
360 meam" etc. [Mal 3:1]. Aliter legitur in euuangelistis hinc, et super Malachiam habetur hec Glosa: Notandum quod Dominus uel Euuangeliste uel alii Apostoli cum de hoc propheta uel de aliis testimonia proferunt, non secuntur uerbum uulgatarum translationum, sed habentes scientiam Hebree lingue, ex Hebreo transferunt, non curantes
365 de sillabis et punctis uerborum, dummodo sententiarum ueritas transferatur.

7 De ewangelistis

"Vade sathana" [Mt 4:10], Glosa: A potestate quam habebas retro. Ieronimus super Matheum: Petro dicitur "Vade retro me sathana"

370 [16:23], id est sequere me, quia contrarius es uoluntati mee. Hic uero
audit "Vade sathana" et non ei dicitur "retro" ut subaudiatur in ignem
eternum qui preparatus est tibi et angelis tuis [cf. Mt 25:41].

In Luca [5:7]: "Impleuerunt ambas nauiculas ita ut mergerentur."
Glosa: Implete merguntur, id est in submersionem premuntur. Hinc
375 patet quod "pene" non est in littera, sed est suppletio magistralis.

"Erant Iosep et Maria mater Ihesu mirantes" [Lc 2:33], non dicatur
"erat" singulariter sed "erant" pluraliter, propter hoc plurale "mirantes"
cum quo construitur.

"Ne timeas habens in utero filium Dei" [cf. Lc 1:30-33], dicunt quod
380 "habens" hic extenditur ad futurum, quia coniungitur cum uerbo futuri
temporis, ut sit sensus habens, id est cum habueris in utero Filium
Dei. Alii euidentius dicunt: Ne timeas, habebis in utero Filium Dei.
Constat quod in hoc uerbo angeli nondum concepit, sed postea cum
credidit et consensit dicens "Fiat mihi secundum uerbum tuum" [Lc
385 1:38].

"Quinimmo beati qui audiunt uerbum Dei et custodiunt illud" [Lc
11:28]. Quinimmo una dictio est, et est "quin" sillabica adiectio, et
idem est quinimmo quod immo, sicut idem est quinpotius et potius;
et ponitur hic "quinimmo" pro potius, et ideo simul pronuntientur
390 "Quinimmo beati," non facta distinctione post quinimmo sicut nec fieret
post immo. Sed dicatur "Quinimmo beati" quasi potius beati, id est
beatiores, "qui audiunt uerbum Dei, et custodiunt illud»; et beatior
fuit ipsa Virgo ex hoc quod uerbo Dei credidit et obediuit, quam quod
Dominum in uentre portauit. Vnde Glosa super Lucam: Quasi non
395 solum laudanda est Virgo quia Verbum portauit in utero, sed maxime
quia precepta Dei seruauit in opere. Alii postquam distingunt quasi
non est mirum si hec beata, immo quod maius sunt beati qui audiunt
uerbum Dei et custodiunt illud, sed hoc non approbant magistri nostri.

"Erat autem uentus contrarius illis" [Mt 14:24]. Hoc non habetur
400 in euuangelio quod legitur dominica quarta post Epiphaniam sed in
euuangelio illo ubi legitur Petrus ambulare super mare [Mt 8:23-7].

Elisabet dici debet per s et non per z. Sabee enim interpretatur
satietas, et Elisabeth, Dei mei saturitas. Vnde in historiis [Jos 19:2]
Sabee per sin Hebreum scriptum septimum uel iuramentum sonat et
405 asperius stridet, scriptum uero per sima Grecum satietate<m> signat
et mollius sonat.

8 De prefationibvs

<"Te, Domine, suppliciter exorare ... > ut eisdem rectoribus guber-

netur"; <"Quia per incarnati ... > per hunc inuisibilium amorem
410 rapiamur." Est enim karitas currus igneus.

<"Qui cum unigenito Filio ... > Cherubin quoque ac seraphin, qui
non cessant clamare iugiter," non "cotidie" qui semper Deum laudant,
et non sunt plures dies in patria sed una dies continua de qua scriptum
est [Ps 83:11]: "Quoniam melior est dies una in atriis tuis super milia."

415 Item: <"Per quem maiestatem ... > celi celorumque uirtutes ac beata
seraphin," quia seraphim per m, clausis labiis, masculini generis est,
seraphin per n, que continue sequitur m in alphabeto, neutri generis
est.

Explicit De erroribvs clericorvm.

420 *Incipit De erroribvs laicorvm.*

Est autem error laicorum in hiis et huiusmodi:

Laicus credit se de fornicatione sua satisfecisse cum concubinam
suam duxerit in uxorem.

Fornicariam egrotantem usque ad mortem non credunt posse saluari
425 nisi nubat, cum melius sit decedere in statu uiduali quam coniugali.

Credunt quidam melius esse de decimis suis dare pauperibus et egenis
quam prelatis opulentis.

Sal non suplet uicem baptismi, nec cespis locum eucharistie, neque
etiam panis benedictus.

430 Credunt consuetudinem quamcumque locum habere rationis uel
autoritatis.

Cum inciderint in canonem late sententie non credunt se excomu-
nicatos sed dissimulant.

Credunt sortilegiis, et spem ponunt in illis.

435 Dixit laicus aliquis, "Clerici otiosi sunt." Responsio: Opera spiritualia
precellunt operibus corporalibus et pluribus conferunt ut orationes et
misse.

Dixit aliquis quem conscientia arguit de uita transacta, "Mallem
usque modo dormisse, et sompniasse me felicem esse."

440 Putant existentem in mortali per elemosinas mereri, non secundum
Apostolum: Sine caritate nihil sit meritorium uite eterne [cf. 1 Cor
13:3].

Putant elemosinam de furto uel rapina faciendam, cum Dominus
exigat oleum purissimum et lucidum [Lev 24:2]. Item scriptum est [Prov
445 21:27]: "Hostie impiorum abhominabiles que offeruntur ex scelere,"
et iterum [Eccli 34:23-24]: "Dona iniquorum non probat altissimus,

nec respicit in oblationibus iniquorum, nec in multitudine sacrificiorum eorum propitiabitur peccatis. Qui offert sacrificium ex substantia pauperum, quasi qui uictimat filium in conspectu patris sui."

450   Putant licitum esse rem alienam casu inuentam retinere, cum dicat Augustinus: "Si quid inuenisti et non reddidisti, rapuisti"; et intellige "reddidisti" actu uel proposito, et rem ipsam uel equipollens. Item Augustinus: "Si res aliena propter quam peccatum est reddi possit et non redditur, penitentia non agitur sed simulatur. Si autem uerasciter
455   agitur, non remittitur <peccatum> nisi restituatur ablatum, si restitui potest."

Hostiam quam sacerdos in altari eleuat ad benedicendum adorant tanquam Christum.

Sacerdos ad fontem baptismi patrinis iniungit ut baptizatum doceant
460   orationem dominicam et simbolum id est "Pater noster" et "Credo," et ipsi ex negligentia omittunt, nunquam non delinqunt?

Mulier que infantem oppressit, hoc solum sacerdoti confitetur et recedit tanquam mundata ab omnibus peccatis suis.

Excomunicatus cum absoluitur recedit tanquam mundus sit ab
465   omnibus peccatis suis, cum retento uno mortali peccato nullum peccatum remittatur.

Cum quis in clericum iniecerit manus uiolentas, incidit in canonem late sentencie. Deinde forsitan clerico satisfecit, dando ei pecuniam uel alio modo, et credit hoc sibi sufficere cum nondum absolutus sit a
470   summo pontifice uel aliquo eius uicario.

10 De hiis qve cantantvr in ecclesia

In festo sancte Trinitatis sit transpos<it>io antiphonarum, et in festo sancti Pauli et sancti Laurentii. Prima sit contra hereticos, qui Spiritum sanctum quasi minorem aliis Personis postponebant; secunda fit contra
475   pseudoapostolos qui Paulum aliis Apostolis minorem dicebant; tertia contra Hebreos conuersos qui nullum martirum nostrorum Stephano conferebant. Quasi Spiritum sanctum quem heretici postponunt nos aliis Personis comparamus, Paulum cui pseudo derogant nos aliis apostolis parificamus, Laurentium etiam Stephano equiparamus.
480   <"Equi>paratio" enim hic dicitur parificatio eo tropo quo plus dicitur et minus significatur.

Feria sexta in ieiunio quatuor temporum in mense septima, post communionem habetur hec oratio: "Quesumus omnipotens Deus ut de preceptis muneribus gratias exibentes beneficia potiora sumamus."
485   Item, Ps. cxvii [118:65] "Teth"; Glosa in hac undecima littera: Gratias

Deo agit de humiliatione. Item super euangelium Iohannis [6:11] ubi
agitur de edulio quinque panum dicitur in Glosa de Domino: Gratias
agit docens nos gratias agere de omnibus beneficiis. Item in ueteribus
missalibus ita habetur: "Miserere quesumus Domine animabus omnium
490 benefactorum nostrorum, et de beneficiis que nobis largiti sunt in terris,
premia eterna consequantur in celis." Item in uulgari locutione gratiarum
actio redditur de exenio misso, non pro. Item nonne competentius
dicitur "de semine colligitur fructus" quam "pro semine." Semen
quidem est opus bonum, fructus est uita eterna. Item secundum
495 quosdam mala opera nostra signum sunt et uia et causa ad dampnationem, bona opera signum et uia sunt ad beatitudinem non causa;
secundum hoc ergo non congrue dicitur "ut pro beneficiis que nobis
largiti sunt in terris premia eterna consequantur in celis." Item Deo
gratias agere est Deo seruire, sed ut aiunt magistri saniores, non est
500 seruiendum Deo pro temporalibus. Non igitur agende sunt gratie Deo
pro temporalibus, licet de beneficiis temporalibus iam collatis gratiarum
actiones persoluende sint propter ingratitudinem uitandam. Item in
festo unius confessoris post communionem habetur hec oratio: "Presta
quesumus omnipotens Deus ut de perpetuis muneribus gratias exibentes
505 intercedente beato confessore tuo, beneficia potiora sumamus." Item
Apostolus in secunda ad Corinthios [9:15] ait: "Gratias Deo super
inenarrabili dono eius." Glosa, Augustinus: Id est de caritate quam
suis donat. Et nota quod in omnibus hiis est de materiale, beneficia
namque Dei sunt nobis materia laudis diuine.

II.3

Tractatus metricus
de septem sacramentis ecclesie

This metrical treatise offers another example of the importance of verses and versification in William's school. In the form in which it has come down to us, the *Tractatus metricus* consists of 291 lines of verse and a prose-compendium of the Apostles' and Prophets' contributions to the twelve articles of faith. It begins with verses on the seven sacraments, in the sequence: baptism, confirmation (no verses), eucharist, marriage, holy orders, extreme unction, and penance (nos. 1-43). These are followed by verses of interest to the preacher and teacher. The "Words of the Apostle Paul concerning prelates of the church" (no. 44) summarize Paul's teachings in 1 Tim 3:1-6; the verses are quoted by Raymund of Peñafort in his *Summa*.[1] Next come two poems concerning the vice of gluttony (no. 45), and two detailing the pains of hell (nos. 46 and 47). The versification of the Ten Commandments (no. 48) is found in Peter Riga's *Aurora*, a versification of the Bible. The list of the ten plagues of Egypt and the interpretation of these plagues (nos. 49 and 50) is also associated with manuscripts of Peter Riga's work. The verses comparing Cain's and Abel's sacrifice that conclude number 50 are an example of a popular classroom exercise, but also point an important moral.[2] The next eight couplets (no. 51) describe the seven vices, first in general, and then by likening each to a specific bird.[3] The final section (no. 52) assigns each of the statements of the Creed to one of the Apostles and notices a foretelling of each in the writings

---

[1] *Summa sti Raymundi de Peniafort ... De poenitentia, et matrimonio ...* (Rome, 1603; rpt. Farnborough, 1967), p. 258, 3:1.

[2] See A.G. Rigg and David Townsend, "Medieval Latin Poetic Anthologies (V): Matthew Paris' Anthology of Henry of Avranches (Cambridge, Univ. Library MS. Dd.11.78)," *Mediaeval Studies* 49 (1987) 352-390.

[3] No source for these verses has been identified; see Morton W. Bloomfield, *The Seven Deadly Sins* ([East Lansing]: Michigan State College Press, 1952), Appendix I, pp. 245-252.

of the Old Testament prophets. This convention became quite popular in the thirteenth century and is represented in the visual arts as well as in written texts.[4] None of the schemata featuring this doctrine corresponds exactly to that in the *Tractatus metricus*.

The *Tractatus* has a tenuous existence; it survives complete in only one manuscript, and a fragment of the text is preserved in another. There is little to differentiate it from numerous collections of *notabilia* made by students and scribes in this period. It is to be hoped that further manuscript copies will be discovered, perhaps some containing a complete set of glosses or explications of the verses. Until that time it is hazardous to make any firm assertions about the nature of the work.

As it stands, this treatise can be compared with the collection of didactic verses that Samuel Presbyter collected in William's school (below, II.15), and with the interesting "catechism" that Alphonse de Poorter published from a thirteenth-century manuscript in Bruges.[5] Like the former collection, this treatise could have served as the basis for *collationes* or informal lectures in William's school. Like the latter, it summarizes in brief compass and in metrical form many of the teachings of the twelfth- and thirteenth-century schools.

This handy compendium of verses that circulated in the school of William de Montibus forms an important adjunct to our understanding of the theological/pastoral education there. No description of late-twelfth and thirteenth-century scholastic training — whether legal, theological, or scientific — can be complete without a consideration of verses and versification.[6] We have in this "treatise" an early example of their use in conveying the essentials of scholastic doctrine to those who would preach, teach, and exercise the *cura animarum*.

---

[4] Cf. the "catechism" from Bruges, edited by Alphonse de Poorter, "Un catéchisme du XIIIᵉ siècle," *Revue d'histoire ecclésiastique* 28 (1932) 73-74; Innocent III, *De sacro altaris mysterio*, PL 217: 773-914; Lionel J. Friedman, *Text and Iconography for Joinville's "Credo"* (Cambridge MA: Medieval Academy of America, 1958); H.W. van Os, "Credo," in *Lexikon der christlichen Ikonographie*, ed. Engelbert Kirschbaum (Rome: Herder, 1968), 1: 461-463. For the motif of the Apostles and the Creed (without the prophets) see Curt F. Bühler, "The Apostles and the Creed," *Speculum* 28 (1953) 335-339; James D. Gordon, "The Articles of the Creed and the Apostles," *Speculum* 40 (1965) 634-640.

[5] "Un catéchisme du XIIIᵉ siècle," pp. 70-74.

[6] Much work remains to be done on this topic. See the older studies by Joseph de Ghellinck, "Medieval Theology in Verse," (1914), pp. 336-354, and Lynn Thorndike, "Unde versus" (1955), pp. 162-193; more recently: Siegfried Wenzel, *Verses in Sermons: "Fasciculus morum" and Its Middle English Poems* (1978).

AUTHENTICITY AND DATE

Neither manuscript copy of this work names William de Montibus as its author. The complete copy in MS *B* follows immediately after the excerpts from William's *Distinctiones* in the manuscript, and is written in the same hand. It is, however, on the basis of internal evidence that the work can be attributed to William.

The most striking link between this treatise and William de Montibus is in the section on the sacrament of penance (nos. 25-43) which consists of all the verses of William's *Peniteas cito peccator*. Indeed, the penitential verses found in this treatise on the sacraments correspond in number and verse-order to the early, ascribed copy of the *Peniteas cito* in Cambridge, University Library MS Ii.1.26.

Other poems in the *Tractatus metricus* are also found in William's *Versarius* — one poem on baptism (no. 3), three on the eucharist (nos. 6 and 8), two on marriage (nos. 16 and 18), and one listing the ten plagues of Egypt (no. 49). Three of these (nos. 6, 16, and 18) are ascribed explicitly to William in the *Summa Qui bene presunt*.

When William's student, Richard of Wetheringsett, came to compose his *Qui bene presunt* he seems to have had something like this treatise on the sacraments before his eyes. Of the first thirty-three poems in the *Tractatus metricus* Richard quotes, in the same order, all but four.

In both content and style this treatise is very like William's other verse-collections. He followed the prevailing custom of the twelfth-century schools in composing *quaestiones* on the seven sacraments (II.13); his fondness for didactic verses as a basis for classroom teaching admits a certain plausibility to the suggestion that he also composed a verse-treatise to serve as the basis for lectures or *collationes* on these sacraments.

Nothing in the text allows us to assign a date of composition, but it seems reasonable to suggest that the *Tractatus metricus* was composed before the *Peniteas cito peccator*, or, more precisely, that the *Peniteas cito* had no independent existence before being extracted from this metrical treatise on the seven sacraments.

SOURCES

As with William's other verse-writings, the sources of these poems can only be described, broadly, as the common theological and poetic inheritance of the twelfth-century schools. One poem (no. 11) is borrowed from Hildebert of Le Mans's *De mysterio missae*, and another (no. 45) is from the same author's biblical epigrams. A poem listing the Ten Commandments (no. 50) is found in the first edition of Peter Riga's *Aurora* (1170 x 1200) and may well derive from that source. Other borrowings will, no doubt, be detected, but no direct sources for the other poems have been identified thus far.

Manuscripts

1. *B* = Oxford, Bodleian Library MS Bodley 419, fols. 103va-105rb. Mid 13th century. Printed below.

2. *D* = Oxford, Bodleian Library MS Digby 20, fol. 92r. 14th century.
    Inc. Txt.: *Septem sunt sacramenta ecclesie scilicet baptismus, confirmacio, heucharistia, penitencia, ordo, coniugium, extrema unccio. Et dicitur baptismus sacramentum intrancium*
    Expl. txt. (incomplete): *Vt sic mens munda, caro casta, refulgeat acctus* (sic).

This fragmentary text, in a fourteenth-century hand, is copied into the blank space following the end of Ambrosius Autpertus's *De conflictu uitiorum atque uirtutum*, ascribed here to Pope Leo, and written in an early-thirteenth-century hand. It preserves only the prologue, poems 1-4 and 6 of the *Tractatus metricus*, but it adds to the verses a bit of explanatory material missing from MS *B*. This fragment suggests that the *Tractatus metricus* originally included both verses and expositions.

The text of the *Tractatus metricus* is printed here in its entirety from Oxford, MS Bodley 419 (siglum *B* in the edition below). The readings of the fragmentary copy MS Digby 20 (siglum *D*), are reported in the *apparatus criticus*. Small capitals are used here to indicate the topical headings. References to other works where these poems are quoted or cited are found in the *apparatus parallelorum locorum*; the following abbreviations are used:

PenCito = *Peniteas cito* of William de Montibus

Vers = *Versarius* of William de Montibus.

Qbp = *Qui bene presunt* of Richard of Wetheringsett (MS HM 19914 of the Huntington Library, San Marino, California).

Aurora = *Aurora Petri Rigae Biblia versificata: A Verse Commentary on the Bible*, ed. Paul E. Beichner, 2 vols. (Notre Dame IN: University of Notre Dame Press, 1965).

IC = Hans Walther, *Initia carminum ac versuum medii aevi posterioris latinorum*. Göttingen: Vandenhoech and Ruprecht, 1959

162   WRITINGS

PS = idem, *Proverbia sententiaeque latinitatis medii aevi*. 6 vols. Göttingen: Vandenhoech and Ruprecht, 1959.
  Hildebert = Hildebert of Le Mans, *De mysterio missae*, PL 171: 1177-1194.
  HildEpig = A.B. Scott, Deirdre F. Baker and A.G. Rigg, "The *Biblical Epigrams* of Hildebert of Le Mans: A Critical Edition," *Mediaeval Studies* 47 (1985) 272-316.

Tractatus metricus
de septem sacramentis ecclesie

Tractatus metricus de septem sacramentis ecclesie que sunt Baptismus intrantium, Confirmatio pugnantium, Viaticum peregrinantium, Penitentia redeuntium, Matrimonium coheuntium, Ordo ministrantium, Vnctio migrantium.

> Tractatus ... migrantium] Septem sunt sacramenta ecclesie scilicet baptismus, confirmacio, heucharistia, penitencia, ordo, coniugium, extrema unccio. Et dicitur baptismus sacramentum intrancium, confirmacio pungnancium, eucharistia intrancium, penitencia redeuncium, coniugium laborancium, ordo ministrancium, unccio exeuncium, quod sic potest retineri: Intrant et pungnant, pergunt, redeunt, abeuntque/Scandunt, seruantur, per septem sacra fideles. *D*

> Cf. *Qbp*, fol. 133rb.

1 SEPTEM SACRAMENTA PER HOS DVOS VERSVS SVBSEQVENTES

Tinctio, crisma, caro, dolor, unctio, lectus et ordo,
Mundat, alit, pascit, renouat, leuat, ornat et unit.

> Septem ... unit] Sacramenta eciam et effectus sic possunt retineri: Tinctio, crisma, caro, dolor, unccio, lectus et ordo / Mundat, alit, pascit, renouat, leuat, ornat et vnit. *D et post* Intrant ... fideles.

> Cf. *Qbp*, fol. 133rb (omitted in MS HM 19914, but included in London, BL MS Royal 9.A.xiv, fol. 64r).

2 AD IDEM

Intrant et pugnant, pergunt, redeunt, abeuntque,
Scandunt, seruantur per septem sacra fideles.

> *Qbp*, fol. 133rb; *IC* no. 9502.

3 QVE SVNT NECESSARIA IN BAPTISMATE.

Flatus, crux, et sal, sputum cum crismate, uestis,
Et cere facula sunt in baptismate signa,
Set dant esse latex, intentio, debita forma.

> *Vers*, no. 71; *Qbp*, fol. 133va.

4 DE PERFECTIS BAPTISMATIS.

Imprimit, adnichilat, aperit, confertque relegat
Baptismus signum, culpam, celum, bona, planctum.

Qui mentem, sensus, actus bene rexerit est rex,
Ad quod inunguntur pectus, uertex, scapuleque.

5 Vngitur, induitur intinctus, luce potitur,
Vt sit mens munda, caro casta, refulgeat actus.

> 3-4 *ante* Qui ... scapuleque] In baptisme iniunguntur pueri tamquam
> reges, scilicet vt bene se regant. Vnguntur enim in pectore ut bene regant
> uoluntates et cogitaciones cordis, cuius sedes est circa pectus. In uertice
> scilicet anteriori parte capitis, scilicet ut bene regant sensus suos qui sunt
> in capite. In scapulis, feruntur onera ibi ergo inunguntur ut dirigant opera.
> Unde uersus *add. D*   5-6 *ante* Vngitur ... actus] Qualis autem debeat
> esse baptizatorum conuersacio figuraliter ostenditur post inunccione et
> immersione in aqua; nam crismali induitur et candela ei datur, cuius
> misterium sic patet *add. D*

> 1-2 *Qbp*, fol. 133va; *PS*, no. 11621.
> 2-4 *Qbp*, fol. 133vb.
> 5-6 *Qbp*, fol. 133vb.

Explicit DE BAPTISMA.

Confirmatio tantum episcoporum est et multum ualet contra fantesias,
unde sunt pueri confirmandi infra annum, uel aliter uertitur parentibus
in periculum.

> Cf. *Qbp*, fol. 134ra.

DE SACRAMENTO ALTARIS.

5 QVE SVNT SVBSTANTIALIA IN HOC SACRAMENTO.

Verborum forma, uinum cum mixta sit unda,
Panis triticius, intentio presbiterorum
Missam perficiunt, ornatum cetera signant.

> *Qbp*, fol. 134ra.

6 QVIDAM SANCTVS.

Constat in altari carnem de pane creari,
  Iste cibus Deus est, qui negat hoc reus est;
Nam sacrum pignus nullus capiat nisi dignus,
Qui capit indigne diro cruciabitur igne.

5 Sub specie uini panisque datur caro Christi
Ne mens horreret crudas carnes set haberet
Nostra fides meritum ne fiat ridiculosum.

Pondus ibi, color, atque sapor, si queritur an sint,
Sunt et forma simul, tantum substantia transit.

> 1-4 *Vers*, no. 413; *Qbp*, fol. 134rb: "De premissis Cancellarius Lincolnie:
> Constat in altari ..."; *IC*, no. 3214; *PS*, no. 3219.
> 6-7 *Qbp*, fol. 134rb; *IC*, no. 18671.
> 8-9 *Vers*, no. 408; *Qbp*, fol. 134ra.

7 SOLVTIO AD OBIECTIONEM QVE POSSET FIERI,
QVOD SACRAMENTVM NON MVTATVR PROPTER PERSONAM.

Hoc sacramentum numquam licet esse sinistrum
Quamuis per prauum celebretur sepe ministrum.
Sicut deterius non fit pro deteriori,
Sic non fit melior pro presbitero meliori.

> *IC*, no. 8340; *PS*, no. 11057.

8 DE EFFECTV HVIVS SACRAMENTI.

Roborat, augmentat, hoc sacrum delet et unit.

> *Vers*, no. 96 (line 4); *Qbp*, fol. 134vb.

9 MISTICE:

Tres partes fracte de Christi corpore signant,
Prima suam carnem, defunctos altera, uiuos
Tertia pars tincta; tres ecclesiasque figurant,
Hinc labor, hinc requies, coquit hanc clementior ignis.

> *Qbp*, fol. 135ra; cf. *Hildebert*, c. 1191; *HildEpig*, p. 311 no. 68.

10 QVOD TOTVS CHRISTVS EST SVB QVALIBET PARTE ET IN OMNI ECCLESIA.

Vt uox, lux, anima simul hic ibi, sic caro Christi.

> *Qbp*, fol. 134rb.

11 MISTICE:

Tempore quo felix assistit presbiter aris
  Mactaturque Patri Filius ipse manens,
Ethra patent, celestis adest chorus, ima supernis
  Iunguntur, fiunt auctor et actus idem.
5 Cetibus hiis anima dum mens dum uita ministra
  Concordant, grates indubitanter agunt.

> 2 Patri] pater *MS*   manens] manes *MS*   3 patent] patet *MS*
> 6 grates] gentes *MS*
>
> *Qbp*, fol. 135ra; *Hildebert*, c. 1182:
> Tempore quo supplex assistit presbyter aris,
>   Mactaturque Patri Filius ipse manens:
> Aethra patent, coelestis adest chorus, ima supernis
>   Junguntur; fiunt actor et actus idem.
> Coetibus his dum mens, dum vox, dum vita ministri,
>   Concordant, grates indubitanter agit.

12 QVOD HOC SACRAMENTVM ROBORAT CONTRA SEPTEM CAPITALIA VITIA, ET QVALIS DEBET ESSE HOSTIA.

Candida trititia, tenuis, non magna, rotunda,
Expers fermenti, non mixta sit hostia Christi.

> *Qbp*, fol. 135rb; *IC*, no. 2350.

13　SEPTEM VITIA.

Nam uenus, bilis, gula, fastus, accidie uis,
Liuor, auaritia sunt a nobis remouenda.
Inscribatur, aqua non cocta, set igne sit assa,
Mentis ut ardorem signet Dominique timorem.

> *Qbp*, fol. 135rb.

14　QVOD PROPHETATVM FVIT IN LEGE.

Man pluit e celis ad plebis uota fidelis,
Panis uitalis typus inclitus ac specialis.

Agni paschalis notat esus quomodo, qualis,
Accedas aris ut Christi carne cibaris.

5　De quibus et quando comedatur pascha uideto,
Quomodo, cur, et ubi fruiturus corpore Christi.

In Domini mensa quid sumis sedule pensa,
Viuere siue mori confert quod porrigis ori.

> 1 Man] Nam *MS*
>
> 1-2 *Qbp*, fol. 135vb.
> 3-4 *Qbp*, fol. 136ra.
> 5-6 *Qbp*, fol. 136ra.
> 7-8 Cf. *IC*, no. 8901.

15　MISTICE DE ORNAMENTIS.

Ara crucis, tumulique calix, lapidisque patena,
　　Sindonis officium candida bissus habet.

> *Qbp*, fol. 135ra; these verses are printed in *Hildebert*, c. 1194, with the
> editorial note: "Hi duo in editis erant ad marginem, quos, ut eumdem
> sensum exprimentes, inter alios inferendos duximus, licet in nullis mss.
> eos legerimus."

DE MATRIMONIO.

16　DE EFFECTV MATRIMONII ET VBI ET QVANDO
ET A QVO FVIT INSTITVTVM.

Coniugium mundat, fecundat, mutat et unit,
　　Pollens auctore, tempore, lege, loco.

Ex auctore, loco, medicina, tempore, signo,
Causa coniugii patet excellentia casti.

> 1-2 *Vers*, no. 751; *Qbp*, fol. 142rb: "... ut docuit bone memorie cancel-
> larius Lincolnie"; the verses are quoted also in William's *Tropi*, and
> *Numerale*.
> 3-4 *Qbp*, *om*. HM 19914; see London, BL MS Royal 9.A.xiv, fol. 87v.

17 QVE DEBENT INQVIRI IN MATRIMONIO FACIENDO.

Hec inquirantur in coniugio faciendo:
Stricta fides, si sint coniuncti proximitate,
Ordo sacer, de fonte sacro susceptio, uotum,
Viuat an in claustro casteue, libido parentum,
5 Que facit affines, cultus, consensus, et etas.

> *Qbp*, fol. 142vb.

18 QVE IMPEDIVNT MATRIMONIVM.

Arriditas, error persone, conditionis,
Etas et uotum, cognatio, cultus, et ordo,
Grandis culpa, furor, inhonestas, arsque maligna,
Susceptus habitus, uiolenta coactio nuptis
5 Coniugium dirimunt uel inire uolentibus obsunt;
Hec si canonico uis consentire rigori
    Te de iure uetant iura subire thori.

> 4 Susceptus] uel *add*. MS
>
> *Vers*, no. 752; *Qbp*, fol. 142vb-143ra: "Impedimenta ... que sic complexit
> cancellarius Lincolnie: ... ."

19 QVE NOTANTVR PER CANDELAM IN MATRIMONIVM.

Mistica quinque tibi candela significantur,
Cera, calor, lux, stuppa, cinis, signantur in istis
Carnis munditia, dilectio mutua, purum
Cor, uite breuitas, dubie meditatio mortis.

> *Qbp*, fol. 143ra; cf. *IC*, no. 8901.

20 QVOD VIR DEBET ALIQVANDO ABSTINERE AB AMPLEXIBVS.

Quinque modis peccat uxore maritus abutens,
    Tempore, mente, modo, conditione, loco.

Quando non debet coiens ardenter abutens,
　　Festa sacerque locus, ieiunia, menstrua, partus.
5 Vt prolem capiat ius reddat, uitet iniqua
　　Si delectatur nimis, aut non impetuose.

> 1-2 *IC*, nos. 12030-1; *PS*, no. 25342.
> 3-6 *IC*, no. 6471; cf. *PS*, no. 25346.

*Explicit **DE MATRIMONIO**.*

*Incipit **DE ORDINIBVS**.*

21 QVE DEBENT INQVIRI AB ORDINANDIS.

Corporis integritas, sine crimine, sexus et etas,
Littera, libertas, baptismus, uita, uoluntas,
Fama, fides, titulus, intentio, forma, potestas,
Tempus: in ordinibus faciendis ista requiris.

> *Qbp*, fol. 143va; *IC*, no. 3357.

22 QVE IMPEDIVNT ORDINARI.

Symon, coniugium, sententia, publica noxa,
Etas, uis, saltus indignos ordine reddunt.

> saltus] finis *MS*

> *Qbp*, fol. 143va; *PS*, no. 29642a.

23 MISTICE DE SEPTEM ORDINIBVS IMPLETIS IN CHRISTO.

\<HOSTIARIVS\>
Dum reicis merces, Ihesu, templumque coherces,
Ordo clauigerii sacer exit in hostia cleri.

\<LECTOR\>
Carnis amicta toga deitas legit in synagoga,
Quo datur ostendi facto sacer ordo legendi.

\<EXHORCISTA\>
Demonium triste cum tollit uox tua Christe,
Est exhorciste sacer ordo traditus iste.

\<ACOLITVS\>
Se docet expresse Christus mundi iubar esse,
Hinc datur ut cernis gestandis ordo lucernis.

<SVBDIACONVS>

Vas fert Christus aque lauacrumque manu dat utraque,
Vasis custodem sacrat ordine presul eodem.

<DIACONVS>

Dans preter mortem Christus cum carne cruorem,
Res monet illicitas debere cauere leuitas.

<PRESBYTER>

Curat monstrare Christus se dans crucis are
Qualis primatus sit in ordine presbiteratus.

> *Qbp*, fol. 143vb; For the tradition of linking each of the orders with
> the life of Christ see Roger E. Reynolds, *The Ordinals of Christ from
> Their Origins to the Twelfth Century* (Berlin: W. de Gruyter, 1978).

*Explicit **DE ORDINIBVS**.*

*Incipit **DE EXTREMA VNCTIONE**.*

24 <DE EXTREMA VNCTIONE>

Vngor in extremis ut sit mihi gratia maior,
   Vt morbus leuior et mea culpa minor.

> *Qbp*, fol. 144rb.

25 DE HIIS QVE NECESSARIA SVNT IN CONFESSIONE.

Peniteas cito peccator cum sit miserator
   Iudex. Et sunt hec quinque tenenda tibi:
Spes uenie, cor contritum, confessio culpe,
   Pena satisfaciens, et fuga nequitie.
5 Vt dimittaris, aliis peccata remittas,
Hiisque satisfacias quos te lesisse fateris.

> *PenCito*, ll. 1-5, 7-8

26 QVE SVNT VITANDA IN HOC SECVLO.

Sperne uoluptates, luxus, spectacula mundi;
Desere consortes prauos populique tumultum,
Secretasque preces et opus pietatis amato.
Omnia peccata plangat contritio uera.

> *PenCito*, ll. 10-12, 14

27 QVALITER INQVIRENDE SVNT CIRCVMSTANTIE.

Scrutans etates, sensus, loca, tempora, membra.
Deplores acta, nolens committere flenda.
Plangas amissa cum commissis et omissis,
Offensasque Dei, quod fratres dampnificasti.

> *PenCito*, ll. 15, 17-19

28 QVALIS DEBET ESSE CONFESSIO.

Vera sit, integra sit, et sit confessio munda.
Sit scita, firma, frequens, humilis, spontanea, nuda,
Propria, discreta, lacrimosa, morosa, fidelis.
Peniteas plane si uere peniteat te,
5 Non per legatum, non per breue, set refer ipse.

> *PenCito*, ll. 20-25

29 QVOD PENITENS DEBET QVERERE SVPERIORES PRELATOS
IN ARDVIS CONFITENDIS SET CVM LICENTIA.

Compatienti, plus sapienti, dic meliori.
Presbiteris multis prodest si confitearis;
Dicere si pudeat semel uni dicito saltem
Quod si non iteras non iterabis idem.

> 1-2 *PenCito*, ll. 27-28
> 3-4 *PenCito*, l. 29 variant readings of MS *O*

30 QVOD SACERDOS DEBET PREDICARE IN GENERE
SVBDITIS PECCATA CAPITALIA VITANDA.

Corporis ut maculas anime sic crimine pandas.
Carnea sunt periuria, crapula, furta, libido;
Mente latet liuor, odium, tumor, ira, cupido.
Precipue pestes septem memores capitales,
5 Non solum fontes set riuos inde fluentes.
Fonte suo riuus magis est quandoque nociuus;
Vnde Loth incestus peior fuit ebrietate,
Atque Caym grauior cedes fraterna furore.

> *PenCito*, ll. 31-38

31 SEPTEM PECCATA CAPITALIA.

Culparum fontes sunt fastus, liuor, et ira,
Accidie neuus et auaritie, gula, luxus.

neuus] venus *MS*

PenCito, ll. 40-41

32 QVOD PENITENS DEBET OMNIA ET VNI DICERE.

Cum singillatim mortalia dixeris uni,
Cuncta simul quecumque grauant comitantia culpas,
Dic citra facta committere que uoluisti.
Dic uenialia, dic que sunt a mente relapsa,
5 Dic tua delicta, generaliter ista reuela.
Nam reus in multis quando peccata fatetur,
Vel queuis dicat, uel nil dixisse uidetur.
Postremum crimen si pure quis fateatur,
Ille tacere potest quicquit redit et comitatur.

PenCito, ll. 43-51

33 IN QVIBVS CASIBVS PECCATVM AGGRAVATVR.

Aggrauat ordo, locus, peccata, scientia, tempus,
Etas, conditio, numerus, mora, copia, causa,
Est modus in culpa, status altus, lucta pusilla.

PenCito, ll. 53-55

34 QVOD LABORANS IN EXTREMIS OMNIA PECCATA SVA DEBET DETEGERE REITERANDO, NEC TAMEN IMPONENDA EST EI PENITENTIA SET INSINVANDA.

Eger peniteat et crimina confiteatur.
Non imponetur huic pena, set insinuetur;
Hanc tamen explebit si firma salus sibi detur.
Si migret, absoluat contritum presbiter egrum;
5 Huncque preces releuent, ieiunia, dona suorum.
Vt sit pena rubor uel uilis ut efficiaris,
Doctior ut fias, iniungitur ut fatearis.
Iudicio teget extrema confessio culpas,
Ne uideat Dominus aut demon uel qui facit illas.

PenCito, ll. 57-61, 63-64, 66-67

35 Qvod omnis prelatvs debet esse mitis et compatiens svbditis svis.

Confessor mitis, affabilis atque benignus,
Sit sapiens, iustus, sit dulcis, compatiensque.
Vt crimen proprium celet peccata reorum.
Sit piger ad penas, sit uelox ad miserandum,
5 Et doleat quotiens facit illum pena ferocem.
Infundat mulcens oleum uinumque flagellis
Nunc uirgam patris, nunc exerat ubera matris.
Sibilet et cantet, stimulet cum cogit oportet.

    8 stimulet] rumilet *MS*

    PenCito, ll. 69-76

36 Qvaliter debet inqvisitio fieri in confessione.

In primis querat contritus quomodo credat;
Si credit corde sane fateatur et ore.
Post hec rimetur peccantis uiscera caute.
Contra naturam culpam non exprimit ullam,
5 Ne super enormi si simplex conueniatur,
De quo nil sciuit ad agendum sic moneatur.

    6 sic] si *MS*

    PenCito, ll. 78-79, 81-84

37 Qvod cavte agvnt cvm nvptis ne possint comprehendi.

Vxor adulterii rea confessore perito
Sic luat admissum ne sit suspecta marito.
Sepe sibi moneat confessos ne recidiuent,
Siue relabantur confestim confiteantur
5 Et uitent causas ad lapsum allicientes.
Solliciti penam complere satisfacientem,
Os seruent caute, sensus cum pectore, renes:
In prauos casus horum procliuior usus.
Hoc est difficile magis et seruare necesse.
10 Vt fori iudex pro pecunia prohibetur
Flectere iudicium, medicus uariare medelas,
Sic anime iudex odio caueat uel amore

Confessos penis onerare uel alleuiare;
Ecclesie morem uel patrum scripta sequantur,
15 Sitque modus pene iuxta moderamina culpe.

PenCito, ll. 86-94, 96-101

38 QVIA CONTRITIO EST PARS MAXIMA SATISFACTIONIS.

Et tanto leuior quanto contritio maior.
Vt medici curant uario medicamine corpus,
Non sanat febrem quod uulnus siue tumorem,
Sic anime uarias egre poscunt medicinas.

PenCito, ll. 102, 104-106

39 CONTRARIA CONTRARIIS CVRANTVR.

Opponas igitur anime contraria morbos:
Propria det cupidus, se castret luxuriosus;
Inuide liuorem depone, superbe tumorem;
Sobrietasque gulam, patientia comprimit iram;
5 Amoneat Iesus rancorem, tedia mestus;
Potus aque redimat excessus ebrietatis;
Carnis delicias castiget uirga flagellas.
Vt bene peniteat ablatum predo reponat.

PenCito, ll. 107-114

40 AVGVSTINVS:
NON DIMITTITVR PECCATVM NISI REDDATVR ABLATVM.

Ex uiridi ligno limphas calor exprimit ignis,
Sic de corde pio lacrimas iacit ardor amoris.
Nos quia peccati medicina semper egemus,
Contra peccatum medicinam semper habemus.
5 Culpa reo nox est, contrito gratia lux est.
Obtenebrat culpa, dat lucida gratia corda.

Sunt extrema crucis contriti quatuor ista:
Spes Dominique timor ac festinatio, finis.

PenCito, ll. 115-122

41 Qvibvs pvnitvr peccatvm.

Sit tibi potus aqua, cibus aridus, aspera uestis,
Dorso uirga, breuis somnus durumque cubile.
Flecte genu, tunde pectus, nuda caput, orans,
Hereat os terre, mens celo, lingua loquatur,
5   Cor dictet. Sit larga manus, ieiunia crebra,
Mens humilis, simplex oculus, caro munda, pium cor,
Recta fides, spes firma; duplex dilectio semper
Ferueat; assiduis precibus, iustis tamen, ora.
Hec age peccator quem uere penitet. A te
10 Tu potius penas peccatis exige dignas
Quam te perpetuis addicat iudicis ira.

PenCito, ll. 123-134

42 Sex opera caritatis.

Vestio, poto, cibo, tectum do, uisito, soluo,
Comodo, compatior, conuerto, dono, remitto,
Arguo, supplico, consulo, do quodcumque talentum.
Flecto genu, uigilo, ieiuno, laboro, flagellor,
5   Vestio dura, pedes nudor, tero cor, peregrinor.
Peniteo, lego, ploro, precor, caro sic maceratur.
Hiis que confessis sint iniungenda notabis.

PenCito, ll. 136-142

43 Qvod pena debet esse qvandoqve occvlta et qvandoqve manifesta.

Publica sit pena, fuerit si publica noxa;
Si lateat licet enormis, lateat quoque pena.
Hoc est, qui peccat oculte, peniteat clam.
Singula confessor prudentius ut moderetur,
5   Affectus causa, uitium, persona notetur.
Mos, cumulus, mors et morbus, rubor acta fatendi,
Difficilisque salus, purgatio dura per ignem,
Detenta culpa tardanti sunt metuenda.
Accelerent nos conuerti, deflere reatus:
10 Horror duritie, grauitatis, mortis et ignis,
Plausu, Tartarei confusio multa ministri,

Temporis ac operum lucrum cum celicolarum
Et fuga Cochiti felix, et adoptio celi.
Ad Dominum festinandi sunt hee tibi cause:
15 Ignis purificans, mors, egritudo ruborque,
Et cure grauitas, et consuetudo, ruina.

Fercula, festa, canes et equi, numerusque clientum,
Vestibus et uasis, domibus curaque parentum
Excelsus superesse negant bona danda potentum.

1-16 *PenCito*, ll. 143-152, 154, 153, 155-158

Explicit **De penitentia**.

Incipit **De verbis apostoli Pavli de prelatis ecclesie**.

44 ⟨De verbis apostoli Pavli de prelatis ecclesie⟩

Prima precipitur quod sit sine crimine presul,
Monagamus, sobrius, prudens, ornatus et hospes,
Casta docens, non percussor, non litigiosus,
Non cupidus, bene prepositus, non neophitusue,
5 Talis apostolica quod presit regula iussit.

IC, nos. 14624 and 14636; *PS*, nos. 22391 and 22400d.

45 Qvot modis qvis peccat edendo.

Est certum quod quinque modis gula dampnat edentem:
Dum nimium comedit, uel edendi preuenit horam,
Querit delicias, parat escas deliciose,
Vel sumit cupide quod non est deliciosum.

5 Abstinet eger, egens, cupidus, gula simia uirtus.

1-4 *HildEpig*, no. 15, p. 284.
5 *IC*, no. 210; *PS*, no. 222a.

46 De qvindecim penis inferni.

Nix, nox, uox, lacrime socii, sitis, phulfur et ignis,
Malleus, stridor, spes perdita, uincula, uermes,
Esse carere Deo, carcer, confessio rara.

47   Ad idem.

Vita set inuita, uermes et uincula, carcer
Et sitis atque fames, Dominique carentia, frigus,
Et calor ac ignis, fumus, conquestio, stridor
Et lacrime, nullum meritum, non ordo set horror,
5 Ira, tremor, tenebre, fetores perpetuique.

48   Decem precepta legis.

Sperne deos, fugito periuria, sabata serua;
    Sit tibi patris honor, sit tibi matris amor;
Non sis occisor, mechus, fur, testis iniqus,
    Vicinique thorum resque caueto suas.

Aurora, 1: 106.

49   Decem plage Egipti.

Sanguis, rana, culex, musce, pecus, ulcera, grando,
Brucus, caligo, mors pignora prima necando.

Vers, no. 1046; cf. *Aurora*, 1: 98.

50   Moraliter exponvntvr.

Est homo sanguineus cui non colitur Deus unus.
Rana loquax heresis nomen reprobat deitatis.
Vt cinifes errant qui sabata sacra prophanant.
Ille cynomia fit qui patres ut canis odit.
5 Fit pecus et moritur quasi brutus adulter habetur.
Feruor uesice feruens furor est homicide.
Fur rapit exterius, Deus illum grandinat intus.
Dente locusta nocet, falsus testis male mordet.
Cor patiens tenebras rapit uxores alienas.
10 Prima perit proles fore si male quis cupit heres.

Sacrum pingue dabo, non macrum sacrificabo: Abel.
    Sacrificabo macrum, non dabo pingue sacrum: Caym.

1-10 Cf. *Aurora*, 1: 98, where these lines are reported as insertions in
three manuscripts of Peter Riga's work. They are also found on folio
50r of MS Lyell 8, Bodleian Library, Oxford.
11-12 *IC*, no. 17014; *PS*, no. 27064

51 <De septem vitiis>

A litibus septem, septem signantur abyssi
  Que sordent animas alliciuntque sibi.

Svperbia:

Pauo rotans caudam, uibrans, sua sidera portans,
  Voce sathan fastus portat in orbe typum.

Ira:

5 Ira coquit coruum, coctus color indicat iram,
  Erumpitque foras fellis amara lues.

Invidia:

Infelix cuculus tanto liuore laborat
  Vt uolucrum perdat perditus ille domos.

Accidia:

Turpis, iners, segnis, nebulose noctis amicus,
  Bubo tristitie signifer esse potest.

Avaritia:

10 Perdis quod sepelis, parua monedula, perdit
  Et sibi quas querit questor auarus opes.

Lvxvria:

Non tenuis tenuem, non paruula, paruule passer,
  Te uenus irritat, sollicitatque iecur.

Gvla:

Vultur edax uentri indulget, feruet et ardet
15   Illius ingluuies perniciesque gule.

    15 gule] gulos *MS*

52 Qvod dvodecim prophete predixervnt dvodecim articvlos fidei qvos dvodecim apostoli concordantia eorvm sic postea scribendo composvervnt.

Ieremias	Patrem inuocabitis me [Ier 3:19; cf. 23:24]
Petrvs	Credo in Deum patrem omnipotentem creatorem celi et terre
Daniel	Filius hominis ueniet [Dan 7:13]
5 Andreas	Et in Ihesum christum, filium eius unicum, dominum nostrum

Isaias	Ecce uirgo concipiet [Is 7:14]
Iacobvs (minor)	Qui conceptus est de Spiritu sancto, natus ex Maria uirgine
10 Ezechiel	Tunc uidebunt in quem crucifixerunt [cf. Io 19:37]
Iohannes	Passus sub Pontio Pilato, crucifixus, mortuus et sepultus
Osee	Morsus tuus ero, inferne [Os 13:14], et in die tertia suscitabit nos [Os 6:3]
15 Thomas	Descendit ad inferna, tertia die resurexit a mortuis
Amos	Qui edificat in celo ascensionem suam [Am 9:6]
Iacobvs	Ascendit ad celos, sedet ad dexteram Dei Patris omnipotentis
Ioel	In ualle Iosaphat iudicabit omnes gentes [Ioel 3:12]
20 Philippvs	Inde uenturus est iudicare uiuos et mortuos
Aggevs	Spiritus meus erit in medio uestrum [Agg 2:6]
Bartholomevs	Credo in Spiritum sanctum
Sophonias	Hec est ciuitas gloriosa que dicit extra me non est aliud [Soph 2:15]
25 Mathevs	Sanctam Ecclesiam catholicam, sanctorum communionem
Malachias	Cum odium habueris dimitte [Mal 2:16]
Simon	Remissionem peccatorum
Zacarias	Suscitabo filios tuos et duplicia reddam tibi [Zach 9:12-13]
30	
Thadevs	Carnis resurrectionem
Abdias	Et erit Domino regnum sempiternum [Abd v.21]
Mathias	Et uitam eternam, amen (id est fiat).

25-26 sanctorum communionem] remissionem peccatorum *add.* MS

II.4

Speculum penitentis

The *Speculum penitentis* is an important example of the type of instruction available to students, priests, and confessors at the beginning of the thirteenth century.[1] It illustrates the careful attention that was being paid to the art of hearing confessions during the years preceding the Fourth Lateran Council's mandate (1215) that all Christians should confess to their proper priest at least once a year.[2]

William's treatise comprises two parts. Part One is unique among the many guides and handbooks produced in this period in its emphasis on the confession of unrecognized and often ignored sins (*peccata magis ignota*, sections 1.1 and 1.5), as well as the more dangerous ones (*peccata magis periculosa*, section 1.2). His discussion of the most common sins among monks, regular canons, and secular canons (section 1.3) perhaps indicates the audience for whom he composed this work. Part One of the *Speculum* also contains an analysis of the types of sins (*De diuersitatibus peccatorum*, section 1.4) based on Peter Lombard's *Sentences*.

The second part of the *Speculum*, sometimes copied as a separate work,[3] is a guide to the actual procedure of hearing confessions (sections 2.1 and 2.2) The priest is instructed to inquire about "carnal" and "spiritual" sins, as well as about "delicts" (sins of omission) and the personal circumstances that aggravate sins. This second part is constructed around an earlier treatise of William's that began: *Sancti estote quia ego sanctus sum* (section 2.2). William has integrated the *Sancti estote* carefully into his new *Speculum penitentis*; the sins that are described in detail in that earlier work are listed succinctly, for

---

[1] The best summary of recent research on such texts is still Pierre Michaud-Quantin's *Sommes de casuistique*; William's *Speculum* is noted in the Appendix. For the scholastic background see Paul Anciaux, *La théologie du sacrement de pénitence au XIIe siècle*.

[2] Canon 21, "Omnis utriusque sexus ..."; *Conciliorum oecumenicorum decreta*, p. 245.

[3] See MSS 4, 8, and 10, below.

ease of reference, in the first five paragraphs of section 2.1. Apparent contradictions between the new and the older work are resolved, and a general conclusion is appended in the last two paragraphs of section 2.2.

The final paragraphs of the *Speculum* (section 2.3) represent a new element in the penitential literature — instructions for the dying. The prayers and practices recommended there found their way into English liturgical manuals by the fourteenth century.[4] They represent one of the earliest manifestations of the *ars moriendi* tradition that would become a crucial element of lay piety by the end of the Middle Ages.[5]

The importance of penitential writings produced before 1215 scarcely needs emphasis. Although few scholars would contend any longer that the flood of penitential handbooks and *summae* written in the thirteenth and subsequent centuries was unleashed by the Fourth Lateran Council's mandate of annual confession, too few of the numerous pre-conciliar treatises have been edited or studied to allow a careful investigation of the beginnings of this phenomenon. William's *Speculum penitentis*, like his *De penitentia religiosorum* and his *Peniteas cito*, is an important witness to the role of penance in the care of souls at the beginning of the thirteenth century.

The *Speculum penitentis* is neither a *summa de penitentia* nor a guide to all aspects of the sacrament of penance. In this treatise William ignores the question of "penances" that the priest should impose as satisfaction for particular sins, a topic that was his primary concern in his *De penitentia religiosorum* (see below, II.5). The emphasis here is on the act of confession. William conceives his *Speculum* as a "mirror" in which readers will be able first to recognize sins,[6] and then to confess these sins or elicit a fruitful confession from others.[7] Such confessional instructions and formularies became commonplace during the thirteenth century, but William's is one of the earliest to ignore completely the older traditions of the "penitentials," and to discuss

---

[4] The prayers "Suscipe me," "In manus tuas," "Ab ocultis," "Delicta iuuentutis," and "Aue Maria" in 2.3 are recommended to the dying penitent in the *Manuale ad usum percelebris ecclesie Sarisburiensis*, p. 112.

[5] See Mary C. O'Conner, *The Art of Dying Well, the Development of the "Ars moriendi"* (New York: Columbia University Press, 1942); the medieval precursors of this tradition still await careful investigation.

[6] "De peccatorum agnitione ... ," the beginning phrase of the introductory paragraph; see below, p. 187.

[7] "Hec sunt de quibus inquisitio facienda est in confessione ... ," the first sentence in Part Two; see below, p. 202.

in detail the new art of confession as it was being understood in the schools.[8]

Although hearing confessions was a duty incumbent on all priests with the care of souls, William's *Speculum* seems not to have been written expressly for the education of the parochial clergy. From William's discussion of particular sins we can infer that he was addressing an audience that had received some formal training in the schools. His exposition of scriptural passages and especially his use of the various scholastic glosses on Scripture to clarify his arguments would have meant little to one who had no experience of this type of exercise.

A more precise delineation of this text's intended audience may be possible. In section 1.3 William outlines the particular sins of three groups: monks, regular canons, and secular canons. Students in William's school at Lincoln were drawn from all three groups, and it is likely that he had these audiences especially in mind when composing his *Speculum*. The longest discussion concerns the specific sins of monks. They are accused of being "disinheritors" of other men, of misappropriating tithes, of appointing unsuitable priests to their appropriated churches, of carrying on business ventures through the agency of laymen, of misappropriating wealth loaned to or deposited in the monastery, of condoning simony, of caring more for their own pigs than for the needs of the poor, and of failing to observe feast days. William's description might apply to all of the cloistered orders, but references to "lay brothers" and *fratres conversi* would apply especially to the Cistercian and the Carthusian houses in England, as well as to the new order of Sempringham — the Gilbertines. St. Hugh of Lincoln, it will be remembered, was prior of the first Carthusian foundation in England (1175) before being elected bishop of Lincoln

---

[8] The most perceptive description of the new types of penitential literature is Pierre Michaud-Quantin's "A propos des premières *Summae confessorum*," *Recherches de théologie ancienne et médiévale* 26 (1959) 264-306. Reservations concerning some of Michaud-Quantin's conclusions are expressed in Joseph Goering, "The *Summa* of Master Serlo and Thirteenth-Century Penitential Literature," *Mediaeval Studies* 40 (1978) 290-311. Examples of confessional instructions and formularies that were perhaps inspired by William's writings are the penitential works of Robert Grosseteste: see Joseph Goering and F.A.C. Mantello, "The Early Penitential Writings of Robert Grosseteste," *Recherches de théologie ancienne et médiévale* 54 (1987) 52-112; idem, "The 'Perambulauit Iudas ... ' (Speculum confessionis) Attributed to Robert Grosseteste," *Revue bénédictine* 96 (1986) 125-168; idem, "Notus in Iudea Deus: Robert Grosseteste's Confessional Formula in Lambeth Palace MS 499," *Viator* 18 (1987) 253-273; Siegfried Wenzel, "Robert Grosseteste's Treatise on Confession, *Deus est*," *Franciscan Studies* 30 (1970) 218-293.

in 1186, and William was also closely associated with St. Gilbert and the Gilbertines.

The sins of regular canons, priests who live in a less formal community and follow a rule such as that of St. Augustine, are described more briefly. They are said to lease their lands out of greed rather than necessity, and to cause scandal in the community by involving themselves in business activities. What particular canons William may have had in mind we cannot say. But his interest in the quality of pastoral care exercised among the canons-regular is displayed not only in this confessional handbook, but also in the model sermons that he composed for an unidentified Augustinian canon (see below, II.16).

In the paragraph entitled DE PECCATIS CANCONICORVM SECVLARIVM William completes this discussion by describing particular sins often attributed to secular canons. Here he strikes most near to home. The secular canons that he had in mind were the clergy serving a large church — a minster or, in William's day, a cathedral. Such were the canons of William's own church, the cathedral of Lincoln. Secular canons are accused of excessive absenteeism, of renting lands unnecessarily, of appointing immoral vicars to stand in for them, and of prattling rather than praying in the choir. William singles out for special comment the wandering habits of certain canons: "When one becomes a canon, the other canons say in chapter: "O how good and pleasant it is for brothers to live together as one" [Ps 132:1]. 'To live', they say, not 'to run'; and 'as one,' not just in one spirit, which is common to all Christians, but in one place, as is proper especially to those who are set apart by a mark of the religious life."

It is perhaps to be expected that William should think first of monks and canons when he composed his *Speculum penitentis*. These men lived together in a milieu that encouraged special discipline as well as learned discourse. They would be more amenable than individual parish priests and lay people to the thoughtful self-examination that William wished to inculcate. Once such audiences had become accustomed to confessing their sins in this new way and to eliciting such confessions from others, it would be only a matter of time before the practice could be extended to other less learned and less disciplined audiences. The seeds of the new penitential discipline that would be embraced by all levels of christian society in succeeding generations were planted in texts such as the *Speculum penitentis*, and nourished among William's students, especially the monks and canons, during these first years of the thirteenth century.

Authenticity and Date

Four of the eleven manuscript copies of the *Speculum* are ascribed to William; no copy is ascribed to another author. Five of the unascribed copies are accompanied in the manuscripts by others of William's authentic works. The work was copied frequently in the thirteenth century; the library of Peterborough Abbey contained at least eleven copies, nine of which are ascribed to William de Montibus.[9] The numerous echoes of William's other writings in this work remove any remaining doubt about his authorship.

No internal or external evidence suffices to date the treatise precisely. William seems first to have composed the treatise *Sancti estote* (section 2.2) and then supplemented this confessional tract with a fuller discussion of the more subtle and more dangerous sins. Both parts were composed by William. He explains that he has purposefully interchanged the order of inquiry concerning carnal and spiritual sins in the two treatises. Having recommended in the *Sancti estote* that one begin by confessing the spiritual, in the new portions of the *Speculum* William lists first the carnal sins. This change, William tells us, is intended to suggest that it is immaterial whether one begins by confessing one or the other; both types should be confessed just as they come to mind.[10] There is no indication that the composition of the *Speculum* long postdates that of the *Sancti estote*. A date of composition for both texts in the thirteenth century (1200 x 1213) seems likely.

Sources

William's source for the materials in the *Speculum* is primarily his own reading in the Bible and its glosses. He uses Scripture thoughtfully, both to reveal and to illustrate various types of sins. Many of the scriptural citations and glosses here are also found in his other works, especially in the *Peniteas cito*, the *Distinctiones*, and the *Prouerbia*.

---

[9] Montague Rhodes James, "Lists of Manuscripts Formerly in Peterborough Abbey Library," *Transactions of Bibliographical Society (Supplement)* 5 (1926).

[10] "Attende etiam quod in tractatu premisso peccata carnalia preposuimus; in eiusdem explanatione illa postponimus, quod ex industria fecimus ad insinuandum quod non multum refert in confessione prius confiteri carnalia quam spiritualia uel uice uersa, cum utrumque oporteat facere secundum quod hec et illa occurrunt memorie," below, p. 209.

William's quotations from patristic authors all derive from the various biblical glosses, from Gratian's *Decretum*, or from Lombard's *Sentences*. His quotations of Aristotle, Ovid, Persius, and other popular authorities can be traced to no intermediate source, but the sentiments are commonplace and used frequently by William as well as other authors.

Manuscripts

1. *C* = Cambridge, Corpus Christi College MS 217, fols. 148r-151r. Early 13th century (above top line).

> Title: *Incipit speculum penitentis editum a Magistro Willelmo de montibus cancellario Lincoln'*
> Inc. Prol.: *De peccatorum agnitione*
> Inc. Txt.: *Attendenda sunt in confessione*
> Expl. Txt.: *Item ante sumptionem eucharistie simbolum fidei reddat, idest Credo in Deum Patrem omnipotentem, et deinceps totum ex ordine dicat.*
> Colophon: *Explicit speculum penitentis.*

References to the biblical citations, using a pre-Langton system of chapter numeration, have been added in the margins.

2. Cambridge, Peterhouse MS 119, fols. 31ra-32vb. Mid 13th century (above top line).

> Title: *Incipit Speculum penitentis*
> Inc. Prol.: *De peccatorum agnitione*
> Inc. Txt.: *Attendenda sunt in confessione*
> Expl. Txt. (imperfect before end of section 2.2): *Item peccat non nunquam qui de bono quod egit penitet et dolet, peccat etiam qui differt confessionem siue conuersionem. Sunt etiam et alia.*

3. Cambridge, Peterhouse MS 255, fols. 128ra-133va. Early 13th century (above top line).

> Title (in plummet): *Incipit speculum penitentis*
> Inc. Prol.: *De peccatorum agnicione*
> Inc. Txt.: *Attendenda sunt in confessione*
> Expl. Txt.: *Item, ante sumptionem eucaristie, cymbolum fidei reddat, idest credo.*

4. Cambridge, St. John's College MS F.4 (141), fols. 44ra-47ra. Mid 13th century (above top line).

> Title: *Ista sunt inquirenda in confessione secundum magistrum Willelmum de monte*
> Inc. Txt. (incomplete, begins with section 2.1): *Hec sunt de quibus inquisitio facienda est in confessione.*
> Expl.: *Item, ante sumptionem eucaristie simbolum fidei reddat.*

The text is followed immediately (fol. 47ra-va) by brief instructions for a confessor: "Cum ad confessionem quis uenerit, sacerdos eum cum tanta humilitate et deuotione suscipiat ... . Huiusmodi uicia precaue artius, quod nobis prestet qui uiuit et regnat." This confessional treatise is not listed in Bloomfield, et al., *Incipits*.

5. Idem, fols. 85ra-88rb. Mid 13th century (above top line).

    Title: (*Incipit speculum penitentis*)
    Inc. Prol.: *De agnicione peccatorum*
    Inc. Txt.: *Attendenda sunt in confessione*
    Expl. Txt.: *Item, ante sumpcionem eucharistie, simbolum fidei reddat*
    Colophon: *Explicit Speculum penitentie.*

The text is written in a cursive hand, different from the text-hand that copied the first copy of the *Speculum* in this codex (no. 4, above). This copy is preceded by a contemporary table of contents, on fol. 85ra, beginning *Incipiunt capitula anime penitentis*, in which the work is divided into sixty-five chapters. The first sixty-three comprise our sections 1.1-1.5; Chapter 64, entitled *De hiis que inquirenda sunt in confessione*, comprises our sections 2.1 and 2.2; and Chapter 65, *De obitu*, corresponds to our section 2.3.

6. *T* = Cambridge, Trinity Hall MS 24, fols. 108ra-112rb. Mid 13th century (above top line).

    Inc. Prol.: *De agnitione peccatorum*
    Inc. Txt.: *Attenda sunt in confessione*
    Expl. Txt.: *Item, ante sumpcionem eucharistie simbolum fidei reddat*

A contemporary table of contents on fol. 108ra divides Part One of the treatise (sections 1.1-1.5) into sixty-two chapters. These are followed by the *Explanatio peccatorum et que inquirenda sunt in confessione* (sections 2.1 and 2.2) and the *De obitu* (section 2.3). This copy of the *Speculum* includes two additions, unique to this manuscript but perhaps authentic, which are printed in the apparatus to the text below, pp. 202 and 203.

7. London, British Library Cotton MS Vespasian D.xiii, fols. 60ra-65vb. Mid 13th century (above top line).

    Title: *Incipit speculum penitentis editum a magistro Willelmo de montibus cancellario lincolniensi*
    Inc. Prol.: *De pecatorum agnicione*
    Inc. Txt.: *<A>ttendenda sunt in confessione*
    Expl. Txt. (imperfect in section 2.3): *deinde generali, vt: Confiteor Deo et beate*

At least one gathering is missing between fols. 65 and 66. The missing pages originally contained the final lines of the *Speculum* and the beginning of a heretofore unidentified copy of the "Synodal statutes for an English diocese" (1222 x 1225?).[11] This copy begins imperfectly on fol. 66ra with the last three words of c. 47 and includes cc. 49-53, 66-69, 54-65 of the Synodal statutes, as well as an unascribed copy of the "Decree for the province of Canterbury" (1225).[12]

8. Idem, fols. 118vb-121rb. Mid 13th century (above top line).

> Title: (*Item eiusdem, unde supra*)
> Inc. Txt. (incomplete, begins in section 2.1): *Hec sunt de quibus inquisicio facienda est in confessione*
> Expl.: *Item, ante sumpcionem eukaristie symbolum fidei reddat, idest Credo, et cetera, et deinde totum ex ordine dicat.*

Fols. 60r-130v of this codex are all written in the same hand. This copy of William's *Speculum* includes only the second part of the treatise. It is preceded, on fols. 115rb-118va, by an ascribed copy of William's *Peniteas cito peccator* (see above, p. 114).

9. London, British Library MS Harley 325, fols. 87r-94r. Mid 13th century (above top line).

> Title: *Speculum penitentie*
> Inc. Prol.: *De agnitione peccatorum*
> Inc. Txt.: *Attendenda sunt in confessione*
> Expl. Txt.: *Item, ante sumptionem eucharistie simbolum fidei reddat*
> Colophon: *Explicit speculum penitentis*

A table of contents, written by the same scribe, is found on fol. 87r. It begins: *Incipiunt capitula speculi penitentis*, and divides the work into sixty-three chapters, the last two being *Explanatio peccatorum et que inquirenda sunt in confessione* and *De obitu*.

10. Oxford, Bodleian Library MS Digby 20, fols. 158r-161r. Early 14th century.

> Inc. Txt. (incomplete, begins in section 2.1): (*De confessione*) *Hec sunt de quibus inquisicio facienda est in confessione*
> Expl. Txt.: *Item, ante sumpcionem eukaristie simbolum fidei reddat, idest Credo in Deum Patrem, et cetera, et deinceps totum ex ordine dicat.*

11. *M* = Paris, Bibliothèque Mazarine MS 730, fols. 65rb-67vb. Mid 13th century.

> Inc. Prol.: *De peccatorum agnicione*
> Inc. Txt.: *Attendenda sunt in confessione*
> Expl. Txt.: *Item, ante sumpcionem eucharistie idest credo symbolum fidei reddat*

---

[11] *Councils and Synods*, 1: 139-154.
[12] Ibid., pp. 154-155.

The *Speculum penitentis* is printed here in its entirety. All of the manuscript copies have been examined; the text below is transcribed from Cambridge, Corpus Christi College MS 217 = *C* (no. 1, above), an early and reliable witness. Selected emendations and variant readings taken from Paris, Bibliothèque Mazarine MS 730 = *M* (no. 11, above), are noted in the *apparatus criticus*. Rubrics in *C* are printed in small capitals, and additional rubrics from Cambridge, Trinity Hall MS 24 = *T* (no. 6, above), are enclosed within angle brackets < >.

The following abbreviations are used to identify sources in the text:

Gl. ord. = Glossa ordinaria; the common marginal gloss to the Bible, as printed, for example, in *Biblia sacra*.

Gl. interl. = Glossa interlinearis; the common interlinear gloss to the Bible, as printed, for example, in *Biblia sacra*.

Gl. Lombardi = *Commentarium in psalmos davidicos*, printed in PL 191: 55-1296; *Collectanea in epistolas Pauli*, printed in PL 191: 1297-1696; 192: 9-520.

HildEpig = Hildebert, *Biblical Epigrams*.

Sent = *Magistri Petri Lombardi Parisiensis episcopi Sententiae in IV libris distinctae*, ed. PP. Collegii S. Bonaventurae, 2 vols., 3rd edition (Grottaferrata: Collegium S. Bonaventurae, 1971-1981).

Decretum = *Decretum magistri Gratiani*, ed. E. Friedberg (Leipzig: 1881).

PS = Hans Walther, *Proverbia sententiaeque latinitatis medii aevi*, 6 vols. (Göttingen: 1963-1967).

Speculum penitentis

Incipit Speculum penitentis editum a Magistro Willelmo de Montibus cancellario Lincolniensi.

De peccatorum agnitione tractatum teximus, penitenti perutilem, cui nomen imponimus Speculum penitentis; hac enim congesta speculantem tum faciem culpe tum faciem anime non est latere.

1.1 Qve sint peccata magis ignota

Attendenda sunt in confessione peccata tum euidentiora, ut fornicationes et adulteria, furta, rapine, et homicidia, tum magis ignota rudibus scilicet hominibus et brutalibus, ut sunt peccata negligentie et ignorantie et pleraque alia.

PRIMVM CAPITVLVM <DE PECCATO NEGLIGENTIE>
Peccata dico negligentie secundum illud [Rom 12:11]: "Sollicitudine non pigri," idest si solliciti estis corde, non sitis pigri opere. "Maledictus enim" ut ait Ieremias [48:10] "qui opus Dei fecerit negligenter."

<DE IGNORANTIA>
Amplius, peccata ignorantie. Vnde super epistolam ad Romanos [*Gl. ord.* in Rom 2:3-4]: "Peccas, o homo, dum tibi impunitatem promittis; grauius peccas quia contempnis bonitatem Dei; grauissime peccas quia ignoras te contempnere." Grauissime, idest periculosissime, sicut periculose egrotat qui morbum¹ ignorat.

<DE CONTINVATIONE PECCATI>
Amplius, continuatio peccatorum. Vnde Ysaias [5:18]: "Ve qui trahitis iniquitatem in funiculis uanitatis, et quasi uinculum plaustri peccatum"; et in Psalmo [30:24]: "Dominus retribuet habundanter facientibus superbiam," Glosa [*Lombardi* PL 191:314]: "Omnes habundanter faciunt superbiam qui non cito² penitent de quolibet mortali peccato." Nota quod dicitur "omnes," ergo non tantum peccantes contra Deum ut contumaces et impenitentes, set etiam peccantes sub Deo, ut qui peccant ex fragilitate carnis et in timore quodam seruili siue naturali, et similiter penitentia naturali.

<DE DILATIONE PENITENTIE>
Amplius, dilatio penitentie. Vnde in Ecclesiastico [5:8-9]: "Non tardes conuerti ad Dominum, et ne differas de die in diem; subito enim ueniet ira illius, et in tempore uindicte disperdet te." Mora quidem ad se trahit periculum.

<DE CONTEMPTV SCIENTIE>
Amplius, contemptus scientie. Vnde Salomon [Prov 19:2]: "Vbi non est scientia anime, non est bonum," suple "eternum"; et in Psalmo [35:4]: "Noluit intelligere ut bene ageret." Item de impiis dicit Iob [21:13-15]: "Ducunt in bonis dies suos, et in puncto ad inferna descendunt. Qui dixerunt Deo: Recede a nobis, scientiam uiarum tuarum nolumus. Quis est omnipotens ut seruiamus ei, et quid nobis prodest si orauerimus eum?"

---

1 morbum] *M*: mortem *C*
2 cito] *M*: scito *C*

<DE SEMINATIONE DISCORDIE>

Amplius, seminatio discordie. Vnde Salomon in Parabolis [Prov 6:12-14]: "Homo apostata uir inutilis, gradiens ore[3] peruerso; annuit oculis, terit pede, digito loquitur, prauo corde machinatur malum, et omni tempore iurgia seminat." Et paulo post [6:16-19]: "Sex sunt que odit Deus, et septimum detestatur anima eius: Oculos sublimes, linguam mendacem, manus effundentes sanguinem innoxium, cor machinans cogitationes pessimas, pedes ueloces ad currendum in malum, proferentem mendacia testem fallacem, et eum qui seminat inter fratres discordias."

<DE EBRIETATE>

Amplius, ebrietas assidua et maledictio frequenter prolata. Vnde Apostolus [1 Cor 6:9-10]: "Nolite errare: neque fornicarii, neque ydolis seruientes, nec adulteri, nec molles, nec masculorum concubitores, nec fures, nec auari, nec ebriosi, nec maledici, nec rapaces regnum Dei possidebunt." Molles autem dicuntur patici, qui patiuntur sodomitas et polluuntur ab eis.

<DE IRA DIVTINA>

Similiter ira diutina. Vnde Apostolus [Eph 4:26]: "Sol non occidat super iracundiam uestram," idest ipsa ira non duret usque ad occasum solis, hoc est non diu duret. Et loquitur hic de ira per uitium, de qua etiam Dominus dicit in Euuangelio [Mt 5:22]: "Omnis qui irascitur fratri suo reus erit iudicio." Non fratri irascitur qui peccato irascitur. Est enim ira per zelum qua quis iuste irascitur uitiis et peccatis, et ad hoc facta est a Deo anima irascibilis.

<DE MENDACIO>

Similiter et mendacium assuetum. Vnde in Apocalipsi [21:8]: "Timidis autem, et incredulis, et excecratis, et homicidis, et fornicatoribus, et ueneficis, et ydolatris, et omnibus mendacibus, pars illorum erit in stagno ardenti igne et sulphure, quod est mors secunda." Timidos dicit eos qui ex timore seruili uel mundano uel humano se chohibent a bono uite eterne meritorio. Incredulos dicit qui non recte credunt seu credere nolunt, ut sit in priuatiuum siue aduersatiuum, uel eos qui desperant. Excecratos uocat excommunicatos. De mendacibus dicit Glosa [interl. ad Apoc 21:8]: "Quibus mendacium est in usu." Et nota quod mors secunda dicitur pena gehennalis, eo quod sit pena nouissima, grauissima, seperans, et superans. Seperans scilicet a uiuis, idest sanctis, et omnino exsuperans hominem, ne de cetero se possit adiuuare

3 ore] *M*: opere *C*

merendo. Vnde [Mt 22:13]: "Ligatis manibus et pedibus, proicite illum in tenebras exteriores." Neque enim poterit dampnatus effectu uel affectu mereri, nec ueniam nec gloriam adipisci. In Ecclesiastico [20:26-27] et scriptum est: "Obprobrium nequam in homine mendacium, et in ore indisciplinatorum[4] assidue erit. Potior fur quam assiduitas uiri mendacis; perditionem autem ambo hereditabunt." Mendacium quidem malignitatis ex duplicitate animi. Illud etiam unicum est mortale peccatum. Vnde [Ps 5:7]: "Perdes omnes qui locuntur mendacium," et [Sap 1:11]: "Os quod mentitur occidit animam." Mendacium uero benignitatis, causa commodi, quale fuit mendacium Raab uel obste-tricum Egiptiarum, secundum Augustinum [3 *Sent* 38.1.3, pp. 213-214] ueniale peccatum est. Mendacium autem hilaritatis, causa ioci, et illud ueniale est nisi in usu fuerit, sicut supra dictum est.

<DE OTIOSA IVRATIONE>

Amplius, otiosa iuratio. Vnde in Exodo [20:7]: "Non assumes nomen Dei tui in uanum." Glosa [*interl. ad loc*]: "Iurando scilicet pro nichilo Dei nomen." Sequitur [Ex 20:8]: "Nec enim habebit insontem Dominus eum qui assumpserit nomen Domini Dei sui frustra." Item in Deute-ronomio [5:11]: "Non usurpabis nomen Domini Dei tui frustra, quia non erit impunitus qui super rem uanam nomen eius assumpserit." Ex hoc autem quod dicitur "non usurpabis" potest intelligi prohibitum esse crebro uel assidue iurare sine causa necessaria, quasi non usurpabis, idest non in usum accipies. Vnde in Ecclesiastico [23:9-10]: "Iurationi non assuescat os tuum; multi enim casus in illa. Nominatio uero Dei non sit assidua in ore tuo," suple ad iurandum, "et nominibus sanctorum non admiscearis," suple in iurando, "quoniam non erit immunis ab eis," scilicet iniuriis sanctorum. Et subintellige hic: non assumendum nomen Dei cum animo iurandi, sicut Aristoles ait in Topicis [6.12; 149b 29-30]: "Non qui clam sumit, set qui uult clam sumere latro est," idest qui animo furandi clam sumit. Vnde secundum quosdam, qui uulgariter et usualiter dicit "per Deum hoc faciam," uel huiusmodi, non iurat set simplicia uerba sunt, nec enim animum iurandi habet. Dominus autem dicens in Euuangelio [Mt 5:34]: "Ego autem dico uobis, non iurare omnino," prohibet iurare serio et animo iurandi de re illicita, otiose, false,[5] dolose, appetere iuramentum, assuescere iuramento, et iurare per creaturas, friuola scilicet oppinione, ut si credat creature numen inesse et presidere, sicut credit ydolatra; uel si credat

---

4 indisciplinatorum] *ed.*: disciplinatorum *CM*
5 false] *M*: falce *C*

se non teneri iurando per creaturam, immo tenetur. In creatura namque iuratur creator.

<DE VERBOSITATE>

Amplius [Ps 139:12]: "Vir lingosus non dirigetur in terra"; Glosa [*Lombardi* PL 191: 1232]: "Si quis uera dicat set preter necessitatem, uir lingosus est." Intellige "dicat" idest dicere consuescat. Item [Mt 12:36]: "Omne uerbum otiosum quodcumque locuti fuerint homines reddent de eo rationem." Super "uerbum otiosum" habetur hec glosa [*interl.*]: "Quod sine utilitate dicitur loquentis et audientis, ut de friuolis et fabulis, scurilia non sunt otiosa set criminosa"; suple: si in usu fuerint.

<DE NVGIS>

Amplius [Bernardus, *Ad Eugenium* 2.13, PL 182: 756]: "Nuge in ore aliorum nuge sunt, in ore sacerdotis blasphemie." Determina: "quasi blasphemie," uel "nuge frequentes et crebre," uel de summo sacerdote hoc dicitur. Item ait Leo papa [*Decretum*, D.32 c.1]: "Omnium sacerdotum tam excellens est electio ut hec que in aliis membris ecclesie uacant a culpa, in hiis tamen habeantur illicita."

<DE CONSENSV>

Amplius, consensus in malum. Hinc Apostolus [Rom 1:32], enumeratis uitiis quibusdam et peccatis, subinfert dicens: "Qui talia agunt digni sunt morte," eterna scilicet, "non solum qui faciunt ea set etiam qui consentiunt facientibus." "Consentire," ut Ambrosius [*Gl. ord., ad loc.*] ait, "est tacere cum possis arguere, uel errorem adulando fouere." Quidam dicunt, "cum possis debito officii," uel "facilitate et facultate debiti"; hoc est dicere "cum possis," idest debeas, "et facile ualeas." Multiplex quidem est consensus, ut alibi diximus.

<DE DELECTATIONE>

Amplius, delectatio morosa, de re scilicet dampnabili, ut de fornicatione et huiusmodi, et post deliberationem et discretionem rationis, et cum continuatione etiam sine consensu in actum. Vnde in Sententiis libro secundo [2 *Sent* 24.12.1, p. 457], de peccato dicitur: "Si diu in cogitationis delectatione teneatur, etsi uoluntas perficiendi desit, mortale est, et pro eo dampnabitur simul uir (Adam) et mulier (Eua) idest totus homo, quia et tunc uir non sicut debuit mulierem cohibuit; unde potest dici consensisse, hoc est, superior pars rationis delectationi sensualitatis, etsi non operi exteriori, quia consentire est nolle corrigere cum possis et debeas." Nota tamen hec esse uerba Magistri set confirmat ea auctoritate Augustini.

<DE CONFIDENTIA>

Amplius, super illum locum Psalmi [77:46]: "Et dedit erugini fructus eorum," legitur [*Gl. ord.*] quod rubigo uel erugo occulte nocens est multum fidere de se, cum se putat aliquid esse cum nichil sit.

<DE ARROGANTIA>

Amplius, Sennacherib quod Dei est uiribus suis ascribit [cf. Is 36], philosophus nature ut naturali ingenio, Pelagius libero arbitrio, moderni[6] heretici industrie et labori suo, qui causam secundariam et cooperantem constituunt principalem et efficientem; contra quod dicitur [1 Cor 13:10]: "Non ego set gratia Dei mecum." Alii omnem[7] fortune attribuunt.

<DE GLORIATIONE>

Amplius, Nabugodonosor gloriatur in edificio, ideo bestia factus homo, idest bestialiter uiuens ad tempus [Dan 4:30].

<DE INSVLTATIONE>

Amplius, captiuitati Israel insultant uicine nationes, ideo et ipse captiuantur [cf. Iudith 5:17-25; Ier 30:16].

<DE VSVRA>

Amplius, dampnatur non solum usura set et superhabundantia. Vnde [Ps 14:5]: "Qui pecuniam suam non dedit ad usuram"; et in Leuitico [25:37] dicit Dominus, "Frugum superhabundantiam non exiges"; et in Ezechiele [18:8,17]: "Vir si ad usuram non commodauerit uel superhabundantiam, et amplius non acceperit, hic iustus est, uita uiuet, ait Dominus Deus." Item in Psalmo super illum locum [54:12], "Et non defecit de plateis eius usura et dolus," [*Gl. ord.*]: "Vsuram committit qui plus exigit in iniuria, uel in qualibet re, quam acceperit." Intellige: exigit ex rancore in iniuria uindicanda; lex enim punit furtum in quadruplum uel amplius.

<DE IMMODERATIONE>

Amplius, qui etiam minimis immoderate herent dampnabuntur, ut habetur super illum locum Apocalypsis [*Gl. interl.* in 18:14]: "Et poma desiderii anime tue."

<DE PAVORE>

Amplius, culpabilis es si digitus hominis pascat te, idest appetitus humani fauoris ad bonum faciendum te impellat, secundum quod

---

6 moderni] *M*: modum *C*
7 omnem] *M*: omen *C*

Persius [*Sat* 1:28] ait: "At pulcrum est digito monstrari et dicier hic est."

\<De impetv\>
Amplius, culpatur qui magis quodam naturali impetu quam ut Deo placeat aliquid agit, et qui plus facit ex naturali dolore quam amore iustitie, ut Israel pungnans contra Beniamin [cf. Iud 20].

\<De intentione prava\>
Amplius, culpantur qui gratia uictualium monachantur, sicut Dominus exprobrat turbe dicens [Io 6:26]: "Queritis me non quia uidistis signa, set quia manducastis ex panibus et saturati estis."

\<De temptatione\>
Amplius, attende quia grauant animam temptare Deum. Vnde [Deut 6:16, Mt 4:7]: "Non temptabis Dominum Deum tuum."

\<De svpplantatione\>
Et supplantare fratrem. Vnde Ieremias [9:4-5] ait: "Vnusquisque se a proximo suo custodiat, et in omni fratre non habeat fiduciam; quia omnis frater supplantans supplantabit, et omnis amicus fraudulenter incedet. Et uir fratrem deridebit, et ueritatem non loquetur."

\<De observatione diervm\>
Peccatum etiam pluribus ignotum, dies obseruare ritu gentilium. Vnde Apostolus Galathiis [Gal 4:10-11] ait: "Dies observatis, et menses, et tempora, et annos. Timeo ne sine causa laborauerim in uobis." Ecce ad auspicium obseruare tempora graue reputat Apostolus.

\<De rapina vel ablatione\>
Peccatum est etiam subtrahere patri uel matri. Vnde in Parabolo [Prov 28:24]: "Qui subtraxherit aliquid a patre suo et a matre, et dicit hoc non est peccatum, particeps homicide est." Et in Euuangelio [Mc 7:11] arguuntur a Domino dicentes patri aut matri "Corban." Et in Ecclesiastico [34:25] legitur: "Panis egentium uita pauperis est; qui defraudat illum homo sanguinis est."

\<De eodem\>
Sequitur ibidem [Eccli 34:26] de peccato pluribus ignoto: "Qui aufert in sudore panem, quasi qui occidit proximum suum." Glosa [*ad loc.*]: "In sudore uultus sui pauper adquirit panem; qui hunc uiolenter tollit quasi interficit."

\<De svbtractione parentibvs\>
Est etiam peccatum graue parentibus egenis necessaria non prouidere.

Hinc Apostolus [1 Tim 5:8] ait: "Si quis suorum et maxime dome-
sticorum curam non habet, fidem negauit, et est infideli deterior." Qui
non habet curam suorum cum possit et debeat, et maxime dome-
sticorum, ut sunt patres et matres, fratres et sorores, filii et filie, et
huiusmodi, fidem negauit operibus, etsi non uerbis, quia proximum
non diligit. Et quodammodo, scilicet in hac parte, deterior est infideli
qui curam suorum naturaliter habet, et quia hic nondum ueritatem
nouit uel promisit, et [Lc 12:47] "seruus sciens et non faciens uoluntatem
domini sui uapulabit multis." Item in Parabolis [Prov 11:17]: "Benefacit
anime sue uir misericors; qui autem crudelis est propinquos abicit."
Et iterum [Prov 30:17]: "Oculum qui subsannat patrem et despicit
partum matris sue, suffodiant eum corui de torrentibus, et comedant
illum filii aquile."

<DE FRAVDVLENTIA IN OPERE DEI>
Amplius, peccatum graue est opus Dei[8] fraudulenter facere. Vnde
Ieremias [48:10]: "Maledictus qui facit opus Dei fraudulenter." Hoc
est ut ibi habetur in Glosa [interl.]: "Vel pro corporalis rei premio,
uel pro laudis uerbo, uel pro humani iudicii gratia." Super illum tamen
locum epistole ad Romanos [Gl. interl. ad 12:11], "Sollicitudine non
pigri," ita habetur ut supradictum est: "Maledictus" etc.

<ITEM DE NEGLIGENTIA>
Amplius, domum scopis mundatam, in baptismo uel penitentia, iam
uacantem a bonis per negligentiam et simulatis[9] uirtutibus ornatam,
repetit spiritus immundus [cf. Lc 11:24-25]. Quippe "manus in manu
non erit innocens malus" [Prov 11:21]. Hoc est, etiam si sit manus
in manu, idest si cesset homo nocere proximo, abstinens a furtis et
huiusmodi, non tamen ob hoc erit innocens, cum anime sue noceat
per pigritiam et negligentiam.

<DE PROVOCATIONE AD MALVM>
Amplius, grauiter peccat qui hominem ad mortaliter peccandum
prouocat. Vt qui mulierem allicit, et ex eius animo consensum elicit,
uel ad fornicandum uel ad mecandum.

<DE PREMVNIRE NOLLE>
Amplius, peccatum est de dampno cauendo proximum non[10] premunire.
Patet hoc in Ezechiele [33:6] de speculatore. Hoc de prelato specialiter

---

8 Dei] M: de C
9 simulatis] M: simulans C
10 non] M: ne C

accipitur. Refert autem quis, quem, de quanto dampno corporis uel anime teneatur premunire.

<DE CESSIONE MALIS>

Peccatum etiam est, siue delictum, peccatum uerbo uel facto non impedire. Vnde Apostolus [Eph 4:27]: "Nolite locum dare diabolo"; locum scilicet intrandi ad nos uel ad alios per cupiditatem uel timorem, que sunt due porte diaboli.

<DE SVBTRACTIONE AVXILII>

Amplius, scriptum est in Parobolis [Prov 24:11-12]: "Erue eos qui ducuntur ad mortem, et qui trahuntur ad interitum liberare ne cesses.[11] Si dixeris, uires non suppetunt, qui inspector est cordis ipse intelligit, et seruatorem anime tue nichil fallit, reddetque homini iuxta opera sua." Hinc super illum locum Psalmi [81:4]: "Eripite pauperem, et egenum de manu peccatoris liberate," dicit Augustinus [Gl. Lombardi, PL 191: 778]: "Hoc minoribus[12] dicitur, per quod ostendit nec illos immunes fuisse a scelere tanto qui permiserunt principibus Christum, cum pro multitudine timerentur, et possent illos a facto et se a consensu liberare. Qui enim desinit obuiare cum potest et debet, consentit."

<DE ACTV INTEMPESTIVO>

Peccant etiam qui tempus congruum non obseruant. Vnde Salomon [Eccle 3:1]: "Omnia tempus habent"; et iterum [Eccle 8:6]: "Omni negotio tempus est et opportunitas," et item [Eccle 3:5]: "Tempus amplexandi, et tempus longe fieri ab amplexibus." Et Apostolus [1 Cor 7:5]: "Nolite fraudare inuicem, nisi forte ex consensu, ut uacetis orationi." Liberis ad cultum Dei procreandis danda est opera, et item continentie. Item legitur in Genesi [7:13]: "Ingressus est Noe, et filii eius, uxor eius, et uxores filiorum eius cum eo in archam"; Glosa [interl.]: "Seorsum uiri, seorsum femine, quia abstinendum est in afflictione." Hinc et Ioel ait sexta capitula [2:16]: "Egrediatur sponsus de cubili suo, et sponsa de thalamo suo"; Glosa [interl.]: "Vt tempore ieiunii non seruiant operi nuptiali, set uacent orationi." Item, super illud Ysaie cxciiia capitula [64:6]: "Quasi pannus menstruate uniuerse iusticie nostre," habetur hec Glosa [Gl. ord.]: "Mene Hebraice, luna Latine, unde menstruate que singulis mensibus solent fluxum sanguinis sustinere, et tunc uiri debent[13] abstinere ab eis. Tunc enim concipiuntur membris dampnati, scilicet ceci, claudi, leprosi, et huiusmodi, ut quia

---

11 ne cesses] M: non sesset C
12 minoribus] M: in moralibus C
13 debent] M: om. C

parentes non erubuerunt misceri in conclaui, eorum peccata pateant cunctis et aperte redarguantur in paruulis." Item in Leuitico [20:18] legitur: "Qui choierit cum muliere in fluxu menstruo, interficientur ambo." Set ibi loquitur de scienter cognoscente palam; qui enim ignoranter, minus puniretur, ut iterum habetur in Leuitico [cf. 15:24].

\<DE CVSTODIA SENSVVM\>
Cauendum est etiam diligenter quia mors ingreditur per fenestras [cf. Ier 9:21], idest mortale peccatum per quinque sensus corporis ad animam habet ingressum. Patet in Eua que suasioni serpentis aurem feliciter accommodauit. Contra quod dicitur [Eccli 28:28]: "Sepi aures tuas spinis, et noli audire linguam nequam." Spinas uocat aculeos timoris Dei uel uerba Dei comminatoria, ut hec [Gen 2:17]: "Quacumque die commederitis ex eo morte moriemini." "Vidit etiam mulier quod bonum esset lignum ad uescendum et pulcrum oculis aspectuque delectabile, et tulit de fructu illius et commedit" [Gen 3:6].

\<DE SECVRITATE IN TERRENIS\>
Amplius, confidere in terrenis et securitatem in eis constituere, et ob hoc ista ambire, culpabile est. Vnde in Apocalypsi [Gl. ord. ad 18:17] leguntur ue dicturi omnes qui in lacum nauigant, "idest qui aliquid certum desiderant habere, ut aliqui episcopatum."

\<QVOD VITIA VIDENTVR VIRTVTES\>
Amplius, ex seruili timore aliquis bonum facit uel malum omittit, et credit se bonum esse et mereri uitam eternam.

Vel in opere suo duos fines constituit finales, diuersos et aduersos. Item [cf. 1 Cor 13:1-2]: "Si caritatem non habeam, nichil sum."

Amplius, uitia uidentur uirtutes esse, ut remissio pietas, etc. "Arta est uia que ducit ad uitam" [Mt 7:14]; de facili declinatur ad dexteram uel sinistram et ita deuiatur. Virtus quidem est medium uitiorum utrimque redactum. Hinc est remissio, hinc seueritas, hinc superhabundantia, idest nimietas, hinc diminutio, idest minoritas. Medio tutissimus ibis, quia modesta est sapientia [cf. Iac 3:17], idest quibuscumque non ultra modum nec infra subsistit. Hoc est ne quid nimis, ne quid minus. Vnde poeta [Horace Serm 1.1.106]: Est modus in rebus etc. Item, pro modico libra flectitur et inclinatur, et tunc perit[14] rectitudo et equalitas.

\<QVOD LAQVEI DIABOLI SVBTILES\>
Subtiles quidem sunt laquei diaboli et abscondite pedice et occulte

---

14 perit] M: om. C

decipule [cf. Iob 18:10], et malum non uitatur nisi cognitum, ideo predicta scienda sunt. Nam ignorans ignorabitur [cf. 1 Cor 14:38], et "simul insipiens et stultus peribunt" [Ps 48:11]. Insipiens est qui nescit, stultus qui non cauet.

<DE CIRCVMSTANTIA PECCATORVM>

Amplius, attendende sunt circumstantie peccatorum, ut tempus, locus, ordo, scientia, etas, status, causa, modus, quantitas, et numerus. Circumstantie enim huiusmodi aggrauant peccatum. Inde est quod Dominus [Ex 34:13] Hebreis, terram promissionis ingressurus, de gentibus ydolatris sic loquens ait: "Aras eorum subuertite, confringite¹⁵ statuas, lucos succidite." Mistice precipit Dominus populo suo fideli, idest christianis, nobis scilicet, ut ydola, idest uitia nostra et peccata principalia, per contritionem et satisfactionem penitus confringamus. Et aras que ydola sustentant, idest facultates et oportunitates et commoditates, que peccatis incitamenta uel fomenta prestant, subuertamus, tollamus et euitemus, ut sunt comesationes, otia, solicitudines. Quod non latuit poetam [Ovid, *Rem am*, 139] dicentem: "Otia si tollas periere cupidinis arcus," et "Quisquis amas, loca sola nocent, loca sola caueto" [ibid., 579]. Precipimur etiam lucos ydola circumstantes, idest circumstantias presertim aggrauantes peccata, confitendo succidere, et ita culturam diabolicam penitus adnullare.

<DE OFFENDERE IN VNO>

Attende etiam quod Iacobus [2:10] ait: "Offendens in uno reus est omnium," idest transgrediens unum preceptum, nullum meritorie obseruat.

<DE RECIDIVATIONE>

Attende iterum et caue tibi ne redeas ad uomitum [cf. Prov 26:11]. Nam in recidiuiante redeunt omnia peccata pristina mortalia que prius erant penitentia dimissa; uel in eo suboritur omnibus equipollens ingratitudo.

1.2 QVE SVNT PECCATA MAGIS PERICVLOSA

Peccata plurimum periculosa et ideo magis cauenda sunt ut illa quibus incidit homo in canonem late sentencie.

Similiter et illa que ex diutina consuetudine fortiter implicant et inuoluunt. De sic peccante dicitur in Iob [18:8]: "Immisit in rete pedes suos, et in maculis eius ambulat implicitus," scilicet obligatus. Difficile

---

15 confringite] *M*: confringe *C*

quidem auellitur homo a peccato quod multo detinuit tempore et multa placuit uoluptate. "Nullique," ut ait philosophus, "remedio locus est, ubi uitia mores fiunt."

Similiter et ista que sequuntur: Defloratio uirginis illicita, ubi non restituitur ablatum.

Heredem ex adulterio procreare, et sic legitimos heredes exheredare.

Consuetudinem grauem inducere, ut in firmis et teloneis.

Item, uix penitet fornicator de prole honesta suscepta.

Item, uix restituitur ecclesia symoniace adquisita.

Item, in lupanari choeunt ignari cum coniugatis uel monialibus uel cum precognitis a leprosis, et sic ipsi lepra inficiuntur, uel cum menstruatis, sicut Ieremias [2:24], tum de synagoga, tum de meretrice corporali, actuali, usuali, et salutaribus moribus[16] obstinata loquens, ait: "Nullus auertet eam. Omnes qui querunt eam non deficient; in menstruis eius inuenient eam." Hoc est, qui querunt eam ad fornicationem non deficient quin inueniant eam etiam in fluxu menstrui sanguinis. Caueat autem predicator in sermone publice menstrua nominare, propter reuerentiam scilicet mulierum uerecundarum, set aliqua circumlocutione honesta quid uelit dicere sic innuat ut detegendo tegat et palliando revelet, presertim cum dicat Apostolus [Col 4:6] "Sermo uester in gratia semper sale sit conditus."

1.3 De peccatis monachorvm

Hec dicuntur esse peccata monachorum quorundam. Homines[17] exheredant. Decimas subtrahunt cum episcopus[18] tributa soluerit pro scandalo uitando. Bigamos uel uiduarum maritos et homicidas ordinari faciunt. Manibus fratrum laicorum negotiationes excercent, sicut Iudei Christum manibus gentilium crucifixerunt. Deposita uel commendata non restituunt, et ita ius naturale omittunt. Fratres conuersi aliquid symoniace adquirunt et prelati dissimulant. Item ad spicas, secundum mandatum legis morale [Lev 23:22], ab egenis colligendas pauperes non admittunt, set ad eas comedendas porcos mittunt, et eis prelati in hoc consentiunt, qui eos non instruunt nec corripiunt. Dies festos non obseruant.

<De qvibvs temptantvr religiosi>
Amplius, hec sunt de quibus temptantur uel uexantur religiosi: hypo-

---

16 moribus] *C*: monitis *M*
17 Homines] *M*: Omnes *C*
18 episcopus] *M*: Christus *C*

crisis, elatio, cupiditas, detractio, inuidia, curiositas, ambitio, murmur, ira, conquestio, indignatio, seminatio discordie, incendium sodome.[19]

De peccatis canonicorum regularium

Hec dicuntur esse peccata canonicorum regularium quorundam. Firmarii sunt forsan ex cupiditate et non ex necessitate; et ita negotiatores, cum negotiatio supponatur cupiditatem et species sit mali, et Apostolus [1 Thess 5:22] ait: "Ab omni specie mala abstinete uos," et in Euuangelio [Mt 18:7]: "Ve illi per quem scandalum uenit."

De peccatis canonicorum secularium

Hec dicuntur esse peccata canonicorum secularium. Minus resident in ecclesia sua et nimis se absentant. Firmarii sunt absque necessitate. Vicarios fornicatores habent. Garriunt in choro ut in foro. Cum quis canonicus efficitur, dicunt canonici in capitulo: "Ecce quam bonum et quam iocundum habitare fratres in unum" [Ps 132:1]. Habitare dicitur, non discurrere, et in unum, non tantum scilicet animo, quod commune est omnibus christianis, set etiam loco, quod speciale debet esse hiis qui aliquo caractere religionis insigniti sunt. Hec autem diximus contra canonicos extrauagantes et girouagantes.

1.4 <De diversitatibus peccatorum>

In omissionibus multum offendimus, ut in scandalo uitando, fratres reprehendendo, elemosinas erogando, talenta multiplicando, et in acceptione personarum. Delicta huiusmodi quis intelligit?

De cupiditate et timore

Porte diaboli sunt cupiditas mala et malus timor. Vnde in Psalmo [30:5]: "Educes me de laqueo"; laqueum uocat insidias et temptationem diaboli, qui per duas portas temptat precipue scilicet et principaliter, scilicet cupiditatis et timoris. Per cupiditatis portam temptauit primo Christum [Mt 4:1-11] tribus modis, scilicet de gula dicendo, "dic ut lapides isti panes fiant"; de auaritia ostendendo regna mundi et promittendo; de uana gloria cum dixit, "mitte te deorsum." Hanc autem portam cum inuenisset clausam, postea temptauit eundem per timorem passionis, quando scilicet in agonia prolixius orauit [Mt 26:36-44], et ita per easdem portas temptat omnes sanctos. Vnde totum corpus Christi, idest ecclesia, dicit: "Educes me de laqueo," etc. De eisdem uero portis habetur ibi [Ps 79:17]: "Incensa igni et suffossa," etc.

---

19 incendium sodome] *M: om. C*

Item peccatur cogitatu, uerbo, opere, quod in tribus mortuis signi-
ficatum est. Tres enim mortuos suscitauit Ihesus: filiam archisina-
gogi in domo [Mt 9:18-26], idest in cogitatione; filium unicum matris
in porta [Lc 7:11-17], idest in uerbo; Lazarum in monumento [Io
11:17-45], idest in opere. Vnde dicitur:

Mens mala mors intus, malus actus mors foris; usus,

Tumba, puella, puer, Lazarus ista notant. [*HildEpig*, no. 66, p. 310]

Item peccat homo in Deum ut blasphemus, peccat in se ut flagitiosus,
peccat in proximum ut facinorosus.

DE CONCVPISCENTIA CARNIS, CONCVPISCENTIA OCVLORVM, ET SVPERBIA VITE

Item Iohannes in epistola canonica [1 Io 2:16] dicit: "Omne quod in
mundo est, concupiscentia carnis est, concupiscentia oculorum, et
superbia uite." Concupiscentia carnis est, cum per tactum uel per
gustum caro delectatur; concupiscentia oculorum est quando uisu
delectatur, ut in pulcris uestibus, argento et auro, et talibus; superbia
uite est omnis ambitio seculi. Prima Ruben primogenitum Israel
dignitate regia priuauit [cf. Gen 49:3-4]. Secunda Iudam a cena magna
Dei exclusit [cf. Apoc 19:17]. Tertia Nabugodonosor regem elatum in
baratrum precipitauit [cf. Dan 4:25-30]. Hiis tribus temptatus Adam
succubuit. Eisdem tribus temptatus Christus triumphauit.

DE PECCATIS ET DELICTIS

Item sunt peccata, sunt et delicta. Vnde Augustinus [*Gl. Lombardi*
in Gal. 6:1, PL 192: 162]: "Delictum fortasse est declinare a bono;
peccatum est facere malum, ut, sicut in laudabili uita aliud est declinare
a malo, aliud facere bonum, quod ammonemur dicente scriptura [Ps
36:27]: "Declina a malo et fac bonum." Ita in dampnabili aliud sit
declinare a bono, aliud facere malum; et illud delictum, hoc peccatum
sit. Peccatum ergo est perpetratio mali; delictum, desertio boni, quod
et ipsum nomen ostendit. Quid enim aliud sonat delictum nisi
derelictum, et quid derelinquit qui derelinquit nisi bonum. Vel potest
uideri illud esse delictum quod ignoranter fit, peccatum quod a sciente
committitur. Indifferenter tamen plerumque ponuntur, et ut peccatum
nomine delicti et delictum nomine peccati appelletur."

Attende etiam quod quedam delicta dampnabilia sunt. Nam in
iudicio delicta legitur Dominus exprobraturus in hunc modum [Mt
25:42]: "Esuriui, et non dedistis mihi manducare," etc. Ait etiam
Dominus [Mt 7:19]: "Omnis arbor que non facit fructum bonum
excidetur" etc.; et Iacobus [2:13]: "Iudicium sine misericordia illi qui
non facit misericordiam."

DE SEPTEM VITIIS PRINCIPALIBVS

Sunt etiam septem uitia principalia siue capitalia, quasi septem gentes Chanaan et septem fontes mortiferi. Hec autem septem sunt inanis gloria siue superbia, ira, inuidia, accidia siue tristitia idest tedium boni quasi ad casum, auaritia, castrimargia idest gula, et luxuria. Et nota quod non dicuntur ista septem uitia criminalia, neque enim omnis ira criminalis est uel omnis accidia, set dicuntur capitalia quia sunt origines peccatorum, sicut scaturigines fontium sunt capita et initia fluuiorum.

DE PECCATO IN SPIRITVM SANCTVM

Est et peccatum in Spiritum sanctum, ubi sunt genera et species. Est enim obstinatio genus, cuius species sunt desperatio et presumptio. Est etiam impugnatio gratie Spiritus sancti genus, cuius una est species impugnatio ueritatis in fratre post Dei agnitionem, uel apostasia; alia species est inuidentia gratie post reconciliationem.

1.5 DE FASTIDIO[20]

Est etiam in quibusdam fastidium manne celestis, idest uerbi diuini, psalmodie, orationum, et huiusmodi, sicut Egiptii et Hebrei in deserto, manna fastidientes, flagrabant desiderio carnium, cuius concupiscentie penam testabantur postea sepulchra concupiscentie [cf. Num 11:1-34].

DE NEGGLIGENTIA IVDICVM

Est et quibusdam negligentia in iudiciis, contra quod Iob [29:16] ait: "Causam quam nesciebam diligenter inuestigabam."

DE NECGLIGENTIA PRELATORVM

Est et aliis negligentia in correctionibus, contra quod Apostolus arguendo Corintheos [1 Cor 5:2] ait illis: "Et uos inflati estis, et non magis luctum habuistis ut tollatur de medio uestrum qui hoc opus fecit." "Inflati estis," non compatiendo fornicatori, idest Corinthio, et "non habuistis luctum" idest dolorem pro peccatis illius quod magis faciendum esset, ut sic scilicet "qui fecit hoc opus," notorium scilicet, "tollatur de medio uestrum," quia omnes estis participes, suple, presertim prelati.

DE INSVLTATIONE MALORVM

Est etiam insultatio peccatum. Vnde Apostolus in epistola ad Romanos [11:18, 20-21], gentili populo conuerso loquens de Iudeis excecatis quasi ramis fractis, ait: "Noli gloriari aduersus ramos. Noli altum sapere,

---

20 De fastidio] *CM*: De tedio uerbi Dei *T*

set time. Si enim Deus naturalibus ramis non pepercit, ne forte nec tibi parcat."

DE INDIGNATIONE
Est etiam peccatum indignatio super diuitiis malorum. Vnde in Psalmo [36:8]: "Desine ab ira et derelinque furorem; noli emulari ut maligneris." Et supra "Noli emulari" [*Gl. interl.* in Ps 36:1]: idest indignari, "in malignantibus," idest in consideratione malignantium quia florent in temporalibus.[21]

2.1 DE CONFESSIONE

Hec sunt de quibus inquisitio facienda est in confessione:

Peccata carnalia ut sunt fornicatio, adulterium, incestus, uel contra naturam, et omnia genera luxurie cum accidentibus suis ut sunt hec: Defloratio uirginis, cognitio meretricis uel ignote cuiusque, et tunc forsitan monialis uel coniugate uel consanguinee uel affinis. Item illusiones nocturne.

Item gula et ebrietas uel immoderata uel assidua. Item furtum, rapina, percussio, uulneratio, homicidium.

Postea uitia spiritualia ut sunt inuidia, ira, inimicitie, odium, cupiditas cum ramis suis ut sunt auaratia, ambitio, appetitus inanis glorie, laudis, et fauoris humani, et huiusmodi.

Item superbia, arrogantia, iactantia, presumptio.

Item locutio praua, ut adulatio, blasphemia, calumpnia, contentio, detractio, exprobratio, fallacia, gloriatio uel de bono proprio uel de

---

21 *post* temporalibus] Iohannes in Apoc. c. xxxvi: "Et inpletum est templum fumo a maiestate Dei." Ibi dicit Ieronimus: "Templum significat corda sanctorum fumus uero compunctionem cordis, qua conpunguntur corda peccatorum usque ad lacrimas." Impletur autem templum fumo quando quorundam corda inplentur penitentie lamento, uerbi gratia audit quilibet peccatorum loquentem predicatorem, et dicentem quod Apostolus dicit: "Neque adulteri neque inmundi, etc. regnum Dei possidebunt." Dum hec audit et considerat que tormenta inferni sibi immineant, compunctus corde effundet fumum, idest compunctionem cordis, dum cum lacrimis confitetur peccatum suum. Fumus quippe multum ignem precedit, quia uidelicet ex confessione peccati et compunctione cordis nascitur ignis caritatis. Prius enim homo confitetur peccatum suum, postea incipit ualde diligere Deum et proximum, et hoc maiestate Dei et uirtute sit, quia Deus sua uirtute illuminat cor illius ut agat penitentiam qui in cordibus hominum confessionem gignit peccatorum. Unde Psalmista: "Confessio et magnificentia in sanctificatione eius," etc. Et alibi: "Qui tangit montes et fumigant," idest mentes secularium hominum, et superborum respectu sue miserationis, compungit, et lamenta penitentie proferunt. Set quamuis ita sit, nemo potest intrare templum, idest nemo potest esse securus de sua conscientia utrum, scilicet indulgentiam consecutus sit. *add. T, fol. 110vb*

malo, iudicium falsum uel temerarium circa actus uel personas, incantatio, mendacium, falsum testimonium, maledictio, murmur contra Deum, nuge, uerbum otiosum, uerbum preceps, periurium, querela, rumorum confictio, suasio ad malum, susurrium, turpiloquium, ua- niloquium.

Item inquirenda sunt: iniustitia,[22] ut merces mercenarii detenta [cf. Tob 4:15], et cuiusque rei aliene detentio, promissi defraudatio, cessio dans locum alii ad peccandum, procuratio peccati, consensus in peccatum alienum, scandalum, coactio uel prouocatio ad malum, uoti fractio, usura uel superhabundantia.

Inquirenda est etiam misericordia uel immisericordia, ut dimissio iniuriarum. Hinc inde inquirenda est etiam penitentia de bono per- petrato, dilatio confessionis.

Item, post confessionem specialem facienda est confessio generalis de delictis, hoc est de omissionibus bonorum faciendorum, de peccatis obliuioni traditis, de multitudine uenialium et incuria,[23] de circumstan- tiis[24] omnibus huiusmodi aggrauantibus. Porro circumstantie sunt etas, ordo, scientia, numerus, locus, et tempus.

Preter hec autem sunt quedam de quibus inquirendum est in con- fessione clerici. Hec autem sunt huiusmodi: Negligentia ministerii, negotiatio in spiritualibus, pactio in spiritualibus, sortilegium, ritus infidelium, caracteres, coniurationes. Inquirenda est etiam symonia cum omnibus speciebus suis. Predictorum autem explanationem in sequenti capitulo reperies.[25]

2.2 EXPLANATIO VITIORVM ET PECCATORVM QVE INQVIRENDA SVNT IN CONFESSIONE

"Sancti estote quia ego sanctus sum Dominus Deus uester." Verba Spiritus sancti sunt in Leuitico [19:2]. Sanctimonia quidem munditia dicitur. Vnde Apostolus [Hebr 12:14]: "Sanctimoniam sequimini sine

22 iniustitia] *M*: iustitia *C*
23 incuria] *M*: iniuria *C*
24 circumstantiis] *M*: circumstantibus *C*
25 in sequenti capitulo reperies] Predictorum autem explanationem inuenies in tractatu qui sic incipit, Sancti estote. Super Amos, malo penitentiam peccatoris quam mortem. Glosa: penitentiam non sanctitati purissime et ecclesie, Christi, que non habet rugam neque maculam, set morti et inferis comparata fit melior. Hec dicimus non ut tollamus spem penitentie, set ut sollicitos reddamus eos et timidiores, qui aperta ianua penitentie, dum sperant futura, perdunt presentia. Et qui absque uulnere potuerunt permanere, incauti uulnus accipiunt ut postea dolore crucientur. *add. T, fol. 111ra*

qua nemo uidebit Deum." Sanctimoniam dicit munditiam et castitatem
mentis et corporis, et consonat illi uerbo Euuangelii [Mt 5:8]: "Beati
mundo corde, quoniam ipsi uidebunt Deum." Igitur Spiritus sanctus,
quia mundus est, munditiam exigit in nobis, quia mundum munda
decent. Spiritus autem immundus locum incolit immundum, ut scrabo
fimum. Spiritus uero sanctus sanctum exigit receptaculum et mundum
diligit habitaculum. Igitur: "Lauamini, mundi estote" [Is 1:16]. Et in
uase mundo balsamum Spiritus sancti, idest eius gratiam, recipite.
Porro, confessio mundat, si tamen ipsa munda fuerit, tunc mundificabit.
Vt autem munda sit et emundans,26 attende quod Dominus in
Euuangelio [Mt 23:25-26] dicit: "Ve uobis scribe et pharisei ypocrite,
qui mundatis quod deforis est calicis et parapsidis, intus autem pleni
estis rapina et immunditia. Munda prius quod intus est, ut fiat quod
deforis est mundum." "Ve" dampnationem innuit eternam. Est enim
ue in gehenna, lamentum in uia, carmen in patria: Ve dampnatorum,
lamentum penitentium, carmen triumphantium. "Intus" inquit, in
conscientia; "pleni estis rapina" idest auaritia, "et immunditia" idest
sordibus uitiorum. "Munda prius quod intus est," cor scilicet et
conscientiam a fraude et concupiscentia, ut postea "fiat quod deforis
est mundum," hoc est ut possis ueraciter ostendere sanctitatem per
opera.
  Iuxta hunc igitur ordinem, si placet, uitia spiritualia prius confiteatur
penitens uel inquirat sacerdos in confessione. Sunt autem uitia spiritualia
huiusmodi:
  Ira, que si diutina fuerit, uertitur in rancorem et odium. Vnde
Apostolus [Eph 4:26] ait: "Sol non occidat super iracundiam uestram."
  Et inuidia, que fel diabolicum est, et uirus antiqui serpentis. Vnde
scriptum est [Sap 2:24-25]: "Inuidia diaboli mors introiuit in orbem
terrarum," et "Imitantur illum qui sunt ex parte eius."
  Item inimicitie et odium. Scriptum est in Leuitico [19:17]: "Ne oderis
fratrem tuum in corde tuo, set publice argue eum, ne habeas super
illo peccatum." Et Iohannes [1 Jo 3:15] ait: "Omnis qui odit fratrem
suum homicida est." Qui enim ex odio insequitur fratrem prouocat
iram et discordiam, et sic quantum in se occidit eum in anima et se
ipsum in anima.
  Item, uitium spirituale cupiditas est, que secundum Apostolum [1
Tim 6:10] radix est omnium malorum. Huius autem rami sunt auaritia
que est ydolorum seruitus, et ambitio que est cupiditas honoris et
appetitus inanis glorie, laudis et fauoris humani, et huiusmodi. Contra

26 emundans] M: emendans C

hec autem ait Apostolus [Gal 5:26]: "Non efficiamini inanis glorie[27] cupidi, inuicem prouocantes, inuicem inuidentes."

Item, uitium spirituale est superbia, que ex angelis demones efficit.

Et arrogantia et iactantia, qualis erat in Phariseo dicente [Lc 18:11]: "Non sum sicut ceteri hominum," etc. Item presumptio, contra quam ait Psalmista [130:1]: "Domine non est exaltatum cor meum," etc.

Post hec autem inquirenda sunt peccata carnalia, ut sunt locutiones praue et huiusmodi. Adulatio, contra quam dicitur [Ex 23:19]: "Non coques hedum in lacte matris," idest non fouebis peccatorem blanditiis et adulationibus. Et Augustinus [*Gl. ord.* in Ps 10:3]: "Alligant animas in peccatis lingue adulantium." Item blasphemia, que ipsi Deo iniuriatur; calumpnia, que proximum offendit; contentio, que amicitias dissoluit; detractio, unde Apostolus [cf. Rom 1:29]: "Susurrones et detractores Deo odibiles sunt." Susurrones sunt qui inter amicos discordias seminant. Detractores sunt qui aliorum bona negant uel inuertunt. Item, exprobratio peccati post penitentiam, contra quod dicitur [Act 10:15]: "Quod Deus purificauit, tu ne commune dixeris," idest immundum. Et iterum [Mt 5:22]: "Qui dixerit fratri suo racha," uel "fatue," ex odio scilicet, "reus erit." Item, fallacia idest deceptio improbabilis et detestabilis. Item, gloriatio de malo, unde [Ps 51:3]: "Quid gloriaris in malitia"; uel de bono, unde Ieremias [9:23-24]: "Non glorietur sapiens in sapientia sua, et non glorietur fortis in fortitudine sua, et non glorietur diues in diuitiis suis; set in hoc glorietur, qui gloriatur scire et nosse me, quia sum Dominus." Item, iudicium falsum, contra quod dicitur [Ps 57:2]: "Recte," uel recta, uel iusta, "iudicate, filii hominum." Et iudicium temerarium circa res uel personas, contra quod dicitur [Mt 7:1]: "Nolite iudicare et non iudicabimini."

Sunt autem quedam media et incerta quo animo fiant, que bene et male possunt fieri. Nescimus etiam qualis futurus est qui nunc apparet malus, de cuius correctione desperare, eumque quasi abiectum reprehendere, temerarium iudicium est. Nolite ergo iudicare uel hominem reprobum esse, uel opera media mala esse, uel mala fieri intentione. De manifestis autem, que bono animo fieri non possunt, permittitur nobis iudicare.

Item, incantatio peccatum est, et sortilegium. Mendacium est, etiam causa ioci uel commodi si fuerit in consuetudine, mortale. Vnde in Apocalipsi [21:8]: "Mendacibus," quibus scilicet mendacium est in usu, "pars illorum erit in stagno ardenti igne et sulphure, quod est mors secunda." Vnicum etiam mendacium malignitatis ex dupplicitate animi

---

27 laudis ... glorie] *M: om. C*

mortale peccatum est. Vnde [Ps 5:7]: "Perdes omnes qui locuntur mendacium," et [Sap 1:11]: "Os quod mentitur occidit animam." Item, maledictio iniusta, ex liuore uindicte, peccatum est. Vnde [cf. 1 Cor 6:10], maledici regnum Dei non possidebunt. Item, murmur contra Deum, propter quod prostrata sunt cadauera Hebreorum in deserto [cf. Ps 105:25-26]. Item, nuge siue scurilitas, que a stultis "curialitas" dicitur, idest iocularitas, que solet risum mouere, si in usu fuerit, grauat. Vnde super illud in Mattheo [12:36]: "De omni uerbo otioso quod locuti fuerint homines, reddent rationem in die iudicii," habetur [*Gl. interl.*] quod uerbum otiosum est quod sine utilitate loquentis dicitur et audientis, ut de friuolis et fabulis. Scurrilia non sunt otiosa set criminosa. Item [Ps 139:12]: "Vir lingosus non dirigetur in terra." Super illud ait Augustinus [*Gl. Lombardi*, PL 191: 1232]: "Si quis uera dicat set preter necessitatem, uir lingosus est." Intellige "dicat" idest dicere consuescat. Item, uerbum preceps peccatum est. Vnde [Eccli 4:34]: "Noli citatus esse in lingua," idest preceps in uerbo; et alibi [Ps 51:6]: "Dilexisti omnia uerba precipitationis lingua dolosa." Periurium etiam prohibetur, unde Dominus [Mt 5:33] ait: "Non periurabis" in nomine meo. Querela etiam iniusta peccatum est. Item, Apostolus [2 Thess 3:12] ait de curiosis: "Denuntiamus hiis ut cum silentio," scilicet non rumorosi, "operantes, panem suum manducent," idest proprii laboris. Item, suasio ad malum peccatum est. Patet in serpente, qui malum male suasit Eue [cf. Gen 3:4-6]. De turpiloquio ait Apostolus [Col 3:8]: "Deponite turpem sermonem," uel turpiloquium, "de ore uestro," quamuis in corde iam conceptus sit. De uaniloquio dicit Psalmista [11:3]: "Vana locuti sunt unusquisque ad proximum suum," etc. Hec autem omnia circa locutionem peruersam attendenda sunt.

Sunt preterea peccata carnalia, ut est fornicatio, que semper plures perdit animas, maris scilicet et femine. Et, ut ait Apostolus [cf. 1 Cor 6:9-10, Eph 5:5], fornicatores regnum Dei non possidebunt. Est et adulterium quod Dominus in decalogo [Ex 20:14] prohibet, dicens: "Non mecaberis." Fornicatio quidem et adulterium lapidatione punie- bantur in lege [cf. Lev 20:10, Dt 22:22]. Est et incestus, uel[28] contra naturam ut masculus choeat cum masculo uel femina cum femina uel cum brutis animalibus. Sunt et fricationes membrorum genitalium usque ad seminis effusionem, que omnia peccata mortalia sunt, et indigna ad loquendum de eis.

Item, a confitente fornicationem querendum est utrum aliquando uirginem deflorauerit, uel meretricem cognouerit. Audiat quid de hiis

____

28 uel] *M*: *om.* C

dicat Apostolus [1 Cor 3:17]: "Si quis templum Dei uiolauerit, disperdet illum Deus," idest in diuersis perdet, scilicet in corpore et anima, quasi sacrilegum. Et [1 Cor 6:16]: "Qui adheret meretrici unum corpus efficitur,"[29] cum ea scilicet. Fornicatio enim ambos socians in culpa unum corpus facit, ut quomodo in natura, sic et in macula unum sint. Accidit etiam ut quandoque, choiens cum ignota, simplicem se credat fornicationem committere, cum tamen cognoscat monialem apostatam uel alterius coniugatam refugam uel propriam consanguineam uel affinem suam.

Nec pretermittende sunt in confessione[30] illusiones nocturne que quidem grauant si ex crapula uel ex premeditatione preueniant. Item, gula primos parentes eiecit de paradiso; ebrietas Loth impulit in incestum [cf. Gen 3:6 et 19:33]. Ait etiam Dominus in Euuangelio [Lc 21:34]: "Attendite ne grauentur corda uestra in crapula et ebrietate." Furtum etiam prohibet Dominus in Euuangelio [Lc 18:20] et in decalogo [Ex 20:15], et Apostolus [1 Cor 6:10] ait: "Neque fures, neque ebriosi, neque rapaces, regnum Dei possidebunt."

Sunt et peccata quandoque grauia: percussio, uulneratio, uel homicidium. Hinc et in lege [Lev 24:17] dicitur: "Qui percusserit hominem uolens occidere, morte morietur." Item [Ex 21:18-19]: "Si rixati fuerint uiri, et percusserit alter proximum suum lapide uel pugno, et ille mortuus non fuerit set iacuerit in lecto, si surrexerit et ambulauerit foris super baculum suum, innocens erit qui percusserit, ita tamen ut operas eius et impensas in medicos restituat." Item [Ex 21:22-23]: "Si rixati fuerint uiri, et percusserit quis mulierem pregnantem, et abortiuum quidem fecerit, si ipsa uixerit, subiacebit dampno quantum expetierit maritus uxoris, et arbitri iudicauerint. Sin autem mors fuerit subsecuta, reddet animam pro anima, oculum pro oculo, dentem pro dente, manum pro manu, pedem pro pede, adustionem pro adustione, liuorem pro liuore." Item, Apostolus [Rom 12:19] ait: "Non uosmetipsos defendentes, karissimi," idest non sitis referientes aduersarios, "set date locum ire," idest iudicio Dei, reseruantes scilicet uindicte Dei, uel ire aduersariorum. In decalogo [Ex 20:13] etiam scriptum est: "Non occides"; et Dominus [Gen 9:6] ait ad Noe et ad filios eius: "Quicumque effuderit sanguinem humanum, effundetur sanguis illius. Ad ymaginem Dei quippe factus est homo."

Inquirenda est in confessione iniustitia, ut merces mercenarii detenta, idest merces operis unde uiuit. "Merces mercenarii apud te non maneat

---

29 efficitur] *M: om. C*
30 in confessione] *M: om. C*

usque mane" [Lev 19:13, Tob 4:15]. Jacobus [5:4] etiam ait: "Ecce
merces operariorum, qui messuerunt regiones uestras, que fraudata est
a uobis, clamat, et clamor eorum in aures Domini sabaoth introiuit."
Iustitia quidem uirtus est reddens unicuique quod suum est. Peccat
etiam qui cedit peccanti cum peccatum impedire possit. Amplius autem
peccat qui peccatum alienum procurat, uel qui in illud consentit. Quia
ut ait Apostolus [Rom 1:32] de peccatoribus peccata mortalia com-
mittentibus: "Digni sunt morte non solum qui faciunt ea set etiam
qui consentiunt facientibus." Peccat etiam qui scandalizat. Vnde [Mt
18:7]: "Ve mundo ab scandalis," que scilicet non cauet. Ille scandalizat
qui dicto uel facto minus recto occasionem dat ruine. Peccant etiam
qui cogunt alios uel prouocant ad peccandum, et qui uota infringunt.
Scriptum est enim [Ps 75:12]: "Vouete et reddite." Vouere uoluntarium
est, reddere necessarium; uouere consilium est, reddere preceptum.

Inquirendum est etiam de usuris. Scriptum est [Ez 18:5, 8-9]: "Vir
si fuerit iustus ad usuram non commodauerit," cuique scilicet quodcumque, "et amplius non[31] acceperit," de quacumque re superhabundantiam quamcumque, "uita uiuet, ait Dominus." Item [cf. *Decretum*,
C.14. q.3. c.3]: "Quicquid sorti accidit, usura est." Hoc est, quicquid
capitali siue catallo superaccrescit, ex pacto scilicet tacito uel expresso,
uel ex petitione[32] commodatoris, intuitu scilicet commodati, usura est.

Inquirendum est etiam de operum misericordie subtractione, ut sicut
potuit non dedit uel minus dedit. Si spicas post messem pauperibus
non reliquid; si sex opera misericordie in Euuangelio [Mt 25:35-36]
exarata non prout debuit exsecutus sit, scilicet "Esuriui et dedistis mihi
manducare," etc. Septimum autem in Tobia [1:20] est sepelire mortuos,
de quo etiam ait Dominus [4 Esd 2:23]: "Mortuos ubi inueneris signans
commenda sepulchro, et dabo tibi primam sessionem in resurrectione."
Sunt etiam alia opera misericordie, ut dimittere iniurias. Vnde [Lc 6:37,
Mt 6:14]: "Dimittite et dimittetur uobis." Et compati, unde [Rom
12:15]: "Flere cum flentibus." Et commodare, unde [Ps 36:26]: "Tota
die miseretur et commodat"; hoc enim de iusto scriptum est; et iterum
[Ps 111:5]: "Iocundus homo qui miseretur et commodat." Dominus
etiam ait in Euuangelio [Mt 5:42]: "Volenti mutuari a te, ne auertaris."
Precellit autem inter opera misericordie animas ad Deum conuertere.
Vnde Dominus ait in propheta [Ier 15:19]: "Si seperaueris pretiosum
a uili, quasi os meum eris," idest animam a mundo uel a diabolo.

---

31 non *M*: *om. C*
32 ex petitione] *C*: expectatione *M*

Item peccat non numquam qui de bono quod egit penitet et dolet. Peccat etiam qui differt confessionem uel conuersionem.

Sunt et alia plura in confessione attendenda et circumstantie peccata aggrauantes, ut subtilissimi laquei tum usure tum symonie, quos ad presens explicare non uacat (maxime quia in Numerale nostro de eis diffusius dictum est).[33] Attende etiam quod in tractatu premisso peccata carnalia preposuimus; in eiusdem explanatione illa postponimus, quod ex industria fecimus ad insinuandum quod non multum refert in confessione prius confiteri carnalia quam spiritualia uel uice uersa, cum utrumque oporteat facere secundum quod hec et illa occurrunt memorie.

In confessione inquirenda sunt septem uitia capitalia cum ramis suis uel riuis. Item, inquirenda est obseruantia decalogi cum appendiciis suis. Item, inquirenda sunt tria que uitium auaritie redimunt; hec autem tria sunt retributio meritorum, restitutio ablatorum, distributio preceptorum.

2.3 De obitv

Hec dicenda sunt in extremis a penitente: "Suscipe me Domine secundum eloquium tuum et uiuam, et non confundas me ab expectatione mea" [Ps 118:116]. "Et nunc que est expectatio mea: Nonne Dominus?" [Ps. 38:8].

"Domine Ihesu Christe, suscipe spiritum meum" [Act 7:8]. Item: "In manus tuas, Domine, commendo spiritum meum," etc. [Ps 30:6]. Item: "Ab ocultis meis munda me Domine," etc. [Ps 18:13]. Item: "Delicta iuuentutis mee et ignorantias meas ne memineris, Domine" [Ps 24:7].

Item, ter dicatur uersus iste: "Dirrupisti, Domine, uincula mea; tibi sacrificabo hostiam laudis," etc. [Ps 115:16-17]. Quia, ut ait Cassiodorus [*Gl. ord.*, ibid.], "hic uersus tante uirtutis a quibusdam esse creditur ut peccata homini dimittantur si in fine uite trina confessione dicatur," idest ter; et intellige hic peccata uenialia, idest penas eorum, nam peccata prius dimissa sunt in contritione uel confessione, prius speciali, deinde generali ut, "Confiteor Deo et beate Marie," et cetera. Item, secundum Augustinum fit in hunc modum: "Deus qui nosti occulta cordis, et opera mea et delicta mea a te non sunt abscondita, quibus ueniam largiaris"; et hic, secundum Augustinum, dimittuntur obliuioni tradita.

---

33 maxime ... dictum est] *C: om. M*

In extrema etiam unctione amplius dimittuntur peccata quo ad penam. Vnde Iacobus [5:15] de unctione dicit: "Si in peccatis sit, dimittentur ei." Dicat etiam agens in extremis "Aue Maria gratia plena, Dominus tecum; benedicta tu in mulieribus" etc. Dicat septem Psalmos si potest, et letaniam, et animam suam Deo commendet. Item, ante sumptionem eucharistie, simbolum fidei reddat idest "Credo in Deum patrem omnipotentem" et deinceps totum ex ordine dicat.

Explicit Speculum penitentis.

II.5

De penitentia religiosorum

William addresses this treatise to a friend who had requested a compendium of penitential doctrine suitable for cloistered monks. The request itself is interesting; it recognizes a distinctive nature to confession and penance in the monastery, and implies that the needs of this group were inadequately addressed by the current penitentials. William responded with this thoughtful exposition of what he had learned "from prudent and discerning theologians about the penance of monks."

This brief text illumines two important and poorly documented aspects of the doctrine and practice of penance in the late twelfth century. First, it tells us something about the adaptation of penitential discipline for use in monasteries. Although the practice of secret confession of sins and penitential satisfaction originated among Celtic monks in the central Middle Ages, few texts have survived to tell us about the practice of that discipline in the monasteries of the twelfth and thirteenth centuries. Frequently we find learned monks advising the secular clergy on the application of penitential doctrine and practice in the diocese,[1] but rarely do they describe the practice within their own monastic walls.[2]

In this text William offers a sensitive adaptation of the techniques for hearing confessions "in the world" to the particular situation of

---

[1] A good example is Senatus, a monk of Worcester, who was appointed to oversee penitential discipline in the diocese. See Philippe Delhaye, "Deux textes de Senatus de Worcester sur la pénitence," *Recherches de théologie ancienne et médiévale* 19 (1952) 203-224, and Mary Cheney, *Roger, Bishop of Worcester 1164-1179* (Oxford: Clarendon Press, 1980), pp. 56-66. Another typical case of a guide written by a monastic author for the use of secular confessors is studied by Pierre Michaud-Quantin, "Un manuel de confession archaique dans le manuscrit Avranches 136," *Sacris erudiri* 17 (1966) 5-54.

[2] One can compare with William's treatise the work(s) on confession written some thirty years later by the secular master Robert Grosseteste to a monastic abbot or prior: See Joseph Goering and F.A.C. Mantello, "The 'Perambulauit Iudas ...' (Speculum confessionis) Attributed to Robert Grosseteste."

those living in the cloister. William specifies in paragraph 2 that the head of the monastery or his delegate should receive the penitent graciously and encourage him to confess the secrets of his heart. He should also warn the penitent that, by virtue of his monastic habit, he is in danger of a greater punishment for his sins than a layman who commits similar transgressions (paragraph 3). Further, he should remind the penitent that his frequent reception of the eucharist exposes him to the grave danger of eating and drinking the body and blood of Christ unworthily; this requires that the monk be even more assiduous than the layman in confessing his sins and in performing the works of penance (paragraph 4). Finally, the monk should be encouraged not to let the fruits of his great labour — his prayers, fasts, and other works — be nullified by some deadly sin (paragraph 5).

When some grave sin is confessed, the monastic confessor is faced with the same necessity as his secular counterpart to use great discretion in consoling the sinner lest he be overly despondent, and simultaneously reproving him lest he commit the sin again (paragraph 6).

A particular difficulty arises for the monastic confessor, however, in the imposition of an appropriate penance for grave but secret sins commited by monks. If he imposes fasts or penances in addition to those already observed in the monastery the secrecy of the confession would be compromised. Moreover, William tells us, it is not customary for monks to undergo as long or as rigorous a penance for sins as that enjoined on laymen because of the onerous observances of their rule which, if observed, cover a multitude of sins. Nevertheless, this brevity and lightness of penance has induced many monks to relapse in their sins. It is therefore necessary to increase the length and severity of penances for those who have often relapsed (paragraph 7).

This introductory discussion of the nature of monastic confession and penance is followed (paragraphs 8-28) by a collection of penitential "tariffs" designed specifically for monks; therein lies the second important contribution of William's treatise to our understanding of medieval penitential discipline. It is well known that lists of tariffs specifying the appropriate penance for particular sins were characteristic of the medieval Church's sacrament of penance.[3] Less clear is the way in which a priest would use such canons, if at all, in the actual

---

[3] See Bernhard Poschmann, *Penance and the Anointing of the Sick*, trans. and rev. Francis Courtney (Freiburg i.B.: Herder, 1964), and Artur Landgraf, "Grundlagen für ein Verständnis der Busslehre der Früh- und Hochscholastik," *Zeitschrift für katholische Theologie* 51 (1927) 161-194.

imposition of a satisfactory penalty. Some have argued that the tariffs became irrelevant during the twelfth and thirteenth century, and were replaced by the free choice (*arbitrium*) of the confessor in imposing an appropriate penance.[4] More recently it has been suggested that the penitential canons or tariffs never really fell out of favour, and that they continued to play a normative role in the practice of penance well into the fourteenth century.[5]

The *De penitentia religiosorum uirorum* lends support to this latter view. William obviously knew the penitential canons well and used them as the basis for his own advice to the monks. Moreover, he demonstrates clearly how the priest's *arbitrium* consists in his adaptation of the authoritative sentences to the particular circumstances of the cases before him. Like other writers, both earlier and later, William perceives the penitential "tariffs" not as rigid and impersonal penalties to be mechanically applied, but rather as a customary framework within which the priest's judgement and discretion can be fruitfully exercised.[6]

William discusses the appropriate monastic penances for sexual sins and drunkenness only, expecting that the confessor will deduce from these the form of imposing penances for other types of sins (paragraph 29). In another work, the *Speculum penitentis* (above, II.4), he describes in greater detail the less obvious sins that monks as well as other clerics and laypeople must confess. His emphasis there, however, is on confession rather than the penitential satisfaction for sins. In the *De penitentia religiosorum uirorum* we find William's advice on the imposition of penances for sins, both those committed in the cloister and, by extension, in the world.

AUTHENTICITY AND DATE

In two manuscripts, (nos. 3 and 5, below), this work is ascribed to William; the other copies are anonymous. Although the ascribed copies

---

[4] See Michaud-Quantin, "A propos des premières *Summae confessorum*," pp. 268, 306. Further examples are cited by Pierre Payer, "The Humanism of the Penitentials and the Continuity of the Penitential Tradition," *Mediaeval Studies* 46 (1984) 340-354, at 350-352.

[5] Payer, "Humanism of the Penitentials"; Joseph Goering, "The *Summa* of Master Serlo and Thirteenth-Century Penitential Literature," pp. 296-297.

[6] See Payer, "Humanism of the Penitentials" for numerous examples from the seventh to the fourteenth century. See also the *De modo confitendi et paenitentias iniungendi* of Robert Grosseteste, edited by Joseph Goering and F.A.C. Mantello, "The Early Penitential Writings of Robert Grosseteste," pp. 52-112.

are from the second half of the thirteenth century and from the fourteenth century respectively they provide independent and uncontradicted testimony to William's authorship. At least three other copies, now lost, are recorded in the medieval catalogues of Peterborough Abbey, where they are also ascribed explicitly to William de Montibus.[7]

The English provenance of the known copies of this work suggest that it was composed after William's return to Lincoln Cathedral in the 1180's. The unnamed friend for whom it was written (*Petisti amice* ...) cannot be identified, but another clue for dating the composition is found in the opening paragraph. William explains that, desiring to meet his friend's request, he will attempt briefly to teach that which he has learned from prudent and discerning theologians (*a theologis prudentibus et discretis*) about the penance of religious. In the writings of his mature years William seldom mentions his teachers, nor does he preface his works with modest disclaimers. It can thus be suggested that the *De penitentia religiosorum uirorum* dates from the 1180's or early 1190's, before William had become an authority in his own right. Nothing in the content or style of the work makes such a date inherently improbable.

SOURCES

This brief text is based on two primary sources, the teachings of "prudent and discerning theologians" of the twelfth century — William's teachers, we presume — and the penitential canons of the Church. Neither source can be identified with precision. None of the published writings of twelfth-century masters of theology is an obvious source of this doctrine concerning the proper form of monastic penance, but further studies in the scholastic writings of this period may well illuminate the background and content of such discussions.[8]

The penitential canons or "tariffs" to which William refers in this treatise can be identified more easily in published collections, but his immediate source(s) are not obvious. Gratian's *Decretum* and Bartholomew of Exeter's *Penitentiale*, two texts known to William, contain canons similar to those quoted here, but neither these works nor any of the other *libri penitentiales* can be identified as the immediate or

---

[7] James, "Lists of Manuscripts Formerly in Peterborough Abbey Library," pp. 39, 66, 67.

[8] The best survey of penitential doctrine in this period remains that of Paul Anciaux, *La théologie du sacrement de pénitence au XIIe siècle*.

exclusive source of William's teachings.[9] Perhaps he was quoting the canons from memory, or referring to one of the small books of penitential canons that every priest was expected to possess, but which have left little trace among the extant writings of the period.[10]

MANUSCRIPTS

1. Cambridge, Corpus Christi College MS 459, fols. 36v-37r. Mid 13th century (above top line).

> Inc. Prol.: *Petisti amice.*
> Inc. Txt.: *Prelatus ergo siue qui uicem eius optinet*
> Expl. (incomplete in paragraph 7): *Quia uiri religiosi multis et uariis obseruanciis regule sue et ordinis onerati sunt ... oportet eis qui sepius relabuntur grauiorem et prolixiorem penitentiam iniungi.*

2. Durham Cathedral, MS B.IV.26, fols. 37v-39r. 14th century.

> Title: *Qualiter religiosi admonendi sunt ad confessionem*
> Inc. Prol.: *Petisti a me karissime*
> Inc. Txt.: *Prelatus ergo siue qui uicem eius optinet*
> Expl.: *Ecce sicut rogasti ... et que penitentie iniungende sunt pro peccatis*
Omits paragraphs 17-23, and 27.

3. *L* = London, British Library MS Royal 8.C.vii, fols. 123v-126r. Later 13th century.

> Title: *Incipit scriptum magistri Willelmi de montibus de penitencia R<eligiosorum>.*
> Inc. Prol.: *Petisti amice.*
> Inc. Txt.: *Prelatus igitur siue uices eius gerens.*
> Expl.: *pro aliis peccatorum generibus.*
> Colophon: *Explicit scriptum magistri W. de montibus de penitencia R<eligiosorum>.*
>   Printed below.

---

[9] On William's use of Gratian and Bartholomew see above, *Peniteas cito*, (II.1). For a general survey of the collections of penitential canons see Vogel, *Les "Libri paenitentiales."* Paragraph 25 of William's text (as well as the words *infra diem tertium* in paragraph 24) are not found in any of the standard collections. Paragraph 26, ascribed here to the "Penitential of Theodore" is usually attributed to the "Roman Penitential," but may have circulated in other texts with the ascription to Theodore; see Joseph Goering, "The *Summa de penitentia* of Magister Serlo," *Mediaeval Studies* 38 (1976) 32 note d.

[10] Thomas Chobham, discussing the books that every priest was required by canon law to know, defines *canones penitentiales* as "libellum quemdam in quo ostenditur que penitentia cui peccato sit iniungenda," *Summa confessorum*, p. 88. See Payer, "Humanism of the Penitentials, pp. 350-352.

4. Oxford, Bodleian Library MS Digby 20, fols. 103v-104v. Late 13th century.

Inc. Prol.: *Petisti amice*

Inc. Txt.: *Prelatus ergo siue qui vicem eius optinet.*

Expl. (imperfect in paragraph 22): *Preterea multa alia vicia maturitate/*

5. *O* = Oxford, Bodleian Library MS Bodley 828, fols. 225r-226v. 14th century.

Title: *Incipit scriptum magistri W. de montibus quomodo religiosi monendi sunt ad confitendum et que penitencia pro peccatis religiosorum est iniungenda.*

Inc. Prol.: *Petisti amice.*

Inc. Txt.: *Prelatus igitur siue qui vicem eius optinet.*

Expl.: *pro aliis generibus peccatorum inponendis.*

Colophon: *Explicit scriptum magistri W. de montibus quomodo religiosi monendi sunt ad confitendum et que penitentia pro peccatis religiosorum sit iniungenda.*

Omits paragraph 23.

The treatise is transcribed in its entirety from MS Royal 8.C.vii of the British Library, London (no 3, above, designated by the siglum *L*), with emendations from MS Bodley 828 of the Bodleian Library, Oxford (no. 5, above, designated *O*). All of the manuscript copies of the text are rather late, and, as is common in practical works of this nature, contain a large number of variant readings. As it is impossible to reconstruct the original text from the extant witnesses, I have presented here the "scribal text" preserved in MS *L*, the most complete witness. Emendations from MS *O* are introduced only when the text of *L* fails to make sense or when the scribe has made some obvious blunder. Sources quoted in the text are identified within square brackets.

De penitentia religiosorum

Incipit scriptum Magistri Willelmi de montibus De penitentia religiosorum.

<1> Petisti amice ut tibi scribendo aliquod doctrine traderem compendium quo scire posses quomodo uiri religiosi admonendi sunt
5 ad confitendum, quomodo audita confessione conueniendi, que peni-

tentia pro quibus peccatis iniungi. Huic petitioni satisfacere desiderans, quod de penitentia religiosorum a theologis prudentibus et discretis didici breuiter docere temptabo.

<2> Prelatus igitur siue uices eius gerens exhibeat se tam affabilem
10 tam benignum uultu et uerbo ut audeat ei penitens secreta cordis sui intimare. Promittat etiam ei, si confiteri et satisfacere uoluerit, plenam indulgentiam et beatitudinem eternam.

<3> Comminetur etiam quod si penitere noluerit duplici pena multabitur quam ille qui in seculari habitu simile peccatum commisit,
15 quia cum ille pro sola transgressione preceptorum dampnandus sit, iste pro transgressione preceptorum et consiliorum, nisi penituerit, duplex in gehenna sustinebit tormentum.

<4> Dicat preterea quod oportet uiros religiosos tanto purius et propensius se per misericordiam et confessionem a peccatis emendare
20 quanto frequentius solent sacrum corpus Christi sumere, et sepius pro se et pro aliis orationibus, ieiuniis, et uigiliis, et laboribus uacare. Quanto enim frequentius corpus Domini indigne manducant et sanguinem eius indigne bibunt tanto frequentius, teste apostolo [1 Cor 11:29], iudicium sibi manducant et bibunt, dum in peccato mortali
25 manentes penitere et confiteri contempnunt.

<5> Preterea quanto magis in orationibus et ieiuniis et in aliis operibus laborant tanto magis studere debent ne fructus tanti laboris per aliquod peccatum mortale amittant. Dum enim est aliquis in mortali, nec per orationes suas nec per alia opera sua potest eternam
30 promereri salutem. Scriptum est enim [Prov 28:9]: "Qui auertit aurem suam ne audiat legem, oratio eius erit execrabilis." Et alibi [Eccli 15:9]: "Non est speciosa laus in ore peccatoris."

<6> Quando uero aliquis confitetur aliquod turpe et grande peccatum, qui audit confessionem eius consoletur eum ne desperet, et corripiat
35 ne recidiuet. Studeat ne consolatio sit nimis blanda aut correptio nimis aspera. Si enim nimis blanda sit consolatio, facile penitens reuertitur ad uomitum; si nimis aspera correptio, facile contingere poterit ut non audeat penitens ei confiteri si in idem peccatum fuerit relapsus. Quocirca quantum est hic habenda discretio ut per mediam uiam incedas ne
40 aut nimia leuitas faciat peccatum iterari aut nimia asperitas ocultari.

<7> Quando autem religiosis uiris pro grauibus et ocultis peccatis penitentiam iniungere debemus in arto positi sumus, attendentes quam difficile sit scire quid uel quantum sit eis iniungendum. Non enim debet

30 Qui] Quod *L*
31 audiat] audeat *L*

eis ieiunium preter id quod communiter a fratribus obseruatur iniungi,
45 nec aliquid aliud unde peccatum suum possit notari. Nec solet eis pro
grauibus et ocultis peccatis adeo grauis ut secularibus iniungi nec tam
longum penitentie tempus, quia uiri religiosi multis et uariis obseruantiis
regule sue onerati sunt que, si obseruate fuerint, magnam penitentiam
possunt implere. Hanc tamen rationem quia multi minime attendentes
50 pro leuitate uel breuitate penitentie ad uomitum reuertuntur, oportet
igitur eis qui sepius relabuntur grauiorem et prolixiorem penitentiam
iniungi sicut in sequentibus docebitur.

<8> Religiosus qui cum muliere semel fornicationem fecerit per
unum annum peniteat hoc modo: Dicat xii psalteria, scilicet quolibet
55 mense unum, et singulis septimanis iii accipiat disciplinas, et singulis
diebus dicat vii psalmos penitentiales cum vii genuflectionibus. Qui
autem bis aut paulo plus talem fornicationem fecerit, iniungatur ei
predicta penitentia cum hac additione, ut cum singulis psalteriis faciat
xxx genuflectiones et dicat xv psalmos cum vii predictis. Qui autem
60 talem fornicationem in consuetudinem duxerit, extendatur ei tota
predicta per iii annos, et si forte diutius in dicto peccato iacuerit, ad
minus tot annis hec penitentia duret quot ipsum peccatum frequen-
tauerit.

<9> Qui semel adulterium commiserit, peniteat per i annum hoc
65 modo: Dicat quolibet mense duo psalteria, et qualibet septimana habeat
v disciplinas preterquam in Natali et in Pasca et in Pentecoste. Item
singulis diebus dicat vii psalmos cum vii genuflectionibus et xv psalmos
cum totidem genuflectionibus. Qui autem bis aut sepius adulterium
commiserit, predictam penitentiam cum hac additione faciat, ut qualibet
70 sexta feria abstineat a companagio, ita tamen ut aliquid inde gustet
pro scandalo uitando. Qui autem adulterium ex consuetudine fecerit,
extendatur ei penitentia proximo dicta per vii annos, preterea iniungatur
ei ut obseruet regulare ieiunium quod communiter obseruari solet a
uiris religiosis per dimidium annum, nec infringat illud aliquo die nisi
75 tempore minutionis aut pro infirmitate corporis aut precepto sui prelati.

<10> Qui mulierem sine uoluntate fornicandi osculatus fuerit, iii
disciplinas accipiat quia malum exemplum dedit. Qui autem cum
uoluntate fornicandi, x disciplinas patiatur cum totidem "Miserere mei,
Deus" [Ps 50]. Si autem in osculando semen effuderit, xv disciplinas
80 sustineat. Si autem super nudam carnem mulieris aut super uestes eius

56 penitentiales] *om.* L
67 diebus *om.* L

fuderit, xxx disciplinas sustineat cum totidem "Miserere mei, Deus," et in sexta feria a companagio abstineat.

<11>   Qui propria manu uel alio turpi motu se semel polluerit, xv disciplinas sustineat cum totidem "Miserere mei, Deus," et dicat vii
85 psalteria. Qui autem hoc uitium in consuetudinem duxerit, peniteat vii annis sic: Quolibet mense dicat iii psalteria, et cum quolibet psalterio faciat xxx genuflexiones, et qualibet septimana v disciplinas capiat cum totidem "Miserere," et singulis diebus dicat vii psalmos cum vii genuflectionibus, et xv psalmos cum genuflectionibus, et qualibet sexta
90 feria abstineat a companagio.

<12>   Qui coierit cum masculo semel, per i annum peniteat sic: Quolibet mense dicat tria psalteria et cum quolibet psalterio faciat xl genuflectiones, et qualibet septimana accipiat vi disciplinas cum totidem "Miserere mei," et singulis diebus dicat vii psalmos cum vii genuflec-
95 tionibus et xv psalmos cum xv genuflectionibus, et qualibet sexta feria abstineat a companagio. Si autem bis aut sepius, extendatur ei dicta penitentia per ii annos. Si autem in consuetudinem duxerit, extendatur ei eadem penitentia per vii annos, et hoc addatur ut quamdiu uixerit feria sexta a companagio abstineat.

100 <13>   Hec autem sit generalis regula ut pro quolibet delicto enormi in consuetudinem ducto iniungatur penitenti preter illam penitentiam que ad certum tempus iniungitur aliqua parua penitentia que duret tota uita sua. Pro qualitate uero personarum poteris predictis penitentiis aliquid addere uel subtrahere.

105 <14>   Notandum quod si quis cum pluribus mulieribus uel cum pluribus masculis cohierit, quia plures animas occidit addendum est aliquid penitentie secundum numerum eorum uel illarum in orationibus et disciplinis uel in abstinentia aliqua.

<15>   Si autem quis non ex proposito uel deliberatione set subito
110 casu et quia mulier se ingessit fornicationem uel adulterium fecerit, multo minor penitentia debet ei iniungi quam illa de qua supradiximus fornicatoribus et adulteris iniungenda.

<16>   Si uero penitens postea confessus fuerit se relapsum in idem peccatum pro quo penitentia ei iniuncta fuerat, iniunge ei ut denuo
115 incipiat, semper tamen cum aliqua additione.

<17>   Qui se inebriauerit, tres sustineat disciplinas et abstineat a companagio uno die.

---

102 penitentia] pene *L*
109 proposito] opposito *L*

<18> Qui per ebrietatem sopitus oblitus est dicere uesperas uel completorium uel aliam horam regularem, faciat dictam penitentiam
120 cum hac additione, ut dicat "Beati immaculati" [Ps 118] usque "Ad Dominum cum tribularer" [Ps 119:1].

<19> Qui per ebrietatem impeditus ad matutinas cum fratribus non surrexerit et eas uel in nocte uel in die sequenti post horam dixerit, iii disciplinis puniatur et tribus diebus a companagio abstineat. Qui
125 per ebrietatem impeditus ad matutinas non surrexerit et eas nec in nocte nec die sequenti dixerit, faciat penitentiam predictam cum additione scilicet ut dicat i psalterium.

<20> Qui ita se inebriauit ut ebrietatem manifestet coram fratribus lapsu pedum uel turpi impedimento lingue uel aliquem percutiendo
130 uel aliter contumelias inferendo uel inonestum iocum faciendo, scurilitate uerborum uel lasciuia cantilene uel turpi motu corporis sui, in capitulo accusetur et grauiter puniatur, ut qui fuit aliis exemplum perditionis fiat omnibus exemplum correctionis.

<21> Si autem predicta signa apparuerint in alico fratre non coram
135 fratribus suis set coram aliis qui nolunt eum acusare, et ipse priuata confessione ipsum peccatum uelauerit, xl disciplinas sustineat, et per totum annum feria sexta a companagio abstineat. Nullum enim uenenum magis detestandum est uiris religiosis sicut ebrietatem que solet miseros mortales in luxuriam et in multa genera peccatorum
140 precipitare.

<22> Preterea, cum multa alia uitia ex etatis maturitate plerumque remedium accipiant, uitio gule nulla potest maturitas etatis mederi, nec potest aliquis ab huius uitii consuetudine se retrahere nisi diuina gratia. Magnam uim faciat carni sue, et certam sibi in potu statuat sobrietatis
145 legem quam non excedat.

<23> Si quis uero per uoracitatem speciem corporis euomerit, lxx diebus peniteat, ut habetur de con. d. ii. [*Decretum*, De cons. D.2, c.28].

<24> Item ex penitentiario Bede [cf. *Barth*, c.102, p.270]: Si quis
150 per ebrietatem infra diem tertium uel uoracitatem eucharistiam euomerit, xl diebus peniteat. Hoc de clericis siue de monachis siue presbiteris intellige, episcopus uero lxx diebus. Si pro infirmitate hoc faciat, vii diebus peniteat.

<25> Si post tertium diem infra octauam hoc egerit, x diebus in
155 pane et aqua peniteat; illud non Bede.

<26> Item ex penitentiario Theodori [*Barth*, ibid.]: Qui per ebrietatem uomitum fecerit, si presbiter aut diaconus, xl diebus peniteat; si monachus, xxx; si laicus, xv; si clericus, xx diebus peniteat.

<27> Qui uero psalterium nescit dicat pro psalterio i psalmum,
160 scilicet "Miserere mei Deus," uel dominicam orationem tot uicibus quot
sunt psalmi in psalterio, scilicet cl.

<28> Hoc autem studeas omnibus modis penitenti persuadere ut ab
actu et uoluntate peccandi cesset et ordinem suum seruet. Si enim hoc
fecerit, remissionem consequi poterit et salutem.

165 <29> Ecce, sicut rogasti, breuiter tibi ostendi quomodo uiri religiosi
admonendi sunt ad confitendum, quomodo audita confessione conueniendi, quomodo penitentia est iniungenda. In hiis ergo habere
poteris formam imponendi penitentiam etiam pro aliis peccatorum
generibus.

Explicit scriptum magistri W. de montibus De penitentia religiosorum.

II.6

Epistola ad moniales

Among the manuscripts formerly in Peterborough Abbey Library were two described in the ancient catalogue as containing "letters of William de Montibus to nuns."[1] Until recently no trace of such letters had been identified. In 1971, however, Albinia de la Mare's painstaking description of MS Lyell 8 in the Bodleian Library, Oxford, revealed what is certainly one letter (perhaps the first in a series) written by William de Montibus to the Gilbertine nuns living at Sempringham.[2]

The letter is a small gem of pastoral instruction. William begins by praising St. Gilbert of Sempringham and comparing his new order to a "paradise of fruit trees, a garden of delights." He introduces himself as a "child" of St. Gilbert who has come to water this garden. Walking through Gilbert's fields, admiring the crops, the flowers, the shrubbery, and aromatic gardens, William breaks out in praises of the monastery of Sempringham. "How awesome is this place!" he exclaims. "This army of virgins is terrifying to the spirits of corruption and the lovers of pollution. In its chastity it terrifies the lustful, in its abstinence it terrifies the dainty, in vigils the indolent, in stability the aimless wanderers, and in monastic life the dissolute."

"Not only is Sempringham a terrifying place," William continues, "but also delightful, pleasant, and sweet like honey. ... Here the unicorn is captured in a virginal embrace. Here the bridegroom rests on a flowery couch of humble conscience; here he pastures his flock among the lilies of the most chaste; here he dallies between the breasts of his beloved."

Having thus captured the nuns' attention, William goes on to warn them against pride and to encourage them in humility by means of

---

[1] See James, "Lists of Manuscripts Formerly in Peterborough Abbey Library." James's number 92 (B.v) is entitled *Epistole W. de Montibus ad Moniales*; his number 85 (S.iv) is described in the old catalogue as containing "Sermones eiusdem [sc. Cancellarii Lincoln.] et Epp. ad Sanctimoniales."

[2] *Catalogue of the Collection of Medieval Manuscripts Bequeathed to the Bodleian Library Oxford by James P.R. Lyell*, pp. 16-20, 324-364, at p. 356 (no. 340).

a catena of proverbs and Scripture sentences upon which the nuns might meditate.

The letter ends somewhat abruptly; it may have been abridged by the compiler of MS Lyell 8, who was assembling a large collection of sermons and sermon materials. The concluding phrase of the text is that of a sermon, not a letter, and would seem to be an editorial device rather than the original conclusion of William's epistle.

William de Montibus had a long and intimate relationship with the Gilbertine Order. The reference in line 18 to his having been a *puer* in Gilbert's household may be only a figure of speech, but it may just as plausibly be a reference to William's own boyhood association with Gilbert of Sempringham in Lincolnshire.[3] Early in the twelfth century Gilbert was the parish priest in his native village of Sempringham. While serving there he spent time teaching boys and girls in his parish, and encouraged seven women to adopt a rule of life based on the Cistercian model.[4] From these humble beginnings emerged the only indigenous English monastic order. In 1139 Gilbert established a second house of nuns, and affiliated lay people (*conversi*) with his houses to assist in the manual labour of the communities. After 1148 Gilbert also founded houses of regular canons (following the rule of St. Augustine) to provide pastoral care for the nuns. By the time of Gilbert's death in 1189 there were nine double monasteries (nuns and canons) and four houses of canons only. The three groups within the order — nuns, priests, and *conversi* — are alluded to in paragraph 3 of William's letter, where he compares the choirs of nuns to gardens, the colleges of canons to orchards, and the communities of *conversi* (*fratrum religiosorum*) to fields.

William de Montibus's high esteem in the eyes of the Gilbertine Order is demonstrated by the part he played in the canonization proceedings for Gilbert.[5] However, this brief letter to nuns is all the evidence that we have at present to indicate that he took an active role in providing pastoral care to the nuns of the order. It is possible,

---

[3] See above, Chapter One, pp. 7-9.

[4] For a history of the Gilbertine Order see Rose Graham, *Saint Gilbert of Sempringham and the Gilbertines: A History of the Only English Monastic Order* (London: Elliot Stock, 1901). See also Eileen Power, *Medieval English Nunneries c. 1275 to 1535* (Cambridge: University Press, 1922); *The Book of St Gilbert*; Giles Constable, "Aelred of Rievaulx and the Nun of Watton: An Episode in the Early History of the Gilbertine Order," in *Medieval Women*, ed. Derek Baker (Oxford: Blackwell, 1978), pp. 205-226.

[5] See Chapter One, pp. 21-22.

even probable, that among the many anonymous sermons *ad moniales* in the Lyell manuscript are other letters by William de Montibus,[6] perhaps part of a longer collection of "Letters to Nuns" such as was reported in the Peterborough catalogue. I have been unable to demonstrate William's authorship of the individual sermons there, but further research in the rich collections of manuscript materials associated with the Gilbertine Order will surely reveal more of the story.

AUTHENTICITY AND DATE

William identifies himself in the address of this letter, thus providing the most secure type of evidence of his authorship. The images he invokes, such as the nesting bird, the garden that is planted and watered by human agency but whose growth comes from God, and the unicorn that is captured by a virgin's embrace, all are familiar themes in William's other writings. The verses and proverbs that he proposes for the nuns' edification are also typical of William's pedagogical method.

William refers to Gilbert of Sempringham as *uere sanctus*. As Gilbert was canonized in 1202, William's letter was probably written after that date.

SOURCES

As one might expect in a pastoral letter, no scholastic authorities are cited. William draws on his own teachings here, and parallel passages for most of the letter can be found scattered throughout his *Numerale*, *Distinctiones*, *Similitudinarium*, *Prouerbia*, and *Versarius*.

MANUSCRIPT

The unique manuscript copy is in Oxford, Bodleian Library MS Lyell 8, fol. 187va-vb. Early 13th century (above top line).

---

[6] See de la Mare, *Catalogue*, p. 18.

Epistola ad moniales

Sacrosantis Dei uirginibus Christo Domino desponsatis, eisque in loco dicto Sempringham, fideliter, diligenter, et hilariter nocte dieque seruientibus, Willelmus de monte, Linconiensis Ecclesie Cancellarius: Puritate casti amoris sponso adherere et eius amore inardescere.

5   Venerabilis ille magister et pater Gilebertus, uere sanctus, sacerdos Dei summi, confessor Christi, negotiator euangelicus strenuus et discretus, prudens et prouidus paranimphus sponsi, querens que sunt Ihesu Christi ut apis argumentosa, Christo Domino seruiuit. Edificauit supra petram Christum. Nidificauit in petra Christo. Pullos plurimos
10 procreauit, cooperante Christo. Deus autem addat ad hunc numerum multa milia, benedicens, fouens, et custodiens in feruore religionis et perseuerantia.

    Plantauerat pater prenominatus paradysum pomorum, ortum deliciarum; immo tot ortos quot sacrarum uirginum choros, tot pomeria
15 quot ueneranda canonicorum collegia, tot uirgulta quot fratrum religiosorum consortia. Ipse inquam plantauit, nos fluentis doctrine rigamus, Deus autem incrementum dare non desinit [cf. 1 Cor 3:7].

    Ego itaque, patrisfamilias predicti puer, transiens per sata eius et plantationes, per areolas illas aromatum, aspiciens, admirans, in laudem
20 monasterii Sempringham prorumpens exclamo: "Terribilis est locus iste" [Gen 28:17], "ut castrorum acies ordinata" [Cant 6:3]. "Vere Dominus est in loco isto" [Gen 28:16], et "Benedicta gloria Domini de loco sancto suo" [Ez 3:12]. Domine Ihesu locum tuum hunc ne dimiseris, dic, Domine, "Hec requies mea in seculum seculi; hic
25 habitabo quoniam elegi eam" [Ps 131:14], et locum, immo potius habitantes in loco [cf. 2 Mach 5:19].

    Terribilis autem est hic exercitus uirginum corrumptionum spiritibus et amatoribus pollutionum. Terribilis est pro continentia libidinosis, pro abstinentia delicatis, pro uigilia pigris, pro inclusione uagis, pro
30 religione dissolutis.

    Nec solum terribilis est locus, set amenus, mellifluus, et iocundus. Hic enim capitur rinoceros amplexu uirgineo. Hic quiescit sponsus in humilis conscientie lecto florido [cf. Cant 1:15]. Hic pascit inter lylya

---

2 Sempringham] Sempingham *MS*
7 sunt *om. MS*
25 immo] imo *MS*

castissimarum [cf. Cant 2:16]. Hic commoratur inter ubera carissimarum
35 [cf. Cant 1:12].

Verum ne in cuiusquam pectoris tumore uel pectore tumorum
excrescat elatio ex ubertate morum, ex habundantia humorum uel et
plus per multa plantata arefiat religio per uiolentiam uel insolentiam,
hec ad presens aspergatur humectatio:

40   Ante mortem ne laudes hominem. Vltima
      Semper expectanda dies dicique beatus
      Ante obitum nemo suppremaque funera debet.
      Vespere detur ei si laus est danda diei.

Non eque glorietur accintus ut discinctus [cf. 3 Reg 20:11], id est
45 pugnans ut trihumphans. Non ait Dominus pugnanti set uincenti, "dabo
manna absconditum" etc. [Apoc 2:17].

Item alia humectatio est humilitatis propositio, ut est hec: Quid habes
quod non accepisti?" [1 Cor 4:7]. Et, "Cum feceritis omnia que precepta
sunt uobis, dicite: Serui (uel ancille) inutiles sumus" [Lc 17:10];
50 bonorum enim nostrorum non eget Deus [cf. Ps 15:2]. Et, "Non sunt
condigne passiones huius temporis ad futuram gloriam" [Rom 8:18],
ad quam nos clementer perducat, qui eternaliter uiuit et regnat, amen,
amen.

36 tumorum] tumoris *corr.* MS
37 humorum] humoris *corr.* MS
38 plantata] diligentiam *add.* MS
43 These four lines of verse are a concatenation of several popular themes; see
Hans Walther, *Proverbia sententiaeque latinitatis medii aevi*, nos. 1146-1147, 32088,
33221. The last three lines are quoted in another sermon found in Lyell 8; see de
la Mare, *Catalogue*, p. 361, (no. 395).
47 Quid] Quis MS

II.7

Numerale

William composed the *Numerale* to introduce students in his Lincoln schools to the discipline of theology. As such it represents an extremely valuable witness to the pedagogical techniques and expectations in diocesan and local schools at the beginning of the thirteenth century. One of William's most popular works, the *Numerale* owes its success to its distinctive combination of scholastic doctrine with theological commonplaces and moral exposition. It remains one of the most accessible and interesting introductions to theology produced in this period.

The introductory sentence adumbrates the purpose and audience of this work: "In introducing the discipline of theology (*facultatem theologicam*) a brief foretaste of some matters will ensure the most competent progress to higher things."[1] In section 2.4, concerning the life of the student (*clericus*), William comments: "The whole of theological study (*summa theologice facultatis*) consists in believing and in acting."[2] The scholastic context of the work, however, is never far below the surface. At the end of section 1.1 it is asked whether one may refer to the saints as gods in scholastic disputations since the Scriptures speak of them as such. William answers: "No, for the mode of Scripture which uses figures of speech is one thing, and the mode of disputation which seeks the naked truth is another."[3]

As the title suggests, the *Numerale* is organized numerically. It begins with short expositions concerning "One God," "One Lord," "One Faith," "One Baptism," and "One Church," and ends with the twelve articles of faith, the twelve hours of the day, and the twelve prerogatives of the Blessed Virgin.

---

[1] "Ad introducendam facultatem theologicam quedam compendiose prelibanda sunt ut competentius ad altiora fiat progressus."

[2] "In credendis quidem et agendis consistit summa theologice facultatis."

[3] See the transcription below, p. 236.

The structure of the *Numerale* has been described as rare and unusual.[4] In fact this artificial method of organizing *sententiae* was already employed by Walter Daniel, an English Cistercian, in his *Centum sententiae* compiled in the second half of the twelfth century.[5] Walter was the biographer of Ailred of Rievaulx, and both Cistercians were in close contact with Gilbert of Sempringham in whose household William de Montibus seems to have served.[6] By the early thirteenth century, perhaps under the influence of William's popular work, a number of other writers produced collections of the same type.[7]

Seen in its historical context, this attempt to organize theological knowledge around the numbers from one to twelve is less unusual than it may appear. William was one of many writers at the turn of the century who was searching for a useful way to organize vast amounts of heterogenous materials.[8] In other writings he experimented with alphabetical organization; here he adopts an even simpler, if less "rational," system. William's *Numerale* should perhaps be compared to Peter the Chanter's *Verbum abbreviatum*. Both are written for similar audiences and contain similar materials; neither is very successful as a coherent *summa* that can be referred to and searched for relevant materials, but each was very successful in its own right.[9]

---

[4] Beryl Smalley and G. Lacombe, "The Lombard's Commentary on Isaias and Other Fragments," *New Scholasticism* 5 (1931) 148.

[5] Talbot, "The *Centum Sententiae* of Walter Daniel," pp. 266-383.

[6] Ibid., p. 274; See above, Chapter One, for William's association with Gilbert of Sempringham.

[7] See the anonymous and unstudied works preserved in London, British Library Royal MSS 10.C.iii, fols. 81v-154v; 12.E.i, fols. 128r-136v; 12.F.xv, fols. 65r-82v; in Lambeth Palace MS 36, fols. 1r-89v; in Leiden, Bibliotheek der Rijksuniversiteit MS Vulc. 48, fols. 122 ff.; and in Oxford, Bodleian Library MS Bodley 897, fols. 38ra-97va. Hugh MacKinnon reports, in his dissertation pp. 261-262, a private communication from Beryl Smalley that suggests a certain Fulgentius also wrote a *Numerale*. He gives the following citation, without specifying its source: "Nam secundum Fulgentium in suo numerali, cap. 7, anima in statu innocentie septem (*sic*) radiis universum decorabat, qui sunt humilitas, veritas, equitas, caritas, virtuosa societas et pacis concordia. Sed sicut tangit Willelmus de Montibus in suo numerali, cap. 26: anima per peccatum correspondenter ad istos radios septempliciter tenebratur ... que sunt superbia, mendacium, homicidium, invidia, iniqua stabilitas, dolorosa duplicitas, et legis discordia. Et hoc probat per scripturam hoc eminente proverbio: Sex sunt que odit Deus et septimum detestat anima eius (cf. below, 7.5).

[8] Rouse and Rouse, *Preachers*, pp. 3-42.

[9] See Baldwin, *Masters*, 1: 15: "The long and short versions [of the *Verbum abbreviatum*] follow a common arrangement of subject matter which exhibits a minimum of logical progression ... . Peter the Chanter obviously had little concern for planning his work on a comprehensive scale. In effect he produced a series of loosely related chapters each of which was suggested by the one preceding. The interest

Just as the Chanter's *Verbum abbreviatum* comprises "a series of loosely related chapters,"[10] so William's *Numerale* presents a number of discrete expositions of theological topics that often are related by a loose, internal logic, but make no pretense to forming a systematic and comprehensive *summa* of theological doctrine. In the first section, for example, William begins with the proposition that "God is one" (1.1). This apparently suggested to him the Pauline text: "One Lord, one faith, one baptism" (Eph 4:5) which provided the topics of the following three chapters (1.2-4). The last item — one baptism — may have brought to mind the text of the *Credo*: "And in one holy, catholic (and apostolic) Church," which immediately precedes the confession of "one baptism" in the ordinary of the Mass, and with which William concludes the first section of his *Numerale* (1.5).

In the second section (2.3) William describes how faith and works are the two things necessary for the adult who has reached the age of reason (*Viatori adulto et discreto*). This leads to a discussion of the two things necessary for the student (*clerico*) (2.4), and for the Christian (2.5). The same theme is resumed in 3.4 — the three things necessary for the sinner — and in 3.10 — the three things necessary for the adult (*adulto et discreto*) to attain salvation. In the same way, each of the topics discussed in 3.13-18 seems to be suggested by the previous discussions.

The popularity of this work, like that of the Chanter's *Verbum abbreviatum*, obviously lay less in its systematic and comprehensive treatment of christian theology than in its thoughtful treatment of discrete topics of contemporary interest. In his conclusion William refers to the work as a *summa*, and such it is.[11] In spite of an organizational framework that, judged by later standards, is awkward and artificial, this work apparently served a generation of English students as a useful introduction to the study of theology.

Authenticity and Date

The *Numerale* seems to have been the most popular of William's longer works. It survives complete in at least eighteen manuscript copies and

---

of the book lies not in its organization, but rather in its wealth of detail and illustrative material."

[10] Ibid.

[11] On the many different types of *summae* composed in the twelfth and thirteenth centuries see Palémon Glorieux, "Sommes théologiques," *Dictionnaire de théologie catholique* (1941), 14: 2341-2350.

extensive portions of the text are copied in another four manuscripts. All are English manuscripts of the thirteenth century, and fifteen of the copies explicitly ascribe the work to William de Montibus. Other writers also borrowed from the *Numerale* and acknowledged William as its author.[12]

Internal evidence demonstrates that this work was composed in England during William's tenure as chancellor of Lincoln Cathedral. He refers explicitly to his *Distinctiones*,[13] and to a collection of his sermons.[14]

Sources

Although the *Numerale* discusses many of the theological commonplaces of the twelfth and early thirteenth centuries, it is not a derivative work and relies on few identifiable sources for its interpretations. The authorities cited are those which were current in the Parisian schools at the end of the century: The Bible and its Gloss, Ambrose, Aristotle, Boethius, Cato's *Distichs* ("in libello ethico paruulis ad morum informationem proposito"), Gratian's *Decretum*, Gregory, Isidore's *Etymologies*, Jerome, *Legenda* of the saints, liturgical readings, Lombard's *Sentences*, Lucan, Ovid, the *Rule of St. Augustine*, Seneca, and Virgil.

Manuscripts

1. Bury St. Edmund's, Cathedral MS 4 [B.357], fols. 88r-95v. 13th century.

 Inc.: *Vnus Deus. Deus unus est. Contra*

 Expl. (imperfect in section 3.16): *plus ab eo exigitur.*

I have not examined this copy.

---

[12] The most extensive borrowings are in Richard of Wetheringsett's *Qui bene presunt* (see above, Part One, Chapters Two and Three).

[13] "Et de hiis plenius diximus in distinctionibus nostris uel in sermonibus" (3.16); "De hac autem plenius in distinctionibus et sermonibus nostris exarauimus" (4.6); "De purificationibus autem, id est remissionibus pretaxatis, planius exarauimus in distinctionibus nostris" (6.2); "Horum auctoritates quere supra de ydriis, et in distinctionibus nostris" (10.5).

[14] "Huiusmodi uero bestie et reptilia uersantur in nemore quod plantauit Abraham in Bersabee ... de quo in sermonibus nostris si quesieris inuenire poteris" (6.1); "sicut radius ex sidere ita Christus ex uirgine. Huius similitudines inuenies in sermone nostro de annuntiatione que sic incipit: Mulier que dampnauit saluauit" (12.1)

2. Cambridge, Fitzwilliam Museum Add. MS 243, fols. 28ra-48va. Early 13th century (above top line).

>Inc. (imperfect): *gloria perpetua superinduenda*
>Expl.: *immediate Deo coniuncta.*
>Colophon: *Hec Deo gratias ... copiosius sunt grata. Explicit.*

The text begins abruptly in section 3.3, following a blank folio in the codex, and at the beginning of a new gathering.

3. Cambridge, Corpus Christi College MS 186, fols. 127ra-173ra. Mid 13th century (above top line).

>Title: (*Incipit numerale Magistri Willelmi de montibus*).
>Inc. Prol.: *Introducendis in facultatem*
>Inc. Txt.: *In primis igitur ut ab hac unitate exordiamur innotescendum est quia scriptum est Deus tuus unus est. Contra*
>Expl.: *immediate Deo coniuncta*
>Colophon: *et hic Deo gracias ... copiosius sunt exarata. Explicit.*

4. Cambridge, Corpus Christi College MS 217, fols. 187v-209r. Mid 13th century (above top line).

>Inc. Prol.: *Introducendis in facultatem*
>Inc. Txt.: *In primis igitur ... Deus unus est. Contra*
>Expl.: *immediate coniuncta.*
>Colophon: *Et hic Deo gracias ... copiosius sunt exarata. Explicit.*

5. Cambridge, Gonville and Caius College MS 138/78, fols. 137va-172ra. Late 13th century.

>Title: (*Hic incipit numerale magistri Willelmi de montibus*).
>Inc. Prol.: *Ad introducendam facultatem*
>Inc. Txt.: *Quia scriptum est in Deuteronomio: Deus est. Contra*
>Expl.: *immediate Deo coniuncta.*
>Colophon: *Hic et Deo gracias ... copiosius sunt exarata. (Hic explicit Numerale magistri Willelmi de montibus).*

6. Cambridge, Jesus College MS Q.B.17 (34), fols. 7ra-9vb. Early 13th century (above top line).

>Title: *Introductiones in theologiam.*
>Inc. Prol.: *Introducendis in facultatem*
>Inc. Txt.: *Unus est Dominus Deus. Set Deus trinus et unus.*
>Expl.: *Hec tria sunt: Gula, gloria uana, cupido.*

This idiosyncratic fragment bears little resemblance to the other copies of William's *Numerale*. Many additional topics are included, and the treatment of shared materials is not verbally identical. This text might be a rough draft for the final version of the *Numerale*, or, more plausibly, a pastiche of selections from William's work with numerous additions from an unidentified source.

7. Cambridge, Peterhouse MS 255, fols. 1r-35r. Mid 13th century (fols. 13r-35r written above top line).

> Title: (*Incipit numerale magistri Willelmi de montibus*).
> Inc. Prol.: *Ingredientibus artem theologicam*
> Inc. Txt. (not clearly marked): *Deus tuus unus est. Deutro. Contra*
> Expl.: *in mediate Deo coniuncta.*
> Colophon: *Et hic Deo gracias ... copiosius sunt exarata.*

8. Cambridge, St. John's College MS F.4 (141), fols. 1ra-42vb. Early 13th century (above top line).

> Inc. Txt.: (*Deus*) *Dicitur Deus essentialiter et naturaliter.*
> Expl.: *in medietate Deo coniuncta.*
> Colophon: *Et hic Deo gracias ... copiosius sunt exarata.*

The beginning of section 1.1 is somewhat fuller than in the version printed below.

9. Cambridge, Trinity Hall MS 24, fols. 102va-107ra. Mid 13th century (above top line).

> Inc. Txt.: (*Vnus Deus*) *Deus unus est. Contra*
> Expl.: *de quibus locuta es gloriosior apparebo.*

The text breaks off in section 3.12. A table of contents for the entire work, written by the same scribe, is found on fol. 102ra-va.

10. Durham, Cathedral Library MS B.IV.20, pp. 91a-183b. Mid 13th century (above top line).

> Title: (*Incipit summa secundum progressum numerorum a magistro Guillelmo lincolniensis ecclesie Cancellario composita*).
> Inc. Txt.: *Deus unus est. Contra*
> Expl.: *immediata Deo coniuncta.*
> Colophon: *Et hic Deo gracias ... copiosius sunt exarata.*

Table of contents on pages 89a-90b.

11. Eton College MS 82, fols. 1r-64r. Early 13th century (above top line).

> Title: *Incipit liber numeralis magistri Willelmi de monte.*
> Inc. Txt.: *Audi Israel, Deus tuus Deus unus est*
> Expl.: *immediate Deo coniuncta.*
> Colophon: *Et hic Deo gracias ... copiosius sunt arata. Explicit* (*Numerale*).

Table of contents on fols. 39v-40v of Eton College MS 76. Chapter 1.1 is somewhat fuller than in the version printed below.

12. Lincoln, PRO MS Ancaster 16/1, fols. 5vb-45rb. Early 13th century (above top line).

> Inc. Txt.: *Audi Israel, Deus tuus Deus unus est.*
> Expl.: *immediate Deo coniuncta.*
> Colophon: *Et hic gracias agendo ... copiosius sunt exarata. Explicit.*

The text is preceded by a table of contents, in the same hand, on fols. 5ra-5vb. Section 1.1 is somewhat fuller than in the version printed above. Sections 3.14 and 3.16 are omitted.

13. *L* = London, British Library, Cotton MS Vespasian E.x, fols. 125v-199r. 13th century (below top line).

    Title: (*Incipit hic nostri pulcrum Numerale magistri, et cancellarii Nichol., de monte Willelmi*).
    Inc. Prol.: (*Ad introducendam facultatem theologicam*).
    Inc. Txt.: *Deus unus est. Contra*
    Expl.: *immediate Deo coniuncta.*
    Colophon: *Et hic gracias agendo ... copiosius sunt exarata. Explicit.*
Followed on fols 199ra-200ra by a table of contents.

14. *H* = London, British Library MS Harley 325, fols. 39r-82r. Mid 13th century (above top line).

    Title: *Magister W. de monte* (*Incipit Liber primus. Vnus Deus*).
    Inc. Txt.: *Deus unus est. Contra*
    Expl.: *immediate Deo coniuncta.*
    Colophon: *Et hic Deo gracias ... copiosius sunt gesta.*
A table of contents is found on fol. 38v.

15. London, British Library MS Royal 11.A.iii, fols. 5ra-34va. Mid 13th century (c. 1245; above top line).

    Inc. Prol.: (*Introducendis in facultatem theologicam*).
    Inc. Txt.: *Deus unus est. Contra*
    Expl.: *immediate Deo coniuncta.*
    Colophon: *Et hic gracias ... copiosius sunt arata. Explicit.*
Section 1.1 is somewhat fuller than in the version printed below.

16. London, Lambeth Palace MS 261, fols. 53r-108v. Early 13th century (above top line).

    Title: *Magistri Willelmi de montibus.*
    Inc. Txt.: *Deus unus est, ut in Deut. capitulo xix, Ysaia cxxx. Contra*
    Expl.: *immediate Deo coniuncta.*
    Colophon: *Et hic Deo gracias ... copiosius sunt exarata.*

17. Oxford, Bodleian Library MS Add. C. 263 (sc. 27646), fols. 55rb-96va. Early 13th century (above top line).

    Title: (*Incipit summa secundum progressum numerorum a magistro Willelmo Cancellario Lincolniensi conposita. Audi Israel, Dominus Deus tuus Deus unus est*).
    Inc. Txt.: *Deus unus est. Contra*
    Expl.: *immediate Deo coniuncta.*
    Colophon: *Et hic Deo gracias ... copiosius sunt exarata. Explicit.*

A gathering is missing between fols. 61 and 62, causing the loss of text from the end of section 3.8 to the middle of 3.16.

18. Oxford, Bodleian Library MS Bodley 897 (sc. 27888), fols. 97va-121ra. Mid 13th century.

> Title: (*Hic incipit numerale magistri Willelmi de Lincolniensisi Cancellarius*).
> Inc. Txt.: (*Unus Deus*) *Deus unus est. Contra*
> Expl.: *immediate Deo coniuncta.*
> Colophon: *Et hic Deo gracias ... opusculis nostris sunt exarata.*

The scribe has omitted section 12.2. A fourteenth-century scribe has compiled an alphabetical subject index on fols. 132r-133r.

19. Oxford, Bodleian Library MS Laud lat. misc. 345 (sc. 1273), fols. 192rb-206vb. Mid 13th century (above top line).

> Title: *Incipit Numerale magistri Willelmi de montibus Lincolniensis ecclesie cancellarii compositum.*
> Inc. Prol.: *Introducendis In Facultatem theologicam*
> Inc. Txt.: (*Vnus Deus*) *Deus unus est. Contra*
> Expl.: *immediate Deo coniuncta.*
> Colophon: *Et hic Deo gracias ... copiosius sunt exarata.* (*Explicit Numerale Magistri Willelmi de montibus*).

A table of contents, written in the same hand, is provided on fol. 192r.

20. Oxford, Bodleian Library MS Lyell 8 (extracts). Mid 13th century (above top line). Fols. 56vb-59va.

> Inc.: (*De quatuor speciebus unguenti*) *De quatuor aromatibus.*
> Expl.: *Golias diabolus est ... ipsi resistitur.*

This extract begins at section 4.4 and extends through section 5.3.

Fol. 143rb-va.

> Inc.: (*De duodecim prerogatiuis beate Marie secundum magistrum W. de montibus in libro numerali*) *Legitur in Apocalipsi*
> Expl.: *immediate Deo coniuncta.*

This extract corresponds to section 12.3.

Fol. 143va.

> Inc.: *Similitudinem trinitatis proferunt*
> Expl.: *in infusione gratie.*

This extract is the final part of section 12.1.

Fols. 169ra-174vb.

> Inc. (imperfect): *tum ecclesie militantis tum ecclesie triumphantis*
> Expl.: *Deo immediate coniuncta. Et hic gracias ... copiosius sunt exarata. Explicit liber qui vocatur numerale.*

This extract begins in section 6.7 and includes all of sections 6.8 to 12.3.

21. Oxford, Balliol College MS 222, fols 48vb-76vb. Mid 13th century.
Title: (*Incipit Numerale magistri Willelmi de montibus canonici Lincolniensis ecclesie ab vno usque ad duodecim*).
Inc. Prol.: *Introducendis in facultatem theologicam*
Inc. Txt.: (*Deus unus*) *Deus tuus unus est, Deut. xix. Contra*
Expl.: *immediate Deo esse coniuncta.*
Colophon: *Et hic Deo gracias ... copiosius sunt exarata.* (*Explicit Numerale magistri Willelmus canonici ecclesie Lincolniensis*).

22. Oxford, Merton College MS 257, fols. 5ra-66ra. Later 13th century.
Title (f. 4ra): (*Incipiunt capitula libri magistri Willelmi de monte qui numerale vocatur*).
Inc. Prol.: *Vnus est Deus et hoc natura docet.*
Inc. Txt.: *Avdi Israel, Deus tuus Deus unus est ... . Contra*
Expl.: *immediate Deo coniuncta.*
Colophon: *Et hic Deo gracias ... copiosius sunt arata. Explicit* (*Numerale*).
A table of contents, written in the same hand as the text, is found on fol. 4ra-vc. The prologue, filling all of fol. 5r, is idiosyncratic and probably was not written by William de Montibus. Section 1.1 is somewhat fuller than the version printed below.

23. Oxford, New College MS 98, fols 1ra-32vb. Early 13th century (above top line).
Title (later hand): (*Incipit summa que vocatur numerale*).
Inc Txt.: *Deus unus est. Contra*
Expl.: *immediate Deo coniuncta*
Colophon: *et hic Deo gracias ... copiosius sunt exarata. Explicit.*

24. San Marino (California), Huntington Library MS HM 19914, fols. 159ra-184rb. Mid 13th century (above top line).
Inc. Prol. (top line cropped): *In primis igitur*
Inc. Txt.: *Deus unus est. Contra*
Expl.: *immediate Deo coniuncta.*
Colophon: *Et hic Deo gracias ... copiosius sunt exarata. Explicit numerale magistri Willelmi Lincolniensis ecclesie cancellarii. Sancta Ositha Deo gracias.*
An extra chapter, *De vitulo Samarie*, has been added between sections 6.4 and 6.5.

Representative portions of the text are transcribed from MS Vespasian E.x of the Cotton collection in the British Library, London (*L*, no. 13 above). Emendations from MS Harley 325 (*H*, no. 14 above) are noted in the apparatus criticus.

Numerale

Ad introducendam facultatem theologicam quedam compendiose prelibanda sunt ut competentius ad altiora fiat progressus. In primis igitur
ab unitate exordiendum est, quia scriptum est:

1.1 Vnvs Devs

Deus unus est [Deut 6:4]. Contra, Apostolus ait [1 Cor 8:5]: Sunt
multi dii, etc. Respondeo: Dicitur Deus essentialiter et naturaliter. Sic
est Deus unus in essentia, trinus in personis.

Dicuntur et dii adoptiue, ut sancti qui per gratiam adoptantur in
filios Dei [Rom 8:14-15]; ut Seth religiosus; et ego dixi dii estis [Ps
81:6]; et dedit eis potestatem filios Dei fieri, etc. [Io 1:12]. Set numquid
angeli qui in Iob [1:6] filii Dei dicuntur dicendi sunt dii? Ita enim
in ystoriis habetur [Gen 6:2]. Potius tamen est ut non dicantur dii
ne credantur esse colendi nec eis exhibeatur latria que est seruitus soli
Deo debita. Contra tamen super epistolam primam Cor. xxxix [8:5-6].

Item nota quia gratia exterior est in collatione operum uel honorum
uel potentie uel glorie; et secundum hoc Iudei dii dicuntur ibi [Ps 81:1]:
Deus stetit in synagoga deorum. Gratia autem interior est, uel in
collatione gratuitorum in presenti, uel in collatione gemine stole in
futuro, et secundum hoc dicuntur sancti dii — nunc semidii, post plene
deificandi.

Dicuntur autem dii potestatiue; hoc est enim ut diximus secundum
gratiam exteriorem. Vnde [Ex 22:28]: Diis non detrahes, id est prelatis;
et: Constitui te deum Pharaoni [Ex 7:1], id est potentem super eum,
uel ut per te potentia diuina declaretur in Pharaone et suis; uel "constitui
te deum," id est timendum ei, quia deus dicitur theos, id est timor.

Dicuntur et dii nuncupatiue uel putatiue, ut demones et ydola. Vnde
[Ps 95:5]: Omnes dii gentium demonia. Sic Ioseph dicitur pater Christi,
putatiue scilicet.

Dicuntur et dii reputatiue uel imputatiue, ad culpam scilicet et ad
penam. Vnde super illud [Ps 80:10]: Non erit in te Deus recens quod
quisque cupit et ueneratur pre ceteris, scilicet hoc illi Deus est. Vnde
[Phil 3:19]: Quorum deus uenter est.

Queritur an in disputatione sancti dicendi sint dii. Respondeo non.
Alia est enim ratio scripture que tropis utitur, alia disputationis que
nudam querit ueritatem.

1.2 Vnvs Dominvs

Vnus Dominus [Eph 4:5]. Contra [1 Cor 8:5]: Sunt multi domini. Respondeo: Dominus dicitur substantialiter ... . Dicitur et Dominus relatiue ... .

1.3 Vna fides

Vna fides, Eph. xiiii [4:5]; Sent. libro tertio, lxxviii [Lombard, 3 *Sent* D.23 c.6]. Contra: Alia fides mea, alia tua; alia fides antiquorum, alia modernorum, quia diuersi sunt articuli quidam; alia fides naturalis, alia gratuita ... . Respondeo: Vna fides; non una numero sed genere ... .

1.4 Vnvm baptisma

Vnum baptisma [Eph 4:5]. Contra: Alius est baptismus Iohannis, alius baptismus Christi; alius baptismus in aqua, alius in spiritu; alius baptismus exterior, alius interior ... . Respondeo: Baptisma Christi instituentis et hodie per ministros exercentis et intus abluentis ... .

1.5 Vna ecclesia

Vna est ecclesia. Vnde: Credo sanctam ecclesiam catholicam. Contra [Ps 67:27]: In ecclesiis benedicite Deo. Respondeo: Vna est ecclesia catholica, id est uniuersalis, et plures sunt ecclesie particulares ... .

2.1 Dvo testamenta

Duo sunt testamenta scilicet scripture, uetus et nouum tum tempore tum effectu; illud terrena conferens, hoc celestia ... . Hec sunt due rote in Ezechiele [10:9] ... duo denarii tum Samaritani [Lc 10:35] tum Vidue [Lc 21:3] ... duo dragmata stateris in ore piscis [Mt 17:26] ... duo ligna in scala Iacob [Gen 28:12] ... duo ubera sponse [Cant 1:12], et duo fontes id est Ior et Dan qui Iordanem conficiunt ... duo gladii [Lc 22:38] ex utraque parte acuti [Apoc 1:16] ... duo cherubin [Ex 37:7] ... duo brachia forcipis [Is 6:6] ... duo cornua tum arietis, tum mitre pontificalis ... duo panni pretiosi in humeris et extremitatibus albe sacerdotalis. Hinc et ita uersifice dicimus:

> Sunt albe panni duo testamenta decentes,
> Sunt stater et scala, sunt forceps, ubera, fontes,
> Denariique rote, cherubin duo cornua et enses.

2.2 GEMINVS MOTVS DILECTIONIS

Caritas Grece dilectio Latine, que duplex est, unus enim motus in Deum dirigitur ... . Alter motus dirigitur in proximum eque meritorius ... .

2.3 FIDES ET OPVS

Viatori adulto et discreto duo necessaria sunt ad salutem, fides et opus ... .

2.4 MVNDITIA ET SCIENTIA

Clerico duo sunt necessaria, munditia uite et sufficientia scientie ... .

2.5 CONSCIENTIA ET FAMA

Christiano duo sunt necessaria, puritas conscientie et odor opinionis bone id est fame ... .

2.6 DEXTERA ET SINISTRA

Due sunt manus et duo sunt opera, id est genera operum. Sunt enim opera nature, quasi manus sinistra, et sunt opera gratie tamquam manus dextra. Tertia manus monstruosum quidem esset in homine, et tertium genus operum, scilicet culpe, detestabile est in quocumque ... .

2.7 REX ET SACERDOS

Due sunt persone quibus sub Deo regitur mundus iste, rex et sacerdos ... .

2.8 DVO GLADII

Duo sunt gladii [Lc 22:38], materialis et spiritualis ... quia distincte et discrete sunt potestates, ecclesiastica scilicet et secularis ... .

2.9 DVE CLAVES

Due sunt claues. Vnde [Mt 16:19]: Tibi dabo claues regni celorum. "Tibi," Petro scilicet et coapostolis ... . Sunt autem claues scientia discernendi et potentia iudicandi. Set obicitur de sacerdote indiscreto.

Respondeo: Quantulacumque scientia in tali, clauis est. Vel clauis est debitum et obnoxietas applicandi se ad discretionem boni et mali, et applicare est usus eius; set secundum hoc symoniacus uel suspensus non habet hanc clauem. Vel clauis est officium discernendi.   Dicunt quidam quod due claues sunt potestas discrete ligandi et potestas discrete soluendi ... . Aliis autem uidetur quod cum dicitur "tibi dabo claues," plurale pro singulari ponitur ... . Est itaque potentia clauis cuius manubrium est scientia, due corrigie sunt ligatio et solutio ... .

2.10 Dve stole

Due sunt stole. Vnde in Apocalipsi [6:11] de sanctis dicitur: Date sunt illis singule stole albe, etc ... . Et est gemina stola, prima est sabbatismus anime, secunda sabbatismus corporis ... quia post mortis occasum gemina stola conferetur ... . Hinc itaque dicitur: O ter quaterque beati, id est in anima uis triplex, et in corpore constante ex quatuor elementis glorificati.

3.1 Tres persone in Trinitate

Tres sunt persone in Trinitate, Grece tria prosopa ... . Sunt etiam tres personales proprietates que scilicet faciunt dici personas uel esse. Nec notetur hic causa efficiens set causa sine qua non ... .

3.2 De tribvs svbstantiis in Christo

Christus trinus est in numero et unus est in numine. Sicut enim in Trinitate sunt tres persone et una substantia, ita in Christo sunt tres substantie, scilicet deitas, anima, caro, et una persona ... .

3.3 De fide, spe, et karitate

Tres sunt uirtutes principales: fides, spes, caritas ... . Hec autem simul infunduntur uel subtrahuntur ... . Contra: ... . Set hoc intellige de fide, spe, et caritate non ex qua, set qua, hoc est non de hiis qualitatibus sed de earum motibus ... .

Sunt autem uirtutes pares in habitu essentia et efficacia ... . Sunt tamen uirtutes impares auctoritate uel dignitate ut dictum est, et etiam in usu, et usus frequentia et euidentia ... .

240 WRITINGS

3.4 De contritione, confessione, et satisfactione

Peccatori tria necessaria sunt ad salutem: contritio, confessio, et satisfactio ... .

3.5 De sobrietate, ivstitia, et pietate

Sobrie et iuste et pie uiuamus in hoc seculo [Tit 2:12]. In hiis tribus aduerbiis comprehenditur summa christiane religionis, et Deus remunerator est aduerbiorum non nominum, uel potius aduerbiorum quam nominum. Sobrie uiuas, hoc ad teipsum, iuste ad proximum, pie ad Deum ... .

3.6 De tribvs mvneribvs Magorvm

Tria sunt munera magorum pretiosa [Mt 2:11] ... aurum etiam primum caritas est ... thus oratio est ... mirra penitentia est ... .

3.7 De tridvo dominice passionis

Est triduum dominice passionis. Vnde [Mt 12:40]: Sicut Ionas in uentre ceti tribus diebus et tribus noctibus, sic filius hominis in corde terre, id est in sepulcro, tribus diebus et tribus noctibus. Perifrasis est, id est tribus naturalibus diebus in quibus sunt tres dies usuales et tres noctes; et preterea hos tres dies naturales accipe sinodochice[1] ... .

3.8 De triplici statv christiane religionis

Est triduum de quo Dominus dicit Moysi [Ex 19:10-11]: Vade ad populum et sanctifica eos hodie et cras, et sint parati in tertium diem ... . Hoc triduum est triplex status christiane religionis: penitentie scilicet, iustitie, glorie. Hos tres status designant tres quinquagene Psalmorum quarum prima terminatur in penitentia ibi: Miserere mei Deus, qui est quinquagesimus et penitentialis ... .

3.9 De triplici sabbato

Triplex est sabbatum: temporis, pectoris, eternitatis ... .

---

1 sinodochice] *H*: sinodoche *L*

3.10 De tribvs necessariis ad salvtem

Adulto et discreto tria sunt necessaria ad salutem: Dei cognitio, et eius glorificatio, et de cognitione gratiarum actio ... .

Vnde svpra
Trinitatis et unitatis notitiam habemus ex creatura per similitudinem ... .

De eisdem
Apostolus de Deo loquens et philosophis ait [Rom 1:21]: Quia cum cognouissent non sicut Deum glorificauerunt uel honorauerunt ... tripliciter est glorificandus corde scilicet et ore, et opere ... .

De tribvs predictis bonis
De Deo scriptum est: Preueniamus[2] uultum eius in gratiarum actione ... . Debemus autem Deo gratias agere de beneficiis presentibus, preteritis et futuris, de generalibus et specialibus, de corporalibus et spiritualibus, de terrenis et celestibus ... .

3.11 De triplici errore

Super Psalmum xciii, scilicet "Deus ultionum," a doctoribus commemoratur circa Deum triplex error blasphemorum. Primus est quo putant Deum hec inferiora et hec mala non uidere; secundus etsi uidet non curare; tertius etsi curet[3] non uindicare ... .

3.12 De tribvs Deo gratis

Tria sunt grata Deo plurimum et accepta. Primum et precipuum est dilectio sincera medullaris et integra: hoc ad Deum. Secundum est circa conuersionem animarum diligens et operosa sollicitudo; hoc ad proximum. Tertium est in bene gestis cordis uel mentis humiliatio ... .

3.13 De tribvs Deo odiosis

Tria sunt que Deus plurimum detestat et odit, et ideo magis cauenda. Hec autem tria sunt desperatio, et in peccatis gloriatio, et apostasia ... . Hiis igitur opponantur remedia: uerba sanctorum et exempla ... .

---

2 Preueniamus] *H*: Preuiamus *L*
3 etsi curet] *H*: *om. L*

Vnde svpra

Dum stulti uitant uitia in contraria concurrunt, et in uitium ducit culpe si caret arte. Diximus Deo plurimum displicere desperationem; huius itaque Caribdim id est uoraginem quidam deuitantes, Scillam id est scopulos presumptionis incurrunt ... . Sunt autem tria que pestem presumptionis procreant et fouent ... .

Secvndvm

Secundum trium preenumeratorum est gloriatio in peccatis sumopere cauenda ... . Fugienda autem hec gloriatio propter tria, scilicet propter diabolice malignitatis in hoc imitationem, propter offense diuine gratuitatem, et propter pene exaggerationem ... .

Tertivm

Tertium preenumeratorum est apostasia, id est auersio uel reuersio uel recidiuatio ... .

3.14 De tribvs famosis persecvtionibvs

Tres sunt famose persecutiones ecclesie quasi tria impedimenta in uia. Primum est aperta rabies et persecutio tirannorum; secundum, fraudulenta seductio pullulantium hereticorum; tertium est corruptio falsorum fratrum ... .

3.15 De tribvs hostibvs anime

Tres sunt principales hostes anime: Mundus, caro, diabolus ... .

Qve remedia contra predicta

Ad trium hostium predictorum infestationem elidendam tria necessaria sunt: Crebra scilicet mortis meditatio, corporalis exercitatio, et uerborum utilium prolatio ... .

3.16 De tribvs infestantibvs hominem
qve svnt ignis, serpens, et mvs

Tria sunt: Ignis in sinu, serpens in gremio, mus in pera. Hec tria suos male remunerant hospites ... .

Vnde vt svpra

Ignis triplex iam pretaxatus, scilicet ire, libidinis, et concupiscientie, male suos remunerat hospites. Nam ira corpus exsiccat, febres generat, rationem turbat ... . Libido uero fedat ... . Porro cupiditas iniuriam infert ... .

Qvod remedivm contra ignem

Ad pretaxatum triplicem ignem extinguendum necessaria est aqua, gratia scilicet, et doctrine uerbum, et uite exemplum ... .

Qvod remedivm contra ignem ire

Igne triplici iam pretaxato quidam comburuntur, alii eo non leduntur, alii ab eo eripiuntur ... . Sane ad cauendum ignem ire necessaria sunt tria: sustinentia, silentium[4] locutionis, et ultionis dilatio ... . Similiter ad ignem libidinis deuitandum cautela est adhibenda ... .

Qve cavtela contra ignem cvpiditatis

Sane ad uitandum exustionem siue lesionem ex cupiditatis igne prouenientem cautela adhibenda est in hunc modum: Circa diuitiarum opulentiam diligenter attendenda sunt onus, obligatio et periculum ... .

Vnde svpra

Sciendum etiam est quod opulentia procreatrix est elationis, et nutrix est uoluptatis et sollicitudinis suffocantis ... .

De eodem

Amplius ad rescindendum cupiditatis uelamen, dicimus quod opum copia uitam non prolongat, nec meritum augmentat, nec certitudinem beat. ...

De serpente

De igne in sinu iam diximus, restat dicere de serpente in gremio. Serpens diabolus est ... .

Qvod remedivm contra virvs serpentis

Serpens iam dictus aditum querens suggerit uel immediate, hoc est per se inuisibiliter, scilicet miro et subtili modo, uel mediate, ut in corpore assumpto ... .

Ad predicta remedivm in doctrina et cavtela

Suggerit et serpens ut dictum est in organis suis, et sic doctrina apponitur ... et etiam cautela ... .

Diabolus serpens est ... . Antiquus enim hostis uel in exordio intentionis ferit et polluit, uel in itinere actionis interficit, uel si nec intentionem uitiat nec in itinere subplantat, in fine actionis durius illaqueat ... .

---

4 silentium] et *add.* L

REMEDIVM CONTRA SERPENTES

Diximus de serpentis antiqui malitia, restat dicere que contra sint remedia, que doctrina opponenda, que cautela adhibenda, ad dolosi fallaciam refellendam et ad malitiosam eius suggestionem elidendam ... .

ITEM DE SERPENTE

Serpens diabolus est. Vnde [Eccli 12:13]: Quis medebitur incantatori a serpente percusso? Incantator est hereticus siue quicumque doctor errans a diabolo deceptus ... . Serpentes etiam dicuntur membra diaboli ... homines dolosi ... homines maledici et iracundi ... homines detractores ... homines parentibus carnalibus uel spiritualibus noxii ... homines astuti, linguosi et seductores ... homines seductores ut heretici et pseudo predicatores et falsi fratres ... homines maligni ... .

VNDE SVPRA

Predictis adicimus quia serpentes sunt parricide et libidinosi ... .

ITEM VT SVPRA DE SERPENTE

Igitur clauus clauum retundat, et serpens Aaron serpentem magicum deuoret [Ex 7:12], hoc est sapientia uincat malitiam, et prudentia superet astutiam ... .

ITEM DE SERPENTE

Vt supra ex parte innotuit, demones serpentes dicuntur ... . Dicuntur et homines serpentes ... . Serpentes etiam uitia dicuntur et peccata ... . Et itaque superbia serpens quia serpit in altum ... . Porro scorpio siue scorpius ... luxuria est ... . Libido chimera est ... . Dipsas genus aspidis est qui Latine dicitur situla ... hec est auaritia ... .

VNDE SVPRA

Sunt plerique serpentes quibus assimilantur demones simul et homines, uitia et peccata, ut Coluber ... . Draco magnus ... . Ydra, draco multorum capitum ... . Basiliscus ... . Iaculus serpens uolans ... . Prester ... . Ipnalis genus aspidis ... .

DE MVRE

Diximus quod ignis in sinu, serpens in gremio, mus in pera, male suos remunerant hospites. De duobus diffusius egimus, de tertio nos breuiter expediamus. Igitur mus Grece sorex Latine dicitur, eo quod rodit et in modum serre precidit. Mures itaque egressi de cauernis suis sunt curiosi scrutatores et detractores ... . Possunt etiam dici mures ipsa uitia seu peccata ut curiositas, detractio, castrimargia, desidia. Hiis itaque perimendis paretur utilis muscipula ... .

3.17 HOSTES HOMINIS QVI SVNT MVNDVS, CORPVS, DIABOLVS

Mundus, corpus, diabolus tres hostes sunt. Mundus hominem peruertit, corpus animam subuertit, diabolus et corpus et animam a creatore auertit ... .

3.18 MOLESTANT IN DOMO FVMVS, STILLICIDIVM, ET MALA VXOR

Tria sunt que molestant hominem in domo, et foras pellunt ut in nugis extra quiescat. Paterfamilias spiritus est, cor domus eius est quia sedes anime est in corde. Tria molestia sunt fumus, stillicidium, et mala uxor. Ex igne uero cupiditatis erumpit fumus arefaciens et lacrimas eliciens. Hec est rapina substantiam pauperum attenuans ... . Ex igne libidinis prorumpit fornicatio ... . Ex igne iracundie prouenit fumus obscurans, turbatio mentis ... .

Porro stillicidium aeris cadens in tectum est suggestio demonis in superiorem uim anime ... . Item stillicidium a tecto cadens in pauimentum est exemplum a prelato in subditos diffusum ... . Est autem uxor mala, sapientia carnis inimica Deo, sicut econtra prudentia dicitur sapientis amica uel sapientia sponsa ... . Item mala coniunx est carnis illecebra ... . Item uxor litigiosa est conscientia cauteriata, remordens, et pungitiua, rationem repugnans et domum cordis conturbans ... .

QVOD SIT REMEDIVM CONTRA PRIMVM MOLESTVM
Ad fumum triplicem iam pretaxatum euitandum remedium est ignis amotio ... .

QVOD CONTRA SECVNDVM
Sane contra stillicidium suggestionis diabolice, firmiter resartiatur quasi duplex tectum, ratio scientie et ratio sapientie, sicut solet in domibus diuitum gemitum supponi tectum, inferius ligneum, superius plumbeum, et ita non timetur stillicidium.

Ad stillicidium autem exempli perniciosi consulatur sapiens architectus qui tectum reparet et reficiat, uel prorsus submoueat et nouum doma culminis superponat. Sapiens architectus ipse Christus est ... .

Porro ad stillicidium uerbi praui fidem et bonos mores corrumpentis, hoc unicum adhibeatur remedium [Mt 5:13; 1 Mach 4:44-45]: Sal infatuatum foras mittatur, et altare profanatum destruatur ... . Hoc est, sacerdos illiteratus[5] uel pseudo uel hereticus amoueatur et officium predicationis ei interdicatur ... .

QVOD CONTRA TERTIVM

Prudentia uero carnis est cum quis intentus et curiosus est in carnalibus, et cum studiosius implet que carnis sunt. Hec uxor ut consanguinea dimittatur et legittima ducatur ... .

Carnis etiam illecebra que et uocatum excludit a cena dominica abiciatur tamquam adultera ... .

Conscientia uero mala corrigenda est ut mulier litigiosa castiganda ... .

3.19 DE TRIBVS GRADIBVS

Tres sunt gradus fidelium in ecclesia, coniugatorum scilicet, continentium, et rectorum ... . In Noe quidem qui archam rexit in undis, prepositos ecclesie; in Daniele qui continenter uixit, continentes uel uirgines; In Iob uero qui in coniugali uita exemplar patientie tribuit, bonorum coniugatorum uitam ostendit ... .

Potest et ita dici primus et inferior gradus, uel ordo, uel status est coniugum, secundus et medius est continentium post lapsum carnis, tertius et superlatiuus est uirginum ... .

Potest et ita distingui: Sunt tres ordines uel gradus in ecclesia Dei, actiui, contemplatiui, et utrorumque prelati.

3.20 DE TRIBVS TEMPORIBVS

Tria sunt tempora, tempus ante legem, scriptam scilicet, et tempus sub lege, et tempus gratie ... .

Ad tria tempora iam pretaxata spectant tres misse in die natalis Domini celebrate. Prima de profunda nocte ... . Secunda in diluculo ... . Tertia in meridie ... .

4.1 DE QVATVOR VIRTVTIBVS CARDINALIBVS

Quatuor sunt uirtutes principales id est ad summum principem ducentes,[6] seu cardinales hoc est ad summum pontificem nos introducentes. Hee uero sunt iustitia, fortitudo, prudentia, temperantia ... .

---

5 illiteratus *om.* L
6 ducentes *om.* L

4.2 De crvce

Crux Christi quatuor habet extremitates quarum dextera significatur obedientia ... . Sinistra designatur paupertas ... . Per partem inferiorem humilitas intelligitur ... . Per partem uero superiorem patientia insinuatur ... .

Crux a cruciatu dicitur. Est autem specialis crux penitentis id est cruciatus penitentialis. Huius crucis profundum est timor cautele ... altitudo est spes uenie ... . Latitudo uero crucis penitentialis caritas est ... longitudo perseuerantia est ... .

4.3 De altari avreo

Quatuor sunt cornua altaris in Apocalipsi [9:13]. Hii sunt predicatores Christi ipsum subleuantes et pro eo mori parati ... . Quatuor autem dicuntur propter quatuor que presertim de Christo predicantur, que sunt natiuitas, passio, resurrectio, et ascensio. Hii sunt potissimi articuli in fide incarnationis Christi, et typum gerunt quatuor rerum que nobis necessarie sunt ad salutem. Prima igitur est natiuitas ad uitam scilicet gratie ... . Secunda est passio ... in corpore scilicet a mundo, carne, diabolo, uel in corde pro proximi scandalo ... . Tertia est lapsorum resurrectio ... . Quarta est ascensio id est profectus in merito ... .

4.4 De confectione vngventi sancti

De quatuor aromatibus, id est aromaticis speciebus ... oleo confectis [Ex 30:22-24] ... . Mirra prima est approbata carnis mortificatio ... . Cinnamomum quod est cinerei coloris est assidua mortis meditatio ... . Porro calamus suaue redolens ... est congrua morum moderatio ... . Cassia quidem odorifera in aquosis nascitur, et crescit in immensum. Hec est deuota cordis compunctio ... . Oleum uero confectionis id est affectum pietatis et ostensionem miserationis ... .

Item de eodem

Possumus etiam predicta quatuor sic intelligere: Mirra precipua est penitentia uera, caritate informata ... . Cinnamomum est humilitas qua homo se cinerem agnoscens sibi uilescit ... . Calamus species odorifera odor est bone opinionis id est fame ... . Cassia aquosa misericordia est reddens cor aquosum per compassionem et oculos aquosos per lacrimationem. Oleum autem nitidum et leue suauitas est conscientie serene ... .

4.5 De compositione thimiamatis

Quatuor species sunt ex quibus componitur thimiama scilicet stacte, onica, galbanum odoriferum, et thus lucidissimum. Thimiama id est incensum ... est oratio ... et quatuor sunt quibus conditur oratio, animi scilicet amaritudo, et cordis humilitas, deuotio mentis, et puritas intentionis ... .

4.6 De qvatvor operimentis tabernacvli, et primo de cortinis

Quatuor erant operimenta tabernaculi [Ex 26], decem scilicet cortine, saga cilicina undecim, pelles arietum rubricate, et pelles iacinctine. Hec sunt quatuor genera fidelium in ecclesia, scilicet confessores, penitentes, martires, uirgines ... . Cortine decem confessores sunt, decalogum id est moralia diuine legis inseruantes et aliis predicantes ... .

De eodem
Saga undecim sunt penitentes; undenarius enim numerus transgressionis qui primus excedit denarium qui numerus perfectus est, et primus limes numerorum ... .

Item de eodem
Sane pelles arietum rubricate martires sunt, pellem pro pelle dantes, pellem scilicet mortalem pro eadem recipienda immortali in resurrectione generali ... .

De qvarto operimento
Quartum operimentum sunt pelles iacinctine colore celum imitantes. Hiis comparantur uirgines propter gradus sublimitatem et celestis conuersationis ... .

4.7 De qvatvor spernendis

Spernere mundum, spernere sese, spernere nullum, spernere se sperni, quatuor optima sunt ... .
Nobis spernenda noscantur quatuor ista: uanitas mundialis, uoluptas carnalis, aduersitas huius seculi, et iugum id est dira et dura dominatio diaboli ... .
Vanitas autem mundi fallax est et pernitiosa ... .

5.1 De quinqve vectibvs

Quinque uectes sunt, id est ordines uectium qui continent tabernaculum [Ex 30:26-27], et quinque sunt que statum ecclesie conseruant. Hec autem quinque sunt doctrina prelatorum, meritum sanctorum, operatio miraculorum, honestas obsequii, et gratia Dei ... .

5.2 De pentapoli

Pentapolim pro flagitio subuertit Dominus [cf. Sap 10:6]. Hoc est regionem quinque ciuitatum, Sodome scilicet et Gomorre, Ademe, Seboim, et Bale siue Segor ... .

Vnde svpra
Quinque etiam in ultionem peccati supradicti reperimus. Hec autem quinque sunt: cecitas, sulfur et ignis, aqua et terre sterilitas ... .
Et nota quod ad exagerationem tum culpe tum pene, faciunt hic ampliatio, grauitas, uniuersalitas, anticipatio, et adiuncta paruulorum perditio ... .

5.3 De fvnda David et qvinqve lapidibvs

Dauid de torrente quinque lapides limpidissimos [1 Sam 17:40-51], id est planos et uolubiles elegit, in pera reposuit ... . Sunt autem lapides uerbum uoti baptismalis ... et uerbum confessionis penitentialis ... et uerbum sancte orationis ... et uerbum predicationis ... et uerbum benedictionis ... . Hii uero lapides electi sunt si sint hec uerba a Deo approbata, caritate informata, et sic uite eterne meritoria. Limpiditas lapidum, uerborum predictorum innuit explanationem et facilitatem absque omni scilicet obscuritate et difficultate ... . Hos igitur lapides assume in pera memorie reconde ... . Porro lapidum in funda rotatio est bonorum predictorum exercitatio ... .

5.4 De qvinqve colvmpnis Tabernacvli

Quinque erant columpne in ingressu tabernaculi [Ex 26:37]. Columpne prelati sunt ... . Et in porticum templi statuuntur due columpne, una uocata iachim, id est firmitas, altera booth, id est in robore. Hii sunt doctores ecclesie per quos alii ingressum habent in domum Dei ... et prelatis quinque necessaria sunt scilicet uita, scientia, facundia, fortitudo, et pastoralis officii sollicitudo ... .

ITEM DE COLVMPNIS

Erant autem quinque columpne pretaxate de lignis sethim deaurate, capita aurea et bases eneas habentes, tentorium id est uelum quoddam a terra in altum suspendentes. Sethim arbor est albe spine similis et est leuissimum lignum et imputribile et incremabile; et prelatus non sit spinosus ex liuore uindicte peccatum puniendo tamquam acute pungendo, nec seuere per excessum rigoris proximum exasperando uel prepropere sententiando ... .

5.5 De qvinqve talentis

Vni seruorum dedit dominus quinque talenta, alii duo, alii unum [Mt 25:15]. Vnde uidendum quid dicatur hic talentum, et quale sit lucrum, et quantum sit meritum, et qualiter intelligendum quod dicitur: Vnicuique secundum propriam uirtutem ... .

DE EISDEM

Quod autem dicitur: Vnicuique secundum propriam uirtutem, intellige secundum propriam dantis, id est secundum benignitatem et misericordiam Domini cui proprium est misereri, uel cuique tradit talentum multiplicandum meritorie scilicet secundum fidem que propria est fidelium ... .

6.1 De senario, primo de operibvs sex diervm

Sex dies sunt in quibus oportet operari [Ex 20:9; Gen 1] ... quia sex etates sunt in quibus oporteat nos a culpa curari et bona operari ut in septima requiescamus a laboribus nostris ... .

DE OPERE PRIME DIEI

Prima quidem die facta est lux. Hec est gratia tenebras, id est uitia, fugans ... .

DE OPERE SECVNDE DIEI

Secunda uero die fecit Deus firmamentum in medio aquarum, quia post illuminationem cordis contriti, necessarium est firmum propositum in bono perseuerandi ... .

DE TERTIA DIE

Tertia die fecit Dominus terram herbas uirentes et arbores fructiferas germinando proferre. Hec autem sunt opera actiue et contemplatiue ... .

DE QVARTA DIE

Quarto die fecit Deus luminaria — solem, lunam, et stellas ... . Sol ... est perfectio caritatis, et perfecta cognitio ueritatis, et in utraque permanentia ... . Facit Deus in microcosmo, id est in minore mundo scilicet homine, lunam, id est mutabilitatem et defectum, maculam sustinens et errorem ... . Facit etiam Deus in microcosmo stellas cum homini confert obedientiam regularem ... .

DE OPERE QVINTE DIEI

Quinto die fecit Deus uolatilia et natatilia ... . Hec aues sunt igitur in homine desideria celestium que per spem eriguntur in altum. Pisces uero qui perambulant semitas maris sunt sollicite cogitationes in profundo cordis ... .

DE OPERE SEXTE DIEI

Sexto die fecit Deus bestias et iumenta et reptilia, tandem creauit hominem horum omnium dominatorem ... . Deus igitur bestias in microcosmo creat cum homini mundi contemptum inspirat; adiungit et iumentum, animal domesticum et mansuetum, cum perfectam confert animi mansuetudinem et fraternam in religione socialitatem ... . Facit et reptile quod totum repit in terra cum summam procreat humilitatem ... .

VNDE SVPRA

Diximus quia Deum in operibus preenumeratis imitari debemus, set qualiter lucem et firmamentum et cetera predicta facere poterimus? Possumus quidem per cooperationem; Deus enim auctor est, homo minister, et liberum arbitrium instrumentum est ... .

6.2 DE SEX YDRIIS

Sex sunt ydrie purificationis Iudeorum [Io 2:6], id est uasa aquatica ad ablutionem Iudeorum exposita. Tropologice uero sex sunt ydrie purificationis Iudeorum, id est confitentium. Hec autem sex sunt: baptismus et penitentia, martirium et misericordia, caritas et sancta eucaristia ... .

ITEM DE YDRIIS

Est etiam baptismus mare eneum fusile et rotundum [3 Reg 7:23] ... . Hoc autem mare eneum est propter sonum professionis in baptismo, ut "Credis in Deum?" "Credo," "Vis baptizari?" "Volo"; et quia uotum baptismale debet esse durabile et nulla uiolari rubigine

culpe. Est et fusile propter gratie infusionem, et rotundum propter orbis
uniuersi purificationem ... .

6.3 DE SEX ALIS

Vidit Iohannes in Apocalipsi [4:6; cf. Is 6:2] quatuor animalia ... et
sunt ale sex ut primum intendat et optet homo placere Deo, secundo
prodesse proximo, tertio proficere in merito, quarto perseuerare in
bono, quinto delectari in Domino, sexto et ultimo frui[7] Deo.

ITEM DE ALIS
De primo dicit Apostolus: Probantes quid sit beneplacitum Deo ... .

6.4 DE SEX ATTENDENDIS

Sex nobis ad cautelam diligenter attendenda sunt, scilicet mundi
uanitas, et corporis iam mortui uilitas, et hostis antiqui astuta
malignitas, uite presentis modicitas, horror mortis, et extremi iudicii
seueritas ... .

6.5 DE SEX INITIALIBVS CHRISTIANE RELIGIONIS

Apostolus ait [Hebr 6:1-3]: Iacientes fundamentum penitentie ab
operibus mortuis, et fidei ad Deum, baptismatum doctrine, impositionis
quoque manuum, ac resurrectionis mortuorum, et iudicii eterni. Hinc
ergo dicimus quia sex sunt initialia et christiane religionis fundamentum
adultis, rudibus, et neophitis in sermone sepius proponenda. Hec itaque
sunt penitentia, et fides, id est simbolum fidei, doctrina baptismatum ... .
Quartum est impositio manuum in baptismo scilicet ad remissionem,
in confirmatione ad roborationem. Quintum est resurrectio mortuorum
ut preterita, capitis, id est Christi, et futura, corporis, id est ecclesie.
Sextum est iudicium futurum quod dicitur eternum ... .

6.6 DE SEX ATTENDENDIS IN OBITV

Sex sunt finalia, id est in fine uite, diligenter obseruanda. Hec uero
sex sunt solutio debiti, sub quo etiam intelligatur restitutio alieni,
compositio testamenti, et confessio peccati, extrema unctio, uiatici
susceptio, et intenta supplicatio ... .

---

7 frui *om. L*

Ad primum uero preenumeratorum spectat quod dicitur: Iustitia unicuique suum tribuit ... .

6.7 DE SEX CONFORTATIVIS

Sex sunt que agentem in extremis confortare possunt. Primum est preparatio per sex, duobus capitulis proximo prepositis declarata [see above, 6.5]. Secundum est fides catholica ... . Tertium est tot suffragiorum, tum ecclesie militantis, tum ecclesie triumphantis, ubertas et habundantia. Quartum est operum bonorum preteritorum recordatio ... . Quintum est iussio diuina, cui prompte parendum est ... . Sextum uero confortatorium est immensa Dei misericordia que uere penitenti statim remittit ... .

6.8 DE SEX ACCELERANDIS

Sex sunt ad que festinandum est, baptismi susceptio, peccati confessio, uerbi diuini predicatio, penitentie iniuncte consummatio, meritorum cumulatio, et status perfectio ... .

AVCTORITATES DE SVPRADICTIS
Porro de festinatione ad baptismum dicitur [Is 55:1]: Omnes sitientes uenite ad aquas ... .

6.9 DE CANTV

Cantus ecclesie per sex sillabas istas disponitur et discurrit: Vt, Re, Mi, Fa, Sol, La; ita et cantus anime id est dilectio eius secundum ista sex discurrat ... . *Vt* abstineatis uos a fornicatione [1 Thess 4:3], quacumque scilicet tum carnali, tum spirituali ... . *Re*sistite diabolo et fugiet a uobis [Jac 4:7] ... . *Mi*serere anime tue placens Deo [Eccli 30:24] ... . *Fa*cite uobis amicos de mammona iniquitatis [Lc 16:9], id est de diuitiis minus licite adquisitis uel retentis, ut cum ueniali peccato ... . *Sol*licitus ambula cum Deo [Mich 6:8] ... . *La*uamini, mundi estote [Is 1:16] ... .

6.10 DE SCACCARIO

Mundum istum quadrifidum scaccario quadrato comparamus, et mundi dilectores ludentibus in scaccis assimulamus. Sicut enim in ludo scaccarii ita et in negotio mundi siue conuersatione mundiali sunt ista

sex: curiositas, cupiditas, et garrulitas, dampnum absque aporiatione,
lucrum sine ditatione, et quedam inanitas delectationis et glorie ... .

6.11 DE STATVA

Legimus in Daniele [2:31-35] de quadam statua ymaginaria quam uidit
Nabugodonosor in sompnis ... . Hanc itaque destruit lapis, id est
Christus, lapis quem reprobauerunt edificantes [Mt 21:42], abscisus de
monte, id est de superba gente Iudeorum, uel de carne uirginis que
mons est ... .

Possunt etiam in statua pretaxata designari sex ista: opulentia
carnalis, excellentia temporalis, potentia secularis, gloria mundi, superbia
elati, et simulatio ficti id est ypocrisis ... .

6.12 DE EVITATIONE PECCATI

Peccatum uitandum est tamquam rete retinens et inuoluens, sicut ignis
ardens et comburens, sicut serpens mordens et ueneno inficiens.
Cauendum est etiam peccatum ut pestis ... ut uulnus siue uulneris
instrumentum debilitans, et ut ipsa mors interimens ... .

Diximus quia peccatum uitandum est sicut ipsa mors; peccatum
quippe mortale morti comparatur et mors appellatur propter sex
causas: Propter uite amissionem ... . Et propter meritorum tamquam
membrorum mortificationem ... . Et propter resurgendi difficultatem ... . Assimilatur etiam morti peccatum propter fetorem, uermescen-
tiam, et incinerationem ... .

6.13 QVOD LVGENDVM EST PECCATVM

Augustinus ait [cf. *Enarr. in Ps.* 29.2.19]: Est confessio peccatorum
et est confessio laudis. Illa luget, hec gaudet; illa medico uulnus ostendit,
hec de sanitate gratias agit. Debemus itaque peccata lugere penitendo-
do ... . Lugendum quidem est propter sex causas, scilicet propter
presentiam peccati et pro absentia sponsi, propter status diminutionem
et temporis amissionem, propter detestandam seruitutis diabolice
uilitatem et doloris penitentialis diuturnitatem ... .

6.14 DE NEGLIGENTIA PRELATORVM

Maledictus qui facit opus Dei fraudulenter [Ier 48:10] siue negligenter.
Negligentia cunctis est uitanda, presertim in prelatis ecclesiasticis

quorum negligentia multiplex est. Maxime tamen in istis sex attenditur, scilicet in loco, libro, altari, sacramento, doctrina, cura ... .

DE CAVTELA NEGLIGENTIE

In suggillationem uero negligentie nostre que ab aliis accepimus ad cautelam in medium ita proferimus. Exemplum: Cum quidam clericus mane ad ecclesiam festinaret ... . Aliud exemplum: Item cum due presbiteri fidei sacramento inter se constringerentur ... .

6.15 DE VITATIONE PECCATI, VEL PENITENTIA

Sex cause sunt precipue cur peccatum cauendum est uel saltem ad emendationem accelerandam. Prima causa est propter uite huius incertitudinem ... . Secunda causa est propter reatus accumulationem ... . Tertia causa est propter mentis obstinationem ... . Quarta causa est propter euitationem grauioris pene presentis siue penitentialis, siue cuiuscumque casualis ... . Quinta causa est ad effugiendam diuturnitatem grauis illius pene purgatorie ... . Sexta causa est euitatio gehenne uel augmenti pene in gehenna ... .

6.16 DE LETITIA

Sex sunt que mentem fidelis spirituali letitia reficiunt. Hec autem sunt innocentia, penitentia, profectus, redemptio generis humani, uisitatio Dei, et promissio Christi ... .

7.1 DE SEPTEM HORIS DIEI

Septies in die laudem dixi tibi Domine [Ps 118:164]. Septem sunt hore uocales quas tamquam pensum cotidianum Deo soluimus ... . Ita sunt et septem hore reales, et illas oportet obseruare ex institutione scilicet ecclesie, et non omittere, que forsan precellunt. Sunt itaque septem hore reales [cf. Mt 25:35-36; Tob 2:7-9]: Esurientem cibare, sitientem potare, hospitem colligere, nudum cooperire, infirmum uisitare similiter et incarceratum. Septimum est mortuum sepelire ... .

7.2 DE SEPTEM BRACHIIS CANDELABRE

Legitur in Exodo [25:31-32] quod septem erant brachia in candelabro. Candelabrum iustus est ... . Ex hastili candelabri procedebant tria brachia ex lateribus hinc et tria inde. Dextera uero significat eternam beatitudinem, sinistra uitam presentem ... . Tria ergo brachia ad dexteram sunt celestium, ut Dei et angelorum et sanctorum ueneratio, deprecatio, et imitatio ... . Sane tria brachia ad sinistram sunt sanctorum sacramentorum ecclesiasticorum susceptio, scientie communicatio, et operum misericordie exhibitio ... . Medium uero brachium id est summa pars stili siue stipitis ipsius candelabri est aurea mediocritas, discretione scilicet moderatione condita ... et uirtus est medium uitiorum utrimque redactum, scilicet inter superhabundantiam et diminutionem, inter nimietatem et remissionem ... .

7.3 De septem donis Spiritvs sancti

Super septem capita brachiorum candelabri equalia ponebantur septem lucerne auree, quasi lampades scilicet ubi oleum accendebatur. Hec autem septem sunt dona Spiritus sancti scilicet timor et pietas, scientia et fortitudo, consilium et intellectus, et tandem sapientia que supremum est in cathalogo [Is 11:2-3] septem donorum ... .

7.4 De septem vitiis capitalibvs

Septem sunt uitia capitalia uel principalia, non dico criminalia seu mortalia set capitalia, quia peccatorum sunt scaturigines et principia. Hec autem septem sunt: inanis gloria, ira, inuidia, accidia, auaritia, castrimargia, luxuria ... .

7.5 De septem qve odit Dominvs

Salomon ait [Prov 6:16]: Sex sunt que odit Dominus et septimum detestatur anima eius ... . Hec itaque septem sunt superbia, mendacium, homicidium, machinatio mali in proximum, festinatio preceps ad quodcumque scelus, falsum testimonium, et discordia siue scisma ... .

8.1 De octo etatibvs

Octo sunt etates, prima ab Adam usque ad Noe, secunda usque ad Habraham uel Moysen, tertia usque ad Dauid, quarta usque ad transmigrationem Babilonis, quinta usque ad Iohannem baptistam uel Christum, sexta usque ad finem mundi ... . Septima etas est dormientium et quiescentium, inchoata secundum quosdam a Christi passione uel resurectione ... . Octaua erit etas resurgentium ... .

8.2 De octo hostibvs anime

Octo sunt hostes anime cuiusque cum satis esset unus. Hii octo sunt
mundus, corpus, diabolus, peccatum, homo ipse, et conscientia remordens, Deus, et sermo Dei ... .

De expvgnatione predictorvm hostivm

Pretaxatos hostes debellare, uel hostilitatem ad pacem conuertere
possumus in hunc modum: Contra mundi odium dilectionem repen-
damus et beneficium ... .

8.3 De octo speciebvs ydropisis spiritvalis

Dominus in Euangelio sanat ydropicum [Luc 14:2-4]. Sunt autem octo
species ydropisis spiritualis. Est enim ydropicus auarus semper egens ...
ambitiosus id est cupidus honoris ... malitiosus ... curiosus ... potator
auidus ... libidinosus ... inflatus id est superbus ... . Est et ydropicus
anelitu fetido maledicus ... . Horum igitur omnium curatio est, simul
cum inductis auctoribus, diuina operatio quasi manus dominice apprehensio. Legitur enim in Euangelio [Lc 14:4] de ydropico quia
Dominus apprehensum sanauit eum ac dimisit.

9.1 De novem vitiis svbtilibvs

Preter subtiles laqueos symonie et usure, sunt quedam in homine uitia
seu peccata adeo subtilia ut ab ipso uel alio uix deprehendi queant.
Huiusmodi sunt ista nouem: rigor, remissio, tenacitas, et prodigalitas,
captatio humani fauoris siue appetitus laudis, ambitio, incauta humilitas,
consensus rationis citra actum exteriorem, et negligentia ... .

10.1 De Decalogo[8]

Psalterium decacordum est decalogus, id est[9] continentia decem mandatorum legis [Ex 20:1-7]. Horum primum est de uno Deo colendo.
Sunt enim tres ypostases, una usia, id est tres persone, una essentia ... .

---

8 De decalogo] Decalogo L
9 decalogus, id est] decalogi L

10.2 De beneficiis Dei

Ne uideamur ingrati et immemores accepti beneficii recolamus etiam in nobis Dei beneficia sepius ea reuoluentes et gratias agentes. Igitur beneficia diuina quasi in quemdam fasciculum colligamus in hunc modum: Occurrunt autem quinque beneficia generalia et communia predestinatis. Hec autem sunt beneficia creationis, sustentationis, redemptionis, signationis, et future glorificationis ... . Occurrunt et quinque beneficia specialia. Hec autem sunt a malis sepe facta liberatio, diuina ad conuersionem expectatio, ab errore reductio, in profectu productio, et talenti commissio ... .

10.3 De debitis Deo reddendis

Reddite que sunt Cesaris Cesari et que sunt Dei Deo [Mt 22:21] ... . Sunt autem decem que Deo reddere debemus. Hec autem decem sunt fides et timor, amor et honor et obsequium, laus, oblatio, uotum, corpus et anima ... .

10.4 De commvtationibvs vel redemptionibvs

Occurrunt ad presens decem commutationes seu redemptiones seu recompensationes licite et utiles. Prima est persone, secunda rei, tertia temporis, quarta loci, quinta cause, sexta forme, septima pene, octaua ritus, nona status, decima uoti ... .

10.5 De remissionibvs peccatorvm

Confide fili, remittuntur tibi peccata tua [Mt 9:2]. Sunt autem decem quibus peccata remittuntur. Hec decem sunt fides, penitentia, baptismus, caritas, misericordia, martirium, tribulatio, oratio, unctio extrema, et sancta eucaristia ... .

11.1 De elemosinis

Date elemosinam et ecce omnia munda sunt uobis [Lc 11:41]. Occurrunt hic undecim genera elemosinarum. Primum est efficaciter penitere ... . Secundum est dare beneficium corporale ... uel spirituale ... . Tertium est debita uel iniurias dimittere ... . Quartum est compati subueniendo siue compatiendo subuenire. Quintum est commodare ... . Sextum est indutias dare ... . Septimum est animas ad Deum conuer-

tere ... . Octauum est ecclesias et domos hospitales edificare ... . Nonum
est loca cenosa siue aquis periculosa pontibus seu ceteris modis peruia
et meabilia facere ... . Decimum est malum impedire ... . Vndecimum
est bonum expedire et promouere ... .

12.1 DE ARTICVLIS FIDEI

Duodecim sunt articuli fidei. Est enim fides sancte Trinitatis qua
creditur Deus esse trinus et unus. Est fides dominice incarnationis qua
creditur Christus de Spiritu sancto conceptus in uirgine ... . Est et fides
natiuitatis qua creditur Christus natus ex Maria uirgine salua matris
integritate et ante partum et in partu et post partum. Est fides passionis
seu mortis dominice qua creditur Christus expirasse in cruce soluta
anima a carne, deitate a neutro. Est fides sepulture dominice qua
creditur corpus Christi unitum deitati iacuisse in sepulcro exanime. Est
et fides descensus Christi ad inferos qua creditur anima Christi armata
deitate inferos debellasse et infernum morsisse. Est fides resurrectionis
qua creditur Christus in corpore et anima reconiunctis rediuiuus a morte
surrexisse. Est fides ascensionis qua creditur Christus in carne et anima
ultra omnem angelicam naturam ascendisse et in dextris siue ad
dexteram Dei Patris sedere; hoc est secundum humanitatem in
potioribus bonis Patris quiescere et secundum diuinitatem equalis Patri
conregnare. Est fides secundi aduentus qua creditur Christus in fine
seculi de celo empireo uenturus in celum aereum et in nubibus, id
est in loco nubium iudicaturus. Est fides generalis resurrectionis qua
credimus corpora nostra a morte resurrectura et perpetua futura. Est
fides finalis retributionis qua credimus premia perpetua danda iustis
et supplicia reprobis. Est fides sacramentalis qua credimus ecclesie
catholice sacramenta ad id quod instituta sunt efficacia, ut baptismum,
penitentiam, sanctam eucaristiam, et unctionem extremam in remissionem peccatorum, confirmationem ad robur, ordinem ad ministerii
dignitatem.

AVCTORITATES
Sane de primo articulo dicitur [1 Io 5:7]: Tres sunt qui testimonium
dant in celo ... .

DE SIMILITVDINIBVS SVPRADICTORVM
Ad predicta similitudines inducimus. Similitudinem Trinitatis prefe-
runt ignis, splendor, calor; fons, riuus, lacus; memoria, intelligentia,
uoluntas, siue mens, notitia et amor ... .

12.2 De dvodecim horis diei

Ait beatus Gregorius [*Hom. in Evang.* 2.21.3]: Dies est uita iusti, nox est uita peccatoris ... . Duodecim sunt hore diei, et duodecim sunt necessaria in uita iusti. Hec autem duodecim sunt fidelitas et prudentia, misericordia et iustitia, dilectio Dei et dilectio proximi, sobrietas et castitas, timor et spes, humilitas et perseuerantia ... .

12.3 De prerogativis beate Virginis

Legitur in Apocalipsi [12:1]: Mulier amicta sole, et luna sub pedibus eius, et in capite eius corona duodecim stellarum. Hec mulier est beata Virgo, ut sit mulier nomen sexus non corruptionis ... . In huius corona sunt duodecim stelle, quia ad eius dignitatem et excellentiam spectant duodecim bona, in quibus patet eius priuilegium seu prerogatiua. Sunt autem ista duodecim fides, caritas, misericordia, patientia, uirginitas et fecunditas, generositas et humilitas, extinctio fomitis in conceptu, immunitas doloris in partu, fortitudo, et supra choros angelorum exaltatio ... . Hec etiam supra choros angelorum canitur exaltata, et creditur immediate Deo coniuncta.

Et hic gratias agendo huius summe finem facimus cui nomen Numerale imponimus. Plura quidem hic omissa in aliis opusculis nostris copiosius sunt exarata.

Explicit.

II.8

Distinctiones theologice

William's *Distinctiones* represents a rich selection of his teachings as a master of theology. Here are displayed the fruits of his studies of sacred scripture, quotations from ecclesiastical and classical authors, examples and similitudes from the world of nature, and the techniques of logical and grammatical analysis as they are to be applied to theological questions. Quickened by William's subtle insight and his faculty of invention, these distinctions exemplify the pedagogical skills that made William one of the most highly regarded teachers of his day.

The literary genre of *distinctiones* reached the height of its popularity in the late twelfth and early thirteenth centuries. A history of the genre has yet to be written.[1] William's *distinctiones* are correctly described in the manuscripts as "theological" rather than strictly "biblical." They include examples of the various meanings of a word in Scripture — its literal as well as its "spiritual" (moral, anagogical, and tropological) senses; but the work as we have it is more a theological textbook or *summa* than a catalogue of biblical usage. William draws not only on Scripture, but on art ("the book of the laity"),[2] on the lives of the saints, the sayings of the Church Fathers, the verses of secular and christian poets, and everyday experience to elucidate the theological significance of a term under discussion.

William's *Distinctiones* resemble other examples of the genre in this period. Some entries lend themselves to schematic or diagrammatic representation (although none are actually diagrammed in the manuscripts). Other entries are more discursive, resembling brief treatises

---

[1] See Rouse and Rouse, "Biblical *Distinctiones* in the Thirteenth Century," pp. 27-37; Wilmart, "Un répertoire d'exégèse," pp. 307-346; Giusberti, *Twelfth Century Scholasticism*, pp. 87-101; Evans, "Alan of Lille's *Distinctiones*," pp. 67-86; Kuttner, *Repertorium*, pp. 208-227.

[2] "LIBER ... Sunt et libri laicales, ymagines ecclesiastice, ubi uisibiles et grosse littere sunt, sculpture et picture edificatorie," Royal 8.G.ii, fol. 46va.

or homilies rather than dictionary entries. They bear comparison to the longer prose sections of contemporary distinction collections,[3] as well as to such amorphous literary works as the *Sententiae* of the school of Laon,[4] and the later *Dicta* of Robert Grosseteste.[5]

Like many of Grosseteste's *Dicta*, these *distinctiones* give the impression of having been composed individually, perhaps on *cedule* or scraps of parchment, and then assembled alphabetically (first letter only) into a continuous treatise.[6] The absence of uniform ordering of entries in the extant manuscripts lends credence to this supposition, as does the absence of internal cross-references in the work. Such cross-references as exist refer the reader either to other books entirely or to an earlier comment within the same entry, never to another entry within the *Distinctiones*.

The forms of the individual entries vary considerably, but some patterns are evident. William frequently begins the entry with a sentence or a didactic verse listing the meanings of a word he intends to discuss. The first entry is typical: "Arcus dicitur Christus, et propitiatio Dei, scriptura, iudicium, robur, intentio, insidie, et dolus."[7] He then proceeds to illustrate each meaning with an apposite verse from Scripture, an example from the natural world or the lives of the saints or from the liturgy, or a theological interpretation.

Another approach is to begin with a Scripture passage, such as "Asperges me hyssopo, et mundabor; lavabis me, et super niuem dealbabor" (Ps 50:9), and then to proceed as above, listing the various ways one is "washed" and explicating each.[8]

Other entries take a more scholastic form. Under "Advent," for example, William describes the various causes of Christ's coming: the efficient cause was the will of the Father in commanding, of the Son in obeying, and of the Holy Spirit in preparing the way. The prayers

---

[3] Manuscripts of Peter the Chanter's *distinctiones* (*Summa que dicitur Abel*), for example, comprise numerous schemata interspersed with longer, prose expositions.

[4] See Valerie I.J. Flint, "The 'School of Laon': A Reconsideration," *Recherches de théologie ancienne et médiévale* 43 (1976) 89-110.

[5] See Thomson, *Writings of Robert Grosseteste*, pp. 214-232.

[6] For an example of this form of composition see the discussion by Yves Lefèvre and R.B.C. Huygens in their edition of Gerald of Wales's *Speculum duorum*, pp. lvii-lxvi.

[7] See the first entry, Arcvs, below p. 268. An example of an entry beginning with a didactic verse is Conivgivm, p. 273, which begins with one of William's favorites: "Coniugium mundat, fecundat, mutat, et unit."

[8] "Asperges me etc. Lauant sanguis, aqua, doctrina, gratia, fides, penitentia, opera, suffragia ... " (Aspersio, below p. 269).

of God's people were a cooperating cause. The final cause was human salvation. Sin, especially that of Adam and Eve, was the cause *sine qua non*. Two other causes are expressed in the present tense as still acting: to give humans something more to be grateful for, and to teach us not only by words (as in the prophets) but also by divine example.[9]

Other entries begin by distinguishing the scholastic "circumstances" — who, what, when, where, etc. For example, William discusses alms in terms of what should be given, to whom, how much, when, why, and how one should give.[10]

Finally, William is fond of beginning his distinctions by recalling the common usage of a term and then proceeding to explore its metaphorical meanings. For example, under "Hunger" he explains: "Physical hunger is that which the poor read daily in the book of experience."[11] The literal or corporeal sense of "Eating" is, again, "that which we read every day in the book of experience."[12]

The variety and heterogeneity of entries precludes simple generalizations about the purpose of these *distinctiones* and the use to which they were put. Although such collections became popular as aides to

---

[9] "ADVENTVS PRIMI QVE SINT CAVSE: Aduentus primi cause sunt uoluntas Dei, desiderium sanctorum, salus hominis, peccata hominis presertim primorum parentum, maior hominis ad gratitudinem obligatio, et plenior hominis per exemplum eruditio. Efficiens quidem causa fuit uoluntas Patris precipientis, et Filii obedientis ... et uoluntas Spiritus sancti habitaculum in uirgine preparantis ... . Sunt desiderium antiquorum causa cooperans et amminiculans ad aduentum Christi ... . Finalis autem causa fuit salus humana ... . Fuit et culpa hominis causa sine qua non ... . Quinta causa est gratitudo ... . Sexta est per exemplum instructio ... ," Royal 8.G.ii, fol. 7va, excerpted below p. 270.
[10] "ELEMOSINA SECVNDO: Date et dabitur uobis [Lc 6:38]. Videndum quid, cui, uel quantum, quando, cur, quomodo dandum. Quid: elemosina ... tum corporalis, tum spiritualis ... . Set cui danda est elemosina, cuilibet quidem indigenti, pro loco, pro tempore, et causa cognita ... . Set quantum dandum est, Tobias ait: Si multum tibi fuerit, habundanter tribue; si exiguum tibi fuerit, etiam exiguum libenter impertiri stude, etc. [Tob 4:9] ... . At quando dare debemus, dum tempus habemus, donec dies est. Venit enim nox, scilicet mortis uel inferni, quando nemo potest operari [Io 9:4] ... . Set cur danda est elemosina? Quia proximo tenetur homo. Vnde ... Quamdiu fecistis uni ex hiis fratribus meis minimis, mihi fecistis [Mt 25:40] ... . Porro si queris quomodo dandum, dicimus quia ordinate, moderate, hilariter, et bona intentione ... ," ibid., fol. 25rb, excerpted below p. 277.
[11] "ESVRIES: Est esuries corporalis quam legunt pauperes cotidie in libro experientie ... . Et est esuries spiritualis triplex. Vna est iustitie, que communis est iustis ... . Altera est sapientie ... . Tertia spiritualiter est prelatorum, que est de conuersione fratris ... ," ibid., fol. 24vb, excerpted below p. 277.
[12] "MANDVCATIO: Est manducatio corporalis quam cotidie legimus in libro experientie. Vnde: 'Manducauerunt et saturati sunt etc.' [Ps. 77:29]. Est et manducatio spiritualis qua comedimus Deum, uerbum Dei, carnem Dei, diabolum, homines, et peccata hominum ... ," ibid., fol. 48va, excerpted below p. 285.

preaching in the thirteenth century,[13] this was not their only use in William's day. Expositions of Scripture and theological arguments, as well as sermons, were built upon the *distinctio* in the schools of William de Montibus and his contemporaries.[14]

Modern readers may find the *distinctio*-format somewhat odd and unwieldy. Nothing in our literary experience corresponds very closely to this unusual genre. This, however, should blind us neither to the popularity and perceived usefulness of *distinctiones* as a literary and didactic form from the twelfth through the sixteenth century, nor to the importance of these texts as witnesses to the intellectual history of their time. The variety of approaches, and of materials adduced, helps to remove the tedium that can be associated with reading this type of literature from beginning to end, as is our habit. In fact, however, most *distinctio*-collections seem not to have been intended for consecutive reading. Rather they represented storehouses of ideas, interpretations, and information on a variety of topics and for a variety of uses. The preacher, the teacher, the student, and the pastor might each find something suitable for their diverse needs.

AUTHENTICITY AND DATE

Nine of the ten extant manuscripts attribute the work to William, and seven of the ascribed manuscripts were written within forty years of his death. Verbal and stylistic similarities to other works written by William confirm the manuscript ascriptions. No specific indication of date is found in the text or the manuscripts, but it was written before the *Tropi* and the *Numerale*, which refer to it. Two internal references to other works written by William cannot be identified with certainty. The first is in the discussion of the "Dove" (COLVMBA), and simply declares that he has treated this subject elsewhere.[15] The second occurs at the end of the distinction on the word "Pro," and refers the reader to his "Questions."[16] The only known work of William's that might

---

[13] See Rouse and Rouse, *Preachers*, pp. 3-90, passim.

[14] See William's use of distinctions in his *Tropi* and *Super Psalmos*, below. See also the perceptive comments of Evans, "Alan of Lille's *Distinctiones*," and of Giusberti, *Twelfth Century Scholasticism*, pp. 87-101, cited above.

[15] "Sancti columbe dicuntur ... de turturibus et pullis columbe, etc. Hec autem alibi tractando declarauimus," Royal 8.G.ii, fol. 13rb.

[16] "Est *pro* locale, ut prelatus sedit pro tribunali, id est in ... . Et est *pro* causale, a causa multiplici. Quere in questionibus," ibid., fol. 65rb; William's *Tropi* also contain a reference to these unidentified "Questions."

be described as *quaestiones* is his *De septem sacramentiis ecclesie*, but no explicit treatment of the topic is found there.

SOURCES

The Bible is the most frequently cited source. In addition to the Vulgate, William refers explicitly to the *Hebraica ueritas* and the "Roman" Psalter. He makes frequent allusions to the lives of the saints, including saints Agatha, Agnes, Anthony, Bernard, Lambert, and Martin. Authorities cited explicitly include Ambrose, Aristotle, Augustine, Bede, Cassiodorus, Pope Leo, Gregory, Hilary, Isidore, Jerome, Origen, Ovid, Seneca, and Pope Symmachus. In addition, numerous pieces of secular and religious verse are quoted anonymously.

MANUSCRIPTS

1. *C* = Cambridge, Gonville and Caius College MS 138/78, fols. 1ra-137rb. Mid 13th century (above top line).
> Title: *Incipiunt distinctiones theologice a magistro Willelmo de Monte collecte.*
> Inc.: *Arcus dicitur Christus.*
> Expl.: *... imitari Christum et Ecclesiam.*

The order of entries under letters "A" and "B" differs from that printed below.

2. Cambridge, Trinity College MS B.16.18 (392), fols. 1ra-172va. Early 13th century (above top line).
> Title: *Incipiunt distinctiones venerabilis Willelmi de Montibus Lincolniensis ecclesie cancellarii.*
> Inc.: *Arcus dicitur Christus.*
> Expl.: (*Verbum*) ... . *Iam nos mundi.*

The text ends abruptly on the last folio of the codex. The order differs somewhat from that printed below, and not all the entries are included in this copy. However seven additional items on penance are preserved only in this manuscript.

3. *L* = London, British Library MS Royal 6.B.x, fols. 43vb-86vb. Mid 13th century (above top line).
> Inc.: *Arcus dicitur Christus.*
> Expl.: (*Desiderium mortis*) ... *sicut et Enoch placuit Deo et transtulit illum Deus mortem.*

The text is incomplete. A table of contents for the entire work is found on fols. 42ra-43va. The last three items listed there are: *Commedere corpus Christi*; *Zelus*; *Zona*.

4. London, British Library MS Royal 8.g.ii, fols. 2ra-92vb. Mid 13th century (above top line).

> Inc.: *Arcus dicitur Christus.*
> Expl.: ... *imitari Christum et Ecclesiam.*
> Colophon: *Expliciunt distinctiones Lincolniensis bone et utiles.*

A sixteenth-century hand, apparently identifying the "Lincolniensis" with Robert Grosseteste, bishop of Lincoln from 1235 to 1253, adds: *vel secundum quosdam W. de montibus.*

5. London, British Library MS Royal 10.A.vii, fols. 1ra-115ra. Early 13th century (above top line).

> Title: *Incipiunt disticiones theologice a magistro Willelmo Lincolniensis ecclesie cancellario collecte.*
> Inc.: *Arcus dicitur Christus.*
> Expl.: (*Xpc*) ... *sicut et cognitus sum.*

A gathering is missing between folios 92-93. A number of brief sermons and theological notes have been interspersed in the last thirty folios. On fol. 87rb, in a sermon for the first Sunday after Ascension, there is a reference to the village of Appleby.[17]

6. London, British Library MS Royal 11.A.iii, fols. 35ra-129vb. Mid 13th century (above top line).

> Title: *Distinctiones theologice a magistro Willelmo Lincolniensis ecclesie cancelario collecte.*
> Inc.: *Arcus dicitur Christus.*
> Expl.: ... *imitari Christum et Ecclesiam.*

7. Oxford, Bodleian Library MS Bodley 419 (sc 2318), fols. 1ra-103rb. Mid 13th century (below top line).

> Title: *Incipit distinctiones magistri W. de montibus secundum alfabetum.*
> Inc.: *Arcus dicitur Christus.*
> Expl.: (*Zona*) ... . *Sicut zona qua semper precingitur.*

This text consists of excerpts from William's *Distinctiones*, followed in each alphabetical section by additions drawn from miscellaneous sources. The additions are usually marked by the scribe.[18]

---

[17] "... ne detis Scotland pro eppelby, hoc est maximum pro minimo."

[18] For example: "Alia distinctio de A ... de B ... " etc., or as on fol. 8vb: "amplius in alio libro ... ." Many of these additions are from the *Allegoriae in sacram scripturam* (PL 112: 849-1088).

8. Oxford, Bodleian Library MS Greaves 53 (sc 3825), fols. 55r-106v. 13/14th century.

> Title (modern hand): *Distinctiones theologicae Guilielmi de Montibus al. Leycester.*
> Inc.: *Arcus dicitur Christus.*
> Expl.: (*Vanitas*) ... *uel penalis est et misera.*

Excerpts only.

9. Oxford, Corpus Christi College MS 43, fols. 1ra-12rb, 16ra-46. Early 13th century (above top line).

> Title (modern hand): *Distinctiones theologicae Guilelmi de Montibus.*
> Inc.: *Arcus dicitur Christus.*
> Expl.: (*Vanitas*) ... *uel penalis est et misera.*

Excerpts only. A table of contents ending with the titles *Vanitas, Vicium,* is written on the flyleaf of the codex. A copy of Bede's *De schematibus et tropis* interrupts William's *Distinctiones* on fols. 12ra-15rb. Folios 18 and 19 have been torn away and are lost, and many columns have been left blank, presumably to accommodate additional material.

10. Utrecht, Bibliotheek der Universiteit MS 312, fols. 1ra-54vb. 13th century (below top line).

> Title: *Incipiunt distinctiones magistri Willelmi de monte Cancellarii Lincolniensis.*
> Inc.: *Arcus dicitur Christus.*
> Expl.: (*Zelus*) ... *uisitans iniquitatem patrum in filios etc.*

Excerpts only. One half column or more has been left blank after each alphabetical segment, presumably to accommodate additional material.[19]

The first entry, *Arcus,* has been transcribed from London, BL MS Royal 8.G.ii (*L,* no. 3 above). Selected variant readings from Cambridge, Gonville and Caius MS 138/78 (*C,* no. 1 above) are cited in the apparatus criticus. Subsequent entries are represented by their incipits and a few additional words and phrases that indicate the direction of William's exposition.

---

[19] A set of distinctions with a different incipit is ascribed to William de Montibus in Heiligenkreuz MS 90, fols. 1-170: "*Magister Wilhelmus de Montibus, Distinctiones sec. ord. alphab.*" Incipit: *Abyssus multiplex est.* Explicit: *pro zona scilicet gracie funiculus culpe.* See Benedict Gsell, *Verzeichniss der Handschriften in der Bibliothek des Stiftes Heiligenkreuz* (Vienna, 1891), p. 147. This codex has not been examined.

Distinctiones theologice

Incipiunt Distinctiones theologice a magistro Willelmo de Monte collecte.

Arcvs: Arcus dicitur Christus, et propitiatio Dei, scriptura, iudicium, robur, intentio, insidie, et dolus.

Arcus Christus: Hic est arcus positus in nubibus celi, pactum et signum federis inter Deum et hominem [Gen 9:12-17], qui in dictis et factis prophetarum assimilatus est, et in medio doctorum templi quasi in nubibus celi, et in choro apostolorum inuentus est. Cotidie etiam uenit in nubibus, id est predicatoribus. Item in Ecclesiastico [43:12-13]: "Vide arcum et benedic qui fecit illum. Valde speciosus est in splendore suo. Girauit celum in splendore glorie sue. Manus excelsi aperuerunt illum." Et Christus quidem uerus Simon, summus sacerdos quasi "arcus est refulgens inter nebulas glorie" [Eccli 50:8]. Huius arcus uiridis color, immarcessibilis diuinitas; rubeus color, purpurata sanguine humanitas. Set et Ezechiel [1:26-28] ait: "Super similitudinem troni, similitudo quasi aspectus hominis desuper. Et uidi quasi speciem electri uelut aspectum ignis intrinsecus per circuitum eius a lumbis eius et desuper, et a lumbis eius usque deorsum, uidi quasi speciem ignis splendentis in circuitu, uelut aspectum arcus cum fuerit in nube in die pluuie." Hic est Christus in carne, in tempore gratie. Yris etiam in nube, Christus in ascensione et in iudicii die, "Et yris erat in circuitu sedis" [Apoc 4:3], quia Dominus in circuitu populi sui. Yris etiam est pax, et propitiatio Dei que est in circuitu ut protegens.

Dicitur et arcus scriptura, unde: "Arcum suum tetendit" [Ps 7:13], temperato scilicet ueteri testamento per nouum. Per cordam enim noui testamenti duritia ueteris testamenti ut ligni flectitur et domatur. Item: "Suscitans suscitabis arcum tuum" etc. [Hab 3:9]. Item in Apocalypso [6:2]: "Ecce equus albus," id est ecclesia, "et qui sedebat super eum," scilicet Christus, "habebat arcum," id est diuinam scripturam, etc. Huius arcus corda breui loco colligitur, quia uerbum abbreuiatum est preceptum caritatis, in quo pendent lex et prophete [Mt 22:34-40].

Arcus etiam iudicium dicitur, unde: "Vt fugiant a facie arcus" [Is 21:15]; et in Lamentationibus [2:4]: "Tetendit arcum suum, quasi inimicus" etc. In arcu lignum solidum est potentia et fortitudo Dei nunc auersa a percussione. In die iudicii applicabitur et adaptabitur, corda tunc extensa et ostensa. Hec est iustitia iaculans sagittas acutas, id est uerba aspera, asperiora, asperima.

Archus robur dicitur ibi: "Conteram archum Israel in ualle Iezrael" [Os 1:5], hoc est robur decem tribuum. Archus etiam intentio, ut ibi: "Archus fortium superatus est," etc. [1 Sam 2:4]. Item arcus pro intentione et robore ibi: "Posuisti ut archum ereum brachia mea" [Ps 17:35], id est dedisti mihi infatigabilem intentionem bonorum operum, siue irremissibilem fortitudinem. Et est hic similitudo rei que non est.

Arcus etiam dicitur insidie et dolus, unde: "Quoniam ecce peccatores intenderunt archum" etc. [Ps 10:3]; et "Gladium euaginauerunt peccatores, intenderunt arcum suum" [Ps 36:14]. Item: "Quemadmodum patres eorum conuersi sunt in arcum prauum" [Ps 77:57], qui scilicet debilis et flexibilis facile remittitur, et ipsi facile retroibant. Vel arcus prauus est qui non eminus iaculatur set in se, hoc est intendentem se spicula conuertit et ipsum a quo intenditur percutit, et fraudulenter absconsus feram tangentem occidit, hec est malitia dolosorum. Conuersi sunt ergo in archum prauum uel peruersum, id est in animi intentionem peruersam.

ADVERSARIVS: Aduersarius diabolus est ... mundus est ... est caro ... .

ASPERSIO: Asperges me, etc. Lauant sanguis, aqua, doctrina, gratia, fides, penitentia, opera, suffragia ... .

AQVA: Est aqua deficiens, fluens, inficiens, reficiens, sufficiens, sordidans, suffocans, amara, mundans, rigans, dulcis ... .

AQVA: Aqua dicitur Deus ... . Aque etiam sunt angeli ... .

ABLVTIO: Sunt ablutiones exteriores in carne, indifferentes ... . Sunt etiam ablutiones in carne que prosunt et necessarie sunt ... .

ABYSSVS: Est abyssus mundi ... . Est et abissus celi uel iudicii diuini ... .

AD NICHILVM: Dicitur de reprobis, quia ad nichilum deuenerit ... quoad euacuationem diuitiarum et deliciarum ... .

ANTIQVA: Ne memineris iniquitatum nostrarum antiquarum ... . Tribus modis dicuntur peccata antiqua; per traductionem ... .

ADIVTOR: Dominus michi adiutor ... est ante pugnam ... in pugna ... post pugnam ... .

AVARITIA: Inclina cor meum in testimonia tua et non in auaritiam ... . Auaritia dipsas est, ydropis, bitumen est, id est gluten ... .

ASCENSVS PRIMO: Est ascensus tumide elationis ... . Est ascensus sancte gloriationis ... .

ASCENSVS SECVNDO: Ascendit Christus super carnem, in crucem, super mortem, et super seculi uolubilitatem et terrenam felicitatem, et super omnem celi altitudinem, et in cordibus per fidem ... .

ARCHA PRIMO: Est archa saluationis, scilicet archa Noe ... et archa significationis, hec est archa testamenti siue testimonii ... .

ANGELICA VITA: In conspectu angelorum. Vt angeli scilicet conspiciant approbando, et ut angelos conspiciam imitando, psallam tibi ... .

ALTVM: Est altum uirtute ... et potestate ... .

APERTIO ORIS: Os quod est hostium corporis debet esse apertum ad confessionem ... . Claudatur ad laudem propriam ... .

ADEPS: Adeps caritas est, desiderium, sapientia ... . In malo dicitur letitia superbi ... .

ARBOR: Arbor dicitur disciplina utilis ... .

ACCEDERE AD DEVM: Deus ubique est sicut uox in diuersis auribus, uita uel anima in corpore ... .

ANGELVS: Est angelus glorie Christus, scilicet magni consilii angelus ... . Est angelus ut ita dicam nature ... .

ANNVITIO: Est annuitio proditorum et ad proditionem, et ypocritarum ad simulationem religionis ... .

ANNVNTIATIO: Annuntiare debes iniquitatem tui, iniquitatem proximi, et laudem Dei ... .

ADVLATIO: Adulatores sunt uenditores olei ... .

AVIS: Auis dicitur Christus ... . Fulica in baptismo ... Pellicanus in deserto et in triduo passionis ... .

ARIES: Aries dicitur Christus ... humanitas Christi ... Apostoli ... .

AMOR: Vinee amoris illiciti sunt uisus et alloquium, contactus et oscula, factum. Hii sunt gradus descensionis in infernum ... .

ADVENTVS: Specialiter propter gentes uenit Christus; Iudei enim per legem saluabuntur ... .

APPROPINQVARE DEI VEL DEO: Licet Deus sit ubique ... dicitur tamen approprinquare uel prope esse per negationem ... per rationem naturalem ... .

AMICITIA: Amicitiam dissoluunt presertim hec quinque: conuicium, improperium, elatio, secreti commissi denudatio, et proditio ... .

ADVENTVS PRIMI QVE SVNT CAVSE: Aduentus primi cause sunt uoluntas Dei, desiderium sanctorum, salus hominis, peccata hominis ... maior hominis ad gratitudinem obligatio, et plenior hominis per exemplum eruditio ... .

ADVENTVS SECVNDI QVE SINT TESTIMONIA: Aduentum Christi secundum et corporum nostrorum glorificationem testantur corus prophetarum, cetus apostolorum, sapientes gentium, uniuersalis ecclesia fidelium, angeli Domini, Dominus ipse ... .

ABSCONSIO VERBI: In corde meo abscondi eloquia tua ... ut librum in archa, manna in urna, pecuniam in sacco, thesaurum in uasa fictili ... .

ADHERENTIA: Est adherentia nature, ut coherentia corporis et anime ... . Est adherentia culpe ... .

AMARITVDO: Est amaritudo malitiosi ... prelati ... .

ACETVM: Habet acetum suum Booth [= Booz], id est Christus ... . Habet et diabolus acetum suum id est malitiam suam ... .

ARCHA SECVNDO: Est archa Noe typus ecclesie ... .

ALTARE: Ara cordis fides est. Super hanc aram offerenda sunt sacrificia, quedam prima, quedam media, quedam extrema ... .

ANATHEMA: Hermon uel Hermoniim anathema interpretatur ... hec sunt uitia et peccata mundi ... .

BONVM PATRIE: Canticum erit uobis ... . Sunt autem quedam bona patrie: Gemina stola, multitudo triumphantium unanimis, consortium Christi et sanctorum angelorum et hominum ... .

BONA PATRIE:[1] In hoc Psalmo [147]: "Lauda ... Ierusalem, Dominum" ... declarantur bona celestis Ierusalem ... .

BENEDICERE: Benedicit nobis Deus peccatorum remissionem dando, uirtutum augmentum largiendo, uitam eternam prestando ... .

BENEDICTIO PRIMO: Triplici maledictioni Ade opponitur triplex benedictio Christi ... .

BENEDICTIO SECVNDO:[2] Benedicite gentes Deum nostrum. Benedicunt gentes Deum peccata confitendo et gratias agendo, laudando, predicando; benedicunt corde, ore, opere ... .

BEATITVDO: Est beatitudo uanitatis et fallacie ... . Beatitudo enim proprie eternorum est, felicitas temporalium ... .

BIBERE: Bibimus potum usualem ut uinum in fragili uase, fragilis reminiscere uite ... . Bibimus Deum ... et sanguinem Christi ... .

BESTIA: Bestie ad literam dicuntur animalia immitia et ferocia ... . Bestie demones dicuntur ... .

BOS: Est bos historicus ... allegoricus ... tropologicus ... anagogicus ... .

BELLVM: In pugna necessaria sunt arma et scientia, fortitudo et audacia, continentia et abstinentia atque perseuerantia ... .

BRACHIVM: Brachium Patris dicitur Filius ... .

BREVITAS RERVM: Breuitas est in diuinis ... . Breuitas est hic in honore ... .

BONVS EST DEVS: Bonus dicitur Deus in natura ... et in misericordia exhibita ... .

---

1 Bona patrie *ed.*: Bona penitencie *L*: De bonis patrie *C*
2 Benedictio secundo ... opere *om. L*

BENEFICIA: Non sunt recordati manus eius ... . Quasi due manus Dei sunt, potentia et misericordia ... .

CARITAS: Caritas dicitur Deus ... uel Spiritus sanctus ... .
ITEM CARITAS: Et ambulabam in latitudine, id est caritate ... .
CONCORDIA: Sine concordia non ualet abstinentia ... nec sapientia ... nec munificentia ... .
CONFIDENTIA: Non debemus diligere carnem, quia terra es et in terram ibis. Nec in amicis confidere ... .
CONFIDENTIA SECVNDO: Confidendum est in Deo ... non in diuite, non in ingenio, non in sapientia propria uel eloquentia ... .
CONTRITIO: Est contritio culpe ... est contritio penitentie ... .
CONFESSIO: Est confessio peccati ... . Est confessio fidei ... .
CONFESSIO SECVNDO: Est confessio laudatiua elati ... est confessio ficti ... .
CONFESSIO TERTIO: Confessionem utilem et penitentiam impediunt peccati magnitudo ... et superbia ... .
CASTIGATIO: Castigat Deus propter peccata preterita ... propter presentia ... propter futura ... .
CORRECTIO: Corrigit homo uiam, uel non errando ... uel errorem euacuando ... .
CRVCIFIXIO: Simul crucifixa sunt caro Christi ... et lex Moysi ... . Crucifixa sunt etiam mors ... et peccatum ... et diabolus ... .
CANDIDATIO: Libanus interpretatur candidatio. Est autem candor nature, fortune, culpe, glorie, gratie ... .
CONSOLATIO: Consolatur Deus hominem aduentus sui promissione ... . Consolatur redemptione ... .
ITEM CONSOLATIO: Consolatur hominem spes ... scriptura ... uerba sanctorum et exempla, et Dei promissa ... .
CIBVS: Est cibus dulcis et bonus doctrina catholica ... . Est autem cibus amarus et utilis, scilicet penitentia ... .
CALIX: Est calix nature, actualis scilicet et usualis ... est enim iniquitatis et culpe ... .
CORPVS CHRISTI: Quod soli boni debeant conficere uel sumere corpus Christi ita constat ... .
CVSTODIA: Depositum prelatis speciale commisit Dominus, sponsam suam ecclesiam ... .
CELVM PRIMO: Celi dicuntur sancti qui sunt casa Ylios, id est domus solis iustitie ... .
CELVM SECVNDO: Sancti dicuntur celi sublimes conuersatione, pluentes doctrina et tamen celantes misteria canibus scilicet et porcis ... .

Columba: Sancti columbe dicuntur ... .

Corvvs: Coruus teter ales, immundus, cadauerosus, improbus, clamosus, raucas et fractas uoces habens, expers affectionis. Homo peccator est ... .

Cervvs: Cerui sunt fideles ... .

Canis: Canes dicuntur gentiles ... . Sunt et canes boni ... . Hii sunt predicatores seu alii iusti ... .

Cornv: Cornu dicitur potentia et robur ... .

Conivgivm:

> Coniugium mundat, fecundat, mutat, et unit,
> Pollens auctore, tempore, lege, loco ... .

Caro: Nomine carnis intelligitur fragilitas ... humanitas ... .

Cvbile: Est cubile diaboli abyssus ... . Est cubile Christi pectus pacificum ... .

Cingere: Deus qui precinxit me uirtute ... . Nota quia procingimur ituri ... succingimur cursuri ... precingimur ministraturi ... .

Calciamentvm primo: Calciamentum dicitur euuangelium siue euuangelica predicatio ... .

Item Calciamentvm: Prohibe pedem tuum a nuditate et guttur tuum a siti ... . Calciamenta sunt exempla sanctorum predecessorum.

Capvd: Apostolus ait: Caput uiri Christus ... .

Capilli: Capilli dicuntur amici ... . Item capilli sunt fideles ... .

Cor: Preter librorum apertionem id est conscientiarum manifestationem in iudicio etiam in presenti corda patent in confessione ... .

Cogitatio primo: Cogitationes praue sunt musce morientes ... aues descendentes super sacrificium ... .

Cogitatio secvndo: Cogitabo pro peccato meo scilicet inde uilem esse ... .

Circvitvs diaboli: Circuit diabolus ad explorandum ... ad impugnandum ... .

Cvrvatio: Est curuatio nature que patet, et culpe quam pretendit in euuangelio mulier que erat inclinata nec poterat omnino sursum respicere ... .

Casvs primo: Est casus nature corrupte, ut mors ... . Est casus gratie ... . Est casus pene, uel temporalis uel eterne ... .

Concvlcatio: Est conculcatio laudabilis qua scilicet Iacob, id est supplantator uitiorum, calcat supra serpentes et scorpiones ... .

Carcer primo: Est carcer nature scilicet corrupte ... et carcer culpe ... .

Carcer secvndo: Est carcer animarum corpus corruptum. Est carcer corporum mundus iste ... . Est carcer reproborum ... .

COMPEDES: Sunt compedes nature ... et sunt compedes culpe ... .

CARBONES: Carbones dicuntur sancti ... diuina scriptura ... .

CVPIDITAS PRIMO: Radix omnium malorum est cupiditas, plus scilicet habendi quam oportet ... .

CVPIDITAS SECVNDO: Est cupere naturale ... gratuitum ... beatum ... .

CONSVETVDO: Consuetudo praua est porta erea, cathena ferrea ... lapis superpositus Lazaro ... .

CONSILIA REPROBA: Dominus dissipat consilia gentium ... .

CONFVSIO: Est confusio adducens peccatum ... est confusio adducens gloriam et gratiam ... .

CASTRA: Sunt castra Dei et sunt castra diaboli ... .

CHORVS: Chorus est temperata uocum collectio ... translatiue, locus, ut: "Iste habet stallum in choro." ... .

CONTEMPTVS: Est contemptus discipline que dicitur epistemen ... est contemptus discipline que fedia dicitur ... .

CARITAS TERTIO: Est caritas initians, cuius est non nocere ... . Est caritas proficiens, cuius est iuuare ... .

CONFESSIO QVARTO: Est confessio tum peccati tum laudis, quedam culpabilis et reprobanda, quedam laudabilis ... .

CONVERTIT DEVS: Conuertit Deus ab infidelitate ad fidem ... .

COGITATIO TERTIO: Cognitiones hominum uane sunt, id est false ... superflue ... perniciose ... .

CASVS SECVNDO: Adam cecidit in locum lutosum et lapidosum; sic cadenti necessaria est purificatio emundans et penitentia solidans ... .

CIVITAS: Est ciuitas malorum ecclesia malignantium ... . Est ciuitas bonorum ecclesia militantium ... . Est et ciuitas beatorum ecclesia triumphantium ... .

CLAVIS: Clauis dicitur potestas, et scientia, et debitum et obnoxietas discernendi, et auctoritas applicandi se ad discretionem boni et mali. Et applicare eius usus est et officium discernendi et potestas iudicandi, et potestas et scientia ... .

DVLCIS DOMINVS: Quam magna multitudo dulcedinis tue, Domine, etc. Dulcis est Dominus in precepto ... . Dulcior in promisso ... . Dulcissimus erit in premio ... .

DILECTIO DEI: Diligite Dominum omnes sancti eius, etc. Videamus a quo, cur, quantum Deus est et quomodo amandus ... .

ITEM DILECTIO DEI: Dilectio Dei increata est eius essentia uel persona ... .

DARE DEI: Dat Deus bona seculi bonis ad remedium non ad solatium ... .

QVATVOR SVNT DEO RESERVANDA: Quatuor Deo committere et reseruare debemus: ultionem in iniuriis propriis, promotionem in dignitatibus ecclesiasticis, nostri commendationem, et diuinorum secretorum profunditatem ... .

QVATVOR SVNT IN MANDATIS CONSIDERANDA: In mandatis Dei quatuor sunt consideranda: auctoritas precipientis ... equitas ... ydoneitas ... et opportunitas ... .

DOMINVS: Quoniam Dominus excelsus terribilis rex magnus ... . In celo magnus ... . In patibulo abiectus ... . In iudicio excelsus, potens, et terribilis ... .

DOMVS DEI: Domus Dei dicitur celum, mundus, sinagoga, ecclesia, corpus, anima, beata Virgo, corpus Christi, sacra scriptura, mens sancta et deuota ... .

QVATVOR QVE FIVNT IN FABRICA DOMVS: In fabrica domus quatuor fiunt: prius exciduntur ligna, postea eruderantur, post iunguntur, post eriguntur. Ita in corpus Christi ... .

DEDICATIO: In dedicatione fiunt quatuor: Innouatio domus, refectio, exultatio, usus mutatio. Ita in resurrectione Christi ... .

DECOR DOMVS: Decor domus consistit in fundamento firmo, id est in soliditate fidei ... .

DVCERE: Dominus dux est ... . Conducit dominus operarios in uineam ... .

DEDVCTIO: Deduc me Domine ut ambulem cum Deo et transferar cum Enoch ... . Ducuntur ad uiam penitentes ... .

DIRECTIO PRIMO: Est directio cordis, oris, operis, intentionis ... .

DIRECTIO SECVNDO: Deus dirigit auctoritate, homo ministerio, gratia uel liberum arbitrium diriget ut instrumentum ... .

DILATATIO: Est dilatatio bona cordis in serenitate conscientie ... . Et est dilatatio oris ... .

DILATIO GLORIE: Tardum est sanctis esse cum Christo propter illam beatitudinem qua fruentur ... .

DERELICTIO DEI: Dereliquid Deus hominem in penam ad examinandum eius patientiam ... uel ad humilitatem conseruandam ... .

DORMITIO CHRISTI: Dormit Christus in cruce et in sepulcro ... . Dormit Christus in nobis ... .

DIABOLVS PRIMO: Diabolus est serpens tortuosus, sordidus, callidus ... .

DIABOLVS SECVNDO: Diabolus leo rapiens est; leon Grece, rex Latine ... .

DIABOLVS TERTIO: Diabolus leo est in crudelitate, draco malitie immanitate, serpens ueneno inuidie ... .

DOLVS: Quidam habent dolum in lingua et non in corde, ut Hebrei ... . Quidam in corde et non in lingua ... . Quidam in utroque ... .

Devoratio: Est deuoratio nature, gratie, culpe, pene ... .

Dolor primo: Secundum multitudinem dolorum meorum ... . Multiplex est dolor. Est enim dolor desperati ... . Est dolor auari ... .

Dolor secvndo: Dolor formatus est qui eruditionis formam prestat ... . Dolor informis est qui non emendat ... .

Dvrvm: Ostendisti populo tuo dura, etc. Ostendisti, Christe, exemplo et uerbo ... .

Defectvs: Est defectus nature ... et culpe ... et gratie ... .

Dissipatio: Est dissipatio corporalis ... . Et est dissipatio interior per timorem ... et per uarias opiniones ... .

Districtvs ivdex: Non punit hic Deus districte secundum modum cum eternam penam criminali debitam mutat in temporalem ... .

Donec: Donec quandoque positiuum est et inclusiuum omnium temporum ... .

Desertvm primo: In deserto sunt sitis, serpens, ardor, harena. Hec in mundo ... .

Desertvm secvndo: Mundus iste desertum est Ydumee id est terrene uel sanguinee quoad reprobos ... .

Dignitas hominis: Decem sunt in quibus patet dignitas hominis et excellentia. Hec autem sunt corporis pulcritudo et membrorum aptitudo ... .

Decor: Est decor corporis naturalis ... et decor corporis accidentalis ... .

Dies primo: Est dies nature ... uel est usualis ... .

Dies secvndo: Dicitur dies dominica, quia ea die apparuit Christus esse Dominus ... .

Dies tertio: Ecce mensurabiles posuisti dies meos ... . Sunt itaque dies hominis mensurabiles scilicet modici et modiales ... .

Dives: Est diues pecunia in rota fortune instabiliter sublimatus ... .

Divitie primo: Diuitie mundiales sunt bona temporis benedictio sinistre ... .

Divitie secvndo: Ecce ipsi peccatores et habundantes in seculo optinuerunt diuitias ... optinuerunt per uiolentiam ut fenerator, raptor, impostor ... . Alius diuitias habet per laborem et congregationem ut mercator ... . Alius per hereditatem et successionem ... .

Divitie tertio: Quibusdam dat Deus temporalia ad alliciendum ... . Quibusdam dat ad consolandum ... .

Dens: Dens tetris et aureis scribitur literis. Dicuntur enim dentes maledica uerba et peccatorum principes ... . Dentes sunt catholici predicatores

Delectatio: Est delectatio nature ... culpe ... .

DISCERE PRIMO: Discere debemus ut faciamus ... et ut intelligamus ... .

DISCERE SECVNDO: Discere uel docere ut scias curiositas est et superbia ... . Discere ut bene uiuas et proximum instruas ... prudentia et caritas est ... .

DISCERE TERTIO: Moyses et Esdras docent cerimonialia precepta et iudicia ... . Primordialia et prima rudimenta docent Dauid et Salomon ... . Iohannes baptista docet moralia ... .

DESIDERIVM: Desiderium pauperis est esse in unitate ecclesie ... et liberari a malo presenti ... .

DESIDERIVM MORTIS: Cum Deus festinet in mercedem iusti et properet educere illum de medio iniquitatis ... mortem non inuiti set spontanei suscipiamus ... .

DEXTERA: Dextera dicitur Filius Dei ... . Dicitur et dextera beatitudo eterna ... .

DVRITIA: Est duritia hebetudinis ... . Est duritia ingratitudinis ... .

DESERTVM TERTIO: Quotiens exacerbauerunt eum in deserto, etc. Generaliter in deserto Deum exacerbat quicumque in hoc mundo Deum irritat id est in iram prouocat ... .

DVRITIA SECVNDO: Durus est aliquis ad uerbum Dei sicut lapis ad ferramentum ... .

DILECTIO TERTIO: Est dilectio naturalis communis bonis et malis et indifferens ... . Est dilectio reproba et dampnabilis ... .

DIES QVARTO: Est dies incarnationis et redemptionis, hic est dies gratie ... .

DISSIPATIO: Bona Dei dissipat id est destruit qui non congregat ... .

EGESTAS: Egeni sumus in anima per ignorantiam ... .

ESVRIES: Est esuries corporalis quam legunt pauperes cotidie in libro experientie ... .

EXPECTATIO PRIMO: Est expectatio nature ... et culpe ... .

EXPECTATIO SECVNDO: Expectat homo Deum ut subueniat in tribulatione ... .

EXPECTATIO TERTIO: Expectat homo Deum in tribulatione liberatorem ... in obitu saluatorem ... .

ELEMOSINA PRIMO: Elemosina est arma, lapis, aqua, thesaurus, oleum, unguentum, semen, ubertas, redemptio, merces, fenus, solutio, ala, flos, odor, hostia ... .

ELEMOSINA SECVNDO: Date et dabitur uobis. Videndum quid, cui, uel quantum, quando, cur, quomodo dandum ... .

ERVBESCENTIA: Erubescant impii et deducantur in infernum ... . Impii

ut sic in priuatiuum sunt infideles sine scilicet pietate, id est cultu
Dei ... .

EDVCTIO: Educit Dominus ab iniquitate peccati, a uanitate mundi, ab
affectu carnali ... .

ERROR: Errat homo per infirmitatem ... et per ignorantiam ... .

EXTENSIO: Extendit Ihesus manum ad eripiendum ut Petrum de mari,
ad abluendum ut pedes discipulorum in cena, et ad sanandum ut
ydropicum et leprosum ... et ad iudicandum quasi ad docendum ... .

ESCA: Est esca nature, actualis scilicet et usualis, ad sustentionem nature ... .

EPVLE: Diues epulabatur cotidie splendide. In epulis et conuiuiis
uituperabilia sunt nimia auiditas ... .

ERVCTVARE: Eructabunt labia mea hymnum, etc. Eripe me et sic
eructabo post ereptionem scilicet a malis ... .

EFFVSIO: Est effusio operationis diuine ... et laudis diuine ... .

EXCELSA: Sunt excelsa nature, scilicet naturalia bona, ratio, ingenium,
etc ... .

ELEVATIO MANVS DEI: Eleuat Deus manum comminando ... et per-
cutiendo ... et exhibendo beneficium ... .

EXTOLLERE CORNV: Dixi "Ego Deus": in scripturis, et in predicatoribus
iniquis, id est hiis qui aduersantur equitati, tum iuris naturalis tum
iuris diuini ... .

EXALTATIO: Exaltantur mali in gloria et honore, in potentia et
dominatione, in superbia, elatione, et in diuitiarum possessione ... .

EXVRGERE DEI: Exurgit Deus per aduentum Filii ... et per auxilium ... .

EGRESSVS CHRISTI: Est egressus Christi eternus ... .

EXITVS CHRISTI ET CHRISTIANI: Exit Christus de sinu Patris, ex utero
matris, de actione ad contemplationem ... .

EXALTATIO CHRISTI: Exaltatus est Christus per predicationem ... et
per miraculorum operationem ... .

EXERCITATIO: Est exercitatio corporalis, spiritualis, mixta ... .

EMVLATIO: Emulatio dicitur indignatio ... . Dicitur et inuidia ... .

EQVVS: Equus est animal immundum ... indiscretum ... impetuo-
sum ... .

EXVLTATIO: Exultant iniusti in uoluptate carnali ... . Exultant et in
uanitate mundi ... .

ECCLESIA: Ecclesia ante legem statuta fuit per fidem, sub lege instituta
per eruditionem, tempore gratie constituta per duorum parietum
coniunctionem, id est iudeorum et gentium, in fide Christi conuenien-
tium ... .

EVCHARISTIA: Dominus ait: Caro mea uere est cibus et sanguis meus uere est potus. Hic est cibus pauperum et mitium ... .

EVGE: Est euge irrisorum, quod ex modo proferendi percipitur et ex pronuntiatione dinoscitur ... .

EXCITATIO: Excitatus uel suscitatus est Dominus: In incarnatione, ad redemptionem ... .

ELECTIO DEI: Eligit Dominus pastores, piscatores, simplices, humiles, ignobiles, et minores ... .

ELOQVIVM: Eloquium Domini inflammauit eum. Eloquium est Spiritus sanctus inspirans et misteria reuelans ... .

FIDES PRIMO: Fides est uirginitas ecclesie, quam nisi quisque integram inuiolatamque seruit absque dubio in eternum peribit ... .

FIDES SECVNDO: Fidem Christianam probant scripture, miracula, martiria; roborant rationes; declarant similitudines; predicatio proponit ... .

FIDELIS: Fidelis est Deus in commissis et promissis ... .

FORTITVDO: Est fortitudo nature creantis ... . Et est fortitudo nature create ... .

FIRMAMENTVM: Firmamentum dicitur Deus ... . Dicuntur et apostoli, uirtute ex alto inditi et uerbo Domini firmati et Spiritu oris eius roborati, firmamentum ... .

FVNDAMENTVM: Fundamentum ecclesie dicuntur prophete ... . Fundamenta etiam ecclesie dicuntur apostoli ... .

FONS: Fons dicitur Deus Pater ... . Fons est euangelium uel ecclesiastica predicatio et doctrina ... .

FLVMEN PRIMO: Flumen dicitur tum Pater tum Filius tum Spiritus sanctus ... .

FLVMEN SECVNDO: Quidam sunt extra flumina Babilonis ut mundi contemptores qui corpore et mente mundum relinquunt ... . Quidam sunt super flumina ... .

FILIVS: Dicitur quis filius per naturam ... et per gratiam et adoptionem ... .

FRATRES CHRISTI: Fratres habet Christus secundem carnem ... . Habet etiam fideles fratres per dilectionem ... .

FACIT DEVS: Dicitur Deus facere in materia et in similitudine ... .

FABER: Faber dicitur Deus ... diabolus ... homo bonus ... .

FORNAX: Est fornax nature in quam missi martires uegetiores et puriores exierunt. Est fornax gratie caritas scilicet perfecta ... .

FERRVM: Ferrum dicitur tribulatio ... .

FODERE PRIMO: Incensa igni et suffosa. Est ignis superbie ascendens ... .

FODERE SECVNDO: Fodit Deus uel prelatus ecclesiasticus ut sapiens architectus ... . Fodit diabolus suggerendo ... .

FOVEA: Est fouea actualis in quam deccendit sapientia cum Ioseph ... .

FVR: Est fur actualis scilicet ad litteram ... . Fur est diabolus ... .

FRAVS: Est fraus siue fallacia mala ... . Est fraus licita ... .

FVNES: Funes sunt compedes, uincula, laquei, uel nature ... .

FAMES: Est fames corporalis uel execrabilis ... uel est miserabilis ... .

FESTINATIO PRIMO: Est festinatio peccantis, penitentis, recidiuantis, obedientis, predicantis, impedientis, succurentis, etatis, et temporis ... .

FESTINATIO SECVNDO: Est festinatio nature ... et culpe ... .

FINIS PRIMO: Finis dicitur consumptio ... et consummatio ... .

FINIS SECVNDO:[3] In finem Psalmus Dauid. Sepius hoc nobis inculcat Esdras in titulis Psalmorum ut semper oculum habeamus dextrum in fine consummationis, sinistrum ad finem consumptionis ... .

FORNICATIO: Super illud Apostoli ad Romanos: "Repletos omni iniquitate, fornicatione," dicit Origenes: "Fornicatio est omnis usus carnalis commixtionis preter legittimum connubium." ... .

FVGA: Est fuga corporis, et hec uel est tutele ... uel est cautele ... uel est pietatis et misericordie ... .

FLOS: Flos est gloria, uel uana ... uel uera et stabilis ... .

ITEM FLOS: Est flos sine fructu mundana scilicet felicitas et carnalis prosperitas ... . Est flos cum fructu ... .

ITEM FLOS: Floret homo carnis nitore ... et iuuentute ... .

FLOS QVARTO: Est flos humanus ut iuuentus, et mundanus ut prosperitas, et philosophicus ... et flos theologicus ... .

FOLIA: Folia sunt operimenta mendacii et uerba excusationum ... . Folia sunt uerba pacifica ... .

FACIES: Est facies nature in qua Deo similes creati sumus ... .

FREQVENTATIO ECCLESIE: Frequentamus ecclesiam ut Deum laudemus ... uel ut oremus ... .

FESTVM PRIMO: Qui diem festum agit in puplico sollempnizat, ab opere seruili uacat, Deum laudat ... .

FESTVM SECVNDO: Est festum cogitationis in mentis scilicet iocunditate et cordis hilaritate ... .

GLADIVS: Gladius dicitur ipse Deus, et Filius Dei, et uerbum Dei, et potestas iudiciaria ... .

---

3 Finis secundo *om.* L

GLADIVS SECVNDO: Christus gladius est, cuius capulus ... in crucem terminans humanitas est ... .

GRAVITAS PRIMO: Est grauitas nature corrupte ... et grauitas gratie ... . Est grauitas culpe ... .

GRAVITAS SECVNDO: Est grauitas nature ... gratie ... culpe ... .

GENERATIO PRIMO: Est generatio carnalis uel in utero — hec est conceptio ... uel ex utero — hec est in lucem editio ... .

GENERATIO SECVNDO: Est generatio carnalis omnibus communis qua generamur ad culpam et penam ... .

GEMINATIO: Geminatio notat firmitatem ... ueritatem ... utilitatem ... .

GRANVM PRIMO: Granum frumenti dicitur Christus propter precellentiam ... .

GRANVM SECVNDO: Granum sinapis est predicatio euuangelii, uel fides, uel corpus Christi ... .

GRADVS: Sunt gradus officiorum ... . Sunt gradus dignitatum ... . Sunt gradus premiorum ... .

GLORIA PRIMO: Est gloriatio malorum mala, peior, pessima. Est gloriatio bonorum bona, melior, optima ... .

GLORIA SECVNDO: Glorificat uel clarificat Deus hominem ut homo glorificet Deum ... .

HOMO PRIMO: Homo est sperma uilissimum, uas stercorum, et cibus uermium, umbra, spuma, lutum solidum ... .

HOMO SECVNDO: Homo est dignissima creatura Dei ... .

HVMANA INDIGENTIA: Humana indigentia multiplex est, scilicet infirmitas id est fragilitas ... et ignorantia ... .

HYPOCRITA: Hypocrita est uas uacuum set signatum, calamus extra nitidus intus uacuus, pomum pentapolis ... .

HABVNDANTIA: Est habundantia temporalium ... . Est habundantia spiritualium ... .

HOSTIA PRIMO: Est hostia pro peccato ... . Et est hostia pacifica ... .

HOSTIA SECVNDO: Tollite hostias et introite in atria eius ... . Est autem hostia cordis, oris, operis, et hominis ... .

HONOR PRIMO: Nimis id est ualde honorati sunt amici tui Deus. Amicus quasi animi custos uocatur ... .

HONOR SECVNDO: Honorati sunt amici Domini, id est apostoli, in Domini electione ... .

HONOR TERTIO: Est honor nature ... . Est honor felicitatis mundane ... .

HVMILITAS: Est humilitas in habitu exteriori ... et in uultu ... .

HILARITAS: Hilaritatem mentis parit caritas ... et munditia conscientie ... .

HAMVS: Hamus est Christus ... uerbum ... peccatum ... .

INVITATORIVM: Est inuitatorium superborum ... persecutorum ... luxuriosorum ... .

ILLVMINATIO PRIMO: Dominus illuminatio uel lux mea, contra ignorantie tenebras erroris et culpe ... .

ILLVMINATIO SECVNDO: Faciem tuam illumina super seruum tuum ... . Sol irradiat quod non illuminat, ut cecum ... .

INTELLECTVS: Est intellectus ex auditu mandati ... et ex opere ... .

IEIVNIVM PRIMO: Accesserunt ad Iesum discipuli Iohannis ... et ait illis Iesus: Numquid possunt filii sponsi lugere (Mattheo, et Luca: "ieiunare") quamdiu cum illis est sponsus? Ad huius capituli euidentiam prelibanda sunt hec ... .

IEIVNIVM SECVNDO: Multiplex est ieiunium. Est ieiunium auari propter lucrum, et hypocrite propter fauorem humanum ... .

IEIVNIVM TERTIO: Est ieiunium hypocrite ... . Est auari ... . Est et ieiunium medici ... . Est et christiani ... .

IVGVM: Est iugum diaboli eius scilicet dominatio ... . Est iugum Christi ... .

IVVENTVS: Est iuuentus nature siue etatis ... . Est iuuentus culpe ... .

IVSTITIA: Est iustitia conferens; hec est diuina essentia ... .

INDVMENTVM: Est indumentum corporale, actuale, usuale, quo Christus in paupere induendus est ... .

INDVMENTVM SECVNDO: Sunt indumenta ad tegendam nuditatem corporis, uel ad operienda pudenda, uel contra algorem, uel contra calorem, uel doloris et tristitie, uel iocunditatis et letitie ... .

INDVMENTVM CHRISTI: Confessionem et decorem induisti ... . Dicitur indumentum Christi caro ... et uirtutes ... .

INNOCENTIA: Est innocentia qui nec sibi nec alii nocet, qui nec miserum facit nec miserum deserit ... .

IVDEI: Iudei aspides sunt insidiosa temptatione ... . Leones sunt mortis Christi inclamatione. Torrentes sunt ... .

IVMENTA: Iumenta dicuntur peccatores propter stoliditatem ... .

INGRATITVDO: Ingratus dicitur qui sibi tribuit quod ex se non habet, ut philosophi dicentes, labia nostra a nobis sunt ... .

IGNORANTIA DEI: Dicitur Deus ignorare uel nescire aliquid per experientiam ... et Deus ignorare secundum hominis opinionem ... .

INIMICVS: Habemus inimicum contra nos scilicet carnem propriam ... iuxta nos scilicet proximum ... .

INIQVITAS: Ab omnibus iniquitatibus meis erue me ... . Est enim iniquitas uenialis ... occulta ... .

ILLVSIO: Illudit et illuditur Deus, diabolus, homo bonus, et homo malus ... .

ILLVSIO SECVNDO: Draco iste quem formasti ad illudendum ei ... . Illuditur autem diabolo ... .

IRA DEI PRIMO: Irascitur Deus bonis corripiendo ... . Irascitur et malis non ulciscendo ... et malis hic puniendo ... .

IRA SECVNDO: Est ira zelantis in corde ... . Et hec quandoque prorumpit in uocem ... .

IVDICIVM PRIMO: Iudicabunt cum Domino patriarche et prophete et apostoli ... .

IVDICIVM SECVNDO: Est iudicium discretionis hic animo et merito, in futuro etiam loco ... .

IVDICIVM TERTIO: Quia neque ab oriente neque ab occidente, etc.; Gregorius iudicium falci comparatur ... .

INFERNVS: Infernus, herebus, auernus, tartarus, orcus, gehenna, baratrum idem est ... .

IGNIS: Ignis dicitur Deus ... . Ignis Filius Dei ... .

INCREPATIO: Increpat Deus reprehendendo et terrendo ... .

INDIGENTIA: Humana indigentia multiplex est, scilicet infirmitas id est fragilitas ... .

IN IVSTIS EST DEVS: Deus est in iustis per inhabitantem gratiam ... . In qualibet re est per essentiam ... .

ID IPSVM: Est id ipsum culpe, ut uanitatis et erroris, sicut in hereticis ... .

IN LIBRO VITE SCRIBETVR ALIQVIS: Dicitur aliquis scriptus in libro uite, id est notitia Dei, per predestinationem ... uel per presentem iustitiam ... .

IRE AD DEVM: Dicitur aliquis ire ad Deum, id est ad similitudinem Dei ... . Dicit et usualiter amicus amico recedenti, "ad Deum uadas," hoc est in Dei custodiam ... .

INVITATORIVM SECVNDO: Inuitat Christus ad conuiuium et requiem ... .

LIBERTAS: Est libertas nature. De iure nature omnes liberi sunt ... .

LAVS DEI PRIMO: Videndum est qualiter laudandus sit Deus, quantum uel quotiens, qui ydonei sint laudare, quando uel quare ... .

LAVS DEI SECVNDO: Omnes creature creatorem laudant, uel immediate ut rationalis creatura, angelus, homo ... uel mediate ut irrationalia et inanimata ... .

LAVS: Laudem debitam uel plenam impediunt grauedo carnis, cura temporalium, consortium malorum, fomes peccati, suggestio diaboli, imperfectio cognitionis ... .

LAVDIS DEFECTVS: Deficiunt in quibusdam laudes Dei propter eorum iniquitatem ... .

LACVS: Est lacus nature ... gratie ... .

LVTVM: Est lutum nature condite uel corrupte ... . Est caro nostra lutum ... .

LIQVEFACTIO PRIMO: Liquefactio fit per solem, uentum, calorem, amaritudinem ... . Ita et per Christum et per Spiritum sanctum liquefiunt peccata ... .

LIQVEFACTIO SECVNDO: Liquefacta est terra ... . Liquefit anima ad uerbi iocunditatem ... .

LIBIDO: Libido in Leuitico est ulcus in cute, lepra in carne, frangens et deformans ... .

LAQVEVS: Laqueus est prelatus malus ... . Laqueus est mulier praua ... .

LABOR PRIMO: Est corporalis uel spiritualis labor culpe, nature, pene, gratie ... .

LABOR SECVNDO: Laborauit Christus cordis anxietate super obstinatione perfidorum, super incredulitate infidelium et duritia cordis ... .

LABOR TERTIO: Est labor nature ... et culpe triplex — cordis, oris, operis ... .

LEO: Leo tetris et aureis scribitur litteris, hoc est et in bono et in malo accipitur ... .

LVNA: Luna dicitur ecclesia ... .

LACRIME PRIMO: Sunt lacrime nature, gratie, fortune, culpe, pene ... .

LACRIME SECVNDO: Lacrima est aqua ignem seu gehennalem seu purgatorium extinguens ... .

LACRIME TERTIO: Lacrime culpe sunt uel libidinis ... uel sunt inuidie et indignationis ... .

LIBERARE DE TRIBVLATIONE: Liberat Deus iustos a tribulatione, ne scilicet penam sentiant ... .

LEVARE PRIMO: Leuat iustus ad Deum oculos ... . Leuat et uocem ... .

LEVARE SECVNDO: Erige aures ad uerbi Dei auditionem. Leua oculos interiores per spiritualium rimationem et celestium contemplationem ... .

LOQVI:[4] Credidi propter quod loqutus sum ... . Tacent quidam ex timore ... uel pudore ... .

LIBER: Est liber nature duplex, scilicet uisibilis creatura ... uel inuisibilis memorie ... .

4 Loqui] Laquea L

Scribi in libro vite: Dicitur aliquis scriptus in libro uite, id est notitia Dei, per predestinationem ... [as above, In libro vite scribetur aliquis].

Lex:[5] Calix in manu Domini est lex ordinata in manu mediatoris, id est in potestate Christi, ut staret dum uellet uel cessaret cum uellet ... .

Lvcerna: Lucerna dicitur Christus ... . Dicuntur etiam sancti lucerne ... .

Item Lvcerna: Lucerna uerbi uiam ostendit ut columpna nubis et ignis ... .

Lac: Est lac malorum ut praua suasio, blanda adulatio ... .

Lavs Dei: Ego autem semper sperabo et adiciam super omnem laudem tuam. Inter spem et timorem tanquam inter duas molas moli debet omnis Christianus ut fiat esibilis Deo ... .

Materia lavdis: Sumitur quandoque materia laudis a diuina essentia ... . Quandoque ex operibus spiritualibus ... .

Lignvm:[6] Lignum dicitur homo ... . Sunt autem ligna campi: rustici, mites, et humiles ... . Sunt et ligna paradisi ... .

Mensa: Est mensa figure spiritualem refectionem presignans non prestans, hec est mensa tabernaculi ... .

Mandvcatio: Est manducatio corporalis quam cotidie legimus in libro experientie ... .

Mvltiplicatio: Multiplicantur mali numerositate personarum, quia "multi uocati." ... .

Manvs: Est manus beneficia, ut manus Dei ad nos missa, sanans, erigens, sustentans, producens, inducens, et remunerans ... .

Mensvra: Est mensura siue peritoria fidei ... sicut Deus diuisit mensuram fidei et caritatis ... .

Commvtatio: Est commutatio Christi prima in incarnatione ... .

Mvndvs: Mundus in maligno positus spiritualis est Egiptus, Jerico, Sodoma, Babilon, forum, stadium, exilium, stabulum ... .

Macvla: Est macula corporis ... . Macula ecclesie mali sunt ... .

Mons: Mons dicitur diuinitas ... . Mons dicitur Pater ... .

Mane: Est mane mundi ... . Est et mane temporis ... .

Martires: Martires sunt in ueteri testamento qui pro lege Dei mortui sunt ... .

Martires secvndo: Ait chorus martirum, "testimonia tua meditatio mea est." Grece martiria que meditata mitigant dolores ... .

---

5 Lex] Calix *L*
6 Lignum] Lingnum *L*; *positum est post* testamenta *in* CL.

Mvtvs: Mutus est quis ex casuali infirmitate, ignorantia, erubescentia, cupiditate, timore, impotentia ... .

Mors: Mors dicitur dissolutio corporis et anime, secundum phisicos uero extinctio uitalis caloris in corde ... .

Mors secvndo: Mors est falx qua homo mane sicut herba secta transeat, etc. Hic est cetus absorbens tandem euomens ... .

Mors Christi: Mors Christi dicitur sompnus siue dormitio propter spontaneam eius uoluntatem ... .

Mare primo: Mare mundus est ... . Hec mare tempestuosum est aduersitate, salsum est amaritudine uel sterilitate ... .

Mare secvndo: Alii sunt supra mare, scilicet mariambuli, ut mundi contemptores ... .

Mirabilis Devs: Mirabilis Deus in sanctis suis. Mirabilis est Deus in se ... in sapientia ... misericordia ... .

Misericordia primo: Misericordia Dei magna est in se ... magna etiam apparet in effectu ... .

Misericordia secvndo: In uia est misericordia Dei flagellans et corrigens ... .

Misericordia tertio: Misericordia quandoque dicitur eternitas dans misericordiam ... . Quandoque miseratio, id est effectus misericordie quantum ad nos accipientes ... .

Misericordia qvarto: Misericordia Dei magna est ... in essentia ... in potentia ... .

Misericordia qvinto: Est misericordia parua, ut in collatione bonorum corporis ... . Misericordia maior est in corporum glorificatione ... .

Memoranda in mandatis Dei svnt qvatvor: In mandatis Dei quatuor sunt consideranda: Auctoritas precipientis ... .

Memor: Memor esse debet homo officii sui, presertim prelatus ... .

Memor secvndo: Dominus memor est bonorum in presenti benefaciendo ... .

Magnificatio Christi: Domine Deus meus magnificatus ... . Deus non magnificatur in se set in nobis id est in cognitione nostra et dilectione ... .

Maria Magdalena: Maria Magdalena non apparuit uacua coram Domino. Detulit in corde fidem, in ore deuotionem ... .

Mvlieris prerogativa: Multiplex est prerogatiua et excellentia mulieris. Attenditur enim dignitas mulieris in hoc quod prima mulier de materia digniore et uenustiore formata est ... .

Medicina primo: Officium medicine siue effectus primus est morbum sanare, secundus sanum saniorem efficere, tertius sanitatem conseruare, quartus sanitatem confirmare ... .

MEDICINA SECVNDO: Non curatur homo uel propter imperitiam medici ... uel propter inutilitatem et inefficaciam medicine ... .

MANSVETVDO: Humilitatem et mansuetudinem coniungit Dominus dicens, "Super quem requiescet spiritus meus nisi super humilem et quietum," id est mansuetum ... .

MEDIVM: Est medium communitatis ... . Est medium manifestationis ... . Est medium equalis distantie ab extremis ... .

MEMORIA HOMINIS: Duplex est memoria, pungitiua et exhilaratiua ... .

ITEM MEMORIA HOMINIS: Homo memor esse debet opificis et operum id est creatoris et creaturarum ... .

SEX MEMORANDA: Rememorari debemus peccatum proprium ... et Dei preceptum ... .

NOMEN DEI: Nomen Dei dicitur Filius Dei ... et gloria et honor Domini ... .

NOBISCVM DEVS: Deus nobiscum est consortio nature ... et cooperatione ... et presentia carnis ... .

NOVACVLA: Nouacula dicitur persecutor ... . Est et nouacula suggestio diaboli ... .

NEGOTIATIO: Est negotiatio actualis, usualis, circa commercia rerum temporalium, multas sollicitudines afferens et animam a Deo retrahens ... .

NVMERATIO: Numerat Deus discernendo siue distinguendo ... et disponendo ... .

NECESSITAS: Sunt neccesitates corporis ... ut esurire, sitire, et huiusmodi ... .

NOVVM: Nouus rex, noua lex, noua facta sunt omnia ... . Nouitas fuit in Christi incarnatione ... .

NOTVM: Dexteram tuam sic notam fac, id est propitiationem, eam nobis exhibendo; Christum, eum clarificando; eternam beatitudinem, eam nobis conferendo ... .

NVBES PRIMO: Est nubes nature actualis scilicet et corporalis ... . Est nubes culpe ... .

NVBES SECVNDO: Nubes dicuntur predicatores propter eleuationem, discursum, irrigationem, et refrigerationem ... .

NOX PRIMO: Nox dicitur tribulatio et aduersitas ... .

NOX SECVNDO: Nox presens seculum dicitur ... .

OLIVA PRIMO: Ego autem sicut oliua fructifera etc. Verba sunt populi fidelis ... .

OLIVA SECVNDO: Olea arbor est, fructus oliua, succus oleum. Quandoque tamen arbor oliua dicitur ... .

OLEVM: Est oleum adulationis ... . Oleum etiam dicitur delectatio peccati ... .

OLLA: Deus quasi figulus est ... . Est et olla tribulationis ebulliens et feruens ... .

ORATIO PRIMO: Oratio uentus est, auicula, thus, thimiamata. Hic est uentus urens, siccans mare rubrum ... .

ORATIO SECVNDO: Oratio efficax et uiolenta iures exercet in celo. Precibus publicani uincitur Deus ... .

ORATIO TERTIO: Oratio infima iacet cum pro terrenis fit ... .

ORATIO QVARTO: In tribulatione maius est desiderium orantis ... et gratior misericordia exaudientis ... .

ORATIO QVINTO: Ego uero orationem meam — ad te Domine, supple — dirigebam. Directionem autem et uiam parant orationi, penitentia, elemosina, abstinentia, et continentia ... .

ORATIO SEXTO: Quare oratio non exaudiatur cause sunt indignitas, indiscretio, maior hominis utilitas, et iusta Dei uoluntas ... .

ODOR: Odor dicitur uirtus ... . Odor etiam dicitur opus ... .

OBEDIENTIA: Est obedientia necessaria qua tenetur subditus obedire prelato intuitu subiectionis etsi non respectu presidentis, consideratione tamen preficientis id est Dei ... .

OBLIGATIO: Est obligatio nature corrupte qua primi parentes obligant nos originali peccato ... .

OPERA DEI: Memor fui operum Dei ... . Sunt opera potentie, opera nature scilicet opera creationis ... .

OCCIDIT DEVS: Occidit Deus animam a corpore separando ... . Occidit et gratiam subtrahendo quasi uitam uirtutis perimendo id est non conseruando ... .

OCVLI: Oculi mei semper ad Dominum ... . Oculi sapientis in capite eius; caput uiri Christus. Oculi stultorum in finibus terre ... . Oculi interiores sunt ratio et intellectus ... .

OS: Per os quod est hostium corporis duo egrediuntur scilicet sputum et uerbum ... . Per os duo ingrediuntur ... .

OBSCVRITAS SCRIPTVRE: Apostolus de Hebreis loquens ... "Hec omnia in figura contingebant illis." ... Tum propter rei magnitudinem ... .

OTIVM CORPORIS: Est otium corporis et negligentie ... . Est otium uoluptatis et luxurie ... . Est otium contemplationis et sapientie ... .

OBLIVIO: Est obliuio peccantis ... . Est obliuio penitentis ... .

PASSIO CHRISTI PRIMO: Passio Christi dicitur calix ... et potio iocunda ... et potio amara ... .

PASSIO CHRISTI SECVNDO: Passio Christi seu martiris dicitur calix, continens pro contento id est potio calida, iocunda, amara, mensurata, cito transiens ... .

PASSIO CHRISTI TERTIO: Christus est holocaustum passus in corpore et anima ... .

PRETIVM: Est pretiositas uel pretium nature ... . Est et pretium culpe ... .

PERSECVTIO: Multi qui persequntur me ... . Vox est generalis iusti id est ecclesie. Sunt autem multi, nam tyranni ... heretici ... .

ITEM PERSECVTIO: Persequntur Absolom Dauid, Iudas Christum, falsi fratres ecclesiam, illiciti motus animam ... .

TERTIO PERSECVTIO: Percutit Deus debilitando ... . Percutit Deus temporaliter puniendo ... .

PAVPERTAS: Ego sum pauper et dolens. Christus pauper fuit substantia ... et pauper spiritu, id est humilis ... .

PATIENTIA: Patientia prima est cum quis equanimiter sustinet reddi sibi malum pro malo ... .

PARATVS: Paratus sum et non sum turbatus ... . Paratus est iustus ad custodiam mandatorum, ad tolerantiam aduersorum, ad credendum et confitendum, ad operandum et proficiendum, ad legis diuine inuestigationem et ad predicationem ... .

PEREGRINVS: Sancti dicuntur hic peregrini propter laborem quem sustinent ... et propter paupertatem ... .

PERFECTIO PRIMO: Sicut tres sunt limites numerorum scilicet denarius, centenarius, millenarius, ita et triplex est perfectio. Prima est sufficientie que est in obseruatione decalogi ... .

PERFECTIO SECVNDO: Est perfectio comprehensionis scilicet intelligentie ... . Est et perfectio apprehensionis scilicet gratie ... .

PECCATOR: Dicitur quis peccator pro originali ... et pro pronitate peccandi ... .

PECCATVM PRIMO: Opposuisti nubem ne transeat oratio. Hec sunt minora mortalia peccata que tamen afflatu spiritus dissoluuntur ... .

PECCATVM SECVNDO: Peccatum supra hominem est, infra, iuxta, circa, coram, contra, post ... .

PECCATVM TERTIO: Quidam peccant ex adipe id est habundantia ... . Quidam peccant ex macie id est inopia ... .

PERIRE: Perit aliquid per errorem ... et per desitionem ... .

DE PENIS GEHENNALIBVS: Sunt autem pene gehennales separatio a consortio sanctorum, attenuatio, miseria scilicet et inopia, carentia uisionis Dei, tenebre, fames et sitis, ardor et algor, fetor, dolor, exprobratio demonium ... .

PROFVNDVM: Est profundum Dei, scripture, hominis, diaboli ... .

PVTEVS: Est puteus Deus, Dei, seculum, seculi, homo, hominis, diaboli ... .

EFFECTVS PECCATI: Peccata grauant, inquinant, uilificant, laborem, dolorem, et uermem conscientie procreant ... .

EFFECTVS PECCATI SECVNDO:

> Aggrauat et fedat peccatum uilificatque
> Mestificat, lassat, corrodit, pungit et urit,
> Obruit atque ligat, tundit, cecat perimitque ... .

EFFECTVS PECCATI TERTIO: Ex continuatione peccatorum subrepit contemptus ... et desperatio ... .

EFFECTVS PECCATI QVARTO: Peccata concludunt et comprehendunt, inquinant et ligant, spoliant et uulnerant, excecant et necant ... .

PENITENTIA PRIMO: Beati quorum remisse sunt iniquitates gratis scilicet a Deo dicente, "Ego sum qui deleo iniquitates." ... .

PENITENTIA SECVNDO: Pro hac orabit ad te omnis sanctus. Pro remissione scilicet facta, et pro impietate tollenda ... .

PENITENTIA TERTIO: Penitenti necessaria sunt dolor, erubescentia, confessio, satisfactio, timor ... .

PENITENTIA QVARTO: Penitentia est principium sermonis tum precursoris tum saluatoris tum apostolorum. Aiunt enim Iohannes et Dominus in initio predicationis sue: Penitentiam agite ... . Hec est uia Domini ... uia recta ... arta uia ... .

PENITENTIA QVINTO: Conuertimini simul in corpore et anima ad me ... in ieiunio sanctificato et fletu ... .

ITEM PENITENTIA:[7] Penitens dolere debet, et dolere et gaudere, confundi et confidere, timere et sperare, satisfacere, perseuerare ... .

ITEM PENITENTIA: Similis factus sum pellicano, etc. Verba sunt penitentis in Psalmo penitentiali. Penitens itaque pellicanus macer est abstinentia.

ITEM PENITENTIA: Si dicebam motus est pes meus, etc. Insinuatur hic qualiter agenda sit penitentia, scilicet per oris confessionem ... .

PENITENTIA: Venite adoremus et procidamus ante Deum (uel Dominum), etc ... . Dauid penitere docet exemplo et uerbo ... .

ITEM PENITENTIA: Penitenti necessaria est oris confessio, carnis maceratio, et societatis malorum deuitatio, uigilie, peccati recordatio et lamentatio, humilitas cordis, sedulitas operis, crebra oratio seu gratiarum actio ... .

---

7 Item Pentitentia ... Pulvis *om. CL; add. Cambridge, Trinity College* MS *B.16.18 (392).*

ITEM PENITENTIA: Similis factus sum pellicano, etc. Verba sunt penitentis in Psalmo penitentiali. Penitens pellicanus est triduo contritionis, confessionis et satisfactionis ... .

EXEMPLA PENITENTIE: Exemplaria penitentium sunt Adam, Dauid, Magdalena, Petrus, Paulus ... .

PVLVIS: Puluis multitudinem significat ... . Puluis modicitas dicitur ... etiam dicitur subtilitas intellectus ... .

PVTREDO: Est putredo nature corrupte ... . Est et putredo casualis in rebus ... .

PENNE PRIMO: Habet iustus alas gemine dilectionis ... . Habet et iustus pennas aliarum uirtutum ... .

PENNE SECVNDO: Quis dabit mihi pennas sicut columbe. Et nomine et re uox Christi est, qui habet pennas defensionis et protectionis, occultationis, calefactionis et fomenti ... .

POTESTAS: Potestas dicitur ipse potens et id unde quis potest, dignitas, prelatio, excellentia, dominium, uis naturalis ... .

PREROGATIVA PAVLI: Prerogatiua et excellentia Pauli consistit in mirabili eius conuersione, in eximia humilitate, serena uirginitate, multiplici labore, in misteriorum cognitione, in doctrine profusione et profunditate, in martirii claritate ... .

PRELATVS ECCLESIE: Sunt in ecclesia pastores humiles qui potius uolunt ministrare quam ministrari ... . Sunt et mercenarii ... .

PREDICATOR: Predicatori necessaria sunt honestas conuersationis et claritas bone opinionis et excellentia utriusque, puritas etiam intentionis, copia scientie, strenuitas officii, et discretio predicationis ... .

PREDICATIO PRIMO: Est predicatio fallax et subdola ... . Est uana et superba ... . Est et questiosa ... . Est et predicatio officiosa, pertinens scilicet ad officium prelati ... .

PETITIO: Voce mea ad Dominum clamaui ... . Et notentur hic que in petitione attendenda scilicet sunt discretio petitionis ... .

PANIS: In pane attenduntur tria: farina, aqua, et ignis quo coquitur. Farina est bona operatio ... .

PRINCIPES PRIMO: Sunt principes terrarum rectores corporum ... . Sunt principes ecclesiarum rectores animarum ... .

PRINCIPES SECVNDO: Sunt principes angeli boni ... et angeli mali ... et homines boni ... .

PROSPERITAS: Est prosperitas temporalis pluribus nociua ... . Prudentibus uero qui sciunt habundare et penuriam pati utilis est et congrua prosperitas temporalis ... .

PRIVILEGIATA: Plura priuilegiata precelsa pollent prerogatiua: Deus trinitas pre omnibus diis ... .

Plvvia: Est pluuia nature ... . Est pluuia miraculosa ... .

Pingvedo: Est pinguedo terrena ... . Est pinguedo carnalis ... .

Pver: Puer etate ... . Est puer humilitate, innocentia, puritate ... .

Prolongatio: Est prolongatio culpe ... . Et est prolongatio pene ... .

Pietas: Est pietas nature increate ... . Est pietas nature create ... .

Protegit Devs: Protegit Dominus uitam nature ... et uitam gratie ... .

Protegit Devs secvndo: Protegit nos Deus contra pericula ne incurramur, contra tormenta ne succumbamus ... .

Pro: Est *pro* locale ... materiale causale ... .

Prope: Dicitur autem Deus prope esse per naturam ... et per misericordiam ... et per penitentiam ... .

Parvitas: Est paruitas nature ... . Est et paruitas gratie ... .

Par vel paritas: Vocabulum paritatis siue equalitatis puta nomen uel aduerbium ... designatiuum est equalitatis, communitatis, aggregationis, conformitatis ... .

Pes: Pedes Dei dicuntur apostoli ... . Pedes sunt ministri ... .

Propitivs: Propitius est Deus peccanti ... ad conuersionem expectando ... et penam differendo ... .

Predicatio secvndo: Bucinate in neomenia tuba ... . Buccina id est tuba predicatio est. Videndum igitur qui debent buccinare, quales, qualiter, et quando, et quis sit effectus siue utilitas buccinationis ... .

Qverere Devm: Queritur Deus per fidem et sacramentorum susceptionem ... . Exquiritur per scientiam, cognitionem et contemplationem ... .

Qvies pigritie: Est quies pigritie ... . Est quies innocentie ... .

Redimit Devs: Redimit Deus per causam et per effectum ... .

Redemptio: Copiosa aput Dominum redemptio propter misericordie habundantiam ... et propter pretii sufficientiam ... .

Remissio peccati: Remittitur peccatum per sacramentum, martirium, fidem, misericordiam, caritatem, orationem, et forsan per pontificalem relaxationem ... .

Remissio peccati secvndo: Beati quorum remisse sunt iniquitates, in contritione ut Magdalena in confessione ut latro et Dauid ... .

Reqvisitio sangvinis: Requirit Deus sanguinem id est ultionem propter effusionem sanguinis de manu interficientis ... .

Retribvtio: Retribuit Dominus peccantibus presertim superbis et obstinatis ... .

REFRIGERIVM: Transiuimus per ignem et aquam et eduxisti nos in refrigerium. Est refrigerium a pena temporali in uia; hoc est solacium temporalium ... .

RESVRRECTIO:

Corpora quod surgent declarant uerba, figure,
Exemplum, simile, ratioque fides generalis
Sponsio ueracis ac summa potentia Christi ... .

RENVNTIARE: Renuntiare debemus peccato ueniali uoluntate etsi non possumus omnino re. ...

REDVCTIO: De abyssis terre, id est de profundis concupiscentie ter-renorum, uel concupiscentie carnis que terra est et in terram ibit ... .

REVERSIO: Titulus Psalmi cxi habet, "Alleluia, reuersionis Aggei et Zacharie." ... Est autem reuersio in baptismo ... .

RENOVATIO PRIMO: Emitte Spiritum tuum sanctum paraclitum, et eo immisso creabuntur homines in bonis operibus ... . Renouat autem Dominus in baptismo ... .

RENOVATIO SECVNDO: Templum Dei sanctum est quod estis uos. Hoc templum renouatur in presenti per gratiam ... .

RECEDERE: Recedit Deus per gratie subtractionem ... et per flagelli suspensionem ... .

ROBVR: Est robur nature quo quis male utitur ... . Est robur nature quo quis bene utitur ... .

REVELATIO: Christus est lumen ad reuelationem gentium. Et dextera manus Patris iam aperta est ... . Reuelatus est Christus per incarna-tionem et natiuitatem ... .

REPVLSIO: Deus repulisti nos et destruxisti nos, etc ... . Repellit Deus bonos, id est passionibus exponit ... .

RESPONDERE: Christi precentor est cui respondendum est ... in concordia caritatis per patientiam ... .

RESPICERE: Quandoque respicimus terram propter humilitatem ... .

ROS: Ero quasi ros ... . Ros Spiritus sanctus est ... .

ROTA: Rota in rota. Mandata enim noui testamenti continentur in ueteris testamenti exemplis, uel uerbis figuralibus, uel moralibus, uel metaforicis, uel manifestis ... .

REGES: Sunt reges animarum prelati scilicet ecclesie ... . Sunt et reges tenebrarum, umbrarum, uitiorum ... .

REGERE: Qui regis Israel intende. Christus tum per se tum per rectores ecclesie regit Israel id est uidentes se ... .

RVMOR: Reperiuntur in sacra scriptura uarii rumores, alii boni qui letificant, alii mali qui mestificant ... .

Rota secvndo: Est rota nature, id est uolubilitas huius uite ... . Est rota fortune ... . Est rota scripture ... .

Respondere secvndo: Abel qui luctus uel uapor interpretatur precentor est lamenti, cui respondeat penitens ... . Christus autem precentor est gaudii ... .

Redemptio tertio: Redimit Christus per causam in cruce ... . Redimit per effectum in conuersione. per fidem, per contritionem ut baptismo uel penitentia, imperium iustificando ... .

Regio: Est regio longinqua dissimilitudinis ... . Regio etiam dicitur infernus ... .

Sacra scriptvra: Sacra scriptura gazophilatium est, thesauro sapientie et scientie plenum ... .

Qvot modis Moyses scripsit de Christo: Dominus ait, "Si crederetis Moysi, crederetis forsitan et mihi." ... Scripsit autem Moyses de Christo locutione dubia siue obscura, ad litteram etiam et manifeste ... .

Sacrificivm legis: Est sacrificium nociuum, spontaneum, pacificum seu salutare ... .

Sacrificia legis: Sacrificia legis non uult sibi Deus offerri ... quia non sunt ei necessaria ... .

Sacrificia oris: Sacrificia oris sunt confessio, oratio, laus, lectio, disputatio, predicatio, et huiusmodi ... .

Sabbatvm: Est sabbatum temporis quod septem dierum reuolutione sepius iteratur ... . Est sabbatum pectoris ... .

Silentivm: Est silentium hominis bonum ... . Est silentium hominis malum ... .

Stvltitia: Tres sunt stultitie generales et admirande que seculares fere uniuersos inuoluunt. Vna est quod nemo sibi pene cauet alterius exemplo, cum unius ruina alterius sit doctrina ... .

Stercora: Stercora sunt peccatores ... peccata ... carnales uoluptates ... .

Simvlacra: Simulacra siue ydola dicuntur ymagines ... . Dicuntur et idola uitia, ut auaritia ... .

Svrditas: Est surditas corporalis dupplex, ut uel fortuite infirmitatis, uel nature deficientis ... .

Svperbia: In curru superbie quatuor rote sunt: contemptus Dei, et contemptus proximi, contemptus proprie subiectionis, contemptus ecclesiastice institutionis ... .

Sompnvs primo: Est sompnus nature ... et culpe ... .

Sompnvs secvndo: Mors dicitur sompnus propter pausationem uel corporis uel anime uel utriusque ... .

SOMPNVS TERTIO: Mors Christi dicitur sompnus siue dormitio propter spontaneam eius uoluntatem ... .

SPERNERE: Spreuisti omnes discedentes a iudiciis tuis, etc. Spernit Deus non uisitando ... affligendo ... .

SPERNERE DEI SECVNDO: Spreuisti uel ad nichilum deduxisti omnes discedentes a iudiciis tuis. Penam adnichilat in bono ... . Peccatum etiam adnichilat ... .

SERVITVS: Quidam sunt serui diaboli ... . Quidam sunt serui Dei ... .

SITIS: Cucurri in siti. Est sitis defectus ... . Est et sitis affectus ... .

SENECTVS: Est senectus nature, culpe, gratie. Est enim senectus etatis: desipientie, maturitatis; et hec uel est scientie uel morum ... .

SEPVLCRVM: Est sepulcrum corporale ... . Et est sepulcrum culpe ... .

SEPARATIO PRIMO: Est separatio loco uel animo, in presenti uel in futuro, generalis uel particularis ... .

SEPARATIO SECVNDO: Separatio quedam loco fit, quedam animo, quedam in presenti ... [a longer version of the previous distinction]

SVRGERE PRIMO: Exurge gloria mea ... . Exurge potenter quasi ab imo ad altum, a morte ad immortalitatem ... .

SVRGERE SECVNDO: Exurgat Deus per aduentum Filii ... . Exurrexit Deus Christus in resurrectione ... .

SVRGERE TERTIO: Surge a lecto, id est carnis uoluptate ... .

SOLITVDO: Errauerunt in solitudine. Est solitudo corporis et solitudo mentis ... . Est solitudo iudeorum et est solitudo gentium ... .

SCRVTINIVM: Est scrutinium explorantis ad temptandum et decipiendum, hoc diaboli est ... . Est scrutinium examinantis, ut in consecratione episcopi ... . Est scrutinium penitentis ... .

SVSCIPIT DEVS HOMINEM: Suscipe me Domine ... . Suscipit Deus hominem in prima conuersione, paruulum quidem per baptismum ... .

SVSCIPIT HOMO DEVM: Suscipit autem homo Deum in incarnatione, sic suscepit beata Virgo ... . Suscepit et cum susceptorem in sacramenti altaris participatione ... .

SVAVITAS: Suauis est Deus bonis in exemplo, promisso, et premio, precepto ... .

STARE DEI: Stat Deus per manifestationem, unde: Deus, factus homo scilicet, stetit in sinagoga deorum ... . Et nos in lectione euuangelii stamus tum scilicet obedire, et ministrare parati ... tum uerba euuangelica ad bellum contra mundum, carnem, diabolum, excitati ... .

SEDES DEI: Est sedes Dei scilicet angeli, qui sedes super cherubim ... . Sedes etiam deitatis corpus Christi proprium ... .

SESSIO: Est sessio humilitatis uel penitentialis uel alicuius tribulationis seu deuotionis ... .

STATVS: Status presens gratie melior apparet quam status paradisi fuisset quo scilicet ad humani generis excellentiam ... .

SAL: Sal dicitur humana sapientia ... . Sal sterilitatem innuit ... .

SAGITTA: Sagitta Christus est ... . Sagitta est euuangelista ... .

SOL: Sol dicitur corpus solare ... . Sol dicitur claritas solis ... .

STELLE: Stelle dicuntur sancti ... .

SONVS: Est sonus penitentie et confessionis ... . Est sonus predicationis ... .

SEMEN: Semen inspiratum est gratia, seminatum uerbum Dei, operatum uoluntas ... .

STATERA: Est statera negotiationis actualis et usualis. Est statera negotiationis spiritualis ... .

SANGVIS: Sanguis et sanguinarius dicitur homicida spiritualis et corporalis ... .

SANGVINIS REQVISITIO: Requirit Dominus sanguinem de manu occisoris ... et de manu prelati ... et de subdito ... .

SANGVIS CHRISTI: Christus sanguine suo nos redemit ... .

SIMILITVDO: Est similitudo nature increate id est diuine ... . Est similitudo creationis siue nature create ... .

SALVS TEMPORALIS: Est salus temporalis, communis bonis et malis, in presenti ... . Est spiritualis interna scilicet remissio peccatorum siue iustificatio ... .

SPES: Spes dicitur confidentia siue presumptio ... . Spes dicitur pia et deuota expectatio glorie future ... .

SALTVS: De sponso dicit sponsa in Canticis, "Ecce uenit saliens in montibus transcendens colles." Christus enim omnes sanctos excedens ... exiliens de celo in uirginis uterum, de utero in presepe, de presepi in crucem ... .

SATIETAS: Est satietas mala, ut que castrimargie est ... . Est et satietas bona ... .

SPERNERE DEVS TERTIO: Spernit Deus hominem a facie sua eiciendo ... .

SINGVLARITAS: Est in Deo singularitas Domini et excellentie ... . Est in diabolo singularitas elationis et superbie ... .

SVAVITAS: Suauis et dulcis est Dominus in reficiendo ... in instruendo ... .

SAGENA: Est sagena bona ... est sagena bona et mala ... .

TEMPTATIO PRIMO: Temptat Deus Abraham et Iohannem ... Iob et Tobiam ... . Diabolus Euam et Christum de tribus uitiis principalibus,

scilicet concupiscentia carnis, concupiscentia oculorum, superbia uite ... .

TEMPTATIO SECVNDO: Temptat Deus hominem probando et manifes-
tando, sic Abraham eius fidem et obedientiam ostendendo ... .

TEMPTATIO TERTIO: Est modica temptatio qua non mouetur homo ... .
Est et temptatio qua mouetur homo uenialiter ... .

TEMPTATIO QVARTO: Temptatio in sola suggestione est ad profectum ... .

THESAVRVS PRIMO: Thesaurus absconditus in agro Christus est ... .

THESAVRVS SECVNDO: Est thesaurus pecunie de quo filii non thesaurizant
parentibus ... . Est thesaurus culpe uel pene ... .

THESAVRVS TERTIO: Est thesaurus pecunie ... . Est thesaurus sapientie ... .

TABERNACVLVM: Tabernaculum dicitur ecclesia presens in qua militamus
et dimicamus. Mundus, caro, demonia diuersa mouent prelia ... .

TEMPLVM PRIMO: Templum dicitur illud salomonicum in Regum et
in Paralipomenon edificatum ... .

TEMPLVM SECVNDO: Est templum Dei materiale, terrenum, actuale,
manuale ... . Est et templum celeste ... .

TRANSIRE: Est transitus Dei, diaboli, mundi, hominis, uel anime ... .

TRANSITVS: Est transitus de malo ad bonum, de uitio ad uirtutem ... .

TRANSILIENS: Generalis yditum id est transiliens eos scilicet habitantes
in terra ... . Hic inquam yditum Christus est de quo scriptum est, "Ecce
iste uenit saliens in montibus, transiliens colles." ... .

TRANSCENDERE: De summo yditum, id est Christo, scriptum est, "Ecce
uenit saliens ... ." Saltus quidem de celo fecit in uterum, de utero in
presepe, de cruce in sepulcrum, de sepulcro rediit in celum ... .

TOLLERE: Dicitur aliquid tolli, id est de loco ad locum transferri ...
et in altum ferri ... .

TEMPORA ANNI: Estatem et uer tu plasmasti ea. Sunt autem quatuor
tempora in anno, sic et quatuor genera hominum in ecclesia. Hyemps
sunt qui torpent gelicidio malitie ... .

TEMPVS PRIMO: Dicitur tempus gratie, reuelate scilicet exibite et
habundantis ... .

TEMPVS SECVNDO: Distinguitur tria tempora, scilicet ante legem, sub
lege, et post legem ... .

TEMPVS TERTIO: Attendenda sunt tria tempora: preteritum, presens,
et futurum ... .

TEMPVS NATVRE: Est tempus nature ... . Est tempus culpe ... .

TERRA: Terra dicitur machina mundialis ... . Et terra centrum mundi ... .

Torrens: Est torrens penalitatis ... et predicationis ... .

Tedivm: Est tedium ex dilatione propter longam scilicet expectationem ... et ex despectione ut dicatur tedium contemptus misere uite ... .

Tronvs: Tronus sedes regis est, cathedra doctoris, tribunal iudicis ... .

Tvrris: Est turris elationis, hec est turris Babel ... .

Tympanvm: Tympanum dicuntur carnalia ... . Alibi dicitur tympanum ... castitas uidualis uel uirginalis ... .

Tvba: Tuba dicitur sacra scriptura ... . Tuba dicitur predicator ... .

Timere: Omnes timent in morte quia omnis homo naturaliter horret mortem ... . Set et Christus in morte timuit. Mali quidem timent de morte id est pro carnis et anime separatione quam sequitur mors eterna ... .

Item Timere: Timendum est pro culpa et pena ... .

Timor: Timor debet esse homini de peccatis preteritis ne scilicet relabatur ... .

Tradere: Tradidit Deus hominem diabolo ad probandum, ut Iob ... .

Tenebre: Tenebre secundum quosdam remotiue dicuntur absentia lucis ... . Dicuntur et tenebre peccata ... .

Tristitia: Tristitiam pariunt aporiatio, rei dilecte amissio, recordatio peccati, formido supplicii, confusio, desperatio, presentia miserie, carentia glorie ... .

Tvrbatio: Est turbatio sensualitatis ... et rationis ... .

Tempestas: Est tempestas cordis, mundi, maris, mortis, iudicii, supplicii ... .

Tribvlatio: Contra tribulationes remedium est diuinorum mandatorum meditatio ... et deuota oratio ... et multiplici tribulationis utilitate recordatio ... .

Item Tribvlatio: Tribulatio uulnus est ... .

Item Tribvlatio tertio: Ignis quedam consumit ut fenum, quedam examinat et purificat ut argentum, quedam probat et ostendit ut aurum purum ... .

Tabescere: Tabescere dicitur quis ex liuore ... ex infirmitate ... et ex dilectione ... .

Tangere: Tangit Deus per infirmitatem ... per compunctionem ... .

Testamenta: Duo testamenta sunt due rote que ad auditores circumquaque, id est in prosperis et aduersis, uoluuntur ... .

Tvrris: Est turris Babel in campo Sennaar quod est fetor uel excussio dentium. Hii sunt lateres id est cupiditas terrenorum et bitumen id est tenacitas ... .

VIA: Via dicitur opus quod uehit ad metam ...Est autem uia dupplex, una uia iniquitatis, mortis, lata; altera uia ueritatis, uite, arcta ... .

VIA SECVNDO: Vias meas enuntiaui ... . Via Chaim est iniustitia ... . Vie Lamech adulterium et homicidium ... .

ITEM VIA: Deus meus impolluta uia eius. Vt sit fides sine errore et heresi ... .

ITEM VIA: Alii ducuntur ad uiam, ut filius prodigus ... . Alii autem ducuntur in uia, ut proficientes quibus timor est presidium et pedagogus ... . Alii sunt supra uia, ut qui supererogant ... .

VOLATVS PRIMO: Quis dabit mihi pennas sicut columbe et uolabo et requiescam. Vox Christi est qui habet pennas defensionis et protectionis, occultationis, calefactionis et fomenti ... .

ITEM VOLATVS: Est uolatus penitentis ... . Est uolatus post penitentiam proficientis ... . Est uolatus predicantis ... .

VINEA: Vinea est synagoga ... . Vinea est ecclesia ... .

VINVM PRIMO: Est uinum nature quod non bibunt Nazarei neque Rechabite. Est uinum culpe ... .

VINVM SECVNDO: Est uinum corporale quod luxuriam prouocat ... . Est uinum culpe ut ydolatrie ... . Est uinum gratie ... .

VINVM TERTIO: Est uinum culpe quod prohibentur bibere sacerdotes Domino ministrantes ... .

VINVM QVARTO: Est uinum nature quod sumendum est moderate ... .

VERBVM DEI: Verbum Dei lucerna est lucens in loco caliginoso donec dies illucescat ... . Hec est stella preuia magos ducens ... . Hec est margarita ... . Hec est speculum sponse ... .

VERBVM: Eloquium Domini inflammauit eum. Verbum Dei igne Spiritus sancti examinatum facula ardens est ... .

ITEM VERBVM: Et ne auferas de ore meo uerbum ueritatis usquequaque. Tollitur uerbum de ore ab auibus celi, per malam conscientiam ... .

VVLNVS ANIME: Vulnus anime letifer est mortale peccatum ... .

VIRGA: Virga dicitur Deus, Christus, regnum Christi, beata Virgo, ecclesia, populus, stabilitas humani generis, uita patrum, iustitia, doctrina, custodia, regimen et directio, disciplina et correctio ... .

ITEM VVLNVS SECVNDO: Est uulnus actuale, scilicet in corpore ... et corruptionis ... et peccati ... .

VINCVLVM: Est uinculum timoris ... et amoris ... .

VETERASCERE: Res ueterascunt propter infirmitatem ... et propter assiduitatem ... et temporis diuturnitatem ... .

VETVSTAS: Est uetustas culpe ... . Et est uetustas pene ... .

VENENVM: Triplex est hominis uenenum, scilicet non cognoscere

WRITINGS

---

se ... et indignari peccata confiteri ... et bona que quis habet dicere ex se habere ... .

Vitivm: Est uitium ex homine siue in homine, quod nascitur ab ipso homine, quod dicitur occultum ... .

Venter: Venter dicitur castrimargia ... et carnalis sensus ... .

Vter: Vter uetus est homo carnalis qui recusat uinum nouum spiritualis uite ... . Vter est cor discentis ... .

Vanitas: Vanus est homo in existentia ... in cogitatione ... .

Vltio: Deus ultionum Dominus. Deus ultionum libere egit, uel fideliter ... .

Velatio: Reuela oculos meos, etc. Velantur oculi exteriores per obscuritatem ... et ex senectute ... . Ita et interiores oculi uelantur ... .

Velvm: Est uelum culpe quod texit suggestio demonis et consensus hominis ... .

Vmbra: Est umbra nature ... . Vt igitur ordinatius sub epilogo iam dicta colligamus, dicimus quia est umbra corporalis, quam nature diximus, et est umbra gratie, glorie, figure, culpe, ignorantie, mortalitatis, instabilitatis, glorie inanis, memorie, criminis, spiritus infernalis, peregrinationis, protectionis, diuine incomprehensibilitatis, theologice obscuritatis.

Vmbracvlvm: Vmbraculum necessarium est ad refrigerandum in uia, et contra iacula, et estum, et tempestatem. Ita et Dominus diuitias umbraciles prestat in uia ... .

Vvlpes: Vulpes dicuntur heretici. Hec sunt uulpes quarum capita disperata, caude colligate, quia secte hereticorum diuerse sunt set in uanitate conueniunt ... .

Vngventvm: Est unguentum curationis contritio scilicet unguentum pungitiuum et incutiens dolorem, quod in mortariolo conscientie conteritur et conficitur ex plurimis et uilissimis speciebus scilicet peccatis ... .

Vertex: Vertex fides est, oleum pingue deuotio est, balsamum caritas est. Vngitur itaque uertex crismate ut habeat fides deuotionem et sit operans per dilectionem ... .

Venatio: Est uenatio cupiditatis, crudelitatis, uoluptatis, necessitatis, caritatis ... .

Vox: Est uox sanguinis que clamat ad Dominum de terra, et uox fletus que penitentie est ... .

Vigilia Dei: Est uigilia Dei ad faciendum ... . Vigilat etiam Deus ad custodiendum ... .

Volvcris: Super ea uolucres celi habitabunt de medio petrarum uel nemorum dabunt uocem ... . Volucres celi id est spirituales, siue uiri, siue femine. Hee sunt columbe simplices et gementes, sociales, felle carentes ... .

VITE DVE: Preter uitam nature due sunt uite; una est culpabilis, altera laudabilis; una est uita culpe, altera est uita gratie ... .

VITA SECVNDO: Vita est corporis uegetatio per animam ... et uiuicatio anime per gratiam ... .

VIRTVS: Virtus dicitur potentia et fortitudo corporis ... . Virtus autem gratuita, catholica, theologica, caritate informata, uite eterne meritoria ... .

VIRTVS SECVNDO: Sicut quatuor elementa constituunt mundum, qui Grece cosmos dicitur id est ornatus ... ita patientia, penitentia, benignitas, et caritas animam ornant ... .

VIRTVS TERTIO: Fuerunt in gentibus uirtutes quamuis naturales, politice, informes, sicut Cato sobrius erat, Seneca continens, Titus liberalis. Set Christianorum sunt uirtutes gratuite, theologice, meritorie ... . Sunt autem quatuor precipue uirtutes Christiane scilicet fides ... spes ... caritas ... humilitas ... .

VIRTVS QVARTO: Sunt uirtutes autonomasice dicte scilicet fides, spes, caritas. Sunt que dicuntur cardinales scilicet iustitia, fortitudo, temperantia, prudentia ... .

VERAX: Dicitur homo uerax non ex se set a Deo, et ea ueritate que falso opponitur ... .

VIRGINITAS: Virginitas priuilegiata est, cuius prerogatiuam indicant hec octo: carnis soliditas, corporis et animi libertas ... .

VISITARE: Visitat Deus ut puniat ... ut sanet ... ut corrigat ... .

VNVM PRIMO: Ecce quam bonum et quam iocundum habitare fratres in unum: corpore, mente, loco, animo ... .

VNICVS: Vnicus est qui non distrahitur per hereses et scismata ... et qui non distrahitur per diuersas dignitates ecclesiasticas et officia diuersa diuersarum ecclesiarum ... .

VNVM SECVNDO: Est una Marthe, quia omnia eius opera que uaria sunt tendunt ad unum finem ... .

VITVLVS: Vitulus dicitur Christus ... . Vitulus dicitur Lucas in uisione Ezechielis. Vituli sunt noui populi, uel innocentes, uel predicatores, uel martires, uel quicumque fideles ... .

VITVLVS SECVNDO: Est uitulus aureus conflatilis in deserto. Hic est aliquis pomposus in monasterio ... .

VT: Vt est temporale ... et qualitatiuum ... et affectiuum ... .

VELLE: Est uelle rationis et uelle sensualitatis ... .

VESTIS: Est uestis artificalis et usualis ... . Est et uestis glorie ... uestis culpe ... .

Vsvra: Est usura pecunie prohibita ... . Est et usura spiritualis, et hec uel est culpe, uel iniurie, uel pene, uel gratie, uel glorie ... .

Vvltvs: Vultus dicitur uetus testamentum quo uoluntas Dei declaratur ... .

Vincere: Vicit leo de tribu Iuda. Christus uicit, Christus regnat, Christus imperat ... .

Venitvr ad Devm: Venitur ad Deum per internam inspirationem ... . Venitur etiam per fidem ... per spem ... per caritatem ... per baptismum ... .

Vinea: Vineam, id est ecclesiam uel animam, exterminat aper, porcus siluestris, spurcus in lege ... .

Verbvm: Verbum Dei est sacrum in se sanctum et sanctificans ... .

Beata Virgo: Beata Virgo castellum est, cuius fossa humilitas ... .

Vinea: Vinea est ecclesia que muro fidei cingitur ... .

Xpc: Christus ab eterno fuit rex, et admirabilis semper in deitate, magnus et laudabilis in incarnatione quidem et natiuitate, in uirginis utero et in presepio paruus et amabilis ... .

Item Xpc: Christus magister est, dominus, et pater noster, mater, nutrix siue nutricius, amicus, sponsus, dux, athleta, pastor, medicus ... .

Xpc tertio: Christus nobis et frater et pater est, ecclesie dominus et sponsus, idem rex et regnum, magister et liber, conuiuium et conuiua, sacerdos et hostia, redemptor et pretium, saluator et salus ... .

Xpc qvarto: Christus latet in altari sub nubilo panis et uini ... . Christus latet in uirtute sacramenti et in corde iusti ... .

Item Xpc: Christus homo dicitur celum ... propter celsitudinem ... et propter celationem ... et propter deitatis inhabitationem ... .

Item Xpc: Christus dicitur Dauid propter nominis interpretationem, agnus propter significationem, uitis uera propter similitudinem in proprietatibus, homo et Deus propter ueritatem nature.

Cena: Est cena culpabilis, ut cena Herodis. Est cena laudabilis, hec est gratie, ut sancte eucharistie ... .

Item Xpc: Christus est panis coctus in clibano, id est uirginis utero ... .

Item Mandvcare secvndo:[8] Manducare corpus Christi proprium et personale, traductum de uirgine, est manducare sacramentaliter id est sub forma sacramentali ... .

8 Item ... secundo] Manducare corpus christi *C*

ZELVS:[9] Zelus dicitur inuidia ... .
Zelus indignatio uel amor ... .
Bonus enim zelus est feruor animi et ardor caritatis ... .
ZONA:[10] Est zona humilitatis ... et penitentie uel mortificationis ... et fidei et iustitie ... et nequitie ... .

9 Zelus] *ex Oxford, Bodleian Library* MS *Bodley 419 et Utrecht, Bibliotheek der Univ.* MS *312: om.* CL
10 Zona] *ex* MS *Bodley 419: om.* CL

II.9

Similitudinarium

This unusual *summa* is a systematic compendium of images, metaphors, similes, and examples for use in all kinds of theological discourse. In his *Proverbia* William created an alphabetical repository of authorities; in his *Distinctiones* he did the same for "reasons" or arguments. Here in the *Similitudinarium* he organizes under alphabetical headings the *similitudines* and *exempla* that will help students, teachers, and preachers to understand theological doctrine, and to transmit this understanding to the people in their care.

William describes the purpose of these similitudes in his prologue:

> For explaining an argument in any kind of discourse we have collected similitudes whencesoever God gives them, knowing that examples and similitudes lend credence to arguments raised and elucidate authorities and reasons.

The similitudes collected here are for use not only by the preacher but also by the teacher, who will employ them along with authorities and reasons in his theological discourses. Similitudes played an important role in early scholastic theology, and William's *Similitudinarium* represents the largest systematic collection of these that has been identified.[1]

Similitudes, for William, can be distinguished from examples (*exempla*) in that the latter are drawn from human history and the former from the world of nature. For instance the entry for MARIA explains that no historical *exemplum* of the virgin birth can be found, but it does have a *similitudo* in the nature of things:

---

[1] For the importance of similitudes in scholastic education, see Fritz Peter Knapp, *Similitudo: Stil- und Erzählfunktion von Vergleich und Example in der lateinischen, französischen und deutschen Grossepik des Hochmittelalters* (Vienna: Wilhelm Braumüller, 1975). For their importance in practical discourse, see d'Avray, *The Preaching of the Friars*, pp. 225-239; Fritz Kemmler, *"Exempla" in Context*, pp. 60-69.

Ego quasi uitis fructificaui suauitatem odoris [Eccli 24:23], ac si aperte dicat: "Partus quidem meus non habet exemplum in sexu mulierum, set habet similitudinem in naturis rerum." Queris quomodo uirginitas genuit saluatorem? Sicut flos uitis odorem.[2]

This distinction between *exemplum* and *similitudo*, however, is not rigidly observed. Although many of William's similitudes are drawn from the world of nature, not a few include historical examples, and when Richard of Wetheringsett composed his *Qui bene presunt*, he introduced many of William's similitudes with the generic designation: *exemplum*.

The second sentence of the prologue specifies the particular form that William chose for his work:

That we might be able to find a simile pertinent to an argument more quickly and easily, we have taken pains to organize this treatise on similitudes in alphabetical order; we give this work the name *Similitudinarium*.

One sees here a clear expression of the new attitudes toward books and theological learning that, during the thirteenth century, resulted in the invention of the fully alphabetical table of contents, subject index, verbal concordance, and numerous other conveniences designed to make written texts effective and efficient educational tools.

The individual entries in this compendium take various forms. Many are quite brief, and read like *bon mots* from the schools:

Controversy: We are dwarfs on the shoulders of giants and small birds on the wings of eagles.[3]
Merit: Just as light and the power of sight work together for seeing, so grace and free choice work together for meriting.[4]
Secular: St. Malachy was no more influenced by his barbarous homeland than are the fish of the sea by their salty home.[5]

Other entries are more discursive:

Preaching: ... Some say that the sum of all preaching is this: "Do good, and it will be well with you." But this is as if one said to a traveller seeking directions: "Always follow the right road and you will reach your

---

[2] Oxford, New College MS 98. fol. 134ra (*O* = no. 13, below).

[3] "CONTENTIO: Nos nani sumus in humeris gigantum, et auicule super alas aquilarum," ibid., fol. 126rb.

[4] "MERITVM: Sicut lux et uisus concurrunt ad uidendum, ita gracia et liberum arbitrium cooperantur ad merendum," ibid., fol. 133vb.

[5] "SECVLARIS: Sanctus Malachias de natali barbarie nichil traxit, non magis quam pisces maris de sale materno," ibid., fol. 139rb.

destination." Does this suffice? Again, some say: "I know the sum of all preaching: avoid evil and do good." This is as if he said: "I have learned the whole of physic and all of medicine: avoid illness and preserve your health." Is it enough to say this?[6]

The importance of such similitudes in late-twelfth- and early-thirteenth-century theology should not be underestimated. It is difficult to find any scholastic dispute from the time of Peter Comestor until well into the thirteenth century that does not employ one or more similitudes to bolster or to develop the argument. When removed from their context and collected independently, as in William's *Similitudinarium*, they appear somewhat facile and unpersuasive; but the purpose of this work is not to persuade, it is to serve as a reference work in which teachers and preachers can find the materials with which to construct cogent arguments.

The direct influence of William's *Similitudinarium* on preaching and teaching cannot be established until this and many other texts have been edited or studied.[7] Stephen Langton may have been familiar with William's collection, and the author of the *Moralia super Evangelium* has been shown to have borrowed from the *Similitudinarium*.[8] The importance of this collection, however, is not only to help clarify the lines of dependence among early scholastic writers, but also to illustrate the value they placed on apt similes and examples in constructing their arguments. The collections of *exempla* for preachers that proliferated in the thirteenth century are only one example of the widespread interest among theologians, and William's *Similitudinarium* may be seen as one of the earliest attempts to make such materials easily accessible to the master and his students.

AUTHENTICITY AND DATE

In five of the thirteen manuscript copies this work is ascribed to William de Montibus, and four of the unascribed copies retain the descriptive

---

[6] "Aiunt aliqui, summa totius predicationis hec est, bene fac et bene habebis. Set hec est ac si uiatori uiam querenti dicatur: Recta semper uia gradere, et sic poteris ad metam peruenire. Numquid sufficit hoc dictum? Item dicunt quidam: Scio totam summam predicationis: Declina a malo et fac bonum. Hoc est ac si dicat: Noui totam fisicam uel uniuersalem medicinam: Caue egritudinem et conserua sanitatem. Sufficit hoc dicere?" ibid., fol. 135rb.

[7] See Bataillon, "*Similitudines* et *Exempla*," pp. 191-205.

[8] See, Roberts, *Sermons of Stephen Langton*, pp. 89-94; E.J. Dobson, *Moralities on the Gospels: A New Source of "Ancrene Wisse"* (Oxford: Clarendon Press, 1975), pp. 93-96.

prologue (*Ad declarandum in sermone* ...) that is characteristic of several of William's writings. Three of the ascribed copies date from the early thirteenth century, and one, no. 3 below, is an early redaction of the text wherein the second series of similitudes has not yet been ordered alphabetically. The ascription of the third series (Series C) to Stephen Langton in MS no. 6 is yet to be fully investigated, but *prima facie* grounds exist for excluding it from William's writings: that series is copied separately in MSS nos. 2, 3, and 6, and is entirely absent in nos. 5, (8), 12, and 13.

No firm date of composition can be assigned to this work. All of the manuscripts appear to be of English provenance, suggesting that the treatise was first published after William arrived in England (after 1180). It appears that he first issued an alphabetical collection (Series A), and then a supplement (Series B) that was not arranged alphabetically, but neither series can be assigned a precise date of publication. The selection of materials for these collections must have taken place over a long period, probably extending back to William's Parisian period and forward into the thirteenth century.

SOURCES

The proximate sources of these similitudes, whether sermons, bestiaries, theological/exegetical writings, or William's own observation and imagination, are not obvious. Richard Hunt noted that several of William's similitudes occur in the sermons of Alexander Neckam, but whether Alexander was a source for William or William for Alexander is still moot.[9]

Explicit reference is made to the following authorities: Cicero (*Tullius*), Eusebius of Emesa, Gregory the Great, Lucan, Origen, Ovid, Peter of Ravenna, Porphyry, St. Remi (*Remigius*), and Virgil.

MANUSCRIPTS

The manuscript tradition of this work is extremely complex. Three distinct series of similitudes can be identified:

Series A. Probably William's original collection, it includes a prologue and an alphabetical arrangement of entries. It is represented in all of the manuscripts.

---

[9] Hunt, *The Schools and the Cloister*, p. 84.

Series B. Probably an addition to his original collection. It circulated as a distinct series in both a non-alphabetical form (Peterhouse MS 255 = no. 3), and an alphabetical form (Bodleian MS Add. 263 = no. 10). At least part of this series, too, is represented in all of the manuscripts.

Series C. The *Similitudines* of Stephen Langton. Such a work was attributed to Stephen by early bibliographers, and a number of the entries in the series ascribed to Langton in MS Ancaster 16/1 (= no. 6) are found verbatim in his sermons.[10] This series also is copied, without ascription, in Peterhouse MS 255. Neither copy is arranged alphabetically. At an early date this work was absorbed into some copies of William's *Similitudinarium*, but it is not represented in all the manuscripts.

These three series have been copied, excerpted, and rearranged in each of the manuscripts. In the following list the de Montibus material (Series A and B) is distinguished from the "Langton" series (C) where possible, and general observations on the nature of each collection are offerred.

1. Cambridge, University Library MS Add. 6757, fols. 1r-49r. Mid 13th century (above top line).

> Title: *Liber iste apellatur Similitudinarium uerborum.*
>
> Inc. Prol.: *Ad declarandum in sermone*
>
> Inc. Txt.: (*De ruina angelorum et de subpletione hominum*) *Ciconia post pullorum auolatum.*
>
> Expl.: (*Xpianus*) ... *Membrum tamen diaboli et non Christi. Sicut caseus signitus est signo crucis. Ita malus Xpianus.*

An amalgam of Series A, B, and C into a single, alphabetically arranged series (like MSS nos. 9 and 11, below). The rubrics or titles in the early part of the text are somewhat idiosyncratic. A quire is missing between fols. 48/49.

2. Cambridge, Peterhouse MS 119, fols. 33ra-40va. Mid 13th century (above top line).

> Title (15th-century hand): (*Similitudinarium*)
>
> Inc.: *Falcones a falcando*
>
> Expl.: (*Contra diuicias superfluas*) ... *Magni misera est custodia census.*
>
> Colophon: *Explicit Similitudinarium.*

Excerpts only. Series A and Series B were apparently copied from alphabetically arranged exemplars, although the rubrics are idiosyncratic

---

[10] See Roberts, *Sermons of Stephen Langton*, pp. 89-94; The examples of Langton's similitudes given by Roberts are all from the "C" Series.

and thus do not now evince this alphabetical organization. Series A ends on fol. 36ra with "*Xpc: Xpc pons est ... sic Christus de Virgine.*" Series B begins immediately with: "<*Acceleratio:*> *Quidam in maturo desiderio.*" The last entry of Series B occurs on fol 37rb: "*Contra ypocritas: Simea ueste humana induitur ... membrum tamen diaboli est et non Xpi.*" Excerpts from the C or "Langton" Series follow without notice. The first is: "<Xᴘɪᴀɴᴠs:> Qui mortaliter peccauit ... ." Series C is not arranged alphabetically.

3. Cambridge, Peterhouse ᴍs 255, fols. 84r-127r. Early 13th century (above top line).

    Title: (*Incipit prologus Similitudinarii magistri Willelmi cancelarii*).
    Inc. Prol.: *Ad declarandum sermonem*
    Inc. Txt.: (*Amor tractatus principium*) *Amor terrenus inuiscat animam*
    Expl. Txt.: (*Confessio*) *... pertingitur ab angustia confessionis.*
    Colophon: *Explicit Similitudinarius magistri Willelmi de monte.*

All three series are copied here. Series A, arranged alphabetically, apparently ends on fol. 99v or 100r following the entry "*Xpc: Xpc pons est ...*", but the precise demarcation is unclear. Series B, in non-alphabetic order, ends on fol. 107r/v: "*Principatus: ... quia nudus ingreditur, nudus egreditur.*" The C or "Langton" Series, in non-alphabetic order, begins there with "Iɴꜰᴇʀɴᴠs: Ita sunt anime in infer-no ... ."

4. Cambridge, Trinity Hall ᴍs 24, fols. 70r-85vb. Mid 13th century (above top line).

    Inc. Prol.: *Ad declarandum in sermone*
    Inc. Txt.: *Amor terrenus inuiscat animam*
    Expl.: (*Xpianus*) *... membrum tamen diaboli est et non Xpi.*

The material in this copy has been organized into two alphabetical series. The first corresponds to Series A, with a few entries from Series B inserted under the appropriate letter of the alphabet. This series ends on fol. 79ra: "*Xpc trahit: ... quia aque multe, populi multi.*" A table of contents for this series is found on fol. 70r. The second series here consists primarily of the "Langton" Series (C) with a few entries from Series B inserted under the appropriate letters. It begins unannounced, with "Asᴄᴇɴsɪᴏ Xᴘɪ: Si ad domum alicuius iturus esses ... ." The final entry (see Explicit, above) is from Series B, the penultimate entry is from the "Langton" series: "Xᴘᴄ ᴘᴠᴇʀ: Si quis cum Ludouico ... qui dicit omnibus affluenter et non inproperat."[11]

---

[11] Cf. ibid., pp. 92-93.

5. *E* = Eton College MS 82, fols. 66r-88r. Early 13th century (above top line).

> Title: *Incipit liber similitudinarii magistri Willelmi de monte.*
> Inc.: *Amor terrenus inuiscat animam*
> Expl.: (*De dominio*) ... *quia nudus ingreditur nudus egreditur.*
> Colophon: (*Explicit*)

Series A and Series B are combined into a single alphabetical series. Additional items are copied into the margins of the text, on scraps of parchment inserted into the codex, and on fols. 88r-90v. A table of contents is found on fols. 64v-65v.

6. *A* = Lincoln, PRO MS Ancaster 16/1, fols. 53ra-76ra. Early 13th century (above top line).

> Title: (*Similitudines secundum magistrum Willelmum Lincolniensis ecclesie cancellarium in sermonibus edite*)
> Inc. Prol.: *Ad declarandum in sermone*
> Inc. Txt.: *Amor terrenus iuniscat animam*
> Expl.: <*Principatus*> *Apostoli in uia ... quia nudus ingreditur et nudus egreditur.*

Series A and Series B combined into a single alphabetical series. It is followed on fol. 76rb by a copy of Series C explicitly ascribed to Langton: "Similitudinarium magistri Stephani Cantuariensis Archiepiscopi. "INFERNVS: Ita sunt anime in gehenna ... ." The text ends on fol. 92rb: "CONFESSIO: Introite portas ... pertingitur ab angustia confessionis." This series corresponds to the unascribed copy in MS no. 3, fols. 107v-127r.

7. London, British Library Cotton MS Vespasian B.xiii, fols. 90va-110va. Early 13th century (above top line).

> Title (15th-century hand): *Hic incipit liber qui dicitur Similitudinarium.*
> Inc.: *Amor. Amor terrenus inuiscat animam*
> Expl.: (*Dilatio uindicte*) ... *quanto diucius distulit ultionem.*

This copy, like that in MS no. 4, is arranged in two alphabetical series. The first comprises the text of Series A, with some additions from Series B. It ends on fol. 101va: "*Xpc trahit: ... quia aque multe populi multi.*" Fols. 90va-91vb, at the beginning of the text, are much disordered. The prologue occurs on fol. 91ra under the title BENEFICIVM DEI. A table of contents for this first series similar to that in MS no. 4 is found on fols. 89vb-90rb.

A second series begins unannounced with: "ASCENSIO XPI: Si ad domum alicuius ... ." It is comprised primarily of entries from the "Langton" Series (C), with some additions from Series B, and is very like that in MS no. 4.

8. London, British Library MS Royal 8.D.iv, fol. 113vb. Mid 13th century (above top line).

>   Title: *Hic incipiunt similitudines*
>   Inc. Txt.: *Amor terrenus inuiscat animam*
>   Expl.: *<Aues rapaces> ... Aquile magnarum alarum sunt potentes huius seculi qui potenter*

This single-column fragment corresponds to the beginning of Series A.

9. London, Gray's Inn MS 13, fols. 56ra-101rb. Late 13th century (below top line).

>   Title: *Prologus super Similitudinarium Magistri Willelmi de montibus.*
>   Inc. Prol.: *Ad declarandum in sermone*
>   Inc. Txt.: *(Angelus) Ciconia post pullorum auolatum*
>   Expl.: *(Xpianus) ... membrum tamen diaboli est et non Xpi.*

An amalgamation of Series A, B, and C into a single alphabetically arranged text, this copy is similar to that in MSS nos. 1 and 11.

10. Oxford, Bodleian MS Add. C. 263 (sc 27646), fols. 96vb-113rb. Early 13th century (above top line).

>   Inc. Prol.: *Ad declarandam in sermone*
>   Inc. Txt.: *Amor terrenus inuiscat*
>   Expl.: *<Xpianus> ... membrum tamen diaboli est et non Xpi.*

Excerpts only, from Series A, B, and C. No rubrics or headings have been provided for alphabetical arrangement, but both Series A and B have been copied from alphabetically arranged exemplars. Selections from the first series end on fol. 110vb: "*<Qualiter Xpc ex Virgine:> ... sic Xpc de Virgine.*" The second series begins with "*<Barba:> Capro similis est qui barbam habet ... *", and ends on fol. 113rb with "*<Xpianus:> ... membrum tamen diaboli est et non Xpi.*" Excerpts from the third or "Langton" series begin there, without notice: "*<XPIANVS:> Qui mortaliter peccant et tum se Christianos appellant ... .*" Selections from this series end on fol. 115ra: "*<EFFECTVS PECCATI:> Si princeps aliquis perrexisset ... sic de quolibet sensualitate.*"

11. Oxford, Balliol College MS 222, fols. 3ra-27vb. Mid 13th century (below top line).

>   Inc. Prol.: *(Incipit proemium) Ad declarandum in sermone*
>   Inc. Txt.: *(Exemplum ciconie) Angelus. Ciconia post pullorum auolatum*
>   Expl.: *(Cristianus) ... membrum tamen diaboli est et non Xpi.*
>   Colophon: *(Explicit Similitudinarius)*

Series A, B, and C have been combined into a single alphabetical series, as in MSS nos. 1 and 9 above. A table of contents for the entire work is found on fol. 2r-v. Some idiosyncratic rubrics have been added;

the original titles often appear in black ink at the beginning of the entry, as in the incipit of the text, quoted above.

12. *M* = Oxford, Merton College MS 257, fols. 68ra-104vb. Later 13th century.
>   Title: (*Incipit liber similitudinarii magistri Willelmi de monte*)
>   Inc. Txt.: (*Amor est quasi viscus*) *Amor terrenus inuiscat animam*
>   Expl.: (*De dominio*) *Apostoli in uia ... quia nudus ingreditur, nudus egreditur.*

Series A and B are combined in a single, alphabetical series, as in MSS nos. 5, 6, and 13. A table of contents is found on fol. 67ra-vc: "*Incipiunt capitula libri Similitudinarii Magistri Willelmi de monte secundum alphabetum.*" The last entry, DE DOMINIO, is followed without a break in the manuscript, by numerous fables and similitudes, including a number of entries from Series C (fols. 104vb-108rb); these are not listed in the table of contents.

13. *O* = Oxford, New College MS 98, fols. 123vb-141vb. Early 13th century (above top line).
>   Inc.: (*Amor*) *Amor terrenus inuiscat animam*
>   Expl.: (*Xpc est lapis conterens*) ... *impius pena perpetua punietur.*

Series A and B are combined in a single, alphabetical series.

Only a complete collation of all the manuscripts will allow an accurate description of the contents of this work. The following provisional account presents a particular stage in the manuscript tradition as represented by MSS nos. 5, 6, 12, and 13. In these manuscripts the contents of two distinct series of William's similitudes have been combined into a single alphabetically organized collection. The third series that was often conflated with William's work, the similitudes ascribed to Stephen Langton in MS no. 6, are not included in this version of William's *Similitudinarium*.

The following has been transcribed from Lincoln PRO MS Ancaster 16/1 = *A*. Selected variants are noted from Eton College MS 82 = *E*, Merton College (Oxford) MS 257 = *M*, and New College (Oxford) MS 98 = *O*. The first ten items of William's *Similitudinarium* are transcribed in full; the remainder of the work is represented here by transcriptions of the topical rubrics and the incipits of each similitude.

Similitudinarium

Ad declarandum in sermone quocumque propositum similitudines undecumque Deo donante collegimus, scientes quia propositiones in medium prolatas probant seu dilucidant auctoritates et rationes, exempla et similitudines. Vt autem facilius et citius aliquod simile spectans ad propositum reperire ualeamus, tractatum presentem de similitudinibus secundum ordinem alphabeti disponere curauimus; huic operi Similitudinarium nomen imponimus.[1]

AMOR:[2] Amor terrenus inuiscat animam ne possit ad superna uolare. Vnde Augustinus: Amor rerum terrenarum uiscus est spiritualium pennarum.[3] Set amor diuinus superueniens uiscum illum soluit sicut ignis ceram.

ADVENTVS CHRISTI: Omnipotens sermo a regalibus sedibus uenit, a sinu patris nec tamen patrem deserens, sicut nec splendor ignem, uel radius solem, nec uox os, nec cogitatio cor ab eo progrediens.

APIS: Apis illa sapiens cum aeris motus suspectos habeat, lapillis sepe sublatis per inania nubila se librat, ne leue alarum remigium precipitent flabra uentorum.

ANGELI: Ciconia post pullorum auolatum nidum terra replet, et Deus ruinam angelorum hominibus suplebit, et tu nidum cordis absentata elatione terra id est memoria mortis et peccati grauem redde, ne uento tiphonico dispergatur ex uitio negligentie.

ADAM: Apud Deum iustum est ut arbor in ramis seruet amaritudinem quam traxit ex radice; hoc est, sentit adhuc proles quod commisere parentes.

APOSTOLI: Apostoli fugabantur, Iudei remanserunt;[4] set apostoli tanquam faces ardentes quocumque ueniebant accendebant; stulti Iudei quando illos de Ierosolimis fugabant carbones ignis in siluam mittebant.

---

1 Ad declarandum ... imponimus] *A*: *om. EMO*
2 Amor] *AO*: Amor quasi viscus *EM*
3 Vnde ... pennarum] *EM*: *om. AO*
4 Apostoli ... remanserunt] *EM*: Apostoli remanserunt, ceteri fugabantur *AO*

AMOR SECVLI: Vis ut intret mel. Vnde acetum nondum fudisti; funde quod habes ut capias quod non habes. Ideo prima renuntiatio est huic seculo et deinde conuersio ad Deum. Qui renuntiat fundit, qui conuertitur impletur.[5]

AVARITIA: Auarus est terra harenosa et mundi salsugine imbuta. Auarus uir inferno similis est. Infernus quantoscumque deuorauerit non dicit satis est, sic et si omnes thesauri terre confluxerint in auarum non satiabitur.

Nostri essemus si illa lucra nostra non essent. Contempnenda est auaritia que uelut ignis quanto plus accipit tanto amplius querit.

ACCIDIA: Vereor ne nos, sicut bruta furfure seu farragine farsita et lutosis adaquata, dapes celestes electuarium et nectar diuinum fastidiamus et nos tangat illud. Omnem escam abhominata est anima eorum, et ideo apropinquerunt usque ad portas mortis.

AFFECTVS: Pes inquinatur etsi nondum corpus, ita affectus polluitur etsi nondum opus immundum sequitur.

AVES RAPACES:[6]
 FALCO: Falcones a falcando quia in falcis ... .
 GIROFALCO: Girofalcones in girum falcando ... .
 ACCIPITER: Accipitres sunt mansueti, rapaces ... .
 NISVS: Nisi diaboli sunt ... .
 MILVVS: Milui domesticis auibus insidiantes ... .
 AQVILA: Aquile magnarum alarum sunt potentes huius seculi ... .
AVES BIFORMIS NATVRE: Aues biformis nature sunt quas alietos uocant ... .
 CICONIA: Ciconie toto brumali tempore ... .
 CICADE: Sunt cicade quedam alate uolantes ... .
 FENIX: Fenix resurgit ex cinere, exurgat ... .
ALE: Ale caritatis et penne uirtutum sarcine sunt non onerantes set decorantes ... .
ACCELERATIO: Quidam in maturo desiderio euanescunt sicut plumascentes in nido pulli ... .
 Sicut alites ut se in aera pennis surrigant ... .
 In anteriora nos extendamus arietum more ... .[7]

5 Amor seculi ... impletur] *EO*: *om. AM*
6 Aves rapaces] *AEM*: De auibus *O*
7 Acceleratio ...] *EMO*: *om. A*

BONVM EST OCCASIO MALI: Messis propria cadit ubertate ... .

BONA IMPERFECTA SVNT OCCVLTANDA: Baculus arundineus rex Egypti ... .

BREVITAS VITE: Dies mei uelocius transierunt ... .

BENEFICIVM DEI: Memoria beneficii diuini scutum est ... .

Vis ut intret mel in uas unde acetum nondum fudisti ... .[8]

BARBA: Capro similis est qui barbam habet in mente ... .[9]

BELLVM: Non est nobis colluctatio aduersus carnem ... .[10]

CARITAS: Sicut ignis ceram sic caritas cor emollit ... .

Tunica Christi indiuisa est pax et unitas uel caritas ... .

Tota lex caritati innititur ... .

Gemina itaque dilectio due ale sunt ... .

Sicut ignis scintillas emittit et fumum ... .

Ex commemoratione beneficiorum tanquam expressione lignorum ... .

COMPASSIO: Radix uerbi est uirtus operis ... .

Sic propheta[11] captiuo populo consedit ... .

CONTEMPLATIVVS: Alia ligna fructus proferunt esibiles ... .

Trocus inter medios cleros dormiens ... .[12]

Cum radius solaris percurrit superficiem aque ... .

CORREPTIO: Si sani tactu digitorum inuicem tangunt ... .

CORRECTIO: Audire debemus errores et abicere ... .

COGITATIO: Quid prodest in loco quies et inquietudo in corde ... .[13]

Auicula contundit ollam ... .

COGITATIO: Mare significat mentem hominis ... .

Ne ut in te spinas et tribulos crescere ... .[14]

CONFESSIO: Sit confessio nuda, aperta non operta ... .

Beati quorum sic tecta sunt peccata ... .

Tu munda prius quod intus est calicis ... .

Non erubescite uulnus detegere ... .

CONTRARIA CONTRARIIS CVRANTVR: Clauus clauo retunditur ... .

CVSTODIA ANIME: Thesaurus in uase est anima in corpore ... .[15]

CVSTODIA: Quid prodest si tota ciuitas custodiatur ... .

---

8 Vis ... fudisti] *EM*: *om. AO*

9 Barba ...] *EMO*: *om. A*

10 Bellum ...] *EMO*: *om. A*

11 propheta] *AO*: Ezechiel *EM*

12 Trocus ... dormiens] *EMO*: Trocus flaggellandus piger est *A*

13 Quid prodest ... corde] *EMO*: *om. A*

14 Ne ut ...] *AEM*: *om. O*

15 Custodia ...] *EMO*: *om. A*

CVLTVRA ANIMI: Vt dicit Eusebius Emissenus, Qui ieiunat ... .

CONFIRMATIO SANCTORVM: Thronus Dei est anima iusti. Sicut gutta aque infusa[16] lagene uini ... .

CONSTANTIA: Si prudentiam amplecteris ubique idem eris ... .

CONCORDIA: In ecclesia actuali lapides coaptati sunt ... .

CONVERSIO: Sponsam suam uir quisque prius blandimentis dulcibus fouet ... .

CANTICVM NOCTVRNVM: Nos cum Philomena diurno nocturnum canticum copulemus ... .

CAVTELA: Deuita foueam in quam uides alium cecidisse ... .

CANDELA: Sicut apposito igne licinium et cera consumuntur ... .

CASTITAS: Status uirginalis excellentie uiduali castitati prefertur ... .

CASTVS OPERE ET MENTE: Qui castus cupit esse de opere ... .[17]

CALCIAMENTVM: Calciamentum tegit et calefacit, ornat ... .

CVPIDITAS: Diabolus uel fenerator uel raptor perdix est ... .

    Homo dum mergitur que tangit apprehendit et retinet ... .

    Cupiditas et consuetudo et libido uiscus diabolicus est ... .

    Esca in muscipula lucrum est in fraude uel usura.

    Sicut puluis pulices sic cupiditas ... .

    Nichil tam contrarium fortitudini quam lucro uinci ... .

CENSVS: Christus laudem uirginitatis uel continentie seu coniugii quasi aureum uel argenteum siue ereum denarium ... .

CRVX: Quasi geminas lanceas dicimus lignum scientie et lignum crucis ... .

COLVMBA: Vigor in alis columbe fortitudo est ecclesie ... .

CONTENTIO: Nos nani sumus in humeris gigantum ... .

COLLOQVIVM ET CONTENTIO: Ex collisione prosilit ignis ... .

COGNITIO DEI: Sicut oculus carnis cum ex natura facultatem habeat uidendi et audiendi auris ... .[18]

CARITAS EST IGNIS: Ignis in ligno uiridi primo quidem difficile apprehendit ... .[19]

    Compagnatio domus Dei mutua dilectio est ... .

    Anima cum se totum effudit in amorem ... .[20]

CONTEMPLATIO: Aliquis bene currens indiget uerbis exhortatoriis ... .[21]

CLERICI: Literas mortis sue defert ... .[22]

---

16 gutta ... infusa] *EMO: om. A*
17 cupit esse de opere ...] *EM*: debet perseuerare ... *AO*
18 Cognitio ...] *EMO: om A*
19 Caritas ...] *EMO: om A*
20 Compagnatio ...] *E: om. AMO*
21 Contemplatio ...] *O: om. AEM*
22 Clerici ...] *EMO: om. A*

CATECHISMVS: Cathecismus est preparatio quedam que magis reddit idoneum baptismo, sicut politio lapidis ... .[23]

CONVERSIO: Sicut solsequium se claudit ad noctem ... .[24]

CONSVETVDO: Nolite dicere sequemur consuetudines patrum nostrorum ... .[25]

CVPIDITAS: Narcisus umbram uanam et decorem falsum captat in aquis ... .

Qui festinat ditari non erit innocens ... .[26]

DEVS: Qui non ferunt solem in rota uideant saltem in radio ... .

Sicut lapis ille qui dicitur magnetes ... .

Mouet Deus et mouetur quasi sitiens sitiri ... .

Deus per se ipsum qui lux est pias mentes illuminat ... .

DEVS EST VBIQVE: Deus est ubique sicut in pluribus locis lux solis ... .

Deus est in omni creatura sua sicut uita in toto corpore.

DIVES: Abraham arietem uisum post tergum ... .

Sic moritur diues in opulentia sicut mus pleno ore in muscipula.

Diuites quasi salamandre in igne degunt ... .

DIVITIE ET CVRE: Spina in pede sunt diuitie in affectu ... .

DIVITIE: Tu diues sarcinam diuitiarum pauperi in itinere ... .

Fluxus sanguinis ex superfluitate prodit ... .

Junonem diuitiarum asserunt deam ... .

Melius est modicum iusto super diuitias peccatorum multas ... .

DIABOLVS: Deus sathan uidet nec tamen sathan Deum uidet ... .

Deus demones ad temptandum laxat et permittit sicut canes ... .

Licet diabolo semel a Deo accepta potestate ... .

Demones canes sunt ... .

Ab angelis et sanctis illuditur hosti tanquam cani ... .

Spiritus immundus uersatur in mundo sicut scarabeus ... .

DE DIABOLO ET EIVS TEMPTATIONE:[27] Abeunt demones iuxta quod scriptum est ... .

DIABOLVS EST CARCERARIVS:[28] Diabolus est similis carcerario ... .

THELONARIUS: Item diabolus simul est thelonario ... .

---

23 Cathecismus ...] *O: om. AEM*

24 Conuersio ...] *EO: om. A:* Conuersio. Aquila ut aiunt pullos suos cum plumescere uidet ... *M*

25 Consuetudo ...] *EMO: om. A*

26 Cupiditas ...] *EMO: om. A*

27 De ... temptatione] *A: om. EMO*

28 Diabolus est carcerarius] *O:* similis carcerario *A:* Diabolus similis est carcerario *EM*

PHARAO: Item diabolus est sicut Pharao persequens ... .

AMALECH: Item similis est diabolus Amalech ... .

MILVVS: Item diabolus miluus est insidiando ... .

CORVVS: Item diabolus coruus est ...

AQVILA: Item diabolus aquila est in altum uolans ... .

VRSVS: Item diabolus ursus est palo ligatus ... .

LVPVS: Item diabolus lupus est ... .

FORTIS ARMATVS: Item diabolus est fortis armatus ... .

SERPENS: Item diabolus est serpens ... .

LEO: Item diabolus est leo seuus et fortis ... .

DRACO: Item diabolus est draco occulte insidians ... .

Elephanti pauenti sub aquis insidiatur ... .

Auctor mortis fonti rudi humani generis ... .

Sicut rusticus fune porcum tenet, ita diabolus ... .

DETRACTOR: Detractor est hedus[29] asper in pilis ... .

DISCORDIA: Discordes in ecclesia corde dissone sunt in cithara.

DISCIPLINA: Mater eruditionis est instantia ... .

DILATIO PENE: Deus penam differens uel diabolus ad tempus se subtrahens aries est retrocedens ut fortius irruat ... .

DILATIO: Si aurum tibi offeram non dicis mihi cras ueniam ... .

DIES IVDICII: Nondum apparuit quid erimus. In hieme sunt arbores sine decore ... .

Congrue iudicium arcus dicitur ... .

Quis enim uel in montem uel in murum ... .

Inter iustos et impios quantum ad homines discretio non apparet ... .

DESIDERIVM CELESTIVM: Arbor directa in altum ... .[30]

DIVITIE: Diuitie spine sunt quas qui amplectitur ... .[31]

ELEMOSINA: Elemosina est aqua extinguens ignem ... .

Elemosina unguentum est ... .

Per iniuriosos iustorum spoliatores pascit Dominus pauperes ... .

De conceptu uere compassionis nasci solet elemosina ... .

Sol obscuratus est in morte Christi ... .

Si quando repentinus ignis habitaculum assumit ... .

Vberior est nummus e paruo quam thesaurus e maximo ... .

---

29 hedus] *AO*: hircus *EM*
30 Desiderium ...] *O: om. AEM*
31 Diuitie ...] *O: om. AEM*

Sicut sinapi caput forte curandum est ... .

Abstinentia sine misericordia sicut lampas sine oleo ... .

ECCLESIA: Ecclesie dicuntur naues ... .

EXCVSATIO: Perizomata sibi faciunt qui excusationes in peccatis pretendunt.

EPISCOPVS: Populus hic labiis me honorat ... .

EBRIETAS: Bacus dicitur Liber quod etiam serui ebrii ... .

Sicut piscis cum auidis faucibus properat ut glutiat escam ... .

HEDVS: Hedus animal fetens est ... .

EXCOMMVNICATVS:[32] Sicut membrum amputatum ... .

EDIFICIVM:[33] Strenuum esse in operibus affectu infidum ... .

FIDES: Anulus in digito est fides in opere discreto ... .

FIDES CVPIDITAS: Fides sic est in anima ut radix bona ... .

FIDELITAS:[34] Hii qui in stadio currunt ... .

FORTITVDO: Fortitudo leonis est in pectore ... .

FVGA:[35] Hec sunt arma iusti ut cedendo uincat ... .

FRAGILITAS: Si uitrei essemus nimis casus timeremus ... .

FALLACIA:[36] Sicut aliquotiens tristem frontem amicus ... .

FLVMEN BABILONIS: Recordemur Syon ut sedeamus flentes ... .

FORTITVDO: Sicut rami et flagella uitium ilico tabescunt ... .[37]

GRATIA: Demissio funis et eius apprehensio extrahunt hominem a puteo ... .

Ad radium solis aperi ostium cordis.

Nemo de uiribus presumat ... .

Est gratie infusio uelut roris uel pluuie irrigatio ... .

SVBTRACTIO GRATIE: Peccanti Deus gratiam subtrahit sicut ingrato tignum.[38]

GLORIA PATRIE: Erit in patria memoria culpe ... .

Nemo sane mentis pro quantacumque pecunia sibi sustineret oculos erui ... .[39]

Mensuram bonam et confertam et coagitatam ... .

In patria nulli superiori ullus inferior inuidebitur ... .

32 Excommunicatus] *AEM*: Excommunicati non participant suffragiis ecclesie *O*
33 Edificium] *AEM*: Fides *O*
34 Fidelitas] *AEO*: Fraus *M*
35 Fuga] *AEO*: Fuga uincitur libido *M*
36 Fallacia] *AO*: Falsitas *EM*
37 Fortitudo ...] *EMO*: *om. A*
38 Subtractio gratie ...] *AO*: *om. EM*
39 Nemo ...] *A*: *om. EMO* (*cf. infra*, Gratitudo)

Id etiam beata illa ciuitas magnum ... .

Spe premiorum tollerabilius ... .[40]

GLORIFICATIO CORPORIS ET ANIME: Circa rationem anime attenduntur scientia et ignorantia ... .

Item corpus de terra mortalitatem habet ... .[41]

GENEROSITAS: Ne uelitis dicere inter uos, "Patrem habemus Abraham" ... .

GVLA: Sicut piscis sub auiditate cibi recipit hamum ... .[42]

GRATITVDO: Nemo sane mentis pro quantacumque pecunia sibi sustineret oculos erui ... .[43]

HVMILITAS ET CARITAS:[44] Arborem attendite, prius petit deorsum ... .

HOMO BONVS:[45] Nummus probate monete et nomine regis insignitur et ymagine.

HOMO FACIT MINISTERIO: Dominus[46] edificator et custos ... .

HOMO LVXVRIOSVS ET DIABOLVS:[47] Sicut scarabeus in fimo uolutatur ... .

Sicut ursus[48] ad palum ligatus gressu terram territ ... .

HOMO MALVS:[49] Falsus Christianus nummus reprobus est.

Homines porcis similes sunt ... .

Malos homines diabolus tamquam malleos ... .

HORREVM:[50] Triticum congregabit Dominus in horreum suum ... .

HYPOCRITA: Gaudium ypocrite ad instar puncti ... .

Hypocrita simia est Bel, histrio ... .[51]

HOMO: Homines sunt ut poma mandragore ... .[52]

HVMILITAS: Forus est pisciculus qui propter exiguitatem ... .[53]

Arduum est quo ascendere molimur ... .

---

40 In patria nulli ...] *AEO: om. M*
41 Item ...] *AEM: om. O*
42 Gula ...] *AO: om. EM*
43 Gratitudo ...] *OEM: om. A*
44 et caritas] *AO: om. EM*
45 Homo bonus] *AO: om. EM*
46 Dominus] *AO:* Christus *EM*
47 et diabolus] *AO: om. EM*
48 ursus] *EM: om. AO*
49 Homo malus] *AEM:* Falsus Christianus *O*
50 Horreum] *AO:* Triticum *EM*
51 Hyprocita ...] *AEM: om. O*
52 Homo ...] *EM: om. AO*
53 Humilitas ...] *AEM: om. O*   Forus] Aphorus dicitur secundum Ysidorum *add. E in marg.*

HONOR SECVLI: Sic agunt qui mundi huius appetunt honores quomodo pueri qui secuntur papiliones ... .[54]

HYPOCRISIS: Golda uulgariter dicitur herba quedam ... .

INCARNATIO CHRISTI: Sicut miles qui ab omnibus timetur in prelio ... .

IVBILVS: Scimus quoniam hii qui multum ebrii sunt ... .

INTENTIO:[55] Farina si in uento portatur a uento dispergitur ... .

IEIVNIVM: Sicut equis sunt imposita frena, ita ieiuniorum ... .

IMITATIO CHRISTI: Imago resultans in speculo conformat se ei qui speculum intuetur ... .

IMAGO: Imagines sanctorum libri sunt laicorum.

IMMISERICORDIA: Parentibus uictualia subtrahens uipera est ... .

IRA: In mente turbida non lucet Dei imago idest ratio ... .[56]

    Iracundiam quidem uelud equum indomitum et ferocem ... .

INFESTATIO PARENTVM: Qui parentes molestant, pediculis assimilantur ... .

INVIDIA: Gregorius: Mens inuidi[57] cum de alieno bono affligitur ... .

    Sicut erugo ferrum ita inuidia ... .

    Canes beneficii memores uideas ... .

INGRATITVDO: Ingrati parentibus et benefactoribus uermibus carnis assimilantur ... .

INIVRIA: Sicut est equus qui recalcitrando percutit, mordet et hinnit ... .

INVIDIA: Sicut aridam quamque fragilemque materiem ... .

    Sicut rubigo proprie ferri corruptio est ... .

    Sicut uultures iocunda queque et amena loca transeunt ... .

IACTANTIA: Licinii superhabundantia religionis est iactantia proicienda.

INVIDIA: Invidia malitie pestis est et uiperea mater ... .

INCARNATIO CHRISTI: Nota quia Christus dicitur lignum uite ... .

IGNIS: Ignis tenaces materias dissoluit ut ligna et lapides ... .

INCARNATIO CHRISTI: Sicut ros descendit et flori infunditur ... .

INSTABILITAS: Triticum non rapit uentus ... .[58]

---

54 Honor ...] *AEM: om. O*
55 Intentio] *AO*: Ignis *EM*
56 imago ...] *AEO*: iracundia *M*
57 Mens inuidi] *AO*: Omnis inuidus *EM*
58 Instabilitas ...] *O: om. AEM (cf. infra*, Stabilitas)

Lvxvria: Quanto detestabilius est infringere sacrosanctam ecclesiam ... .[59]

Lectio: Sepe inter cotidianas delicias etiam uiliores cibi ... .

Labor: Lucta Iacob benedictionem promeretur ... .

    Secari et uri se permittit homo ... .

    Mercatores ut diuitias uenturas adquirant ... .[60]

Lvx: Sicut egris et incarceratis et nauigantibus ... .

Locvtio:[61] Sit tibi collum ardee ne sis preceps in sermone ... .

    Multiloquium non declinat peccatum, fluuius exundans cito colligit
lutum ... .

    Alliga sermonem tuum ne luxuriet ... .

Locvtio prava:[62] Sic uerba proximorum audiendo cotidie ... .

Lappa: Lappa alligat et alios adherentes sibi impedit ... .

Limbvs inferni: Vt speculum absque luce ... .

Libido: Ferreas mentes libido domat et sanguis hircinus dissipat
adamantem ... .

    Quomodo si aliquis carbones ignis apprehendat ... .

    In Tullio, Venus quod ad omnia ueniat legitur ... .

    Cur amor Veneris dicatur filius nullus ignorat ... .

    Anteus gigas erat, filius terre ... .

Lvxvria: Homo spurcus porcus est; fornicaria sanguisuga est ... .

    Porcus idest spurcus celum non respiciens est fornicator... .

    Quanto detestabilius est infringere sacrosanctam ecclesiam quam
plebiam domum ... .[63]

Libido: Sicut ad cotem ferrum exacuitur ... .

Lux:[64] Tempus huius seculi quasi nox est ... .

    Sicut pre nimio solis fulgore splendor stellarum ... .

    Augustinus de Iudeis qui magis iudicant Christum fuisse nasciturum
in Bethleem ... .[65]

Labor: Sustinens laborem attende mercedem ... .[66]

Libido: Rosa que ruboris intensi deliciis aspectui gratiosa est ... .

    Flamma crescit iniecta pinguedine ... .[67]

---

59 Luxuria ...] *AO: om. EM*
60 Mercatores ...] *A: om. EMO*
61 Locutio] *EM*: Loqui *AO*
62 Locutio praua] *AO: om. EM*
63 Quanto ...] *EMO: om. A*
64 Lux *ed.: om. AEMO*
65 Tempus ...] *AME: om. O*
66 Labor ...] *EMO: om. A*
67 Libido ...] *EM: om. AO*

Misericordia Dei: Per ineffabilia diuine pietatis uiscera ... .

Post redemptionem a corruptione quid restat nisi corona ... .

Misericordia Christi:[68] Illud quomodo non accusas quod et cum publicanis manducabat ... .

Misericordia:[69] Homo immisericors coruus est ... .

Qui ut faciat misericordiam optat esse miseros ... .

Augustinus: Noli misericordie pontem[70] subuertere quem transisti ... .

Mvnditia: Sicut studet quis officiorum suorum uasa munda seruare ... .

Meritvm: Sicut lux et uisus cooperantur ad uidendum ... .

Margarita: Margarite pisces sunt qui de rore concipiuntur ... .

Monachvs: Hirundines uolando apes capiunt ... .

Omnes qui ad usum huius uite quaslibet artes excercent ... .

Sicut miles plurimo onere pregrauatus prepeditur ... .[71]

Mali:[72] Cardui asperi et acuti sarculo preciduntur et abiciuntur ... .

Memoria peccati: Sicut umbram corporis mortalis ... .

Memoria mortis:[73] Surculis generosis, idest sanctorum exemplis ... .

Mors:[74] Falci succidenti et furi suffodienti ... .

Mors anime: Sicut plerumque uisibiliter in domo integra ... .

Mvndvs: Mundus ad similitudinem oui est dispositus ... .

Decor seculi quasi flos lilii ... .

Mvndana diligere: Quidam more infantilis stultitie diligunt ... .

Quedam mulieres grauide affectant ... .[75]

Meretrix: Meretrices ab obscenitatis et odoris ac rapacitatis similitudine lupas uocamus ... .

Maria virgo: Ego quasi uitis fructificaui ... .

Que habitas in ortis amici, etc. Poma carpimus ... .[76]

Medicina: Clauus clauum expellit et antidotum uenenum absorbet ... .[77]

Mvtva dilectio: Compaginatio domus Dei mutua dilectio est ... .[78]

Anima cum se totam effuderit in Dei amorem ... .[79]

---

68 Christi] *AO*: Dei *EM*
69 Misericordia] *AO*: Inmisericordia *EM*
70 pontem] *AO*: fontem *EM*
71 Omnes ...] *EMO*: om. *A*
72 Mali] *EM*: Monasterium *AO*
73 Memoria mortis] *AEM*: Mors et timor *O*
74 Mors] *AO*: om. *EM*
75 Quedam mulieres ...] *EM*: om. *AO*
76 Que habitas ...] *EM*: om. *AO*
77 Medicina ...] *O*: om. *AEM*
78 Mutua ...] *AEM*: om. *O*
79 Anima ...] *EM*: om. *AO*

MVTATIO OFFICIALIVM: Musce que ueniunt recentes acrius pungunt ... .[80]

NATIVITAS: Natus est Christus de uirgine sicut radius de sydere ... .
NAVIS: Velum spiritu plenum est corpus dominicum malo crucis appensum ... .
NEGLIGENTIA: Ne efficiamur illis similes qui causa querendi necessaria uictui ad ciuitatem pergentes ... .

ORATIO: Desiderium intensum clamor est ad Deum ... .
   Tardius exaudiuntur quorundam orationes ... .
   Oratio subtilis auicula est ... .
OBLATIO: Ostendit quis dominum suum temporalem ... .
OPVS: Exemplum uiatici colligendi artificiose mellificandi in nido ecclesie ... .
HOMO FACIT MINISTERIO: Dicitur architectus domum illuminare ... .
OBLIVIO:[81] Flos expansus cito deciduus ... .
OTIOSITAS: Iuuenis in otio quasi iumentum[82] sine iugo ... .
OBITVS: Qui bona defuncti suscipiunt et consumunt ... .
   Non est uita humana sicut ludus puerilis ... .

PRELATVS: In primogeniti conuiuio Sathan obruit filios Iob ... .
   Sicut aqua baptizans in ima descendit ... .
   Per obliquas fenestras lumen intrat et fur non ... .
   Tanquam e luto sub die formatus ... .
   Ex arsi et thesi idest eleuatione et depressione stellarum ... .
   Sol magis calefacit ualles remotiores quam montes propinquiores ... .
   Qui recte buccinare intendit spiritum attrahit ... .
   Christus in humanitatis susceptione cera humanitatis apposita igni deitatis ... .
   Quanto maior honor tanto maiora pericula ... .
   Super cathedram Moysi sederunt scribe et pharisei ... .
   Pro patribus tuis nati sunt tibi filii ... .
PREDICATOR: Predicator docens et non faciens es sonans est ... .
   Pascit coruus Heliam ... .
   Corda campane est mensurata uita predicantis ... .

---

80 Mutatio ...] *AEM*: *om. O*
81 Obliuio] *A M*: Nesciat sinistra quid faciat dextera *O*: *om. E*
82 iumentum] *A O*: iuuentus *EM*

Qui recta dicit et non agit ut arcus prauus in se iacit.

Dum cecus cecum pascit ... .

Cos in se hebes est, aciem tamen ferri magis acutam reddit ... .

PREDICATIO: Verbum in ore polluto diuinum radius solis est in loco immundo ... .

Si infirmis uno in tempore exhortationis sermo fuerit ... .

Paulus Corinthios quos in omni uerbo ... .

Necesse est semper ut sermo predicationis cum auditorum debeat qualitate formari ... .

Aiunt aliqui summa totius predicationis hec est: bene fac et bene habebis ... .[83]

Sicut ferrum ex lapide ita sermo ex corde lucis scintillas elicit.

Sicut qui oculos dolent solis lumen accusant ... .

Cur non sapientie sicut cythare et tibie impenduntur labor et studium ... .

PREDICATIO ET ORATIO: Sicut ex escis carnalibus alitur caro ... .

PROTECTIO DEI: Scuto circumdabit te ueritas ... .

Protectio Dei scutum est ... .

Scuto circumdabit te ueritas eius. Scutum supra dilatatur, infra angustatur ... .

PROMISSIO DEI: Mel promissionis Dei dulce sapit palato fidei.

PROSPERITAS FALLAX: Piger cantat cum cicada in estate ... .

PRVDENS VIATOR:[84] Boni sic utuntur temporali subsidio sicut uiator utitur umbra ... .

PROSPERITAS:[85] Stulti quasi per amena prata ad carcerem... .[86]

PECVNIA: Puteorum aqua si frequentius hauriatur ... .[87]

PROFECTVS: Non possis oculo quantum contendere linteus ... .

Informis minus solidis idest argillosis ... .

PASSIO CHRISTI: Duo sunt que foramen faciunt in petra ... .

A terra est exaltatus omnia ad se attracturus ... .

Christo passo in carne et uos eadem cogitatione armamini. Tamquam elephanti inspecto sanguine uue ... .

POTESTAS: Vis non timere potestatem? Fac quod bonum est ... .

PERSEVERANTIA: Fimbriam uestimenti dominici tangere ... .

PECCATOR: Sicut pila rotunda uolubilis ima petit ... .

Pulli aquile degeneres a luce solari lumina deflectunt ... .

---

83 Aiunt ...] *EMO: om. A*
84 Prudens uiator] *AEM*: Pecunia uel prosperitas *O*
85 Prosperitas] *EO: om. AM*
86 Stulti ...] *EMO: om. A*
87 Pecunia ...] *EMO: om. A*

De peccatore dicitur in Iob, leuis est super faciem aque ... .

Ratio peccatorem reuocet, mitiget spes ... .

Ciuitatem et castrum domini sui hostibus citra sanguinis effusionem ... .

Inuidus assimilatur musce ... .

PRAVVS HOMO: Nonne ouis trahitur cui esurienti herba monstratur? ... .

PIGER: Homo ignauus nauci et officiperdi fucus est ... .

PIGRITIA IN PROSPERIS:[88] Piger in prosperis exultans ... .

PERICVLA TEMPORIS: Est autem corpus graue, tempus breue ... .

PECCATVM: Sicut ponderosa ad centrum tendunt ... .[89]

PECCATVM: Fugientes quidem peccatum sicut bruta animalia ... .

Sicut statere momentum si in unam partem depresseris ... .

Quisquis non uult igniri exilientem igniculum non sinat ... .[90]

Peccatum est mus, serpens, ignis, quia rodit, pungit, et urit ... .

Peccatum in primo parente quasi uermis fuit in radice ... .

Fundamentum aliud nemo potest ponere ... .

Sicut asinus carduos comedit ... .

Later quasi luter a luto, cum recens est potest aqua dissolui ... .

Nos sumus quasi musce, peccata retia, diabolus aranea ... .

PONDVS PECCATI ET CARITAS:[91] Plumbum et lapis ima petunt ... .

EFFECTVS PECCATI:[92] Nemo prius alii quam sibi nocet ... .

Qui uult nocere proximo similis est ei qui attemptat alium percutere gladio ... .

PENA PECCATI: Annus pro die imputabitur ... .

PECCATORVM FVGA:[93] Circumspice omnia et cauta intentione considera ut effugias sicut damula ex laqueis et sicut auis ex retibus ... .

PENITENTIA:[94] In puteo cordis sit aqua contritionis ... .

De stilla populi congregabitur Iacob; apparet in stellicidiis que gelu constricta in superioribus pendent ... .

In medicamento penitentiali, herba predominans est elemosina ... .

Omnia ligna cupiditatis consumit ignis caritatis.

Sic sacerdos peccatum dimittet sicut baculus percutit uel oculus uidet ... .

88 in prosperis] *AEM*: et labor *O*
89 Peccatum ...] *O*: *om. AEM*
90 Sicut statere ...] *EMO*: *om. A*
91 Pondus peccati] *EM*: Peccatum *AO*
92 Effectus peccati] *AO*: Peius leditur dampno innocentie quam pecunie *EM*
93 Peccatorum fuga] *AEM*: Fuga peccati *O*
94 Penitentia] *AEO*: Contritio *M*

Sal uulnus curat, animam sapientia sanat.

Sicut nauem exhoneramus ita quedam dispensamus ... .

Redeat Agar ad dominam suam ... .

Item exeat Abraham a Caldea, Loth a Sodoma ... .

Tabule penitentie firmiter hereas ... .

In nebula patent aranee et in penitentia culpe.

Sicut patienter tolerat egrotus quando in eo putridas carnes urit ... .

Qui in peccatis excusationes pretendunt, malorum suorum aduocati fiunt.

Via regia nobis est ut funambuli linea ... .

Fumus spissus et humidus euaporat ... .

Medicus ad egrum ueniens in ferro et igne putridas carnes urit et secat ... .

Qui plurima peccata habet si omnia dimittat preter unum similis est illi qui, ligatus multis catenis, omnes preter unam rumpit ... .[95]

Mensura honeris pro mensura debet esse gestantis ... .

Per amarum poculum confectionis peruenitur ad gaudium salutis.

Sicut sol post pluuiam clarior fulget ... .

Lauamini lauacro scilicet penitentie ... .

Penitentia non sit nouacula superficiem tantum abradens ... .

Nostis quod fera uel auis illaqueata fame cruciatur et moritur ... .

Labor precedat requiem et resurrectionem gloriosam sicut parasceue sabbatum et diem dominicum ... .

Lacrima aqua est; faciem humectat ... .

Turtur amisso coniuge sedet in arido ... .

Peccatum uulnus est ... .

Adhibenda est post lapsum cautela ... .

Puer ustulatus ignem ueretur ... .[96]

Potio amara est dum sumitur, cauterium pungit cum incidit... .

Maria cum tympano canit ... .

Qui plangit peccatum et iterum admittit peccatum quasi si quis lauerit laterem crudum ... .

Cum ergo nos a Deo uideri non credimus ... .

PENITENTIE EFFECTVS: Sicut sol noctis tenebras fugat et non nubeculas ... .

PENITENTIE DILATIO: Dicit aliquis homo: Iuuenis sum; facio quod me delectat ... .

PEPLVM CROCEVM IN VETVLA: Sicut est peplum croceum in uetula ... .

95 Qui plurima ...] *EMO: om. A*
96 Puer ...] *EM: om AO*

PENITENTIA: Post scopam flatus plenius mundat aream ... .

   Quamdiu ferrum est in uulnere non est malagma apponere ... .

PREDICATIO CHRISTI: Ex Syon species decoris eius ... .

PASSIO CHRISTI: Arbor splendorem solis habens in se ... .

PROTECTIO DEI: Scutum est protectio Dei, in temporalibus angustum ... .

PREDICATIO: Ex tenui fistula et gracili uox dulcior sepius emittitur ... .

   Preco uerbi Dei dicitur predicator ... .

PREDICATIO PECCATORIS: Qui bene loquitur et non operatur est sicut
sunt tibicines ... .

   Luna, idest ecclesia uel anima, terra interposita amore terrenorum,
patitur eclipsim.

PERSEVERANTIA: Nolite similes esse sambuco ... .[97]

PRESVMPTVOSVS: Presumptuosus similis est ei qui uidet athletam
pugnantem ... .[98]

PASSIO CHRISTI: Myrra masticata fetori oris ex uitio stomachi proce-
denti medetur ... .[99]

PREDICATIO: Apostoli de Ierusalem fugati quasi ligna ardentia ... .[100]

PECCATA: Nemo prius alteri nocet quam sibi, peccatum enim simile
est facule ... .

   Sicut lepra sic peccata ... .[101]

PECCATOR EST MOLA:[102] In circuitu impii ambulant; mola quippe ... .

PECCATVM DIABOLI: Iudicauit Dominus crimen demonis ... .[103]

PENITENTIA: Sicut agnita resurrectione Domini gauisi sunt discipuli,
sic anima resurgente ... .[104]

PROSPERA ET ADVERSA: Stelle tantum in nocte lucent, in die la-
tent ... .[105]

   Gregorius, Moralium libro xxi: Iniustus ad debitam mortem currens ... .[106]

PRELATI: Sol admirationem parit intuentibus ... .[107]

---

97 Perseuerantia ...] *EM: om AO*
98 Presumptuosus ...] *EM: om. AO*
99 Passio ...] *EM: om. AO*
100 Predicatio ...] *EM: om. AO*
101 Sicut lepra ...] *EM: om. AO*
102 Peccator est mola] *A*: Peccator *E: om. MO*
103 Peccatum diaboli ...] *EM: om. AO*
104 Penitentia ...] *E: om. AMO*
105 Stelle ...] *AO: om. EM*
106 Gregorius ...] *EM: om. AO*
107 Prelati ...] *EM: om. AO*

Qvidam prosvnt aliis et non sibi: Quid dicam de infidelitate iudeorum ... .

   Similes facti fabris arche Noe ... .

   Quis dum in domo est que comburitur ... .[108]

Qvomodo Filivs nascitvr a Patre: Ponamus aliquid natum super
aquam uelut uirgultum aut herbam... .

Qvaliter Christvs nascitvr ex Virgine: Sicut auis ex ligno bernaca,
scilicet de abiete sine mixtura maris et femine ... .[109]

Resvrrectio mortvorvm: Qui costam edificauit in mulierem ... .

Renovatio: Renouabis faciem terre tollendo faciem culpe ... .

Remedivm contra accidiam: Caput grauatum manus sustinet ... .

Recidivatio: Pharaonitici sunt qui post plagam ... .

Rapina: Mirmicoleon Latine dicitur formicarum leo ... .

Item Rapina: Aliqui rapiunt non sua qui uel tanquam lupi siluestres
uel tanquam accipitres ... .

Raptor: Raptor similis est baculo ... .

Remedivm contra temptationem: Dixit senex: Mulier quando uult
ablactare filium suum ... .[110]

Rapina: Ericius si inuenerit poma in terra prostrata ... .[111]

Spiritvs sanctvs: Columba non requiescit in palude ... .

   Sicut odor ex arbore aromatica ... .[112]

   Spiritus sanctus sicut apis fauum mellis incolit ... .

   Aqua ex fonte et riuo profluens ... .

   Spiritus sanctus tanquam auis celica ... .

Sapiens: Humilis sapiens est aluear, extra luteum, intus melle plenum.[113]

Stabilitas: Triticum non rapit uentus nec arborem ... .

Scientia: Scientia luci uel Deo assimilatur ... .

   Ad radium solis in domo uidentur attomi ... .

   Pila scientia est inutilis absque motu ... .

Salvs: Sicut animus melior est corpore ... .

Psallere: Psallam et intelligam ... .

Scriptvra: Scriptura est tela: historia stamen est, figura subtegmen.

108 Quis ...] *EM: om. AO*
109 Qualiter ...] *EM: om. AO (cf. infra, Xpc de Virgine)*
110 Remedium ...] *EM: om. AO*
111 Rapina ...] *EM: om. AO*
112 Sicut odor ...] *AEM: om. O*
113 Sapiens ...] *AO: om. EM*

Cui uerbum sacri eloquii nisi lapidi simile dixerim ... .

Quando possumus de diuinis operibus que leguntur ... .

SEMEN: Mirum quidem est quomodo desperamus de eternis ... .

SPES: Canticum est itinerantis spes uespertine quietis et uberrime refectionis ... .[114]

SVBVENIRE: Membra in constitutione corporis sibi inuicem subueniunt; lapides in fabrica ecclesie ... .

SINVS ABRAHE: Sinus Abrahe uel superior locus erat inferni ... .

SANCTI NON COMPATIVNTVR DAMPNATIS IN INFERNO: Licet pater filium, uel filius patrem, uel mater filiam ... .

SIMILIA SIMILIBVS CVRANTVR: Sathanas sathanam expellit, clauus clauo retunditur, draco draconem uorat ... .

SENEX: Inueteratus dierum malorum incorrigibilis est sicut confracta testa uetus irreperabilis est.

SENECTVS: Qui thesaurum fodiendo querit ... .

SECVLARIS: Sanctus Malachias de natali barbarie nichil traxit, non magis quam pisces maris de sale materno.

SVPERBIA: Olla uento inclusa crepat in fornace ... .

Omne pomum, omne granum, omne frumentum, omne lignum habet uermem suum ... .

Superbia est apotheca peccati.

Ventus tiphonicus fructus deicit ... .

Pauo pulcherima auis est ... .[115]

SECVLARIS: Harena salsugine maris infecta fructum non facit ... .[116]

SVGGESTIO ET PREDICATIO: Ex collisione erumpunt scintille ... .

SERPENS: Serpens quidam accessurus ad fontem prius uenenum euomit ... .

Serpens ut dicitur per angustum foramen transire nititur ... .

SENSVALITAS: Sensualitas lia lippa dicitur et sepe in iudicio fallitur, sicut rectum in aqua fractum et curuum reputatur.

SENECTVS: Senes similes sunt ebriis ... .[117]

TRINITAS: Vt contorta trium candelarum insimul lucentium, trinitas est personarum.

Exemplum trinitatis et similitudinem qualemcumque assignare poterimus in sole, radio, feruore ... .

114 Canticum ...] EMO: Canticum etiam inter algores in ore itinerantis A
115 Pauo ...] EMO: om. A
116 Secularis ...] AO: om. EM
117 Senectus ...] AEM: om. O

TIMOR:[118] Aquila per naturam nimii est caloris ... .

TIMOR DOMINI:[119] Si multitudini ramorum non pepercit Deus ... .

TIMOR: Qui timore compulsus et in extremis coartatus testamentum componit ... .

TIMOR SERVILIS: Supra Psalmum xciii dicitur quod irreuerenter et aperte peccans similis est leoni ... .

TROPVS: Pessimo quasi lucra dare est dampna non inferre ... .

TRIBVLATIO: Nec miles equum odio habet quem calcaribus urget ... .[120]

   Pro Iuda turbabatur nauis Petri.

   In naribus galline uel auce penna posita ... .

   Cum multe sint tribulationes iustorum ... .

   Sicut pueris insensatis ad lutum ludentibus ... .

   Aurifex uas necessarium facere uolens ... .[121]

   Origines: Sicut caro si sale non aspergitur ... .[122]

   Dominus dedit, Dominus abstulit ... .

   Quod lima ferro, quod flagellum grano ... .

   Sicut solaris radius lucens emicat in facie aque ... .

   Sic electorum desideria dum premuntur aduersitate proficiunt ... .

   Manet dissimilitudo passorum etiam in similitudine passionum ... .

   Non pari motu exagitatum exhalet horribiliter cenum ... .[123]

TEMPTATIO: Carduus si nascatur in uia ... .

TRIBVLATIO: Terrores quos cernimus sequentis ire precones sunt ... .

ITEM TRIBVLATIO: Pretiosior est gutta mirre que sponte manat ... .[124]

TEMPESTAS: Fluctus dicti sunt quod flatibus fiant ... .[125]

TRIBVLATIO: Attende quicumque ob iniustas quereris uexationes, ferrum igne decoctum emollitur ... .[126]

VOLVNTAS DEI: Voluntas Dei regula scriptoris est, uel cementarii funiculus ... .

VERBVM DEI: Contemptor uerbi Dei aspis surda est ... .

   Sicut pigmentum in ore frequenti reuolutione dulcescit ... .

   Semen uerbi diuini necat estus cupiditatis ... .

---

118 Timor] *AEM*: Timor uel uerbum Dei *O*
119 Timor Domini] *AEM*: Time *O*
120 Tribulatio ...] *AEM*: *om. O*
121 Aurifex ...] *EM*: *om. AO*
122 Origines ...] *AO*: *om. EM*
123 Non pari ...] *EM*: *om. AO*
124 Item Tribulatio ...] *AEM*: *om. O*
125 Tempestas ...] *AEM*: *om. O*
126 Tribulatio ...] *AEM*: *om. O*

Verba apostoli cibus anime sunt ... .

Sicut ex carnalibus escis alitur caro ... .

Grossa materies utilior est in structura domus ... .

VNITAS ECCLESIE:[127] Multi radii, rami, riui, unus sol, unum robur, unus fons ... .

Sicut rami in stipite, membra in corpore, corde in cithara, ita nos simus in unitate.

VNITAS ECCLESIASTICA: Obsecro, inquit Apostolus, uos fratres ... .

Quomodo enim solis multi radii set lumen unum ... .

VNANIMITAS SANCTORVM IN PATRIA:[128] Concordia sanctorum est ut oculorum quo unus aspicit ... .

VIRGINITAS: Minorem locum habebit mater in regno celorum quoniam maritata est ... .

VOTVM: Pharaonitici sunt qui egritudinibus ut plagis tacti prompte promittunt ... .

VOLATVS: Non pigrescamus set de terrenis consurgamus ... .

VERBA: Verba sunt uehicula sensuum, folia fici ... .

VIA:[129] Sicut hiis quibus per districtos in excelso funes incedere disciplina est ... .

Transiuimus, inquiunt fideles, per ignem et aquam ... .

VITA PRESENS:[130] Esca in muscipula est dulcedo uite presentis ... .

Mundus est locus peregrinationis et exilii ... .

Item mundus forum est in quo sancti se et sua pro Deo uendunt ... .

VTILITAS EST IN VILIBVS: Sunt herbe uiles set utiles ... .

VINDICTA: Qui lutum percutit se ipsum inquinat ... .

VTI SVGGESTIONE DIABOLI: Sic male bono utitur reprobus et bene malo utitur probus ... .

VOLVPTAS: Esca in muscipula uoluptas est in culpa.

Voluptas uiscus est.

VITIA: Super aspidem id est negligentiam ... .

Coagulatum est sicut lac cor eorum ... .

VOLVPTAS:[131] Auersum a matre pullum galline uel auce ... .

Scuto circumdabit te ueritas eius ... .[132]

---

127 ecclesie] *EM*: *om. AO*
128 Vnanimitas] *AO*: Vnitas *EM*
129 Via] *AO*: Via per quam itur *EM*
130 Vita presens] *A*: Vite dulcedo *EM*: *om. O*
131 Voluptas] *EM*: *om. AO*
132 Scuto ...] *AEM*: *om. O*

Voluptas: Multe facies hominum sic et corda diuersa ... .[133]

Verbvm Dei: Ad calorem solis, id est dilectionem Dei manna liquefit ... .

   Verba Dei sunt quasi species aromatice ... .

Verbvm: Sicut est superior lanugo cardui lenis ... .[134]

   Lucem diei bubones non sustinent ... .[135]

   Arbor plerumque ab ubertate fructus destituitur ... .[136]

Verbvm Dei: Cithara Dei diuina doctrina est ... .[137]

Xpc: Christus pons est utramque ripam attingens ... .

   Christus apis, mel proferens in primo aduentu ... .

   In sole calor et splendor in uno radio sunt ... .

   Vt musicus melos tonis dulcibus reddat, pariter tria adesse uidentur:
ars, manus, corda ... .

   Quod uirga nuces produxerit ymago est dominici corporis ... .

   Quemadmodum medicum tunc maxime admiramur cum uidemus
eum difficiles hominum ualitudines curantem ... .

   Ille qui quasi apis in conceptione ... .

Xpc de Virgine:[138] Sicut auis ex ligno bernaca ... .

Xpc est lapis conterens: Lapis Christus est, olla homo est ... .

Xpc: Christus prius quasi sol in rota non poterat uideri ... .

Xpc trahit omnia: Omnia ad me traham id est amor mei omnia ad
se trahet ... .[139]

De dominio:[140] Apostoli in uia tractant de eorum maioritate ... .[141]

---

133 Voluptas ...] *O: om. AEM*

134 Sicut ...] *EMO: om. A*

135 Lucem ...] *AEM: om. O*

136 Arbor ...] *A: om. EMO*

137 Verbum Dei ...] *AEM: om. O*

138 Xpc de Virgine] *O:* Qualiter Christus ex uirgine *A: om. EM (cf. supra,* Qualiter
Christus ...)

139 Xpc trahit ...] *AEM: om. O*

140 De dominio] *EM:* Principatus *A: om. O.*

141 Apostoli ...] *AEM: om. O*

II.10

Proverbia

William's *Prouerbia et alia uerba edificatoria* comprises what we would call a florilegium, or an encyclopedia of quotations, for use by preachers, teachers, and students. He has collected here the pithy wisdom of the Bible and the liturgy, classical authors, the Church Fathers and their ecclesiastical successors, and the common people.

Reference works like this one have a long history, but William's collection stands at the beginning of a golden age in which they enjoyed unparalleled popularity. During the thirteenth and subsequent centuries a great deal of energy was devoted to the collection, organization, and presentation of the *dicta* and wise sayings of ancient (and not-so-ancient) authorities. A librarian at the end of the fifteenth century summed up the usefulness of the genre in his comments on another compendium very similar to William's:

> This book contains diverse extracts ... gathered into one collection from the diverse "wheatfields" of the authorities. Within its covers one finds promptly at hand the material that one could scarcely find in searching through many separate volumes. One finds listed here in alphabetical order, like a concordance, the more important and commonest topics that arise in both lectures and sermons, and, indeed, those topics which might be helpful to a person in all things.[1]

William's *Prouerbia* is a significant, and hitherto largely unnoticed, contribution to the florilegia-literature of the Middle Ages.[2] It is

[1] This description of Thomas of Ireland's *Manipulus florum* in the shelf-list of the Salvatorberg catalogue (now Weimar MS qu 22) is quoted by Richard H. Rouse, "Backgrounds to Print," p. 42.

[2] In general, see H. Marie Rochais, "Florilèges spirituels," and Philippe Delhaye, "Florilèges médiévales d'ethique," in *Dictionnaire de spiritualité* (1962), 5: 435-475; B. Munk Olsen, "Les classiques latins dans les florilèges médiévaux antérieurs au xiii siècle," *Revue d'histoire des textes* 9 (1979) 47-121, and 10 (1980) 115-164; Rouse and Rouse, *Preachers*; idem, "Florilegia of Patristic Texts," in *Les genres littéraires dans les sources théologiques et philosophiques médiévales: Definition, critique et exploitation*, Actes du Colloque international de Louvain-la-Neuve, 25-27 mai 1981 (Louvain-la-Neuve, 1982), pp. 165-180.

distinguished from contemporary collections by its length, its organization, and its comprehensiveness; not until the early years of the fourteenth century would a comparable work, the *Manipulus florum* of Thomas of Ireland, be produced.[3] The text of William's *Prouerbia* is divided into 281 subject categories which are organized alphabetically (first letter only) to facilitate the use of this work in scholastic and pastoral education. Previous florilegia had been organized according to author with all the quotations from a single author, on whatever topic, grouped together or divided into a very few topical categories. William's choice of several hundred topics, most of them familiar to the readers of his other writings, made his work more accessible to scholars and preachers who wished to find apposite quotations for their own uses.[4]

More than 5,000 Latin proverbs and quotations are grouped under these 281 topical headings. One of the limitations of William's work was its casualness regarding attributions of authority. Few of the quotations specify the particular work of an author in which they might be found, and many even fail to specify the author. Nevertheless the range of authorities included in William's *Prouerbia* is impressive (see below, *Sources*). Earlier collections had drawn on one or two types of literature — the classical poets and/or philosophers, or the Church Fathers, for example. William's *Prouerbia* encompasses a much wider field. He includes pagan and christian writers of both poetry and prose, as well as edifying *dicta* of the popes and councils of the Church, quotations from saints' lives, and even popular proverbs. An example of this last type of material, one that has come down unchanged to our own day, is the first entry under the rubric "On Guests," namely, "Guests, like fish, begin to smell after three days."[5]

Subsequent generations would refine and improve on William's techniques for constructing a dictionary of quotations. Alphabetization of subject entries by the whole word rather than the first letter only was introduced during the thirteenth century. Cross references by means of "dummy" or empty headings and reference symbols would be provided to guide the reader in his or her search. More care would be taken to specify accurately the author and work from which

---

[3] Rouse and Rouse, *Preachers*, pp. 113-161.

[4] Rouse and Rouse, ibid., pp. 7-42, discuss the historical development of this type of organization, and its importance in the *Manipulus florum* (pp. 117-121).

[5] "DE HOSPITIBVS: Hospites triduani incipiunt fetere ut pisces ... ," Oxford, New College MS 98, fol. 86rb = *O*, no. 3 below.

quotations derived, and to introduce the reader to the *originalia*, the complete works of the authorities quoted.[6] But the basic innovations that characterized this important kind of reference tool are already evident in William's *Prouerbia*.

AUTHENTICITY AND DATE

All three of the extant manuscript copies ascribe the work to William de Montibus; all the ascriptions date from the first half of the thirteenth century. The style of the work, including the brief prologue, is typical of William's other writings. The text's division into numerous, alphabetically arranged topics is unusual in florilegia of this period, but corresponds precisely to William's organization of his *Distinctiones*, *Similitudinarium*, and *Versarius*; nearly all of the topic headings can be found in one or more of these authentic works. The most recent authorities are from the middle of the twelfth century (Gratian, Bernard), and are of no use in dating the work. The English provenance of the extant manuscript copies suggests that it was written in Lincoln, perhaps at about the same time as the similarly organized *Distinctiones* and *Similitudinarium*.

SOURCES

The authorities quoted in the *Prouerbia* are extremely diverse. They include classical and late-antique authors (both poets and "philosophers"), the Church Fathers, lives of saints, conciliar decrees, papal pronouncements, and more recent ecclesiastical writers such as St. Anselm, Hildebert of Le Mans (of Lavardin), and St. Bernard. William did not excerpt all of these quotations from the original writings of the authors. He undoubtedly drew on several of the extant florilegia and scholastic collections circulating at the end of the twelfth century. Many though not all of the quotations from ancient authors, for example, are found in such collections as the *Proverbia* and *Sententiae philosophorum*,[7] the *Florilegium Gallicum*,[8] and the *Florilegium An-*

---

[6] All of these refinements are discussed in Rouse and Rouse, *Preachers*, passim.

[7] Edited by Eduard von Wölfflin in *Caecilii Balbe De nugis philosophorum* (Basel, 1885), pp. 18-43.

[8] See R.H. Rouse, "Florilegia and Latin Classical Authors in Twelfth- and Thirteenth-Century Orleans," *Viator* 10 (1979) 131-160; Rosemary Burton, *Classical Poets in the "Florilegium Gallicum"* (Frankfurt M.: Peter Lang, 1983).

gelicum.[9] No single collection, however, can be shown to be the source from which William drew his authorities.

Quotations from the Bible and its glosses may have been excerpted by William himself. So, too, the occasional references to twelfth-century writers and to lives of saints may be the fruits of his own reading. The ubiquitous quotations of Hildebert of Le Mans (*Episcopus Cenomanensis* in the manuscripts), however, suggest a pre-existing collection of his *sententiae.* All of the quotations from popes, bishops, Roman law, and Church councils, and many from the Church Fathers seem to have been excerpted from Gratian's *Decretum*; indeed, Gratian himself is cited occasionally. These may be the fruits of William's own reading, but we might better infer from them the existence of one or more legal/canonical florilegia that served as the sources of William's citations.

In addition to the Bible and the Gloss, William cites by name the following authorities (names have been anglicized here, but occasionally are given in their more familiar Latin forms):

Alcuin, Albinus, Alexander (the Great), Pope Alexander ɪ, Ambrose, Pope Anacletus, Anselm, Arator, Aristotle, Augustine, Basil, Basilissa, Bassus, Bede, Bernard, Boethius, Cassiodorus, Cato, Pope Celestine ɪ, Caesarius (of Arles), Cicero (and *Tullius*), Claudian, Pope Clement ɪ, Codex (of Roman Law), Constantine the Bishop, Cyprian, Cyril, Digest (of Roman Law), Diogenes, Egidius (Life of), Ephraem (Syrus), Epicurus, Pope Eutychian, Eusebius, Pope Evaristus, Fabius Verricosus, Pope Felix, Gilbert (of Poitiers?), Gratian, Pope Gregory (the Great), Haymo, Hesychius, Hilary, Hildebert of Le Mans, Horace, Isidore, Jerome, John Chrysostom, Pope John vɪɪɪ, Josephus, Juvenal, Lambertus, Pope Leo ɪ, Lives of the Fathers, Lucan, Lucretius, Manefranes, Martial, Pope Nicholaus ɪ, Council of Orleans, Ovid, Abbot Palladius, Pope Paschasius, Pope Pelagius, Persius, Plato, Plautus, Pliny, Prosper (of Aquitaine), Prudentius, Publi<li>us (Syrus), Pythagoras, Secundus the Philosopher, Seneca, Sidonius, Simonides, Pope Siricius, Pope Sixtus, Socrates, Statius, Pope Stephen v, Symmachus, Bishop Tarasius, Terence (*Comicus*), Theophrastus, Council of Toledo, Pope Urban ɪɪ,

---

[9] See R.H. Rouse and M.A. Rouse, "The *Florilegium Angelicum*: Its Origin, Content, and Influence," in *Medieval Learning and Literature: Essays Presented to R.W. Hunt*, ed. J.J.G. Alexander and M. Gibson (Oxford: Clarendon Press, 1976), pp. 66-114. This work was used by Gerald of Wales as a source for many of his classical quotations; he may have made its acquaintance during his sojourn in Lincoln in the 1190's. See Goddu and Rouse, "Gerald of Wales and the *Florilegium Angelicum*," pp. 488-521.

St. Vincent (Life of), Virgil, Zeno. Quotations of popular proverbs
are scattered throughout the work.

MANUSCRIPTS

1. *J* = Cambridge, Jesus College MS Q.B.17 (34), fols. 48ra-62vb. Early
13th century (above top line).

> Title: (*Incipiunt prouerbia et alia uerba edificatoria a magistro Willelmo
> Lincolniensis ecclesie cancellario in ordinem disposita*)
> Inc. Prol: *Ad edificacionem animarum*
> Inc. Txt: (*De amore uel amicicia uera uel ficta*) *Beda super Tobiam*
> Expl. Txt: (*De diuiciis*) ... *hoc est possessiones iam senes querimus.*

Incomplete; text ends on the fourth line of column b, and the remainder
of fol. 62vb is blank.

2. *T* = Cambridge, Trinity Hall MS 24, fols. 86va-101ra. Mid 13th
century (above top line).

> Title: (*Incipit liber prouerbiorum excerptus a magistro Willelmo de
> monte*)
> Inc. Prol: (*Incipit prologus*) *Ad edificacionem animarum*
> Inc. Txt: (*De amore uel amicicia uera uel falsa*) *Beda super Tobiam*
> Expl. Txt: (*De inpetu*) ... . *Numquid apud parthos, armeniosque latet.
> Iam cras istud habet priami uel*

Incomplete; the remainder of fol. 101 is blank. A table of contents
for the complete work is found on fol. 86r.

3. *O* = Oxford, New College MS 98, fols. 59va-123vb. Early 13th
century (above top line).

> Title: (*Incipiunt prouerbia et alia uerba edificatoria a magistro Willelmo
> Lincolniensis ecclesie cancellario in ordine disposita*)
> Inc. Prol.: *Ad edificacionem animarum et morum informationem*
> Inc. Txt.: (*De amore uel amicicia uera uel falsa*) *Beda super Tobiam*
> Expl. Txt.: (*De Xpiano*) *Ieronimus* ... . *Fidelis male uiuens oculos habet
> in luce clausos, et infidelis bene uiuens oculos habet in tenebris apertos.*

The prologue and the 127 citations that comprise the first entry,
De amore uel amicitia uera uel falsa, are transcribed in full from
Oxford, New College MS 98 (*O*), the only complete copy, with selected
variants from Cambridge, Jesus College MS Q.B.17 (*J*) and Trinity Hall
MS 24 (*T*). The topical rubrics of the subsequent entries are printed,
and are followed by numbers within square brackets indicating an
approximate count of the quotations under that heading.

Prouerbia

Incipiunt Prouerbia et alia uerba edificatoria a magistro Willelmo Lincolniensis ecclesie cancellario in ordine disposita.

Ad edificationem animarum et morum informationem undecumque[1] excerpta utilia proferimus ex omnibus escis que mandi possunt in archam inferentes, ubi etiam flores reperies ad oblectandum, margaritas ad ornatum, fauos ad[2] esum, et ad confortandum electuaria salubria. Que autem ab omnium[3] bonorum largitore Deo accepimus, ad ipsum referimus, ipsi in omnibus gratias agentes, et eius honori et utilitati publice studium et operam impendentes.

DE AMORE VEL AMICITIA VERA VEL FALSA[4] [127]
BEDA SVPER TOBIAM: Sunt amici carne nominis non hominis inimici anime. IDEM super Iudith: Qui ueneni poculum porrigit, labium calicis melle tangit, ut quod dulce est presentiatur ne quod mortiferum est timeatur.[5]

Amor carnalis infatuat et mortificat creaturam spiritualem,[6] uel languere facit.

ANSELMVS: Affectus carnalis infatuauit in me saporem spiritualium; amor terrestrium extinxit in me delectationem celestium.

Facilius uitaretur aperta inimicitia quam occulta. Ille enim difficile uitatur, qui in labiis bona portat et in corde mala occultat.

Quos amplexus mundi implicant, minus ad celestia hanelant.

Iudei licet pleni essent eorum uentres aqua de petra, tamen aride erant mentes; adaquauit eos Dominus quasi pecora non homines, quia non egerunt grates: "Et dilexerunt eum in ore suo, et lingua sua mentiti sunt ei" [Ps 77:36].

Anima adultera plus diligit anulum quam sponsum, id est dona Dei quam Deum.

Amicus non est qui particeps fortune non est.

Ita amicum habeas ut posse fieri hunc inimicum putes.

---

1 undecumque] *JT*: unumcumque *O*
2 ad] *JT*: in *O*
3 omnium] *JT*: omni *O*
4 falsa] *OT*: ficta *J*
5 timeatur] *JT*: timantur *O*
6 spiritualem] *JT*: spiritualis *O*

SENECA: Per absentationem et dissuetudinem unius[7] ad alterum claudicat affectio, et est amor incidens, et leuius remittitur. IDEM:[8] Amicitia nec maiorem effert, nec minorem secludit, set utrumlibet in parem admittit et socium. IDEM: Si uis amari, ama. IDEM: Sunt amicitie quas temporarias populus apellat, que utilitatis causa assumpta est; tam diu placebit quam diu utilis fuerit. IDEM: Possis dicere quandam esse insaniam amicitiam. IDEM:[9] Conciliari nisi[10] turpi ratione amor turpium non potest. IDEM: Consortium rerum omnium inter nos facit amicitia; nec secundi quicquam singulis est nec aduersi; in[11] commune uiuitur. Nec potest quisquam beate degere qui se tantum intuetur, qui omnia ad utilitates suas conuertit: alteri uiuas oportet si uis tibi uiuere.

EPISCOPVS CENOMANENSIS: Iustum est ut aduersa communicent qui prosperis coutuntur. IDEM: Vicem mihi rependes si ames me et ores pro me. IDEM: De tua memoria quid loquar que meum[12] pectus altius irrupit, latius occupauit, stabilis possidet, uiuenti conuiuit.[13] IDEM: Locorum uel temporum[14] incommoda, sanctus amor ignorat. IDEM: Maximum duco atque habeo quod mihi uestre sacrarium familiaritatis aperuisti. IDEM: Negligenter cauetur hostis cuius ingressus pacificus expectatur.

CATO: Parce laudato, nam quem tu sepe probaris, una dies qualis fuerit monstrabit amicus. IDEM: Demissos animo et tacitos uitare memento; quod flumen placidum est forsan latet altius unda. IDEM: Qui simulat uerbis nec corde est fidus amicus; tu quoque fac simile, sic ars deluditur arte.

POETA (VIRGILIVS):[15] Quid non speremus amantes? IDEM: Omnia uincit amor, et nos cedamus amori. IDEM: Quis fallere possit amantes?

ALIVS POETA (STATIVS):[16] Nil transit amantes. IDEM: Nichil flagrantibus obstat.

POETA (OVIDIVS):[17] Negligimus spinas cum cecidere rose. IDEM: Heu mihi cur animis iuncti seiungimur undis? Vnaque mens tellus non habet una duos. IDEM: Quos credis fidos effuge tutus eris. IDEM: Vt ameris

---

7 unius] *JT*: unus *O*
8 Idem] *JT*: *om. O*
9 Idem] *J*: *om. OT*
10 nisi] *JT*: non *O*
11 in] *JT*: id est *O*
12 meum] *JT*: mecum *O*
13 conuiuit] *JT*: conuiuet *O*
14 temporum] *J*: temporis *OT*
15 Virgilius] *J*: *om. T*: *in marg. O*
16 Statius] *om. JT*: *in marg. O*
17 Ouidius] *om. T*: *in marg. JO*

amabilis esto. IDEM: Vulgus amicitias utilitate probat, et cum fortuna statque caditque fides. IDEM: Illud amicitie sanctum et uenerabile nomen prostat et in questu pro meretrice sedet. IDEM: Diligitur nemo nisi cui fortuna secunda est. IDEM: Res est solliciti plena timoris amor. IDEM: Quid deceat quid non, non uidet ullus amans. Nobilitas sub amore iacet. IDEM: Vnde hoc compererim tam bene queris, amo. IDEM: Meminerunt omnia amantes. IDEM: Nullus bene celat amorem. Eminet indicio prodita flamma suo. IDEM: Hinc amor hinc timor est, ipsum timor auget amorem. IDEM: Non ueniunt in idem pudor atque amor. IDEM: Nunc male res iuncte calor et reuerentia pugnant. Quid sequitur in dubio est. Hec decet ille iuuat. IDEM: Idem procul insano uictus amore timor. IDEM: Quis enim celauerit ignem, lumine qui semper proditur ipse suo. IDEM: Obsequio plurima uincit amor. IDEM: Heu sero reuocatur amor, seroque iuuentus, cum uetus infecit caua senecta capud. IDEM: Militat omnis amans, et habet sua castra cupido. IDEM: Sompnus non bene prestat amanti. IDEM: Nox et amor uinumque nichil moderabile suadent; illa pudore uacat, liber amorque metu. IDEM: Ludit et interdum prelia miscet amor. IDEM: Arte leues currus arte regendus amor.[18] IDEM: Et leuis est, et habet geminas quibus euolet alas. Difficile est illis imposuisse modum. IDEM: Dulcibus est uerbis dulcis uel mitis alendus amor. IDEM: Militie species amor est, discedite segnes. Non sunt hec timidis signa ferenda uiris. IDEM: Quod iuuat exiguum est, plus est quod ledit amantes. IDEM: Non possunt ullis ista coire modis, scilicet amor et reuerentia. IDEM: Diuitiis alitur luxuriosus amor. IDEM: Non bene conueniunt, nec in una sede morantur, maiestas et amor. IDEM: Tempore[19] creuit amor. IDEM: Notitiam primosque gradus uicinia[20] fecit. IDEM: Conscius omnis abest, nutu signisque loquuntur, quoque magis tegitur, tectus magis estuat ignis. IDEM: Quid non sentit amor? IDEM: Nil certe est quod non effreno captus amore ausit, nec capiunt[21] inclusas pectora flammas, atque moras male fert. IDEM: Facundum faciebat amor. IDEM: Nulla est secura uoluptas. IDEM: Nos cuncta timemus amantes; credula res amor est. IDEM: Suadet amor facinus. IDEM: Spes est que capiat, spes est que pascat amantem. IDEM: Longa uiget assuetudine flamma. IDEM: Quid non amor improbus audet? IDEM: Omnis amans semper quod timet esse putat.

---

18 Arte ... amor] *JT*: *om. O*
19 tempore] *JT*: tempora *O*
20 uicinia] *JT*: uictima *O*
21 nec capiunt] *T*: capiunt *J*: sapiunt *O*

ALIVS POETA (ORATIVS):[22] Ne fidas inter amicos sit qui dicta foris eliminet. IDEM: Archanum neque tu scrutaberis ullius unquam commissumque teges et uino tortus et ira.

ALIVS POETA (IVVENALIS):[23] Aulam resupinat amici, scire uoles secreta domus atque inde timeri.

BOETIVS: Prius carus quam proximus esse cepisti. IDEM: An presidio sunt amici quos non uirtus set fortuna conciliat.[24] Set quem felicitas amicum facit, infortunium facit inimicum.

SENECA: Que pestis efficacior ad nocendum quam familiaris inimicus.

SECVNDVS PHILOSOPHVS: Amicus est desiderabile nomen, homo uix apparens.

SENECA: Amicitie officium est idem uelle idem nolle; secreto ammonere, palam laudare. IDEM: Dissimulare magis humanum est quam dare operam id scire quod te nosse amicus nolit.

AVGVSTINVS: Tantum frigitur bonus quantum amat. Frustra quis pro illo orat qui fratri debitam caritatem negat.

GREGORIVS: Vires quas imperitia denegat, caritas subministrat. IDEM: Plerumque caritas quibusdam occupationibus prepedita, et integra flagrat in corde, et tamen non monstratur in opere. Quia et sol cum nube tegitur non uidetur in terra, et tamen ardet in celo, sic esse occupata caritas solet, intus uim sui ardoris exerit, et foris flammas non ostendit.

Amor Christi martires prodigos sanguinis facit.

DE SANCTO EGIDIO: Iam tunc foris scintillabat indiciis intus succensa lampas caritatis.

AMBROSIVS: Omnia seua et inmania, facilia et prope nulla facit amor.

Angusta est uia laboranti, lata amanti.

Caritas que non proficit deficit,[25] et que nichil adquirit non nichil perdit.

Non minor est uirtus quam querere parta tueri.

Quis ita sollicitus est in spiritualibus ut artifices in secularibus; quis in gratuitis et meritoriis ut illi in mechanicis? Quis tantam dat anime curam ut corpori? Probatio dilectionis est exhibitio operis; inde conicimus eum plus diligere corpus quam animam, qui sepius et sollicitius et libentius consulit in egritudine medicum quam sacerdotem.

Iustum est ut qui Dei feruet amore, omnibus habeatur dignus honore.

---

22 Oratius] *om. T*: *in marg. JO*
23 Iuuenalis] *om. JT*: *in marg. O*
24 conciliat] *ed.*: conciliatos *J*: consiliatur *OT*
25 deficit] *JT*: *om. O*

Tu uero omnia cum[26] amico delibera, set de ipso prius.

MANEFRANES, cum illi diceret quidam ille amicus illius est, cur ergo inquid ille diues est, ille pauper est.

ARISTOTELES: Difficile est in re prospera amicos probare, in aduersa semper facile.

THEOFRASTVS: Expedit magis probatos amicos amari quam amatos probari.

Amicitias immortales esse oportet.

SENECA: Hos omnes amicos habere operosum est, satis est inimicos non habere. Itaque sapiens numquam potentium iras prouocabit, immo et declinabit, non aliter quam in nauigando procellam.

ORIGINES: Quomodo est quidam carnalis cibus et alius spiritualis, et alia carnis potio et alia spiritus, sic est quidem amor carnalis a Sathana ueniens alius amor spiritus a Deo exordium habens.[27]

IERONIMVS: Facilius potest negligentia emendari quam amor nasci.

TVLLIVS, DE AMICITIA: Nulla est excusatio peccati si amici causa peccaueris. IDEM: Hec in amicitia lex sancciatur ut neque rogemus res turpes, neque faciamus rogati. IDEM: Hec lex amicitie sancciatur, ut ab amicis honesta petamus, et amicorum causa honesta faciamus.

Plurimum in amicitia amicorum bene suadentium ualet auctoritas. Verus amicus est is qui tanquam alter idem.

SIMACVS: Mollis est animus diligentis, et ad omnem sensum doloris arguitur. Si negligentius tractes cito[28] marcescit ut rosa; si durius teneas liquescit ut lilia.

SALOMON [Prov 13:20]: Amicus stultorum similis efficietur. IDEM [17:17]: Omni tempore diligit qui amicus est. IDEM [18:1]: Occasiones querit qui uult recedere ab amico. IDEM [18:24]: Vir amicabilis ad societatem magis amicus erit quam frater. IDEM [22:11]: Qui diligit cordis munditiam, propter gratiam labiorum suorum habebit amicum regem. IDEM [27:5-6]: Melior est manifesta correctio quam amor absconditus. Meliora sunt uulnera diligentis quam fraudulenta oscula odientis.

IHESVS FILIVS SIRACH [Eccli 6:1]: Noli fieri pro amico inimicus proximo.

ITEM SALOMON, DE AMICITIA FALSA [Prov 19:4]: Diuitie addunt amicos plurimos; a paupere autem et hii quos habuit separantur.

ITEM IHESVS FILIVS SIRACH [Eccli 6:8]: Est amicus secundum tempus suum, et non permanebit in die tribulationis. IDEM [6:10]: Est amicus

---

26 cum] *JT*: animi *O*
27 habens] *JT*: hominis *O*
28 cito] *T*: negligencius *J*: negligenter *O*

socius mense, et non permanet in die neccesitatis. IDEM [37:1]: Est
amicus solo nomine amicus. IDEM [37:2]: Sodalis et amicus ad
inimicitiam conuertuntur. IDEM [22:25]: Mittens lapidem in uolatilia
deiciet illa; sic et qui conuiciatur amico dissoluit amicitiam.

IEREMIAS [9:4-5]: Vnusquisque se a proximo suo custodiat, et in
omni fratre suo non habeat fiduciam. Quia omnis frater supplantans
supplantabit, et omnis amicus fraudulenter incedet, et uir fratrem
deridebit, et ueritatem non loquetur. Docuerunt enim linguam suam
loqui mendacium; ut inique agerent laborauerunt. ET PAVLO POST [9:8]:
Sagitta uulnerans lingua eorum dolum locuta est. In ore suo pacem
cum amico loquitur, et occulte ponit ei insidias.

ABDIAS, AD EDOM [1:7]: Viri federis tui illuserunt tibi; inualuerunt
aduersum te uiri pacis tue. Qui comedent tecum ponent insidias subter
te.

MICHEAS [7:5]: Nolite credere[29] amico, et nolite confidere in duce;
ab ea que dormit in sinu tuo custodi claustra oris tui.

IERONIMVS: In amicis non res queritur set uoluntas, quia alterum
ab inimicis sepe prebetur, alterum sola caritas tribuit.

29 credere] *JT*: tradere *O*

DE CONSILIO [16]
DE CONSENSV [7]
DE CAVTELA [17]
DE CONTINENTIA [4]
DE CASTITATE [10]
DE COMPASSIONE [9]
DE CORREPTIONE VEL COR-
    RECTIONE [28]
DE CVRIALIBVS [2]
DE CORPORE VEL CARNE [15]
DE CONVIVIO [9]
DE CENA [5]
DE CANTV [6]
DE CONCVPISCENTIA [5]
DE CVPIDITATE [50]
DE CONFVSIONE [3]
DE CONTRARIIS [2]
DE CRVDELITATE [5]
DE CASV [3]
DE CAVSA REI [10]
DE COMPOSITIONE CORPORIS [10]
DE CONSERVATIONE VEL
    CVSTODIA [7]
DE CONSVETVDINE [35]

DE MODO DICENDI [10]
DE MODO DISCENDI[30] [33]
DE DISPUTATIONE [21]
DE DETERMINATIONE VEL
    DISCRETIONE [17]
DE DECIMIS [5]
DE DONIS [44]
DE DIVITIIS [99]
DE DELICIIS [5]
DE DILIGENTIA [2]
DE DESIDERIO [2]
DE DIE IVDICII [22]

DE DETRACTIONE [17]
DE DAMPNO [3]
DE DIABOLO [8]
DE DVRITIA VEL OBSTINATIONE [8]
DE DOLORE ET TRISTITIA [30]
DE DEO [37]
DEVS IN SANCTIS [1]
OMNIA BONA A DEO [73]
DE DEI SCIENTIA [3]
DE DEI MISERICORDIA ET GRA-
    TIA [42]

DE ESV [8]
DE EBRIETATE [23]
DE ERRORE [2]
DE EGRITVDINE [2]
DE EXCOMMVNICATIONE [1]
DE EXCVSATIONE IN PECCATIS [16]
DE ETATE ET TEMPORE[31]
DE ECCLESIA [15]
DE ELEMOYSINA [48]
DE EXEMPLO [10]

DE FIDE [35]
DE FORTITVDINE [4]
DE FAVORE [8]
DE FAMA [22]
DE FEDIA [1]
DE FESTIS [5]
DE FVRE VEL FVRTO [6]
DE FORTVNA [30]
DE FAME[32]
DE FVGA [7]
DE FEMINA [58]
DE FORNICATIONE [12]
FLVERE [1]
FALLERE VEL FALLI [7]

---

30 De modo discendi] *T*: Discere *O*: *sine tit. J*
31 De ... tempore] *in tabula T*: *om. JO*
32 De fame] *in tabula T*: *om. JO*

DE FICTIONE [3]
DE FRAGILITATE [3]

DE GVLA [28]
DE VANA GLORIA [32]
DE PRIMA GRATIA [6]
DE GAVDIO [12]

DE HOMINE [9]
DE HOMICIDIO [8]
DE IPOCRISI VEL HERESI [25]
DE HISTRIONE [2]
DE HOSPITIBVS [7]
DE HVMILITATE [34]
DE HONORE [2]

DE IRA [54]
DE INVIDIA [33]
DE IRRISIONE VEL ILLVSIONE [8]
DE INIVSTO [3]
DE INIVRIA [4]
DE INGRATITVDINE [3]
DE IACTANTIA [3]
DE INFIRMITATE [7]
DE IGNORANTIA [4]
DE IVVENE [8]
DE INSTABILITATE [21]
DE IMPATIENTIA [7]
DE IMPETV VEL ACCELE-
    RATIONE [15]
DE IVDICIO [15]
DE INFERNO [7]
DE IOHANNE BAPTISTA [2]
DE IEIVNIO [18]
DE IVRAMENTO [5]
DE IVSTITIA VEL IVSTO [11]
DE INGENIO [4]
DE INTENTIONE [4]
DE IRE VEL ITINERE [10]

DE LIBIDINE VEL LVXVRIA [51]
DE LITE [22]
DE LABORE [15]
DE LOCO [18]
DE LVDO [5]
DE LETITIA [4]
DE LAVDE [30]
DE LEGE [14]
DE LECTIONE [20]
DE LOQVELA [125]
DE LINGVA [14]
DE LARGITATE VEL LIBERALI-
    TATE [8]
DE LIBERTATE [2]

DE MINISTERIO VEL MINISTRO [3]
DE MILITE CHRISTI [3]
DE MORTE [116]
DE MARTIRIO [16]
DE MIRACVLIS [2]
DE MARIA VEL MVLIERE
    BONA[33] [6]
DE MVNDO [21]
DE MALITIA MVNDI [17]
DE MALO HOMINE [37]
DE MERETRICE VEL MVLIERE
    MALA [24]
DE MENDACIO [17]
DE MALEDICTIONE [6]
DE MORA [1]
DE MATRIMONIA [23]
DE MODO [14]
DE MENSVRA [4]
DE MEMBRIS CORPORIS [1]
DE MAGNITVDINE [3]
DE MEDICINA [6]
DE MISERICORDIA [7]

---

33 De ... bona] *JO*: De moniali *in tabula* T

DE NEGOTIATIONE [2]
DE NEGLIGENTIA [6]
DE NECESSITATE [3]
DE NOBILITATE [23]
DE NATVRA [2]

DE OCVLO [8]
DE OTIO [23]
DE OBPROBRIO [6]
DE ODIO [1]
DE OPERE³⁴ [77]
DE ONERE [2]
DE OBEDIENTIA [11]
DE OBLATIONE [11]
DE ODORE [1]
DE ORATIONE [57]
OMNIBVS OMNIA FACTVS [2]
DE ORDINE [6]

DE PECCATO ET PECCANTIBVS [188]
DE PENITENTIA ET DE PENI-
  TENTIBVS [139]
DE PENA [23]
DE PATIENTIA [59]
DE PRELATIS [167]
DE PRINCIPE [65]
DE PREDICATORIBVS [104]
DE PABVLO ANIME [6]
DE PATRE FAMILIAS [3]
DE PARENTIBVS [3]
DE POTESTATE VEL POTENTIA [7]
DE PRIVILEGIO [1]
DE PVLCRITVDINE [10]
DE PRVDENTIA [6]
DE PROVIDENTIA [4]
PROBATE OMNIA [3]
DE PACE [3]
DE PROSPERITATE VEL FELI-
  CITATE [18]

DE PIGRITIA [10]
DE PRODIGALITATE [9]
DE PAVPERTATE [67]
DE PEDAGOGO [1]
DE PASSIONE VEL MORTE
  CHRISTI [7]
DE POTV [11]
DE PROFECTV [2]
DE PERSEVERANTIA [10]
DE PATRIA [4]
DE PREMIO [5]

DE QVESTIONE [4]
DE QVADRAGESIMA [1]
QVERERE DEVM [7]
DE QVIETE [2]

DE RAPINA [11]
DE RARO [3]
DE RATIONE [1]
DE REGE [6]
DE RVMORE [4]
DE REPREHENSIONE [12]
DE REMISSIONE [2]
DE RISV [5]

DE SOCIETATE VEL SOCIALI-
  TATE [27]
DE SOBRIETATE [9]
DE SPE [13]
DE SCRIPTVRIS VEL SCRIBENTI-
  BVS [15]
DE STVDIO [1]
DE SCIENTIA [32]
DE SAPIENTIA ET SAPIENTE VERO
  VEL FALSO [22]
DE SACRAMENTO [3]
DE SIGNIS [1]
DE SIMONIA [4]

---

34 De opere] *J: in tabula T*: De oracione *O*

DE SVPERBIA [57]
DE STVLTO VEL STVLTITIA VERA
  VEL FALSA [24]
DE SERVO VEL SERVITVTE [21]
DE SVBDITIS [12]
DE SENSIBVS CORPORIS [1]
DE SOMPNO VEL SOMPNIO [11]
DE SENECTVTE [33]
DE SEPVLCRO [6]
DE SOLLICITVDINE [11]
DE SOLITVDINE [5]

DE TIMORE [63]
DE TORPORE [3]
DE TEDIO [3]
DE TRIBVLATIONE [126]
DE TEMPORE [8]
DE TEMPERANTIA [1]
DE TACITVRNITATE [7]
DE TROPO [3]

DE VERBIS DEI [30]
DE VOLVNTATE [11]
DE VOTO [8]
DE VIRGINITATE [14]

DE BEATA VIRGINE [3]
DE VITA [18]
DE VITA ACTIVA ET CONTEM-
  PLATIVA [13]
DE VVLTV [2]
DE VISV [8]
DE VIGILIA[35] [3]
DE VVLGO [2]
DE VESTIBVS [18]
DE VIA VEL PEREGRINATIONE [22]
DE VVLNERE [2]
DE VITIIS [12]
DE VANITATE [2]
DE VOLVPTATE [11]
DE VSVRA [3]
DE VINDICTA [17]
DE VIRTVTE VEL VSV VIRTVTIS [4]
DE VNITATE VEL VNANIMITATE [6]
DE VERITATE [3]
DE VTILITATE [3]
DE VICTORIA[36]

DE XPO [48]
DE XPIANO [3]

---

35 De uigilia] *J*: *in tabula T*: Vigilate *O*
36 De uictoria] *in tabula T*: *om. JO*

II.11

Tropi

The application of the grammatical, rhetorical, and logical teachings of the twelfth-century schools to theology is the aim of this interesting and unusual *summa*. Like Peter the Chanter's homonymous work, *De tropis loquendi*, William's *Tropi* represents the culmination of several decades of theological discussion in Paris. Both writers summed up the consensus of the schools concerning the proper use of the liberal arts for interpreting sacred scripture. William's *summa* is more straightforward and somewhat less technical than the Chanter's, but both reflect the high standards of interpretative skills demanded of theological students in the schools of Paris as well as Lincoln.

William introduces his work with an elaborate similitude:

> We dispense God's gifts. To those banging on the doors of the house we present the keys. To let light into the house we open the windows. We call this house "sacred scripture." Its doors are the authoritative writers (*auctoritates*). The keys and windows are ways of speaking which we call tropes or schemata, that is figures of speech.

An understanding of the principles of grammar, rhetoric, and logic is indispensable for the correct understanding of sacred scripture, and for appreciating the writings of its authoritative interpreters. These latter include not only the Church Fathers, but also councils, popes, theologians, and others whose works had been so assiduously assembled in the twelfth-century collections of theology and canon law. Tropes and figures of speech are the keys to understanding these authorities and the windows by which light can be shed on the Scriptures themselves.

In emphasizing the importance of grammatical, logical, and rhetorical principles for interpreting Scripture, William is in a tradition that goes back at least to Augustine's *De doctrina christiana*. But the immediate context of this work is the theological teachings of the late twelfth-century schools, especially at Paris.[1] In general approach, it bears

---

[1] See especially the suggestive studies by the late Franco Giusberti: *Materials for a Study on Twelfth Century Scholasticism*; and Gillian R. Evans's many studies,

comparison with the first two books of Peter of Poitiers's *Sententiae*,[2] with the theological questions from the school of Odo of Soisson and those of other mid-twelfth-century theologians,[3] and with Alan of Lille's *Distinctiones* and *Regulae caelestis iuris*.[4]

In both intention and conception William's *Tropi* is comparable to Peter the Chanter's *De tropis loquendi*,[5] but the oft repeated assertion that William's work derives from Peter's is a tenuous one. This conclusion was based on the presumption that William was Peter's student in Paris, but this seems very unlikely (see above, Chapter One). Rather it seems that Peter and William studied and taught as contemporaries at Paris, and William may have been the elder. No attempt has yet been made to date the composition of Peter's *De tropis loquendi*, but none of his other scholastic writings has been dated before 1186, when William had already moved from Paris to Lincoln. A comparison of the contents of the two works reveals no verbal dependence of one work on the other; indeed, despite the similarity of their titles, the works follow quite independent lines of approach. The occasional similarities in choice of examples or lines of argument point to their authors' shared training in the Paris schools and to their common reading in the literature of the day, but not necessarily to a literal dependence of one writer on the other. If William's *Tropi* was composed after 1200, it is possible that he had seen a copy of Peter's work (Peter died in 1197), but there is no evidence for the hypothesis that William brought a copy of Peter's *De tropis loquendi* with him when he returned from Paris to England c. 1186.[6] An edition of Peter's work will allow a more accurate comparison of the two treatises; from a purely pedagogical point of view, however, William's *Tropi* is the more clearly organized and the easier to follow.

---

including *The Language and Logic of the Bible*; some of her other works are cited below. A rich collection of logical and grammatical texts from the 12th-century schools, many written by and for theologians, are found in L.M. de Rijk, *Logica modernorum*.

[2] *Sententiae Petri Pictaviensis*, ed. Philip S. Moore, Marthe Dulong, and Joseph N. Garvin, 2 vols. (Notre Dame IN: University of Notre Dame Press, 1943, 1950); cf. de Rijk, *Logica modernorum*, 1: 163-178.

[3] See Giusberti, *Twelfth Century Scholasticism*, pp. 113-145.

[4] The *Distinctiones dictionum theologicalium* is printed in PL 210: 687-1012; the *Regulae* (PL 210: 621-684) have been edited by Nikolaus Häring, "Magister Alanus de Insulis Regulae caelestis iuris," *Archives d'histoire doctrinale et littéraire du moyen âge* 48 (1981) 97-226; cf. Evans, "Alan of Lille's *Distinctiones*," pp. 67-86.

[5] See Evans, "Peter the Chanter's *De Tropis Loquendi*, The Problem of the Text," pp. 95-103; idem, "The Place of Peter the Chanter's *De Tropis Loquendi*," pp. 231-253; idem, "Peter the Chanter's *De tropis loquendi*," in *History of Universities* (1982), 2: 1-14; Guisberti, *Twelfth Century Scholasticism*, pp. 87-109.

[6] Suggested by Evans, "Problem of the Text," p. 100.

William's *Tropi* was written for the students of theology at the cathedral school at Lincoln. Although these students might have received a somewhat less sophisticated preparatory training in the arts than their counterparts in the Parisian schools, they should not be imagined as ignorant of the principles which William applies in this work. William FitzStephen, in his life of Thomas Becket, gives a lively description of student recreation in the London schools of the later twelfth century:

> On holy days the masters of the schools assemble their scholars at the churches whose feast day it is. The scholars dispute, some in demonstrative rhetoric, others in dialectic. Some hurtle enthymemes, others with greater skill employ perfect syllogisms ... . Sophists who produce fictitious arguments are accounted happy in the profusion and deluge of their words; others seek to trick their opponents by the use of fallacies ... . Boys of different schools strive against one another in verse, or contend concerning the principles of the art of grammar or the rules governing the use of past or future ... .[7]

William's book is carefully organized to build on just such skills and turn them to the use of understanding the Bible and the Church authorities. Part One, comprising approximately thirty percent of the whole, deals with individual words (*dictiones*) and their multifarious meanings. Organized alphabetically, it is, in fact, a collection of *distinctiones* intended to clarify by analysis and example the different meanings of a word as it is used in Scripture and in theological or canonical discourse.

Part Two, DE POSITIONIBVS, concerns the positing or substitution of one word, or part of speech, or form of expression, for another. The entries in this part usually take the form: "Ponitur x pro y." The purpose here is sometimes to solve difficulties in the biblical text, for example the presence of a masculine form when one would expect the feminine.[8] Sometimes it is to suggest an interpretation of an obscure passage.[9] Most frequently the purpose is simply to clarify the meaning of a text. For example, William explains that the present tense some-times indicates the near future: "I ascend to my Father" (Io 20:17),

---

[7] Quoted in Edwards, *English Secular Cathedrals*, pp. 188-189.

[8] "GENVS ... . Dicunt filii Eth Abrahe: 'sepeli mortuum tuum,' idest Saram mortuam, et ponitur forsan masculinum pro feminino propter dignitatem generis, et quia post mortem non queritur sexus, quia ex tunc neque nubent neque nubentur ... ," p. 369.

[9] "SICVT PRO PER: Ponitur sicut pro per ut ibi: 'Extendens celum sicut pellem' [Ps 103:2], idest scripturam per predicatores mortales qui sunt sicut pelles Salomonis ... ," p. 368.

and sometimes the distant future: "Behold I come quickly" (Apoc 3:11).[10]

Part Three, DE ATTRIBVTIONIBVS, examines various statements in which an action or passion is attributed grammatically to one subject or object but in reality pertains to another; these entries are introduced by a phrase such as: "Attribuitur x quod est y." For example, in the phrase *O felix culpa*, happiness is attributed to the antecedent — the fault — when it really designates the consequence or result of that fault.[11] So too, when we say that some saint or prelate blesses, or remits sins, or saves, we are attributing to the member of Christ's body that which actually pertains to the head.[12]

Part Four, DE RESOLVTIONIBVS, addresses the problem of seemingly false statements which can be "resolved," according to the techniques of the grammarian and logician, into true equivalents. The entries are introduced by the phrase: "Resoluitur x in y." For example, the negative statement "Not the work but the intention is rewarded" is resolved into an elective one: "the intention, more than the work, is rewarded."[13] Similarly, an affirmative statement is sometimes to be resolved into a negative one: "'God wishes all persons to be saved' [1 Tim 2:4], that is, no one will be saved except by Him."[14]

Part Five, DE MODIS DICENDI, comprises approximately thirty percent of the text. Here William discusses figures of speech that are true statements but which might lead to errors in theological discourse if the student is not aware of the figures employed. The examples, introduced with a phrase like: "Dicitur x quod intelligendum est y," include discussions of speculative theology such as the trinitarian affirmation that "the Father and the Son love each other by the Holy Spirit,"[15] as well as more practical and pastoral issues. In discussing the ways in which one is said to give something to another William

[10] PRESENS PRO FVTVRO, below, p. 370.

[11] "ANTECEDENS PRO CONSEQVENTI: Attribuitur antecedenti quod est consequentis, uel ponitur antecedens pro consequenti, ut ... 'O felix culpe,' idest euentus ex culpa, scilicet occasione culpe ... ," p. 372.

[12] "MEMBRVM: Attribuitur membris quod capitis est, ut cum de sancto aliquo seu prelato dicitur quia sanctificat, remittit peccata, saluat, uel aliquid huiusmodi ... ," p. 373.

[13] "NEGATIVA: Resoluitur negatiua in electiuam, ut 'non opus set uoluntas remuneratur,' id est potius uoluntas," p. 375.

[14] "AFFIRMATIVA IN NEGATIVAM ... . Et 'Deus uult omnem hominem saluum fieri,' id est nullus saluabitur nisi per eum," cf. p. 375.

[15] "PROPTER APPARENTIAM ... . Item 'Pater et Filius diligunt se Spiritu sancto,' id est ostenduntur se diligere per hoc, scilicet quod communiter spirant Spiritum sanctum," p. 382.

raises the question of support for travelling entertainers: "It is one thing to invite minstrels, which is the deed of bad persons, another thing to admit them when they impose themselves, which pertains to the imperfect, and another ... to give them alms along with a reproof, or to repel them entirely, which is the act of the perfect."[16]

The sixth part is an addendum containing various general rules, solutions, and magisterial determinations. These are not systematic principles such as Alan of Lille's *Regulae*. Rather they are precepts and clarifications, recorded in no definite order, and presumably arising out of William's continuing teaching. One rule, under the heading DE MATERIA, explains: "Where the matter is lewd and indecent, or unprofitable, or dangerous, or hidden, or too difficult, one should cease disputing."[17] Another explains that "judgements and proofs must come from authorities, reasons, examples, and comparisons; for teaching by example is effective, but where does it say that proofs should be made with swords and cudgels."[18] Several entries take the form of responses to objections, for example: "To objections concerning the excesses of the saints, one responds 'it was done or said according to the intimate counsel of the Holy Spirit'"; Concerning obscure objections, one responds "'God knows' or ... 'seek not those things which are above you' [Ecclus 3:22], that is, beyond your capabilities."[19]

As these last responses suggest, William's *Tropi* was written with the classroom in mind, one filled with students of theology who might or might not have had a systematic introduction to the liberal arts. The *Tropi* makes little pretence of original speculation. Rather it seeks to make the fruits of several decades of theological and grammatical/logical teaching accessible to students in the Lincoln schools. Like Peter the Chanter's *De tropis loquendi*, this is a pedagogical tool designed

---

[16] "DICITVR ALIQVIS DARE: Dicitur aliquis dare quia permittit aliquid extorqueri uel accipi ... . Vbi tamen notandum quia aliud est ystriones inuitare quod malorum est, aliud est ingerentes se admittere quod imperfectorum est, aliud est eis uendere, idest cum correptione dare uel omnino repellere, quod perfectorum est," p. 380.

[17] "Vbi materia turpis est et indecens uel inutilis uel periculosa uel occulta uel nimis ardua, ibi subsistendum in disputatione," p. 387.

[18] "IVDICIVM: Iudicandum est et probandum est secundum auctoritates, rationes, exempla, similitudines; 'Viua et efficax est doctrina per exempla' [cf. Heb 4:11-12], set gladiis et fustibus facienda probatio ubi legitur?" p. 387.

[19] "DE EXCESSV SANCTORVM: Ad obiecta de excessu sanctorum, respondemus, 'Familiari consilio Spiritus sancti factum est uel dictum est,'" p. 387.

"OBSCVRA: Ad obiecta obscura, respondemus, 'Deus nouit,' uel 'Deus uoluit,' uel 'igni comburatur' [cf. Mt 3:12], uel 'O altitudo' etc. [Rom 11: 33]. Et 'Iudicia Dei abissus multa' [Ps 35:7], et 'altiora te' idest sensu tuo 'ne quesieris' etc. [Ecclus 3:22] ... ," pp. 387-388.

to exercise young theologians in the subtle skill of interpreting texts and formulating arguments.

AUTHENTICITY AND DATE

This work is ascribed to William in eight of the twelve known manuscripts; the other four bear no ascription. An internal reference at the end of Part One informs us that the *Tropi* was written after the author's *Distinctiones*, *Quaestiones* (unidentified), and a collection of sermons. The two Lambeth manuscripts (nos. 6 and 7 below) may witness to an earlier redaction of the text. They both end at the conclusion of Part Five, and omit the reference in the prologue to "rules and other materials" to follow the fifth part.

A casual aside under the rubric DE DVOBVS TESTAMENTIS in Part Six might contribute to the dating of this work. William illustrates different types of permission, and uses as an example: "Permissio specialis et etiam temporalis, ut Anglicos in quarto gradu contrahere." The traditional prohibition of marriage within the first seven grades of relationship was altered by the Fourth Lateran Council in 1215 (c. 50), so that only the first four grades were prohibited. William's example of the English receiving special permission to marry within the fourth grade of relationship clearly antedates 1215, but no record of such a special allowance being contemplated for, or directed to, the English has been identified.

SOURCES

In addition to the Bible and its Gloss, the following authorities are cited explicitly: Ambrose, Aristotle, Augustine, Bede, Boethius, Chrysostom, Constantine (the African), Fortunatus, Galen, Gratian's *Decretum*, Gregory, Hilary, Jerome, Lucan, Nicene Council, Peter Comestor's *Historia scholastica*, Peter Lombard's *Sententiae*. On the relation of William's *Tropi* to Peter the Chanter's *De tropis loquendi*, see above.

MANUSCRIPTS

1. Cambridge, Corpus Christi College MS 217, fols. 169r-187r. Mid 13th century (above top line).

> Title: *Incipiunt tropi a magistro Willelmo lincolniensis cancellario ad theologicam facultatem collecti.*
> Inc. Prol.: *Dei dona dispensamus*
> Inc. Txt.: *In primis dicimus*
> Expl.: *figura conuersionis et transposicionis.*

2. *C* = Cambridge, Corpus Christi College MS 397, fols. 131r-163v. Early 13th century (above top line).

    Inc. Prol.: *Dei dona dispensamus*
    Inc. Txt.: (*De dictionibus*) *In primis itaque dicimus*
    Expl.: *figura conuersionis et transpositionis.*

3. Cambridge, Gonville and Caius College MS 316/712, fols. 119ra-140vb. Mid 13th century (above top line).

    Title: *Incipit summa de diuersa uocabulorum significacione edita a magistro Willelmo de monte.*
    Inc. Prol.: *Dei dona dispensamus*
    Inc. Txt.: *In primis itaque dicimus*
    Expl.: *figura conuersionis et transposicionis.*

4. Cambridge, Jesus College MS Q.B.17 (34), fols. 15ra-43va. Early 13th century (above top line).

    Title: *Incipit summa de diuersa uocabulorum significacione edita a magistro Willelmo de monte.*
    Inc. Prol.: *Dei dona dispensamus*
    Inc. Txt.: *In primis itaque dicimus*
    Expl.: *figura conuersionis et transpositionis.*
    Colophon: *Expliciunt tropi in theologica facultate edita a magistro Willelmo de montibus cancellario lincolniensis ecclesie. Mons iste dicitur a multis mons coagulatus, mons pinguis.*

5. London, British Library Cotton MS Vespasian E.x, fols. 43v-59v. 13/14th century (below top line).

    Title: *Incipiunt tropi in theologica facultate, a magistro Willelmo linc. ecclesie cancellario collati.*
    Inc. Prol.: *Dei dona deprehensamus*
    Inc. Txt.: *In primis itaque dicimus*
    Expl. (incomplete in Part One): (*Mereri*) ... *habere uel uti, pati, uel omittere.*

6. London, Lambeth Palace MS 122, fols. 178ra-198va. Early 13th century (above top line).

    Inc. Prol.: *Dei dona dispensamus*
    Inc. Txt.: *In primis itaque dicimus*
    Expl. (incomplete in Part Five): (*Vnum*) ... *Et petrus meruit martirium, uel anima eius purgatorium.*

7. London, Lambeth Palace MS 199, fols. 226ra-248vb. Early 13th century (above top line).

    Inc. Prol.: *Dei dona dispensamus*
    Inc. Txt.: *In primis itaque dicimus*
    Expl. (incomplete in Part Five): (*Vnum*) ... *Et Petrus meruit martirium, uel anima eius purgatorium.*

8. Leiden, Rijksuniversiteit MS Vulcanianus 48 (E.173), fols. 195ra-212rb. Early 13th century (above top line).

Title: *Incipiunt tropi magistri Giullermi de monte.*
Inc. Prol.: *Dei dona dispensamus*
Inc. Txt.: *In primis itaque dicimus*
Expl.: *figura conpositionis et transpositionis.*
Colophon: *Explicit.*

9. *B* = Oxford, Balliol College MS 222, fols. 27vb-48va. Mid 13th century (below top line).

Title: *Incipiunt tropi magistri W. de montibus canonici ecclesie lincolniensis.*
Inc. Prol.: *Dei dona dispensamus*
Inc. Txt.: (*De dictionibus*) *In primis itaque dicimus*
Expl.: *figura conuersionis et transpositionis.*
Colophon: *Expliciunt tropi.*

10. *O* = Oxford, New College MS 98, fols. 33ra-59rb. Early 13th century (above top line).

Inc. Prol.: *Dei dona dispensamus*
Inc. Txt.: (*De diccionibus*) *In primis itaque dicimus*
Expl.: *figura conuersionis et transpositionis.*

11. Utrecht, Bibliotheek der Universiteit MS 312, fols. 126vb-142va. Mid 13th century (above top line).

Title: *Incipiunt tropi siue modi loquendi secundum magistrum Willelmum de monte.*
Inc. Prol.: *Dei dona dispensamus*
Inc. Txt.: *In primis itaque dicimus.*
Expl.: *figura conuersionis et transpositionis.*

12. Worcester, Cathedral Library MS F.61, fols. 169ra-180ra. 14th century (below top line).

Title: *Incipiunt tropi magistri Willelmi de Monte.*
Inc. Prol.: *Dei dona dispensamus*
Inc. Txt.: *In primis itaque dicimus.*
Expl.: *figura conuersionis et transpositionis.*
Colophon: *Explicit.*

A gathering is missing between fols. 171 and 172, thus eliminating the end of Part One (from the entry on *De*), and all but the last two entries of Part Two.

The following transcriptions from each of the topical headings of the *Tropi* are taken from Oxford, Balliol College MS 222 (*B* = no. 9, above) with selected variants from Cambridge, Corpus Christi College MS 397 (*C* = no. 2, above), and Oxford, New College MS 98 (*O* = no. 10, above).

Tropi

Dei dona dispensamus; pulsantibus claues ostiorum porrigimus; ad dilucidationem fenestras domus aperimus. Domum autem sacram Scripturam dicimus, ostia eius auctoritates, claues et fenestras modos loquendi quos tropos seu scemata idest figuras nuncupamus. Primum igitur de dictionibus hic agimus, secundo de positionibus, tertio de attributionibus, quarto de resolutionibus, quinto de modis dicendi, postremo de regulis et quibusdam aliis.

1 DE DICTIONIBVS

In primis itaque dicimus quia dictio semel posita[1] equiuoce accipitur, ut ibi: "Inclina cor meum Deus in testimonia tua et non in auaritiam" [Ps 118:36]; inclinat enim Deus ad bonum faciendo, ad malum permittendo ... . Item "Christus finis est legis" [Rom 10:4], terminans scilicet figuralia et implens moralia ... .

Quandoque solitaria est dictio nonsensus, ut "Christus non est creatura," scilicet pura, hoc est ita creatura quod non creator. Et "uirgo cogitat ut sancta et corpore et spiritu sit," idest sanctior, siue sancta magis.

ARTICVLVS FIDEI: Porro de dictionibus[2] hic secundum ordinem alphabeti disseramus. Attende ergo quia articulus fidei dicitur enuntiabile, ut uerum, credibile, credendum, creditum, ut "Christum esse passum" uel "Christum fuisse passurum" uel "hoc totum Christum esse passurum," uel patientem uel passum. Itaque Christum esse passum est aliquid quod ego credo quod non credidit Abraham. Sunt enim quidam articuli fidei alii nunc quam tunc, quidam idem, ut Deum esse trinum et unum. Quod autem dicitur "fides eadem tempora diuersa" intelligendum est de simbolo, sicut idem est populus licet alii homines, uel fides eadem est idest de eisdem siue circa eadem, uel creditum est idem.

Vel articulus fidei est euentus, ut passio Christi, que tamen non est, sicut materia Lucani est Cesar qui tamen non est.

---

1 posita] *BO*: posita non ex significatione uel consignificatione, set ex diuersa acceptione *C*

2 dictionibus] *BO*: dictionibus in primis pauca prelibauimus *C*

Et habet fidelis articulos fidei, scilicet enuntiabilia uel euentus in intellectu. Abraham itaque credidit Christum esse passurum quod quondam fuit articulus, hodie non, sicut "ecce uirgo concipiet" [Is 7:14] olim fuit prophetia, modo non.

Vel articulus fidei dicitur res, non euentus, ut "fides passionis portio," portio scilicet simboli habita de Christi passione, non pena eius scilicet patientia uirtute, set passione actiua idest sufficientia uel tollerantia pene. Et "fides Trinitatis est articulus fidei," nec dicitur hic est fides uirtus, set fidei uirtute creditur fides passionis uel fides Trinitatis. Set quid est fides Trinitatis nisi Trinitas credita? Sicut ratio sapientie, superior scilicet pars rationis, quid est nisi sapientia? Admittunt autem quidam quia Trinitas ipsa est articulus fidei.

ADORATIO: Scriptum est: "Dominum Deum tuum adorabis, et illi soli seruies" [Mt 4:10]. Contra, "Abraham adorauit populum terre" [Gen 23:7] ... . Respondeo, Grece liturgia uel latria uel latrensis dicitur seruitus uel seruitium religionis et cultus qui soli Deo debetur. Seruitus autem amoris communis homini et Deo et cuicumque superiori uel pro superiori Grece dulia dicitur. Cum ergo dicitur ab Apostolo "inuicem seruientes" [cf. Gal 5:13], iubemur per caritatem seruire inuicem, quod Grece dulium. Iubemur uni Deo seruire, quod Grece latrium, unde "et illi soli seruies" [Mt 4:10], unde dampnantur ydolatrie, hanc seruitutem scilicet ydolis exibentes ... .

AVREA: Aurea dicitur gloria uite eterne communis. Aureola est perfectio remunerationis scilicet supereminens magnitudo glorie, mensura super-effluens, et incrementum glorie, ut fructus centesimus quale est premium prelatorum, mundi contemptorum, martirum, et uirginum ... .

ANATHEMA: Apostolus ait: "Si angelus aliud euangelizet, anathema sit" [Gal 1:8]. Iosue ait de Iericho: "Sit ciuitas hec anathema et omnia que in ea sunt Domino" [Ios 6:17]. Ibi anathema in malo, hic in bo-no ... .

ADVLTER: Adulter uel huiusmodi dicitur quis actu, ut qui cognoscit alienam credens suam, uel reatu, set quoad oppinionem et conscientiam et quoad equipollentiam, ut qui cognoscit propriam credens alienam; et est aliquis adulter simul actu et reatu scienter cognoscens alienam.

ALIVD:[3] Aliud quandoque melius dicitur, unde Apostolus secunda Corintheo [2 Cor 11:4]: "Si is qui uenit," idest pseudo, "alium Christum predicat," idest excellentiorem, "quam ego" etc. Dicitur et aliud contra-

---

3 Aliud] *CO: om. B*

rium ... in fine symboli misse quod editum est in Niceno concilio subiunctum est "qui aliud docuerit" idest contrarium uel aliter ... . Item differentia substantialis facit aliud, idest differentie substantialiter. Item dicitur et aliud genere, specie, numero, dissimilitudine et uoluntate ... .

AVCTORITAS: Dicitur auctoritas Patris innascibilitas et principalitas; ipse enim est causa et principium omnium, et solus Pater habet auctoritatem in Trinitatem, quelibet uero trium personarum in creaturis. Dicitur et Pater auctor Filii quia genitor, et tum Pater tum Filius auctor Spiritus sancti ... .

AVCTORITAS MORTIS CHRISTI: Auctor mortis Christi dicitur Deus Trinitas approbando ... diabolus suggerendo ... .

BAPTISMVS: Dicunt quidam quia baptismus est ablutio, idest actio abluentis, que licet sit symoniaca et ita mortale peccatum tamen in eo quod est actio est bonum et a Deo, et est sacramentum ecclesiasticum ... . Aiunt alii quod baptismus est ablutio, idest passio abluti ... . Asserunt nonnulli quod baptismus est susceptio sacramenti ... . Plerique perhibent quod baptismus est ablutio, idest aqua abluens ... . Si ergo queritur quamdiu est aqua baptismus, respondeo: Quamdiu durat prolatio uerborum ... . Fatentur nonnulli quia baptismus est quiddam compositum ex actione baptizantis et passione baptizati, et forsan aliis concurrentibus. Set quid sit illud et quod predicamentale non determinant. Dicunt enim non omnia genera rerum comprehendi decem predicamentis Aristotilis; neque enim ibi includuntur consuetudo, silogismus ordo, et plura alia ... . Inquiunt alii baptismus est caracter; set si caracter est sacramentum, cuius rei est signum? Et cui etiam et a quo imprimitur? Quis hic qui baptizat? Dicunt autem alii quod ablutio aque baptismus est signum scilicet interioris ablu ... .

BAPTISMVS: Est baptismus in aqua, in penitentia, in sanguine; hec enim uicem baptismi supplent in articulo necessitatis ... .

BONVM: Bonum dicitur summum bonum, causa et fons et origo boni, unde "nemo bonus nisi Deus" [cf. Mt 19:17], essentialiter, causaliter, naturaliter; et res bone nature ... .

CREDERE: Credere dicitur habere fidem, sic credit paruulus uel dormiens; et uti fide, idest moneri, et sacramentum fidei suscipere, sic paruulus credit quod pro eo patrinus respondet ... .

CONFESSIO: Est contritio uel confessio uniuersalis, habita scilicet uel facta de omnibus peccatis ... . Est et particularis, de peccatis notis et ignotis ... .

COACTIO: Est coactio conditionalis, ut in Petro negante ... . Est absoluta et uiolenta, ut in Marcello papa ... .

CORPVS CHRISTI: Corpus Christi proprium speciale et personale est quod traductum est de Virgine ... . Corpus Christi res est cuius sacramentum dicitur forma panis in altari ... . Corpus Christi misticum et generale est ecclesia[4] ... .

CARITAS: Caritas dicitur Deus Trinitas, unde "Deus caritas est" [1 Io 4:8] ... . Caritas Filius ... . Et caritas magis apropriato uocabulo Spiritus sanctus ... .

CONSCIENTIA: Conscientia dicitur commissorum scientia; comissa uoco opera precedentia ... . Et estimatio idest putatio, ut "iste loquitur contra conscientiam." Et intentio, ut "iste habet cauteriatam conscientiam," idest prauam intentionem et adustam ... .

CONCVBITVS: Est concubitus coniugalis siue nuptialis, causa scilicet prolis generande et regenerande uel causa debita reddendi. Est concubitus fragilis, ut causa incontinentie uel infirmitatis. Est concubitus impetuosus et detestabilis. Primus ex toto excusatur, secundus ex parte, tertius nullomodo, quia est mortale peccatum.

CAVSA: Causa attendenda est. Sepe enim necessitas aliquid cogit, ut uti iuratione infideli per falsos deos, uel mutuatione feneratoris, uel plures habere tunicas siue ecclesias dumtamen non superfluas ... .

CAVSA: Attende etiam quia cum quid prohibetur uel precipitur uel consulitur propter causam, potius causa in dicto est quam propositum, ut "non neophitum, ne" etc. [1 Tim 3:6], et in primitiua ecclesia interdictus est esus sanguinis propter scandalum. Prohibetur etiam assiduitas iurandi propter periurium ... .

CAVSA: Item causa propter quam uel sine qua non fieret parit simoniam, causa sine qua fieri non posset nequaquam. Quandoque etiam redditur predicamentum cause, ut "homo assumptus in Deum clarificatus est," idest persona secundum quod homo, uel secundum humanitatem assumptam ... .

CARO: "Caro et sanguis regnum Dei non possidebunt" [1 Cor 15:50], idest carnales. Contra, "non potui uobis loqui quasi spiritualibus set quasi carnalibus" [1 Cor 3:1]. Respondeo, spiritualis dicitur uel carnalis homo uel uita uel scientia ... .

4 misticum ... ecclesia] *BO*: sacramentum est cuius res est ecclesia uel unitas ecclesie *C*

CAPVD: Apostolus ait: "Omnis uiri capud Christus est; capud autem mulieris, uir" [1 Cor 11:3] ... . Dicitur autem metaforice Christus capud ecclesie, et in omnibus hiis metaforicis supple "quasi," et expone secundum proprietates rei proposite.

DEVS: Dicitur Deus substantialiter siue naturaliter, ut Deus Trinitas scilicet Pater, Filius, Spiritus sanctus ... . Deus dicitur adoptiue, participatione scilicet deitatis ... .

DILECTIO DEI: Hoc nomen dilectio cum de Deo dicitur uel est essentiale, ut sit dilectio Dei eius uoluntas et approbatio ... . Vel est personale, ut cum dicitur "dilectio que est ex Deo Deus est" ... .

DILECTIO HOMINIS: Dilectio hominis interior motus mentis est, scilicet affectus; dilectio exterior exhibitio beneficii scilicet effectus ... .

DIGNITAS: Dignitas dicitur excellentia cause, ut "Deus dignus est laudari," quia in eo est hec dignitas scilicet naturalis eius bonitas. Et dignitas dicitur idoneitas ... .

DEBITVM: Est debitum promissi, secundum quod dicitur "Deus debet dare uitam eternam perseueranti," quia sic promisit ... . Est debitum comissi, secundum quod beata Virgo plus debet Deum diligere quam Magdalena, quia cui plus committitur plus ab eo exigitur. Est debitum dimissi ... debitum iuris ... debitum meriti ... debitum nature ... debitum officii ... .

DENOMINATIO: Denominatio uel nominatio uel appellatio sumitur a predominante secundum naturam, ut "quid natura tale magis tale est," scilicet potentialiter, licet non dicatur usu loquendi, quoniam penes arbitrium est, et ius et norma loquendi, potentia quippe preiudicat actui. Et Constantinus ait in Libro graduum quod nomen rei attribuitur ab ea qualitate que sibi dominatur ... .

DE: Est de uel ex distinctiuum, ut "Filius de Patre." Distinguitur enim persona a persona, tamen est ei consubstantialis. Est de gratuitum uel operatiuum uel potentiale uel affectiuum, ut cum dicitur "Christus incarnatus, conceptus, natus de Spiritu sancto" ... .

EXCEPTIO: Attendende sunt exceptiones, ut hic: dixit Dominus ad Noe, "Finis uniuerse carnis uenit coram me" [Gen 6:13]. Glosa: Omnium mortalium preter eos qui in archa sunt saluandi, quasi seminarium secunde originis ... .

EXTENSIO: Est et extensio figure uel regule licita, ut "tantum facis quantum intendis" a simili, tale, quale, ei, cui, et huiusmodi. Ab una enim regula plures coniciuntur ... .

FACERE DEI: Facit Deus per se, ut cum creat, idest de nichilo aliquid facit. Facit et mediante natura, propagando scilicet et ex similibus similia producendo ... . Facit et Deus per ministrum ... .

FORMA: Forma dicitur natura, ut "Qui cum in forma Dei esset" [Phil 2:6], idest in plena essentia et equalitate Patris. Hec est forma substantialis non accidentalis ... . Dicitur et forma factura ... et forma exemplar ... et forma figura et similitudo ... .

FIDES: Fides dicitur opinio, nam uehementer opinari credere dicitur sicut uehementer credere, scire. Dicitur et fides qualitas naturalis scilicet credulitas, hec est fides naturalis, informis, politica, philosophica; uel qualitas uirtus gratuita, formata, meritoria, catholica, theologica. Dicitur et fides fidelitas ... .

GEMINATIO: Geminatio notat assiduitatem, unde Apostolus, "Exspectatio creature reuelationem filiorum Dei exspectat" [Rom 8:19], idest exspectans creatura assidue, in actu exspectandi est sui gloriam. Item geminatio notat augmentum, ut "exspectans exspectaui Dominum" [Ps 39:2] ... . Et attentionem, ut "Moyses Moyses," "Martha Martha." Et diuersitatem, unde in Ezechiele de Nabugodonosor rege Assyriorum: "faciens faciet ei iuxta impietatem eius" [Eze 31:11], faciens scilicet ex me faciet per se; Deus enim auctor fuit, Babilonius minister ... .

GRATIA: Prima gratia est fides operans per dilectionem; hec gratis data uoluntatem liberat et sanat et preparat ut bonum uelit, et ita est operans; post adiuuat ne frustra uelit, et ita est cooperans ... .

ITEM GRATIA: Gratia autem dicitur quandoque Dei uoluntas ... . Quandoque donum Dei gratuitum ... . Quandoque dicitur gratia eterna beatitudo, et est gratia quia meritum ex gratia, nam: "Quicquid habes meriti preuentrix gratia donat." ...

HERETICVS DICITVR QVIS: Hereticus dicitur quis fidei uiolatione ut Arrius, contumaci scripture expositione ut iudeus, pacis dissentione ut scismaticus, sacramentorum contaminatione ut symoniacus.

INGENITVS: Ingenitus stricte dicitur Pater, et ita hoc nomen ingenitus tantum de Patre dicitur relatiue, cuius correlatiuum quod erit? Numquid hoc totum genitus uel procedens uel aliquid ei equipollens, ut aliunde existens. Ingenitus in ampla acceptione dicitur non genitus, secundum quod et Spiritus sanctus est ingenitus ... .

IVS: Ius dicitur sententia data, et mera iustitia sine scilicet dispensatione. Et consanguinitas, ut queritur "pertinet iste ad te?" ... Dicitur et ius potestas, ut "iste est alieni iuris" idest potestatis ... .

Iustum: Dicitur iustum natura et causa, ut Deus cuius iustitia natura est, ut qui iustificat creaturam. Dicitur etiam iustum participatione iustitie naturalis uel gratuite ... .

Impossibile: Impossibile dicitur secundum superiores causas, uel secundum inferiores, uel secundum has et illas. Item impossibile dicitur difficile ... .

Idem: Idem dicitur genere, specie, numero, equipollentia, similitudine, ut fidelium una est fides et eadem.

Ignorantia: Ignorantia dicitur nescientia uel contemptus sciendi, uenialis uel mortalis. Item ignorantia est mala omissio discendi in eo qui scire tenetur, uel huius delicti reatus; uel est defectus et pena.

Interrogatio: Est interrogatio dubitantis ad scientiam, scilicet circa rem incognitam ... . Et admirationis, ut in re cognita ... . Et increpationis, et dicitur exothema, ut "quare fremuerunt gentes" [Ps 2:1]. Et causa eliciende confessionis ... .

In: In tollit potentiam, ut "angelus est inuisibilis," nec enim in sui natura a mortalibus uideri potest. Tollit et actum, ut cum dicitur uia immeabilis ... .

Littera occidit: Littera occidit [2 Cor 3:6]; intellige per occasionem. Littera enim etiam moralis ut Decalogus occidit culpa occasionaliter, scilicet ex prohibitione ... .

Maior:[5] Virtutes pares sunt essentia, habitu, efficacia; impares usu, auctoritate, dignitate. Hinc dicitur maior horum uel hiis est caritas, et fides gignit spem, spes caritatem ... .

Maioritas caritatis: Dicitur caritas maior radicatione, robore, constantia, deuotione, feruore, affectu, effectu ... .

Meritum: Meritum dicitur causa, unde "merces fidei uita eterna"; et dignitas, ut "beata Virgo meruit portare Christum"; et exigentia, ut "O felix culpa" etc.; et ydoneitas, ut hic meretur promoueri in episcopum, idest ydoneum se facit ad hoc ... .

Mereri:[6] Item mereri dicitur habere, uel uti, pati, uel omittere.

Melius: Melius nomen est uel aduerbium, ut "Deus potest melius facere quam facit." ... Melius nomen ut fiat comparatio non inter personas set inter negotia ... .

5 Maior] *O*: Mater *BC*
6 Mereri] *B*: Item *C*: *om. O*

MEMBRVM CHRISTI: Dicitur quis membrum Christi uel ecclesie per predestinationem ut Saulus, per presentem iustitiam et uite sanctitatem ut Iudas, per sacramentorum participationem[7] ut Symon magus.

MATRIMONIVM EFFECTVS:

    Coniugium mundat, fecundat, mutat, et unit,

    Pollens auctore, tempore, lege, loco.

Mundat, idest mundos facit uel seruat a fornicatione ... .

MEDIATOR: Christus secundum quod Deus est mediator per causam et uirtutem idest potestatem ... . Christus secundum quod homo est mediator per instrumentum et ministerium ... . Item Christus secundum quod est gygas gemine substantie, idest persona dupplicis nature, est mediator substantiali mediatione, que scilicet duas substantias, idest duas naturas, complectitur; neque hac est mediator secundum quod Deus neque secundum quod homo, set secundum quod simul est Deus et homo ... .[8]

NATVRA: Natura dicitur naturale bonum, unde "uidit Deus cuncta que fecerat et erant ualde bona" [Gen 1:31]. Et uitium nature, unde "natura sumus filii ire" [Eph 2:3]. Et infirmitas nature ... .

NECESSITAS: Est neccesitas contracta siue traducta, ut ex originali peccato scilicet quod necesse est nos mori. Est illata, ut illato tibi letali uulnere, necesse est te mori. Et est assumpta, ut monachus ex necessitate abstinet a carnibus ... . Item necessitas dicitur ineuitabilitas ... .

DE EODEM:[9] Secundum Boetium uero due sunt necessitates, simplex una ueluti quod necesse est homines omnes esse mortales, altera ex conditione, ut si aliquem ambulare scias eum ambulare necesse est. Item necessaria dicitur consequens ... .

NISI: Hec dictio nisi excludit excellentiam, ut "Nemo bonus nisi Deus" [cf. Mt 19:17]; solus enim Deus excellenter bonus est, idest summum bonum ... . Excludit et euidentiam ... .

ODIVM DEI: Odium Dei dicitur reprobatio idest non approbatio, uel prescientia dampnationis ... .

ORATIO: Est oratio questuosa, facta scilicet pro questu ... et hii accipient dampnationem maiorem. Est oratio pomposa, ut ypocrite, et hec fit in peccatum. Est et officiosa, ut sacerdotis quia ex officio orat, et hec

---

7 ut Iudas ... participationem] *CO: om. B*

8 simul ... homo] *C: om. BO*

9 De eodem] *B: om. CO*

indifferens est. Est et oratio caritatiua, facta scilicet in caritate et ex caritate, et hec non fit in peccatum set est meritoria uite eterne.

PROPHETIA: Prophetia dicitur preuisio, uel predictio, uel prefiguratio.

PIETAS: Pietas dicitur theosebia siue eusebia, idest diuinus cultus siue bonus cultus. Dicitur et pietas misericordia naturalis uel gratuita ... .

POTENTIA:[10] Est potentia naturalis que uel Deus est uel a Deo. Potestas etiam dicitur ipse potens ... .

PERMISSIO: Permissio dicitur ubi non est prohibitio, ut de minoribus malis que consuetudinis sunt et fragilitatis, ut sunt primi motus ... . Dicitur et permissio tolerantia uel sustinentia uel dispensatio ... .

PREPOSITIO: Preponitur aliquis alicui in meritorum comparatione, ut extraneus religiosus patri nefando; in beneficiorum collatione, ut pater nefandus extraneo religioso; in officiorum executione, ut catholicus heretico; in obedientie exhibitione, ut episcopus proprius etiam flagitiocissimus alieno etiam religiosissimo.

PREPOLLENTIA:[11] Cum queritur utrum prepositorum prepolleat tria consideranda sunt, in quo preeminentia, circumstantia, caritas, et utrum duorum malorum preponderent ... .

PECCATVM: Peccatum dicitur causa peccati, ut "peccatum habitat in carne," idest corruptio causa peccati. Dicitur et peccatum diabolus, auctor peccati ... . Peccatum etiam dicitur fomes peccati ... .

PVNITIO: Item, peccatum punitur, idest peccato pena opponitur, ut scilicet secundum quantitatem culpe sit quantitas pene; homo malus punitur, idest torquetur, homo bonus punitur, idest per penam Deo unitur ... .

PENA: Est pena edificans; hec uel est purgans ut in Maria et in ecclesia expectante, uel est probans seu meritum augmentans ut in Iob. Est pena corrumpens ... .

PATI: Pati dicitur a passione, unde de martiribus dicitur iniuste sunt passi set iuste coronati. Et a patientia ... .

PLEONASMOS:[12] Pleonasmos est ut cuius participatio eius in idipsum: "Et crediderunt in uerbis eius <et laudauerunt laudem eius>" [Ps 105:12].

---

10 Potentia] *CO*: Potestas *B*
11 Prepollentia] *BC*: Prepositorum *O*
12 Pleonasmos] *BC*: *om. O*

POSTQVAM: Postquam notat continuationem subsecutionis, ut "postquam ego locutus fuero tu loquaris"; et idemptitatem temporis, ut "postquam consummati sunt dies octo ut circumcideretur puer" [Lc 2:21], idest in illis consummatis scilicet in octaua die ... .

PER: Per est operatorium, ut "per manus apostolorum fiebant signa"; et cooperatorium, ut "hoc facio per Dei gratiam," idest non ego solus, set gratia Dei mecum ... .

PRECEDERE: Precedit in dicendo quod comitatur in agendo, ut "in principio creauit Deus celum et terram" [Gen 1:1] ... .

QVIS: Quis utrumque sexum complectitur sicut mortuus et proximus, unde pro emorissa dicit Dominus: "Quis me tetegit?," et paulo post, "Tetigit me aliquis" [Lc 8:45-46] ... In hiis itaque et consimilibus nomen masculini complectitur utrumque sexum.

ITEM QVIS: Item, quis notat impossibilitatem, ut "generationem eius quis enarrabit" [Is 53:8; Act 8:33], diuinam scilicet, uel difficultatem si de humana intelligis ... .

QVERERE: Querit quis increpatiue, ut "Adam ubi es?" [Gen 3:9] Queritur etiam ut iudex ... .

QVOMODO: Quomodo nota est dubitationis, ut "quomodo possunt hec fieri"; et admirationis et doloris ... .

RES: Hoc nomen res nunc personaliter accipitur nunc essentialiter, unde Augustinus: "Res quibus fruendum est sunt Pater et Filius et Spiritus sanctus, eadem tamen Trinitas summa res est," etc.

REDEMPTIO: Redemptio nostra facta est in cruce quoad causam, in baptismo quoad effectum ... .

REMISSIO: Remissio peccati est gratia remittens uel delens reatus, tunc primo inest cum peccatum primo abest, et ita peccatum remittitur non habenti sicut gratia subtrahitur non habenti.

SACRAMENTVM: Sacramentum dicitur significatio, unde in Apocalypsen dicit angelus Iohanni: "Ego dicam tibi sacramentum mulieris" [Apoc 17:7]; et sacrum secretum ... . Dicitur et sacre rei signum ... . Et iuramentum ... .

SANCTIFICARE: Sanctificare dicitur sanctum facere uel sanctiorem, uel sanctitatem conferre ... .

SALVS: Est salus eterna Deus causa salutis. Est salus spiritualis, ut gratia in presenti uel gloria in futuro. Est salus corporalis, ut sanitas uel liberatio a tribulatione ... .

SCIRE: Dicitur Deus scire seu cognoscere per prescientiam, ut "nouit Deus qui sunt eius." Et per notitiam, ut "Deus omnia scit." Et per approbationem, ut Moysi dicit: "Te ipsum noui ex nomine" [cf. Ex 6:3], hoc est proprie et specialiter placuisti mihi.

SERVITVS: Seruitus soli Deo debita consistens presertim in excellenti dilectione et sacrificii exhibitione Grece dicitur liturgia uel latria uel latrensis, unde ydolatria que quod soli Deo debetur ydolis datur. Seruitus uero communis homini et Deo et cuicumque superiori uel pro superiori, ut cruci pro crucifixo, Grece dulia dicitur.

STOLA: Stola dicitur uestis talaris, a thelon quod est longum, unde mustela quasi mus longus. Hinc dicitur prima stola gloria anime, ut impassibilitas perpetua. Secunda stola gloria carnis, ut immortalitas ... .

STATVS: Est status innocentie, ut ante lapsum in paradiso, et hic bipartitus scilicet ante gratuita et post gratuita. Est status miserie post lapsum extra paradisum ... . Est status gratie sub Christo ... . Est status glorie cum Christo ... . Item tres status sunt scilicet coniugatorum, uiduarum, uirginum ... .

SIMVLATIO: Est simulatio deceptionis de qua "similator ore decipit amicum suum" [Prov 11:9]; et cautele, ut in angelo comitante Tobiam; et stultitiam simulare loco prudentia summa est, ut simulant Dauid arrepticius, et exploratores Iericho ... . Est simulatio significationis ... . Est simulatio instructionis, ubi non est duplicitas, ut Deus "se finxit longius ire" [Lc 24:28] ... .

TENERI: Dicitur aliquis teneri ratione precepti, legis scilicet naturalis uel scripte, ut "diligere Deum"; et beneficii, ut gratus esse ... . Dicitur et quis teneri uel ratione commissi, ut cure pastoralis secundum quod prelatus tenetur animam dare pro ouibus, idest paratus esse ad hoc.

TRADERE CHRISTVM:[13] Tradidit Christum Pater mittendo, qui proprio Filio non pepercit set pro nobis omnibus tradidit illum. Tradidit se Christus obediendo ... .

VIRTVS GRATVITA: Data sunt naturalia dona gratuita, ut uirtutes caritate informate ... .

---

13 Tradere Christum] *C:* Tradidit Christum *O:* Tacere *B*

VERITAS: Veritas incommutabilis essentie Deus est. Veritas generis et nature est in incomplexis, ut "hec est uera aqua, hic uerus ignis," uel est in complexis, ut "ego ueniam." Hec ueritas logica est attendens compositionem predicati ad subiectum. Hec est ueritas dicti, a qua dicitur quis uerus. Alia est ueritas dicentis, hec est theologica, a qua dicitur quis uerax, cum scilicet non loquitur contra conscientiam. Huiusmodi est ueritas uirtutis et gratie. Aristotiles uerum querit, Christus ueracem. Similiter est falsitas dicti faciens falsum, et est falsitas dicentis faciens fallacem.

Iam de dictionibus aliqua perstrinximus; plura si placet in sermonibus nostris uel distinctionibus, uel in questionibus reperies.[14]

2 DE POSITIONIBVS

Post dictiones de positionibus agamus. Ponitur autem dictio pro dictione, ut ex pro in sicut ibi: "Nemo potest duobus dominis seruire; quicquid facis uel ex amore Dei uel ex seruitute diaboli," suple, "facis" [cf. Mt 6:24]. Potest et hoc de ibi predictis [Mt 6:1-23] intelligi scilicet elemosina, oratione, ieiunio, oculo nequam uel simplici factis, ut "quicquid facis tu seruus constituaris."

SICVT PRO PER: Ponitur sicut pro per ut ibi: "Extendens celum sicut pellem" [Ps 103:2], idest scripturam per predicatores mortales qui sunt sicut pelles Salomonis ... .

NE PRO VT: Ponitur ne pro ut, unde in Ysaia: "Exceca cor populi ne forte uideat," etc. [Is 6:10] ... .

SVPER PRO IVXTA: Ponitur super pro iuxta, uel post, uel de, ut ibi ... "Pharao sompnians putabat se stare super flumen" ... .

SI PRO NON: Ponitur si pro non, ut ... "si noui eum" ... .

SI PRO AN: Ponitur si pro an, ut ibi: "Si est scientia in excelso" idest Deo, idest "scit Deus hoc an non?"

IN PRO CVM: Ponitur in pro cum, ut in epistola Iude ibi: "Ecce uenit Deus in sanctis suis facere iudicium" [Iudae 1:14-15].

IN PRO POST: Et in pro post, ut ibi: "Et uiuet adhuc in finem," idest post finem in inferno.

IN PRO PRO: Ponitur in pro pro, ut "Ora Patrem in abscondito" [Mt 6:6], et "in spiritu et in ueritate oportet adorare" [Io 4:23], idest pro spiritualibus et ueris bonis ad Deum orare ... .

14 Iam ... reperies] *BO: om. C*

IN PRO PER: Ponitur in pro per, ut "iusti intrabunt in eam" [Ps 117:20], idest per eam in celum.

SECVNDVM PRO IN: Ponitur secundum pro in, ut "Christus secundum diuinitatem habuit Deum Patrem." ...

SECVNDVM PRO EX: Ponitur secundum pro ex, ut "Christus secundum humanitatem habet Deum creatorem."

NOMEN PRO ADVERBIO: Ponitur etiam nomen pro aduerbio, sicut "sole recens orto" [cf. Mt 13:6], idest recenter; et "donec illud bibam nouum in regno meo" [cf. Mt 26:29], idest nouo modo ... .

ADVERBIVM PRO NOMINE: Ponitur aduerbium pro nomine, ut "fecerunt Magi similiter," idest similia; et "benefecerunt quia scelus sanguine uendicauerunt," idest bonum opus operati sunt ... .

PRONOMEN PRO NOMINE: Ponitur pronomen pro nomine, siue indi- uiduum pro specie, ut "cur timebo in die malo," etc. [Ps 48:6] Hic enim propheta in persona sua generalem habet causam. Et Iohannes baptista ait ad Dominum: "Ego debeo a te baptizari" [Mt 3:14] idest homo debet per te ab originali peccato mundari ... .

GENVS: Ponitur genus pro genere, ut masculinum pro feminino, ut Genesi xliii [Gen 23:6] dicunt filii Eth Abrahe: "sepeli mortuum tuum," idest Saram mortuam, et ponitur forsan masculinum pro feminino propter dignitatem generis, et quia post mortem non queritur sexus, quia ex tunc neque nubent neque nubentur ... .

NEVTRVM: Ponitur neutrum pro masculino: "Minuisti eum paulo ab angelis" [Ps 8:6], idest faciendo minorem angelis; et "hec tria unum in tres."

FEMININVM: Ponitur femininum pro neutro, ut "unam petii a Domino" [Ps 26:4].

NVMERVS: Ponitur numerus pro numero, ut per silemsim singulare pro plurali ... i Thimotheo vii [1 Tim 4:14], "cum impositione manuum presbiteri," idest presbiterorum, quia minus tribus esse non possunt in ordinatione episcopi, ut fuerunt in ordinatione Iacobi ... .

PLVRALE PRO SINGVLARI: Ponitur et plurale pro singulari, Exodo cxxiiii [Ex 32:31], "fecerunt sibi deos aureos" ... factus est enim uitulus ... .

ANTITHOSIS: Ponitur per anthithosim casus pro casu, nominatiuus pro genitiuo, ut "uterque Christus" idest utriusque nature ... . Et accusatiuus pro genitiuo ... .

TEMPVS PRO TEMPORE: Ponitur tempus pro tempore, presens pro preterito, ut "circumcisio prodest si legem obserues" [Rom 2:25], idest profuit in legis statu, legem spiritualiter obseruanti ... .

PRESENS PRO FVTVRO: Ponitur et presens pro iminenti futuro, ut "ascendo ad Patrem meum" [Io 20:17] ... et etiam pro remoto futuro ... .

PRETERITVM: Ponitur et preteritum pro futuro, "foderunt manus meus et pedes meos" [Ps 21:17] ... .

FVTVRVM: Ponitur et futurum pro preterito, ut ibi: "Super montes stabunt aque" [Ps 103:6], idest steterunt tempore diluuii ... .

FVTVRVM: Ponitur et futurum optatiue, ut "in monte Dominus uidebit," idest uideat; et preceptiue, "diliges proximum" [Mt 19:19], idest diligas.

TOTVM PRO PARTE: Ponitur totum pro parte synodochice, ut in Deuteronomio: "Ostendit Dominus Moysi omnem terram" [Deut 32:52], idest partem omnis terre ... . Item habetur duodecim apostolis pro undecim. Mos enim sacre scripture limites numerorum ponere siue modicum desit siue supersit. Vnde et dicuntur septuaginta interpretes cum tamen essent septuaginta duo ... .

PARS PRO TOTO: Ponitur et pars pro toto, ut Syon pro Iudea ... .

SIMPLEX: Ponitur simplex pro composito per afferesim, ut "populus qui nascetur," idest renascetur, "quem fecit Dominus," idest refecit ... .

COMPOSITVM PRO SIMPLICI: Ponitur et compositum pro simplici, ut "addidit Ionatas deierare" [1 Sam 20:17], idest iurare; set de ibi intensionem notat, ut sit deierare multum iurare.

GENVS PRO SPECIE: Ponitur genus pro specie, ut "predicate euangelium omni creature" [Mc 16:15], rationali scilicet ... .

SPECIES PRO GENERE: Ponitur et species pro genere, idest inferius pro superiori, ut "Deus assumpsit hominem," idest humanum genus redimendum uel humanam naturam sibi copulauit glorificandam ... .

CONTINENS PRO CONTENTO: Ponitur continens pro contento methonomice, ut "In principio creauit Deus celum" [Gen 1:1], per quod continens et contentum accipitur ... .

CONTENTVM PRO CONTINENTE: Ponitur contentum pro continente, ut in Regum [3 Reg 7:23] "fecit Salomon mare," idest laterem. ...

ANTECEDENS PRO CONSEQVENTI: Ponitur antecedens pro consequenti, uel attribuitur antecedenti quod est consequentis, ut "qui diligit iniquitatem odit animam suam" [Ps 10:6], idest nocet ei; et "Deus odit uel irascitur," idest punit.

CONSEQVENS PRO ANTECEDENTI: Ponitur et consequens pro antecedenti, ut ibi: "Conuertit cor eorum ut odirent populum eius" [Ps 104:25], idest Deus benefecit populo suo eum multiplicando, unde Egyptii conuersi sunt ad inuidiam que est odium aliene felicitatis. Potest et ita intelligi, conuertit occasionaliter, uel permisit conuerti ... .

OPVS OPERATVM: Ponitur opus operatum pro opere operante et e conuerso, unde Psalmista: "Ne simul trahas me cum peccatoribus" [Ps 27:3], Glosa: Ipsi operantur iniquitatem, idest meam mortem, hoc est crucifixionem actiue, ex qua mea mors ... .

VNIVERSALIS AFFIRMATIVA: Ponitur uniuersalis affirmatiua pro uniuersali negatiua, ut "quicquid est de ueritate humane nature resurget," et "Christus illuminat omnem hominem" [Io 1:9], idest nullus illuminatur nisi per eum ... .

QVALE PRO QVALITATE: Ponitur quale pro qualitate, ut capilli crispi [cf. Is 3:24] sunt accidentia, idest crispitudo est accidentalis forma ... .

QVALITAS PRO QVALI: Ponitur et qualitas pro quali, ut "supplico clementie tue," idest tibi clementi ... .

ACTIO VEL SVBSTANTIA PRO ACCIDENTE: Ponitur actio uel substantia pro accidente, ut "quoniam non cognoui nego" idest uitia negationis ... .

QVOD PRO QVALE: Ponitur quod pro quale, uel quis pro qualis, unde Apostolus prima Cor. [15:37], "non corpus quod futurum est seminas set nudum granum," idest non quale futurum ... .

SVBSTANTIA PRO QVALITATE: Ponitur substantia pro qualitate uel quali, uel intelligitur cum substantia etiam qualitas, unde Dominus Iudeis: "Et me scitis" [Io 7:28], idest meam humanitatem ... .

RES PRO PREPARATIONE: Ponitur res pro preparatione ad eam uel proposito, quasi scilicet consequens pro antecedenti uel effectus pro causa, ut "qui spernit minima paulatim decidit" [Ecclus 19:1], idest ad casum tendit ... .

FACERE PRO DICERE: Ponitur facere pro dicere, unde Apostolus Ebre [cf. Hebr 1:6]: "Et cum iterum introducit scriptura," idest introducendum dicit ... .

DICERE PRO FACERE: Ponitur et dicere pro facere, unde "dixit Dominus ut appareret in nube," idest hoc fecit ... .

PERSONA PRO PERSONA: Ponitur persona pro persona, ut Adam pro Eua sicut supradictum est; et antiqui pro posteris, sicut parentes in filiis adorant Ioseph ... .

PERSONA PRO PERSONA: Ponitur etiam alio modo persona pro persona, ut scilicet modus pro modo, ut "benedicite aque que super celos sunt Domino" [Dan 3:60], sunt pro estis ponitur, uel benedicite pro benedicant ... .

POSITIVVM PRO COMPARATIVO: Ponitur positiuum pro comparatiuo, ut "bonum est confidere in Domino quam confidere in homine" [Ps 117:8], idest melius, quod et habet Hebraica ueritas.

ADIECTIVVM: Ponitur adiectiuum substantiue preintellecto scilicet articulo, ut malignus et superbus sicut ibi: "Tu humiliasti sicut uulneratum superbum" [Ps 88:11], et de Christo legitur: "Iustus perit, et non est qui recogitet" [Is 57:1], et "iustus autem quid fecit?" [Ps 10:4].

3 DICTVM EST DE POSITIONIBVS.
CONSEQVENS EST AGERE DE ATTRIBVTIONIBVS.[15]

Attribuitur uni quod conuenit alii gratia uicinitatis, ut "sensualitas meretur," idest ratio scientie ei adiuncta. Et Beda super illud Parabolarum: "Timor Domini principium sapientie" [Prov 1:7], seruilem timorem ponit pro initiali.

ANTECEDENS PRO CONSEQVENTI: Attribuitur antecedenti quod est consequentis, uel ponitur antecedens pro consequenti, ut in Ecclesiastico: "Omnia in futuro querentur," idest manifestabuntur et scientur ... . Et "O felix culpa," idest euentus ex culpa, scilicet occasione culpe ... .

CONSEQVENS: Attribuitur consequenti quod est antecedentis ... . Ita et uulgariter dicitur, "Iste uult suspendi," quia uult furari ... .

EFFECTVS: Attribuitur cause quod est effectus, ubi et redditur predicamentum cause, ut "libera me de sanguinibus" [Ps 50:16], idest peccatis que ex corruptione sanguinis ... . Item accedit uerbum ad elementum, scilicet inuocatio efficacie, cuius causa est ex uerbo idest Filio Dei.

EFFECTVS: Attribuitur effectui quod cause est, et quod dicitur redundat in causam, unde Dominus ait: "Verba que ego locutus sum uobis

15 Dictum ... attributionibus] *BC*: *om. O*

spiritus et uita sunt" [Io 6:64], idest a spiritu et uita, hoc est a me a quo habent quod spiritualiter intellecta uiuificent ... .[16]

ATTRIBVTIO SIGNO QVOD EST REI: Attribuitur signo quod rei est, ut "qui plus laborat plus mercedis accipiet," idest qui plus habet caritatis cuius signum est labor ... .

REI: Attribuitur rei quod signi est, ut "maioris potentie uel misericordie est recreare quam creare," idest signum maioris potentie est, quia aliquid obloquitur uel maioris misericordie cum ibi gratia appareat magis. Item "spiritus apparuit," idest columba que erat signum et indicium presentie Spiritus sancti ... . Et "corpus Christi uidetur in altari," idest forma panis que huius sacramenti et rei sacramentum est ... .

INSTRVMENTVM: Attribuitur instrumento quod artificis est uel operis facti in eo uel quod quis in eo patitur uel quod fit eo mediante, ut "crux est salus nostra" idest crucifixus ... .

ARTIFEX: Attribuitur et artifici uel utenti uel operi quod est instrumenti, ut "diabolus excecat," idest peccatum. Et quandoque priuatio uel corruptio Deo attribuitur que peccato conuenit instrumento Dei utentis ... .

TOTVM: Attribuitur toti quod partis est, ut "calcas me" pro pede, "uulneras me" pro manu. Et "ecclesia errat," idest aliqui de ecclesia, particularis ecclesia non totalis, catholica, generalis ... .

PARS: Attribuitur parti quod totius est, ut ibi: "Omnis caro ueniet" [Ps 64:3], idest homo ... .

CAPITI: Attribuitur capiti quod membrorum est, propter scilicet corporis unitatem et capitis auctoritatem, unde de Christo dicitur: "Hic est qui baptizat" [Io 1:33]; ipse enim auctor est et instituit baptsimum, et per ministros exterius intinguit, et per se interius mundat; ipse enim baptizat in Spiritu sancto ... .

MEMBRVM: Attribuitur membris quod capitis est, ut cum de sancto aliquo seu prelato dicitur quia sanctificat, remittit peccata, saluat, uel aliquid huiusmodi ... .

MEMBRA: Attribuitur quibusdam membris quod aliorum membrorum est, unde super illud Marci, in fine, "Qui uero non crediderit condemp-

---

16 et quod dicitur ...] *BO:* Hillarius: "Christus non sensit uulnera," idest non habuit causam pene ... *C*

nabitur" [Mc 16:16]: "Per alios paruuli credunt." Potest tamen intelligi credunt, idest fidem habent uel sacramentum fidei participant ... .

PRIORIBVS: Attribuitur prioribus quod posterorum est, antecessoribus quod successorum est, ut ibi: "Maior seruiet minori" [Gen 25:23; Rom 9:13]; Idumei enim seruierunt Hebreis, non autem Esau Iacob nisi eum persequendo ... .

POSTERIS: Attribuitur posteris quod priorum est, ut "Due gentes in utero tuo sunt" [Gen 25:23], Idumei scilicet et Iudei, idest patres eorum, Esau scilicet et Iacob.

NATVRA: Attribuitur nature quod rei est, ut "diuina natura facta est homo," idest Dei natus siue Deus natus, hoc est Dei Filius factus est homo ... .[17]

RES: Attribuitur rei quod nature est, ut "homo unitur Deo," idest humana natura diuine. Et "homo est assumptus uel coniunctus Deo," uel aliquid huiusmodi ... .

SVBIECTVM: Attribuitur subiecto quod est accidentis siue qualitatis siue proprietatis, ut "homo est assumptus," idest humanitas est assumpta. Et "natiuitas est hodie sancte Marie Virginis," idest sollempnitas natiuitatis.

4 NVNC POST ATTRIBVTIONES AD RESOLVTIONES VENIAMVS.[18]

TEMPORALE: Resoluitur temporale in causale, unde "Exaudi Domine uocem deprecationis mee, dum (idest quia) oro ad te, dum (idest quia) extollo ad templum manus meas," etc. [Ps 27:2]

ACTIVVM: Resoluitur actiuum in passiuum, unde in Exodo xxxvii [33:19], "Vocabo nomine Domini coram te," idest uocabor, set hoc ego faciam ideo "uocabo" posuit ... .

PASSIVVM: Resoluitur passiuum in actiuum, ut "ab isto male legitur euangelium," neque in euangelio mala passio, set is est sensus: Iste male legit euangelium.

VOCABVLVM ACTVS: Resoluitur uocabulum actus in uocabulum apti-tudinis, ut ibi: "Non quia dicitur set quia creditur," idest credibile

---

17 ut diuina ...] *BO*: Sent., unde Hillarius lib. ii, cxxxviii: nature cui contradicis heretice humanitas est ... *C*
18 Nunc ... ueniamus] *BC*: *om. O*

est ... . Et "matrimonium est coniunctio maris et femine indiuiduam uite consuetudinem retinens," idest eius retentiua ... .

VOCABVLVM APTITVDINIS: Resoluitur uocabulum aptitudinis in uoca-bulum actus, ut "corpus Christi post resurrectionem palpabile fuit," idest palpatum ... .

NEGATIVA: Resoluitur negatiua in electiuam, ut "non opus set uoluntas remuneratur," idest potius uoluntas ... .

COMPARATIVA IN ELECTIVAM: Resoluitur comparatiua in electiuam, uel negatiuam, ut "bonum est confidere in Domino quam confidere in homine" [Ps 117:8], idest potius in Domino quam in homine, uel ita in Domino et non in homine; non enim in homine puro ponenda est spes salutis ... .

AFFIRMATIVA IN NEGATIVAM: Resoluitur affirmatiua in negatiuam, ut "Christus aliud est ex matre quam ex Patre," idest non id ex Patre quod ex matre ... . Ita etiam dicitur egro: "Abstine a cibis nociuis et sanior eris," idest minus infirmus ... .

VNIVERSALIS AFFIRMATIVA: Resoluitur uniuersalis affirmatiua in uni-uersalem negatiuam, unde Leuitico de hostia pro peccatis: "Quicquid tetigerit carnes eius sanctificabitur" [Lev 6:27], idest carnes eius non debent tangere aliquid immundum. Et paulo post: "Omnis masculus de genere sacerdotali uescetur de carnibus eius" [6:29], idest nullus nisi masculus.

NEGATIVA: Resoluitur negatiua in affirmatiuam, ut cum de multum lucrante dicitur, "non parum profecit iste," et "non parum diligit qui plurimum benefecit."

NOMEN IN ADVERBVM: Resoluitur nomen in aduerbum, unde "prono-men significat meram substantiam," idest mere. Et "Deus creat animam bonam" [cf. Gen 1:21], idest bene. Et "sacrilegum panem comedit hereticus," idest sacrilege. Et "peccator sibi iudicium manducat et bibit" [1 Cor 11:29], idest dampnabiliter sumit eucaristiam. Et "alio est Pater, alio est Deus," idest aliter Deus, nam relatiue Pater, substantialiter Deus.

5 DIXIMVS IAM DE RESOLVTIONIBVS, RESTAT VT DE MODIS DICENDI ALIQVID DICAMVS.

INDICATIVE: Dicitur indicatiue quod subiunctiue intelligendum est; dicitur enim quid esse non quod est set quod esset si non impediretur, ut "ueniale peccatum bonum adimit." Et "Lucifer beatitudinem amisit," non quam habuit set quam habiturus erat. Et "opus bonum sine caritate minorem penam meretur." Et "iste multum correctus est a malis," scilicet que fecisset nisi manum cohibuisset. Et Iosue ait: "Auferte deos alienos de medio nostri" [Ios 24:23], non forsan qui erant set essent de facili nisi cauerent; uidit enim eos Iosue pronos ad ydolatriam, et ideo precipit cauere. Sic Abrahe iam egresso, corpore non mente et uoluntate, cum haberet animum forsitan reuertendi, dictum est: "Egredere de terra tua" [Gen 12:1], non in qua scilicet erat, set esset nisi Dominus prohibuisset. Item dicit Daniel Nabugodonosor: "Peccata tua elemosinis redime" [Dan 4:24], idest penam que esset futura, si non occurreret elemosina, si tunc rex huic consilio prophete adquiesceret. Item "iusti per misericordiam mente ire uolunt ad positos in tormentis ut eos liberarent, set non possunt." Volunt, idest uellent si possent, si scilicet confirmati non essent. Vellent inquam per misericordiam mente ire, idest compati.

SINGVLARITER: Dicitur singulariter quod indefinite uel generaliter accipiendum est, ut "concupiscentiam nesciebam esse peccatum," etc. Generalem causam in persona sua agit. Et "ego debeo a te baptizari" [Mt 3:14], idest homo, uel conditionaliter et subiunctiue intellige, idest si deberem baptizari, a te baptizarer ... .

SIMPLICITER: Dicitur simpliciter quod intelligendum est conditionaliter cum possibilitate, ut ... "uouete et reddite" [Ps 75:12], idest si uouetis reddite si tamen ualetis ... .

SIMPLICITER: Dicitur aliquid simpliciter quod intelligendum est dictum in respectu, ut "nemo perfectus in uia," respectu scilicet perfectionis patrie ... .

ALIQVID: Dicitur aliquid quia ita est in genere, non in specie, ut "homo est dignum creatura Dei," et "uotum Iepte bonum," et "homicidium maius adulterio."

ALIQVID: Dicitur aliquid quia ita est in radice, ut "peccauimus in Adam" [cf. Rom 5:12], et "Leui decimatus est in Abraham" [cf. Heb 7:9].

ALIQVID: Dicitur aliquid tale ab effectu siue per causam, ut "insanias falsas" [Ps 39:5], et "in signis et prodigiis mendacibus" [2 Thess 2:9], quia scilicet magice fient et fantastice ut prestigia ... .

SVPPLETIO: Dicitur aliquid quod intelligendum est cum suppletione, unde "suple et leges." Et sepe subauditur aliquid uel audiendum est, ut "soli boni remittunt peccata," meritorie scilicet ... . Quandoque subintelligitur conditio, ut "irascimini et nolite peccare" [Eph 4:26], et Apostolus: "Volo autem omnes homines esse sicut me ipsum" [1 Cor 7:7], Glosa: "Omnes tales si fieri posset uolebat esse sicut se ipsum, idest continentes." In omnibus autem iuramentis de futuro et uotis et promissionibus apponitur uel subintelligitur conditio nisi impediat causa urgentissima, uel nisi maturiori consilio mutauero propositum. In omnibus reseruatur auctoritas ecclesie ... . Item quantum ad effectum suple, ut "non conficiunt uel non baptizant heretici," et "non est corpus Christi quod scismaticus conficit," non est scilicet quoad effectum ... . Item suple presertim, ut prelatis dictum est: "Nolite possidere aurum," etc. [Mt 10:9]; si enim cupiditas omnibus inhibita maxime prelatis qui ad contemptum diuitiarum hortantur. Item supple principaliter, ut "Christus fundat ecclesiam uel edificat"; Christus enim maximum et primum fundamentum est, alii secundario dicuntur ... .

In omnibus eclipticis locutionibus aliquid supplendum est, ut ... . "Quicquid potest Pater potest Filius," supplendum est aliquid et intelligendum est hoc de subiectis diuine misericordie.

Item suple quoad hoc uel hoc, ut "Christus passus est pro omnibus," suple quoad sufficientiam ... .

DE FACTO VEL PROPOSITO: Quandoque dicitur aliquid quod intelligendum est de facto uel de proposito uel eius equipollenti, ut "non dimittitur peccatum nisi restituatur ablatum"; restituatur scilicet re uel uoluntate, facto uel proposito, in se uel in equipollenti; et restituatur intellige parti uel toti, idest homini uel ecclesie; et quod ablatum est, iniuste ... .

SIC VEL NON SIC DE IVRE: Dicitur aliquid quod intelligendum est sic uel non sic de iure, ut in Deuteronomio dicitur populo Israel: "Non poteris alterius gentis hominem regem facere qui non sit frater tuus" [Dt 17:15], hoc est non habebis alienigenam set indigenam ... .

PROPTER SOLAM INCHOATIONEM: Dicitur aliquid fieri propter solam inchoationem, ut "domus fit," et "iste iuit Romam," et "uado ad patrem." ... Et "Christus mortem nostram moriendo destruxit," idest destructionem eius inchoauit ... .

VOLVNTAS: Dicitur aliquid fieri quod uoluntate fit, ut in Leuitico ultimo: "Quod si mutauerit" etc. [Lev 27:10], idest mutandi uoluntatem habuerit ... .

LICENTIA: Dicitur aliquid fieri pro licentia faciendi, ut ibi: "De fructu lignorum que sunt in paradiso uescimur" [Gen 3:2]. Et Thomas tangebat Dominum quia ad hoc inuitatus est cum dictum est: "Infer digitum tuum huc" [Io 20:27].[19]

PROPTER AVCTORITATEM: Dicitur aliquid propter auctoritatem, ut "de Patre procedit Spiritus," principaliter secundum Augustinum, proprie et uere secundum Ieronimum. Hec autem dicitur propter auctoritatem Patris; quod Spiritus sanctus procedit et etiam a Filio, hoc ipsum habet Filius a Patre.

PROPTER PRINCIPALITATEM: Dicitur aliquid propter principalitatem, ut "sola eterna sunt diligenda," idest illa ut precipua ... .

PROPTER DEBITVM: Dicitur aliquid esse propter debitum quia scilicet ita debet esse, ut "Credo in Deum," hoc est credere debeo ... .

PROPTER CONTINENTIAM: Dicitur aliquid hoc uel tale, uel fieri uel esse propter continentiam, ut "seculum nequam" et "dies mali" propter malitiam hominum et miseriam, sic "loca mala" ut latronibus plena ... .

PROPTER SIGNVM ET CAVSAM: Dicitur aliquid propter signum et causam, unde Apostolus de Christo: "Qui traditus est propter delicta nostra et resurrexit propter iustificationem nostram" [Rom 4:25]. Augustinus: Mors et resurrectio Christi delicta nostra tollunt, et utraque iustificant, tamen mors Christi sola interitum ueteris uite significat, et in sola resurrectione noua uita significatur ... .

PROPTER EXPEDITIONEM ET EXPRESSIONEM: Dicitur aliquid propter expeditionem et signi expressionem, ut "ubi maior est lucta ibi maior corona"; lucta enim expeditior est ad merendum uel expressius signum meriti.

PROPTER MODICITATEM: Dicitur pro modicitate de aliquo nihil uel non esse, ut "nil habuit Codrus," idest parum; modicitatem enim notat, non rei priuationem ... .

MODICVM PRO NICHILO: Modicum autem quandoque pro nichilo reputatur, ut dicitur: "Mali non sunt," et "Hely non corripuit filios." ...

MODICVM PRO NICHILO: Modicum etiam pro nichilo dicitur, ut "mitissima est pena paruulorum," idest nulla ... .

---

19 Licentia ...] *BO: om. C*

PER IMPOSSIBILE: Dicitur aliquid per impossibile ut sic propositum probetur, ut "si angelus de celo euangelizet uobis preterquam euangelizauimus uobis, anathema sit" [Gal 1:8], quasi impossibile est ... .

PER ANTIFRASIM: Dicitur aliquid uel intelligitur per antifrasim, ut "parce bellum, lucus, situla," et "benedic Deo et morere" [Iob 2:9] ... .

AFFIRMATIVE: Dicuntur aliqua affirmatiue que intelligenda sunt per remotionem contrarii, ut "pena paruulorum," idest non gloria; et "oportet episcopum esse monogamum" [cf. 1 Tim 3:2], idest non bigamum ... .

NEGATIO CVM AFFIRMATIONE: Dicuntur aliqua negatiue cum immutatione contrarii, ut "iste non odit," idest diligit ... . Item uulgariter dicitur "ne moreris" idest cito ueni. Et nota quod in huiusmodi minus dicitur et plus significatur.

Secundum quosdam etiam nomina numeralia dicta de Deo non ponunt set tollunt, et ideo non positiue set remotiue accipienda sunt, ut "unus Deus est," idest non sunt plures dii, et "plures persone sunt," idest non una sola. Et hic resoluitur in negatiuam affirmatiua.

PROPTER SIMILITVDINEM: Dicitur aliquid propter similitudinem, ut Iacob ait: "Ego sum Esau" [Gen 27:24], quia pilose manus similitudinem maioris expresserant ... . Et "Prometheus fecit homines," idest ymagines hominum ... .

PROPTER DISSIMILITVDINEM: Dicitur aliquid aliquorum per dissimilitudinem, hoc est dissimiliter, ut iustitia hominis iustitia Dei dicitur, Dei scilicet dantis, hominis accipientis ... .

PROPTER DIVERSITATEM: Dicitur aliquid quod per diuersitatem intelligendum est, hoc est de diuersis, ut "in manus tuas commendo spiritum meum" [Lc 23:46], idest potestati tue commendo, Pater, cito recepturus ... .

PER DIVERSITATEM MVLTIPLICEM: Porro plerumque quod dicitur per diuersitatem multiplicem accipiendum est, ut scilicet referatur ad diuersitatem temporum, ut cominationes et promissiones prophetales, unde "distinguite tempora et concordabit scriptura." ... .

Sunt et alie uarietates attendende in hunc modum: "Si peccauerit in te frater tuus" etc. [Mt 18:15], intelligenda est pars auctoritatis de peccato occulto, pars de manifesto, sicut pars ad litteram pars mistice cum dicitur fratricidium Caim septima generatione aquis cathaclismi est deletum ... .

GENERALITAS LOCVTIONVM: Igitur, ut ex predictis partim innotuit, generalitas locutionum quandoque restringitur ut intelligatur quid dictum causaliter uel personaliter uel temporaliter uel localiter. Causaliter scilicet tali uel tali causa, ut "non facias sculptile neque similitudinem neque adorabis ea neque coles" [Ex 20:4; Deut 5:8], hac de causa scilicet ut adores, nam et Moyses fecit cherubin et Salomon cherubin et leones et boues ... .

DE GENERALITATE LOCVTIONVM: Sepe in sacra scriptura generalitas locutionum restringenda est ad certam etatem, uel ad modum, uel ad statum, uel ad genus rei. Ad etatem, ut ibi: "Qui crediderit et baptizatus fuerit" etc. [Mc 16:16]; et "Deus reddet unicuique secundum opera sua" [cf. Mt 16:27], hoc enim de adultis et discretis intelligendum est ... .

DIVERSITAS: Adhuc de diuersitate loquimur. Videtur quandoque dici de creatore quod de creatura accipiendum est, ut "non idem est natura quod res nature." ...

SECVNDVM SE DICERE QVOD SECVNDVM ALIVD DICIT: Videtur etiam quis secundum se dicere quod secundum aliud dicit, ut Hyllarius: "Non idem est Deus et quod Dei est." Hoc enim dicit secundum hereticum, uel opponendo dicit non asserendo.

CASVALITER: Videtur etiam dici casualiter quod dicitur occasionaliter, ut "prohibitio Dei fuit causa peccati Ade," idest occasio ... . Item uulgariter dicitur alicui: "Gladio tuo te interficis."

DICITVR ALIQVIS DARE: Dicitur aliquis dare quia permittit aliquid extorqueri uel accipi ... . Sic Christus dedit eucharistiam Iude, et aliquis aliquid dat ystrioni. Vbi tamen notandum quia aliud est ystriones inuitare quod malorum est, aliud est ingerentes se admittere quod imperfectorum est, aliud est eis uendere, idest cum correptione dare uel omnino repellere, quod perfectorum est.

AVFERRE: Dicitur quis auferre non quod fuit set quod esse potuit, ut "qui occidit peccatorem aufert animam Deo." Ita aliquis alii aufert prebendam uel ecclesiam.

AMITTERE: Dicitur aliquis amittere quod non habuit set quod habiturus fuit uel aptitudine uel debito sub conditione, ut "iste perdidit ludum in scaccis," et Lucifer uel Iudas amisit beatitudinem regni celestis.

TEMPORALE: Quandoque quod dicitur temporale est, ut ex pretaxatis elicitur, uel ad certum et determinatum statum referendum est, uel ad certas personas, ut scilicet generalitas locutionis causa cognita restringatur, sicut illud: "Si habueritis fidem sicut granum," etc. [Mt 17:19] ...; hec ad tempus primitiue ecclesie spectant ... .

LOCALE: Plerumque quod dicitur locale est, ut ex supradictis innotuit, quandoque uero conditionale, ut "qui uolunt hinc transire ad uos" [Lc 16:26], idest uellent si possent ... .

SIMPLICITER: Sepius autem dicitur simpliciter quod intelligendum est conditionaliter, ut "uirtutes celorum mouebuntur" [Mt 24:29], idest mouerentur si fieri posset ... .

YPERBOLICE: Dicitur et aliquid yperbolice, ut "frigidius glacie pectus amantis erat et luce clarius," et "candidiores Nazarei eius niue" etc. [Lam 4:7] ... .

POSITIONES: Sicut etiam ex predictis patet sepe indicatiue uel optatiue posita, subiunctiue uel conditionaliter intelligenda sunt, ut ... Christus dicit Patri: "A timore inimici eripe" etc. [Ps 63:2], scilicet ut non eos timeam qui tantum corpus occidere possunt. Set numquid Christus pro se orat ne timeat timore mundano? Respondeo, sic timeret nisi Deus esset; uel hoc orat in persona ecclesie ... .

EX HABVNDANTI: Dicuntur et aliqua ex habundanti, ut ad incutiendum timorem uel ruborem, sicut Nicholaus papa dicit Lothario, "ne duos aut tres testes adhibeamus," etc., Causa xi, q. iii, Precipue.

YRONICE: Dicuntur et alia yronice, ut "Quod facis fac citius" [Io 13:27] ... . Item irrisorie, ut "Si crederetis Moisi, crederetis forsitan et mihi" [Io 5:46]; irrisio enim est increduli, non dubitatio Christi.

VOCABVLVM: Quandoque uocabulum quantitiuum facit in qualitatem non in quantitatem, ut cum dicitur "fructus centesimus," uel "centuplum accipiet" [Mt 19:29], idest spiritualia. Quandoque qualitatiuum facit in quantitatem non qualitatem, ut "uehemens amator proprie coniugis adulter est," et "qui procurant uenena sterilitatis adulteri sunt," quantitate scilicet peccati non qualitate; adeo enim peccant ut adulteri set non ita.

COMPLETIVE: Quandoque quod completiue dicitur completionis notat uicinitatem, ut in Danielis xxiii [Dan 9:2] ibi: "Vt complerentur desolationis Ierusalem septuaginta," hoc est ad completionem desolutionis ... .

INDIRECTA RATIOCINATIO: Dicitur autem nonnumquam aliquid quodammodo loquendi, ubi est indirecta ratiocinatio, ut quando impossibile aliquid probatur tropice, scilicet et ad alterum, ut uidelicet ammota impossibilitate, remaneat ueritas, ut ibi: "Si angelus de celo aliud uobis euangelizet" [Gal 1:8], quasi si esset possibile ... .

PER COMPARATIONEM: Dicuntur et aliqua per comparationem, hoc est respectu, de quo et supra; set repetimus ut aliqua exempla addamus. Legitur in Parabolis: "Non est grandis culpa cum quis furatus fuerit" etc. [Prov 6:30]; Glosa: ad comparationem adulterii, de quo scilicet subdit ... .

PER EXPRESSIONEM; HOC EST EMPHATICE: Dicitur aliquid per expressionem, hoc est emphatice, ut "Darius est impius scelus," quia multum scilicet participat scelere ... . Et Dominus in Ysaia: "Ecce ego creo Ierusalem exultationem, et populum eius gaudium" [Is 65:18], emphasis est. In huiusmodi uero nomen qualitatis que subiectum sibi uendicat et que inter alias preeminet, supponit pro quali. Item "humanitas est passa, diuinitas illesa," idest homo passus. Et ut "in personis proprietas et in maiestate adoretur equalitas," idest persone distincte et equales adorentur; aiunt enim quidam persona est proprietas idest distinguitur proprietate ... .

PER CAVSAM: Dicitur aliquid per causam, ut "Deus penitet," in membris scilicet, hoc est facit nos penitere, uel "mutat quod fecit," antecedens pro consequenti. Et est cum dicitur "Deus penitet" uel "irascitur" et huiusmodi antropospathos ... . Hoc locutionis tropo dicitur dies letus uel tristis, uel demonium mutum, potio uel herba sana, laus iocunda, scriptura sacra, doctrina sana ... .[20]

PROPTER SIGNVM: Dicitur et aliquid propter signum, ut "quam multipliciter tibi caro mea" [Ps 62:2], idest opera que facio ministerio corporis expressa signa sunt quod anima mea sitit ad Deum ... .

PROPTER APPARENTIAM: Dicitur et aliquid esse uel fieri propter apparentiam, ut "hoc est," idest apparet uel uidetur esse. Verbum enim quandoque significat rem suam, quandoque notitiam sue rei, ut "Pyrrus erat talis," idest uidebatur talis esse ... . Item, "Pater et Filius diligunt se Spiritu sancto," idest ostenduntur se diligere per hoc, scilicet quod communiter spirant Spiritum sanctum, sicut proles est indicium amoris parentum ... .

PROPTER OSTENSIONEM: Ex iam dictis patet aliquid dici propter ostensionem, manifestationem et euidentiam, et quod dicitur res fieri

---

20 Hoc locutionis ...] BC: om. O

cum innotescit, quod etiam ex subiunctis liquebit exemplis ... . "Ego indurabo cor Pharaonis," [Ex 7:3] idest quam durum sit demonstrabo ... .

PROPTER INDICIVM:²¹ Preterea propter indicium dicuntur huiusmodi, "lex mortis" [Rom 8:2], indicatiua scilicet et etiam occasionaliter effectiua uel illatiua ... .²²

PROPTER DEFECTVM:²³ Dicitur aliquid propter defectum, ubi est apoiopesis, ut in Geneseo xii [Gen 3:22]: "Nunc ergo ne forte mittat manum suam et sumat de ligno uite" etc., Glosa: apoiopesis que irato uel turbato congruit. Supplendum enim est "eicite eum," unde statim subditur: "emisit eum Deus de paradiso." Alia littera habet: "Videte ne forte mittat" etc., et secundum hoc non est apoioposis ... .

DE RE IN PROPOSITO:²⁴ Dicitur aliquid quod intelligendum est ita esse uel fieri in re uel in proposito, ut "non dimittitur peccatum nisi restituatur ablatum," scilicet re uel proposito. Ita "non saluabitur nisi baptizatus," scilicet re uel uoluntate ... .

PROPTER VNIONEM ET ADHERENTIAM:²⁵ Dicitur aliquid propter unionem et adherentiam, ut ... homo fidelis dicitur catholicus non solum quia habens fidem catholicam set etiam quia iusto catholico, idest generali iusto, adheret caritate, et capiti Christo fide et caritate. Item, "rudis bene credit," idest bene credenti adheret.

DE ESSE VEL FIERI IN MATERIA VEL SIMILITVDINE: Dicitur aliquid esse uel fieri quia in materia uel similitudine uel quia in prescientia Dei, ut "qui uiuit in eternum creauit omnia simul" [Ecclus 18:1], in materia scilicet quoad corpora uel similitudine quoad animas siue specie ... .²⁶

DE MINVS ET PLVS: Quandoque minus dicitur et plus significatur, ut "quia tenebre non obscurabuntur a te" [Ps 138:12], idest tenebrosi peccatores illuminabuntur a te ... .

DE PLVS ET MINVS: Quandoque plus dicitur et minus significatur uel intelligi datur, ut ... . "Exitus aquarum deduxerunt oculi mei" [Ps 118:136], idest effusiones lacrimarum; yperbole est, idest copiosas lacrimas quasi fluenta fontium pro recordatione peccatorum ... .

21 Propter indicium] *BC: om. O*
22 Preterea ...] *BC:* Patet itaque quia sepe dicitur et tropice dicitur res fieri cum innotescit ... *O*
23 Propter defectum] *BC: om. O*
24 De ... proposito] *BC: om. O*
25 Propter ... adherentiam] *BC: om. O*
26 De esse uel fieri ...] *BC: om. O*

DE PARTITIONE: Quandoque partimur inter uerba et sensus, ut "enarrem uniuersa mirabilia tua" [Ps 25:7], idest ut enarrata uniuersa sint mirabilia tua, et "narrabo omnia mirabilia tua" [Ps 9:2], idest quecumque dicam de operibus tuis sint mirabilia; et cum dicitur, "magnificetur Dominus" [Ps 39:17], hoc est nos in eo magnificemur, credendo scilicet confitendo, operando, predicando, et laudando eum magnum ... .

Item partiuntur uerba et sensus cum dicitur, "hic transit per medios enses"; non sunt enim medii enses, set hoc est "hic transit medius per enses." ...

PREDICTIO PER FVTVRVM:[27] Quandoque per futurum fit predictio et preceptio, ut in Deuteronomio lxxxii [Deut 18:15]: "Prophetam de gente tua et de fratribus tuis sicut me suscitabit tibi Dominus Deus tuus, ipsum audies." Vel est preceptio tantum, ita et ibi: "Diliges Dominum Deum tuum" etc. [Deut 6:5].

PER FVTVRVM ORATIO: Quandoque per futurum fit oratio, ut modus pro modo ponitur, ut indicatiuus pro imperatiuo, sicut ibi: "Multiplicabis in anima mea uirtutem" [Ps 137:3], idest multiplica.

ADIECTIO: Predictis adicimus cum quorundam tamen repetitione, quia dicitur de aliquo ipsum esse aliquid uel alicuiusmodi secundum rei ueritatem, ut "Tu es Christus, filius Dei uiui" [Mt 16:16]. Per nuncupationem, ut "omnes dii gentium demonia" [Ps 95:5] ... .

PROPTER IMITATIONEM: Dicitur et aliquid propter imitationem, unde: "Vnus ex uobis diabolus est" [Io 6:71] ... . Dicitur et propter rememorationem et representationem, ut quod offertur a sacerdote et consecratur uocatur sacrificium et oblatio quia memoria est et representatio ueri sacrificii et sancte immolationis facte in ara crucis (quere Sententiis libro iiii, cap. lxx). Christus tamen hostia fuit in cruce et in altari ... .

MEDIATE VEL IMMEDIATE: Dicuntur et alia alicuiusmodi mediate uel immediate, ut "omnia creata sunt ex nichilo," quedam scilicet mediate, quedam immediate ... .

DE NON ESSE: Dicitur aliquid non esse quia non legitur, ut "peccatum in Spiritum sanctum non remittitur" [cf. Mt 12:32], idest non legitur alicui remissum. Ita dicitur Melchisedech sine patre, et sabbatum primum sine uespera.

---

27 Predictio] ed.: Predicacio B: om. CO

Dictvm: Videtur preceptiue dictum quod licentialiter dicitur, ut in Leuitico et in Deuteronomio: "Omne animal tale comedetis" [cf. Lev 11; Deut 14], fas est sub forma precepti.

Vnitas popvli fidelis: Numerosa est unitas populi fidei; sicut enim participatione speciei plures homines unus, ita participatione fidei plures fideles unus. Ad iudicium igitur ueritatis plurimum censetur generalis iustus, nunc singulariter, nunc pluraliter; et ad populum et de populo nunc singularis nunc pluralis fit sermo, quod maxime patet in Deuteronomio, et ibi: "Qui confidunt in Domino sicut mons Sion" etc. [Ps 124:1] ... .

Notandum quod aliter fiunt exceptiones in theologica facultate quam in aliis. Verbi gratia: "Omne peccatum quodcumque fecerit homo extra corpus est," idest extra uinculum carnalis concupiscentie, "qui autem fornicatus" etc. [1 Cor 6:18]; et "omne peccatum et blasphemia remittetur homini, Spiritus autem blasphemie non remittetur" [cf. Mt 12:32], idest omne peccatum remissibile est excepto hoc.

Vnvm: Quandoque plura proponuntur ut unum, ut "malum est nunc ultimo esse iustum." Et "iste bene gaudet de eo quod nunc ultimo peccat." Et "Christus uoluit a Iudeis crucifigi," aut cum peccato Iudeorum uel sine, siue Christus crucifixus est iuste uel iniuste. Et "bonum est seruiliter timere." Et "Petrus meruit martirium" uel "anima purgatorium."

6 Regvle cvm determinationibvs et solvtionibvs[28]

De collatione rervm:[29] Fit quandoque collatio rerum uel personarum uel generum uel statuum in eadem persona uel in diuersis ut inter duo proposita uel propositi ad eius contrarium uel inter causam et effectum et huiusmodi alia, ubi etiam attendenda sunt adiuncta circumstantie et cause plures. Neque enim una circumstantia preeminentiam facere solet propositi ad propositum. Ideoque in argumentatione facienda de collatione que prout sepius ueritatem infert non simpliciter set secundum quid admittendam, respondendum est et soluendum quantum ad hoc, uel secundum hoc, uel in eo quod sic, uel aliquid tale.

Collatio inter debitores: Fit autem collatio inter debitores uel debita uel dimissiones, cum dicitur: "Cui minus dimittitur minus diligit"

---

28 Regule ... solutionibus] *O: om. BC*
29 De collatione rerum] *BC: om. O*

(Lc 7:47), quantum scilicet ad hoc, idest minor dimissio minus obligat ad diligendum quam maior in alio ... .

DE RE: Quandoque etiam solue respondendo "de re uerum, de dicto falsum," uel econuerso, ut "in predestinatum dampnari, prophetiam cassari," et huiusmodi.

ALTERVM PRO ALTERO: Quandoque alterum pro altero ponitur, ut "numquid," quod relinquit sub negatione, ponitur pro "nonne," quod sub affirmatione est, ut ibi, Ieremia li [Ier 12:9]: "Numquid auis discolor hereditas mea michi?"

INTELLECTVS: Quandoque accipitur aliquid per abstrahentem intellectum, et nonnunquam ita est in intelligentia, non in existentia.

LIGNVM: Quandoque qui dirigit tortuosum lignum, nititur in contrarium dum timet reflexum.

DIVERSITAS PERSONARVM: Quandoque solutionem elicimus ex diuersitate personarum, rerum, temporum, locorum, statuum, opinionum, generum, modorum, consignificationum, acceptionum, respectuum, partium, naturarum, etatum. Verbi gratia, ex diuersitate personarum sicut ibi: "Cum occideret eos, querebant eum" [Ps 77:34]. Rerum, ut Iohannes baptista dubitauit dicens: "Tu es qui uenturus" etc. [Mt 11:3], dubitatione scilicet pietatis non tarditatis uel incredulitatis; uel tunc dubitauit non ante. Et est diuersitatis temporum ... .

DE DVOBVS TESTAMENTIS: In utroque testamento sunt precepta, consilia, prohibitiones, permissiones, et dissimulationes. Precepta sunt moralia uel ceremonialia uel mixta ... . Attenditur et similiter generalitas uel specialitas circa consilia, prohibitiones, permissiones, et dissimilitudines. Consilium speciale est: "Vende omnia" [cf. Lc 18:22]. Permissio specialis et etiam temporalis, ut Anglicos in quarto gradu contrahere. Et nota quod permissio dicitur concessio, ut in monachum uesci carnibus, et dispensatio, ut in libello repudii, et sustinentia, ut "Deus permittit peccata per patientiam," scilicet expectans.

DE CAVSA COGNITA: Dicimus et aliquid fieri causa cognita, ubi intelligentia sumenda est ex causis agendi uel permittendi. Est autem causa necessitas, ut non est communicandum hereticis, excommunicatis, ubi scilicet paucitas est. Necessitas tamen cogit ubi est multitudo, ut modo Machometicorum (idest Saracenorum) ... .

IN SE VEL IN EQVIPOLLENTI:[30] Precepta et consilia implentur in se uel

---

30 In ... equipollenti] C: om.BO

in equipollenti uel in maiori, sicut nonnumquam opus impletur in uoluntate, uotum minus in maiori, hores reales in predicatione, septem opera misericordie in spirituali obseruatione uel mundi renunciatione.

Ratio factorvm: Ratio factorum ex causis est intelligenda faciendi; parcitur quidem etati, condescenditur infirmitati, defertur potestati, permittitur ruditati uel nouitati, procuratur sanitas, mulcetur debilitas, sicut promissione terrenorum in ueteri testamento alliciuntur et fouentur infirmi ... .

Ivdicivm propositionvm: Iudicium propositionum uersatur circa subiectum et predicatum, quod innuit Apostolus dicens prima Timotheo i [1 Tim 1:7]: "Neque intelligentes que locuntur, neque de quibus affirmant."

Ivdicivm: Iudicandum est et probandum est secundum auctoritates, rationes, exempla, similitudines; "Viua et efficax est doctrina per exempla" [cf. Heb 4:11-12], set gladiis et fustibus facienda probatio ubi legitur? Secundum Augustinum, non est querendum de statu eorum quorum certa est dampnatio. Non queramus ea que non sunt, ne non inueniamus ea que sunt.

De materia: Vbi materia turpis est uel indecens uel inutilis uel periculosa uel occulta uel nimis ardua, ibi subsistendum in disputatione.

Ivstitia positiva: Dicunt quidam: Nichil solidum est in positiua iustitia, set quod Spiritu sancto inspiratus loquitur homo, iustum est.

Institvtio:[31] Institutioni quandoque derogaretur ob consuetudinem utentium in contrarium et tacito consensu romane Ecclesie.

Lex privata: Lex priuata, priuilegium, superior causa, et lex Dei preiudicant in multis.

De inconsvetis: Ad obiecta de inconsuetis, respondemus: "Alia ratio reformat pactum," uel "frequens est aliquid extra regulam inueniri."

De etate minorvm: Ad obiecta de etate minorum, respondemus: "Iura se applicant ad ea que frequentius fiunt."

De excessv sanctorvm: Ad obiecta de excessu sanctorum, respondemus: "Familiari consilio Spiritus sancti factum est uel dictum est."

Obscvra: Ad obiecta obscura, respondemus: "Deus nouit," uel "Deus uoluit," uel "igni comburatur" [cf. Mt 3:12], uel "O altitudo" etc. [Rom 11:33]. Et "Iudicia Dei abissus multa" [Ps 35:7], et "altiora te" idest

31 Institutio] B: om. CO

sensu tuo "ne quesieris" etc. [Ecclus 3:22]. Et "non plus sapere quam oportet sapere" [Rom 12:3]. Et "qui uehementer emungit, elicit sanguinem" [Prov 30:33]. Et "sicut qui mel commedit multum non est ei bonum, sic qui perscrutator est maiestatis opprimetur a gloria" [Prov 25:27].

KARITAS: "Vbi par caritas, par meritum," uite eterne scilicet, penes caritatem uel uoluntatem omne meritum. Non faciunt in quantitatem meriti sexus, status, numerus, tempus.

CARITAS ET SACRAMENTVM: Adiciunt merito uel premio caritas et sacramentum, opus priuilegiatum ut predicatio et martirium, adicit et gratia Dei.

DE OPERIBVS: Nec operum numerositas nec temporum diuturnitas auget meritum, set uoluntas melior et caritas maior, nisi occasionaliter uel quandoque.

ADIVNCTIO: Attendenda est adiunctio, ut "quisquis eorum alterum uendiderit sine quo reliquum non prouenerit, neutrum non uenditum derelinquit." Et "qui unum dicit, quodammodo multa dicit." Et quotiens duo sese necessario sequntur uel comitantur, posito uno, ponitur alterum; interempto uno, interimitur reliquum. Patet in predestinatione et saluatione, in prophetia et eius euentu ... .

DIVERSA RELATIO: Attendenda est relatio diuersa, ut "mulier que dampnauit saluauit": laxa est relatio; non enim eadem numero set specie et genere, non eadem personaliter, set sexu ... .

PER YPALAGEN DICTVM:[32] Attende per ypallagen dictum; propterea non poterant credere, quia dixit Ysaias: "Excecauit Deus oculos eorum" (cf. Is 6:10); quia enim non poterant credere ideo predixit Ysaias; et est causa sine qua non; et intellige "non poterant credere," idest noluerunt, uel non potuerunt de facili ... .

TRANSPOSITIO SIVE CONVERSIO: Attendenda est et transpositio siue conuersio, ut ... in Exodo cv (Ex 27:5) de arulis altaris dicit Dominus Moysi: "Quos pones subter arulam altaris," idest subter quos pones arulam, et est ydioma Hebreum, sicut "Osanna filio Dauid" (Mt 21:9), uel subter ponitur pro super, sicut altum pro profundo ... . Item secunda Thimotheo ii (2 Tim 1:15): "Auersi sunt a me omnes qui in Asia sunt," hoc est omnes illi qui auersi sunt, idest recesserunt a me, modo sunt in Asia. In lectione uero tum ueteris tum noue legis, sepius occurit figura conuersionis et transpositionis.

32 Per ... dictum] C: *om. BO*

II.12

Versarius

This unique *summa* of mnemonic and didactic verses is one of William's latest and most unusual creations. Organized like his *Distinctiones, Similitudinarium,* and *Proverbia,* the *Versarius* contains nearly 4,400 lines of verse, comprising 1,375 distinct poems or verse-units, distributed under some 900 alphabetically arranged subject headings. William reveals himself, here, not as a great poet but as a skilled versifier of theological doctrine. He transposes *sententiae* from the Bible, the *Glossa ordinaria,* the writings of theologians, naturalists, historians, and from his own prose works, into verse for the use of preachers, teachers, and students in the schools. Many of the poems are accompanied by interlinear glosses, written above the line of verse and keyed to particular words by means of letters and symbols; these add to our understanding of the uses of such didactic poetry in William's school. Mnemonic and didactic verses played an important role in medieval education, and William's *Versarius* represents one of the most ambitious collections of such materials yet discovered.

In a stimulating article entitled "Unde versus," Lynn Thorndike called attention to the numerous mnemonic verses that circulated in manuscripts of medieval scientific writings.[1] Playing on the ambivalence of the Latin word *unde,* he asked the question whence these verses came. With the evidence of William de Montibus's *Versarius* we can begin to answer that question. It seems clear that such didactic verses were composed by medieval masters to reinforce their scholastic teachings. In William's case they seem to have been part of the regular scholastic exercises, supplementing the master's lectures on a set text.[2] Their diffusion, then, was not only literary (scribes copying poems from one manuscript into another) but also oral (students recalling verses that

---

[1] "Unde versus," *Traditio* 11 (1955) 162-193.

[2] See below, the comments on Samuel Priest's *Collecta* of glossed verses from William's school (II.15), where it is suggested that these represent William's *collationes* or *repetitiones.*

they memorized in the schools and copying them into their own works and the works of others).

Because of the unique, alphabetical organization of the *Versarius*, literary borrowings from it can be detected in many poetic anthologies. Peter Binkley has discussed an example in Cotton MS Titus A.xx of the British Library, London.[3] Numerous other manuscripts that include poems from the *Versarius* may have acquired these from other sources. Their authors and scribes might have known William's poems directly, from having studied under him in the schools or having read his works, or indirectly through the medium of other teachers, writers, and scribes who carried on the tradition of conveying scholastic doctrine through mnemonic verse.

The idea of a vast, alphabetically arranged repository for school verses was probably William's own invention. He intended that it be used by readers to locate quickly and easily a summary of theological or moral doctrine on specific topics.[4] The plan of the *Versarius* is like that of William's other alphabetical collections — the *Distinctiones*, the *Proverbia*, and the *Similitudinarium*. In all of these it is the topical rubrics that are alphabetized, and these by first letter only. In the *Versarius* the subjects within each alphabetical division are organized, loosely, according to an older system, that of the "natural" order of things.[5] Thus under the letter "A" William begins with poems relating to God (ADVENTVS, ASCENSVS, etc.) and to angels; then he turns to the world of human/moral action (AMOR, AMICITIA, ANACHORITA, etc.), and finally to the world of nature (AQVA, ARVNDO, ANIMALIA, etc.). The work as a whole also preserves some of this "natural" organization of materials, concluding as it does with the letter "X" and the whole series of poems on Christ (XPC) who is the "end" toward which all activities are ordered.

If, as seems likely, the *Versarius* grew out of classroom exercises in which William sought to reinforce the theological teachings presented in his formal lectures, they offer unique insights into the methods and the content of education in this period.[6] These verses also served to

---

[3] See Peter Binkley, "Unedited Poems from Cotton Titus A. XX With a Note on Chaucer's Sparrowhawk," *Scintilla: A Student Journal for Medievalists*, 2-3 (1985-1986) 66-100. Binkley edits the poems numbered 54, 230, 233, 669, 672, 673, and 674, and the glosses to nos. 672-674.

[4] See William's references to the *Versarius* in his sermons (II.16), nos. 132 and 139.

[5] Cf. Rouse and Rouse, *Preachers*, pp. 34-36.

[6] Compare William's other versified writings, the *Collecta* (II.15), the *Peniteas cito peccator* (II.1), and the *Tractatus metricus de septem sacramentis* (II.3).

recapitulate doctrines presented in William's other writings. For example, poem number 459 presents a mnemonic summary of the *De erroribus laicorum*, Part 9 of his *Errorum eliminatio* (see above, II.2):

> Scito quod a multis laicis erratur in istis:
> Inuentum, decima, sal, cespis et hostia, nupta ... .

The gloss to these verses reads:

> *Inuentum*: Can. xiiii, Q. v. Si quid inuenisti et non reddidisti rapuisti.
> *Decima*: Quam credunt potius alicui pauperi dandam quam sacerdoti diuiti.
> *Sal, cespis*: Credunt sal sufficere pro baptismo, cespitem uel panem purum pro eukaristia.
> *Et hostia*: Credunt oblatam in altari eleuatam statim esse corpus Christi.
> *Nupta*: Si nubit amasio suo fornicaria credunt ex hoc remissum esse peccatum fornicationis. Vel in obitu nubit fornicaria ut saluetur in egritudine.

The gloss to line four of the verses, "Canon, patrinus, suffocans, sorsque solutus," leaves no doubt as to the source of the poem: "Non credunt se excommunicatos cum incidunt in canonem late sententie. Quere in erroribus laicorum."

The importance of mnemonic verses and short poems in many genres of medieval literature has been emphasized recently by Siegfried Wenzel in his *Verses in Sermons*.[7] In William's *Versarius* we have perhaps the most ambitious single collection of such verses produced in the Middle Ages, including more than one thousand "poems" heretofore undescribed in the scholarly literature. This collection provides unique opportunities for exploring not only the question *unde versus*, but *quis, quid, ubi, quibus auxiliis, cur, quomodo*, and *quando* as well.

AUTHENTICITY AND DATE

An attempt to establish the authorship of these ephemeral school verses may be foolhardy. Such verses are part of a common tradition from which authors and scribes drew materials *ad libitum*, and they are ubiquitous in the margins and blank spaces of medieval manuscripts. Nevertheless someone did compose these verses, and the existence of a large compendium like William's *Versarius* allows us to probe their origins in more detail.

---

[7] *Verses in Sermons: "Fasciculus morum" and its Middle English Poems* (Cambridge MA: Mediaeval Academy of America, 1978).

There is no doubt that William compiled the *Versarius*. It is ascribed to him in one copy, and the other, although unascribed, is in a manuscript that contains only William de Montibus's writings. The alphabetical organization of the work as well as cross references in the glosses indicate that the compilation was conceived as a unified *opus*, and the glosses contain accurate references to William's other writings — the *Similitudinarium*, the *Distinctiones*, the *Speculum penitentis*, and the *Errorum eliminatio*. The style and doctrine are consistent with that of his other writings, and many of the verses and glosses appear, verbatim, in his other works.

The authorship of the verses themselves, however, is more problematic. Are they William's own compositions or did he simply draw on the common repertories of school verses for his didactic collection? To answer this question we might first look for evidence that these verses did, in fact, circulate before William's day.

Systematic research on the circulation of such verses has only recently been undertaken, but the volumes of alphabetical indices published by Hans Walther provide a starting point.[8] Of the 1,375 first lines of verse printed below from William's *Versarius*, only 228 are included in Walther's lists. If we eliminate from that number the fifty-eight Walther drew from folios 1r-12v of MS Douce 52 in the Bodleian Library, Oxford, which is almost certainly dependent on William's *Versarius* for its poems, and the two entries in Walther that are taken from the manuscripts of the *Versarius* itself (nos. 4 and 65, below), we are left with only 168 of the 1,379 first-lines for which there is *prima facie* evidence of their circulation independent of William's *Versarius*. Of these only a few can be shown incontrovertibly to have originated before William's day. Numbers 488, 489, and 612 are found in manuscripts dating to the eleventh and early twelfth centuries; number 310 is quoted by John of Salisbury; numbers 114, 165, 869, 1101, and 1286 are attributed by Walther to Serlo of Wilton; num-

---

[8] *Initia carminum ac versuum medii aevi posterioris latinorum* (Göttingen: Vandenhoech and Ruprecht, 1959); *Proverbia sententiaeque latinitatis medii aevi*, 6 vols. (Göttingen: Vandenhoech and Ruprecht, 1963-1967). See also the work of Jürgen Stohlmann, "Nachträge zu Hans Walther, Initia carminum ac versuum medii aevi," *Mittellateinisches Jahrbuch*, 7 (1972) 293-314; 8 (1973) 288-304; 9 (1974) 320-344; 12 (1977) 297-315; 15 (1980) 259-286; 16 (1981) 409-441; and idem, "Nachträge zu Hans Walther, Proverbia sententiaeque latinitatis medii aevi," *ibid.* 12 (1977) 316-329; 13 (1978) 315-333; and Paul Gerhard Schmidt, *Proverbia Sententiaeque Latinitatis Medii ac Recentioris Aevi*, New Series, 7-9 (Göttingen: Vandenhoech and Ruprecht, 1982-1986).

bers 143, 490, 513, 552, 597, 644, 1078, 1299, and 1300 are attributed to Hildebert of Le Mans; and numbers 327, 661, and 698 are assigned to Marbod. To this list should be added the quotations from Ovid (no. 1326 = *Metam* 15.389) and Martial (no. 715 = *Epigr* 8.12), both of which are identified as such in the manuscripts of the *Versarius*, as well as the line from Juvenal (no. 324 = *Sat* 14.207). No doubt more of the verses will be identified as direct quotations or paraphrases of pre-existing poetry (William's penchant for paraphrasing lines from the classical authors is discussed below), but relatively few of the poems constituting the *Versarius* are known to have circulated before William's day.

The bulk of the other verses known to Walther are cited there from later manuscripts and provide no firm evidence that William simply borrowed from already existing poetry to compose his *Versarius*. A few verses in this collection are also found in the writings of William's contemporaries. Most frequent are verses in the *Liber parabolarum* ascribed to Alan of Lille.[9] One verse (no. 159) is quoted in Alexander Neckam's *De naturis rerum*, composed before 1205.[10] Other verses included in the *Versarius* are quoted anonymously by the English Cistercian who compiled the *Distinctiones monasticae*,[11] and by Gerald of Wales.[12] As Alexander and Gerald were close associates of William de Montibus, and the *Distinctiones monasticae* were probably compiled after William's death, we cannot rule out the possibility that they borrowed from William's writings or teaching.

We are left, then, with a very short list of poems in the *Versarius* that definitely were not composed by William. Although the list of verses that can be ascribed to other writers, or that circulated before the later twelfth century and thus could not have been composed by him, will grow with further research, the clear implication is that William is responsible for the bulk of the verses collected here.

---

[9] Above, nos. 25, 26, 105, 166, 229, 325, 504, 626, 802, 912, 982, 1078, 1140, 1170, and 1201. The *Liber parabolarum* is printed in PL 210:581-594. Although the manuscripts of this work are all from the 14th and 15th centuries, Marie-Thérèse d'Alverny defends Alans authorship in *Alain de Lille*, pp. 51-52.

[10] *Alexandri Neckam De naturis rerum libri duo*, p. 329 (2.187).

[11] Below, nos. 85, 118, 1151. Excerpts from this work are printed by J.B. Pitra, *Spicilegium Solesmense* (Paris, 1885), vols. 2 and 3, and by Wilmart, "Un repertoire d'exégese," pp. 307-46. See further, R. W. Hunt, "A Manuscript Containing Extracts from the *Distinctiones monasticae*," *Medium aevum* 44 (1975) 238-241.

[12] Nos. 1025 and 1333 are quoted in Gerald's *Gemma ecclesiastica* 2, 6, p. 191, and *Speculum ecclesiae* 3, 8, p. 170, respectively.

Positive evidence of William's authorship is encountered occasionally. The *Summa Qui bene presunt*, an avowed compilation of William's teachings, quotes many of these verses and sometimes ascribes them explicitly. For example the verses noted below in number 413 are introduced in the *Qui bene presunt* with the words:

> De premissis Lincolniensis Cancellarius sic ait:
> Constat in altari carnem de pane creari ... .[13]

Likewise entry number 751 is quoted thus in the *Qui bene presunt*:

> Coniugium mundat, fecundat, mutat, et unit,
> Pollens auctore, tempore, lege, loco.
> ut docuit bone memorie Cancellarius Lincolnie.[14]

Lines three to seven of number 752 are also quoted and ascribed to William:

> Quedam que impediunt mutuam debiti redditionem, que sic complexit
> Cancellarius Lincolniensis:
> Ariditas, error persone, conditionis,
> Etas et uotum, cognatio, cultus, et ordo,
> Grandis culpa, furor, inhonestas, arsque maligna,
> Susceptus habitus, uiolenta coactio nuptis,
> Coniugium dirimunt uel inire uolentibus obsunt.[15]

A careful study of the manuscripts of the *Qui bene presunt* will disclose further attributions.

Samuel Presbyter in his *Collecta ... ex diuersis auditis in scola magistri Willelmi de Montibus* (see below, II.15) quotes the poems numbered 218, 585, 713, 714, 752, and 826. Of course these verses that were heard in William's school may still have been written by someone other than the master who quoted and glossed them, but good reasons exist for attributing them to William.

The best evidence for William's authorship of the verses is in the integral relation between verse and gloss that is evident in many of the poems. Numerous entries in the *Versarius* are meaningless without the accompanying gloss. For example, number 1198:

> QVE PERIMANT SVPERBIAM:
> Depede, prefati, rumor, fit ruptio tifi

---

[13] London, BL MS Royal 9.A.xiv, fol. 68va.

[14] San Marino (CA), Huntington Library MS HM 19914, fol. 142rb; the verses are unascribed in MS Royal 9.A.xiv.

[15] MS HM 19914, fol. 142vb; the verses are unascribed in MS Royal 9.A.xiv.

becomes comprehensible only through the gloss which explains that the destruction of pride ("tifi" = typhi) involves calling to mind the things noted mnemonically in the first three words:

> *DE*bilitas id est fragilitas commemorata, *PE*ccata, *DE*licta; consideratio *PRE*cedentium ut perfectiorum, *FA*ctus es de limo, *TI*mor Dei qui zelotes est, *RV*ina angelorum, memoria *MOR*tis.

The gloss on number 1337 is similar; it concerns the equality and inequality of the virtues, a topic that William also discusses in his *Numerale* (see above, II.7):

> Prestant equales uirtutes E N E A nobis,
> Has et inequales V A D A dant, elementa notabis.

"E N E A" is glossed: "*E*ssentia, *N*atura, *E*fficacia, h*A*bitus," and "V A D A" as: "*V*sus exterior, *A*pparentia, *D*ignitas, *A*uctoritas." The same doctrine can be found in *Numerale* 3.3.

Also very frequent are the verses that might be called "circumstantial" to designate their use of the classical doctrine concerning the "circumstances" of human acts. These circumstances were expressed in the verse:

> Quis, quid, ubi, quibus auxiliis, cur, quomodo, quando.[16]

The "circumstantial" poems in the *Versarius* ring the changes on this basic conceit, beginning with the first verse, on Advent:

> Quis ueniat uideas, quo, quando, quomodo, quare.

This verse is of little use in itself, but provides the occasion for a gloss that elucidates the meaning of "Advent." Some sixty poems in the *Versarius* are of this type; as they are easily composed and depend for their usefulness on the accompanying gloss, it would be foolhardy to assume that William borrowed them from existing collections. Rather, they have all the marks of the kind of verse a teacher would compose *ad hoc* to illustrate particular points of doctrine.

If we add to these examples the numerous poems and glosses that refer implicitly or explicitly to William's other works, we have considerable evidence that William was an industrious "versificator." William certainly made use of existing poems in his *Versarius*, either by quoting them directly or by paraphrasing them, but until it can be shown that a particular poem in this collection was certainly written by someone

---

[16] Johannes Gründel, *Die Lehre von den Umständen der menschlichen Handlung im Mittelalter* (Münster: Aschendorffsche Verlag, 1963), p. 128.

else, or was in circulation before William began his versifying efforts, his authorship should be granted at least *prima facie* assent.

The only firm indication of a date of composition for the *Versarius* is the references to other of William's writings. These suggest that it was composed after the *Errorum eliminatio, Distinctiones, Similitudinarium,* and *Speculum penitentis,* all of which are mentioned in the glosses. Contemporary events make few appearances here, but the unglossed verses entitled CONQVESTIO CLERICORVM SVSPENSORVM (no. 228):

> Nobis suspensis, Christi suspenditur ensis;
> Quando reuertetur Domini uindicta sequetur

might well refer to the interdict on England in 1208-1213. If so, this would date the composition of the *Versarius* to the end of William's career. The individual poems, however, were doubtlessly written or collected over a long period before being assembled into this reference work.

SOURCES

To speak of William as the author of these school verses may be misleading. The *Versarius* is not a poetic creation like Alan of Lille's *De planctu naturae* or *Anticlaudianus*. Rather it is a versification of theological and moral commonplaces drawn from many sources. These sources include existing poems, passages of Scripture, popular proverbs, and other common materials, excerpted and recast by William to make a particular point. For example, in the verses concerning the divine attributes (no. 254):

> Tu Deus adiutor, medicus, dux, rex, mihi pastor/ ...

the fourth line:

> Tu dominus, tu uir, tu mihi frater eris

is a quotation from Ovid (*Epist Heroid* 3.52). The two verses of no. 514:

> Paulus ait: Carne peccati seruio legi
> Set Deum legi me seruum mente subegi

are simply a versification of Paul's letter to the Romans (7:25): "Igitur ego ipse mente servio legi Dei, carne autem peccati legi." Under the rubric "House guests" (HOSPES, no. 560) William versifies one of the popular sayings that he collected in his *Proverbia*:

Verum dixit anus quod piscis olet triduanus
Eiusdemque more simili fetet hospes odore.[17]

The most frequent sources cited in the glosses are the Bible and
its Gloss, Augustine, Ambrose, Boethius, Claudian, Gregory, Jerome,
Isidore, Martial, and Ovid are invoked, along with Gratian's *Decretum*
and Lombard's *Sentences*, but these authorities appear infrequently.
The only contemporary author to be mentioned is Robertus de
Camera.[18]

MANUSCRIPTS

Two exemplars of the *Versarius* have been identified. Both were carefully copied and corrected. Occasional errors and omissions suggest
that neither is a copy of the other, but a full collation will be necessary
to establish their precise relationship. The Cambridge manuscript (*C*)
presents the poems in a single series, arranged alphabetically according
to the first letter of the text's rubrics. The British Library copy (*L*)
is in two parts, each comprising an alphabetical series of rubrics from
A to X.

1. *C* = Cambridge, Corpus Christi College MS 186, fols. 21r-126v, 1r-
20v. Mid 13th century (above top line).
   Inc. Gloss: *Deus Christus, Ysaias: Deus ipse ueniet et saluabit nos.*
   Inc. Txt: (*De primo aduentu*) *Quis ueniat uideas.*
   Expl. Gloss: *Adversarios.*
   Expl. Text: (*Miracula Christi*) *Firmant et fulgent, Christi miracula
   terrent.*
Verses and glosses to be added to the text are copied on fols. 1r-20v
and marked for insertion by means of letters and symbols written in
the margin. The glosses are interlinear, written above the line to which
they refer. Other notes, in a contemporary hand, are added in the
margins. These include excerpts from William's *Similitudinarium* and
his *Proverbia*.[19]

---

[17] See the *Proverbia*, Oxford, New College MS 98, fol. 86rb: "Hospites triduani
incipiunt fetere ut pisces."

[18] Gloss to no. 563, "Mente, manu, uerbo, causa neco denique rendo": " ... . Ita
et magister Robertus de camera: Per occasionem, familiari consilio Spiritus sancti,
se ipsos occidunt Sampson, Razias, et martyres quidam. Set non sunt hec trahenda
ad consequentiam." On Robert see John W. Baldwin, *Masters*, 1:5, 153-154.

[19] The first entry of both works is copied on folio 24r: "Amor terrenus inuiscat
animam ..." (= *Similitudinarium*); "B<eda> super Tobiam: Sunt amici carne ..."
(= *Proverbia*).

2. *L* = London, British Library MS Add. 16164, fols. 15r-58r, 63r-108r. Mid 13th century (above top line).

Part One:

> Inc. Gloss: *Deus ipse. In hoc ergastulum.*
>
> Inc. Txt.: (*Aduentus Christi primus*) *Quis ueniat uideas.*
>
> Expl. Txt.: (*Domus Christi*) ... *Perflent, ex petra firma stat ista domus.*

Part Two:

> Inc. Gloss: *Deus manifeste ueniet.*
>
> Inc. Txt.: (*Aduentus Christi secundus*) *Regis ad aduentum.*
>
> Expl. Gloss: *Id est hominis, scilicet anima.*
>
> Expl. Txt.: (*Vita et doctrina Christi*) *Conuenit et uite, lingue doctrina perite.*

Another verse: (*Zona*) *Se cingit fortis, humilis, castus, moderatus*, is added on fol. 108v, but the rubric is not included in the table of contents, nor is it found in MS *C*. The fourteen verses of *Vno rinoceros* (no. 1106) are added, without rubric, at the bottom of fol. 108v.

The gloss is written above the line and in the left and right margins. A table of contents on fols. 12r-13v presents the rubrics of both parts in a single, alphabetical list with the A-rubrics of Part One followed by the A-rubrics of Part Two, and so on.

A note on the first flyleaf of the manuscript, in a fourteenth-century hand, reads: *Titulus huius libri: Versarius Magistri Willelmi de montibus Johannis episcopi.* A mid-thirteenth-century hand wrote the following on fol. 11v: *Hunc librum dedit Dominus Iohannes quondam Ardfertensis episcopus Deo et ecclesie sancti Albani.* This is probably John Breton, bishop of Hereford from 1269 to 1275. Folio 14v is blank except for the ascription: *Versus magistri Willelmi de montibus*, in a fourteenth-century hand.

The following is transcribed from Cambridge, Corpus Christi College MS 186 (*C*), and the folio references are to that manuscript. Additional verses were copied on folios 1r-20v of this codex and marked for inclusion in the body of the *Versarius*. These verses are inserted silently in the appropriate place.

Only the first item, DE PRIMO ADVENTV, is transcribed in full, with its gloss. For the rest, the topical headings or rubrics and the first line of each poem under that heading are transcribed. The identification of verse-units or "poems" under each heading has been facilitated by the British Library copy, MS Add. 16164 (*L*), where they are often marked by rubricated initial letters. Additions or emendations from this second manuscript copy are printed within angle brackets < >. The numbers in square brackets [ ] following each first-line of verse indicate the number of lines in that poem in MS *C*. Square brackets are also used to indicate extra syllables. The asterisk (*) immediately following the verse number indicates that the verse is also found in MS *L*. An alphabetical index of the first lines is provided in Appendix B, below.

Versarius

DE PRIMO ADVENTV

1*   Quis^a ueniat uideas, quo,^b quando,^c quomodo,^d quare.^e [1]

   a Deus Christus, Ysaias [35:4]: "Deus ipse ueniet et saluabit nos."
   b In hoc ergastulum. Ergastulum siue ergasterium est operatorium scilicet ubi rei ad opera facienda relegabantur, et significat mundum siue corpus humanum quod cuiusque anime ergastulum est, unde Dominus in Exodo xiii [6:6]: "Ego Dominus qui educam uos de ergastulo Egyptiorum," id est de tribulationibus mundi quibus tribulantur sancti, "et eruam de seruitute" scilicet corporali et spirituali, "ac redimam," scilicet pretioso sanguine filii, "in brachio excelso," scilicet potentia manifesta incarnato filio.
   c Cum uenerit plenitudo temporis, post longa preconia, cum multiplicatis infirmitatibus accelerarent ad medicum.
   d Per uirginem humiliter, per aquam et sanguinem misericorditer.
   e Venit filius hominis querere ouiculam et dragmam perditam, et saluum facere quod perierat.

2   Culpa,^f salus,^g meritum,^h Dominiⁱ clementia, discum^k

   f Causa occasionalis. O felix culpa, etc.
   g Causa finalis. Qui propter nos homines et propter nostram salutem descendit de celis.
   h Sanctorum <sci>licet causa cooperans.
   i "Secundum misericordiam suam saluos nos fecit" [Tit 3:5]
   k Seu lintheum, idest Christum, Actus Apostolorum xxvii, ii [= Act 11:5]: Et uidit celum apertum et "descendens uas quoddam," idest corpus Christi, "uelut lintheum magnum," quia mortuum et sindone inuolutum.

In terram mitti^a faciunt de culmine celi.

   a Hoc est humiliter incarnari

DE SECVNDO ADVENTV

3* Qualis, ubi, quando, quare uel qualiter, unde/ [5]
4* Regis ad aduentum sunt hec uenientis in urbem/ [6]

(21v)

5* Abdita propalans, reproborum pectora turbans/ [2]
6* Adueniet iudex Christus districtus in ira/ [3]

(22r)

7* En iam Christus adest quia tempus transuolat omne. [1]

DE VTROQVE ADVENTV

8* Iudicium, mors, mens, caro, dant Christum uenientem/ [2]
9* Hec mundi finis ac incarnatio, cor, mors/ [2]
10* Iram uenturam recolas, metuas, caueasque. [1]
11* Quis, quotus ascendat, quare, uel quomodo, quando/ [3]

(22v)

ANGELI

12* Celicole sunt castra Dei parere parati/ [3]
13 Seruat et adiuuat, instruit, expedit angelus, istuc/ [5]
14* Vt duo conferret, niue mulcet, fulgure terret/ [2]
15* Ciues celestes cum parent carne recentis/ [2]

ASCENSVS

16* Quis per quem scandat ubi cerne uel unde uel ad quid/ [3]

(23r)

17* Ascensus gradus est primus contempnere mundum. [1]

ASSVMPTIO

18* Quot Deus assumat, unde et quo, quomodo, quando. [1]
19* Antiquus primum nos suscipit hostis ut ursus/ [5]

(23v)

ASSVMPTIO GENTIVM

20* Dextra, capud, uirgo, latro, sanguis, monumentum/ [5]

ANIMA

21* Stuppa caro fragilis, cooperta ligataque pixis/ [4]
22* Vix sine sorde potes participare luto. [1]

(24r)

ADORATIO

23* Inspice cur uel ubi, quis, quo, quem uel quid adoret. [1]

AMOR

24* Sicut amor Domini cunctorum fons meritorum/ [3]

AMICITIA

25* Clarior est solito post maxima nubila Phebus/ [2]
26* Perdimus anguillas manibus dum stringimus illas/ [4]

AMOR BONVS ET MALVS

27* Colloquii lignis sacer et contrarius ignis/ [2]
28* Nutibus et signis internis proditur ignis. [1]

DE AMICIS IOB

29* Iob tres dilecti non recte recta loquuntur/ [2]

ABNEGATIO PROPRIORVM

30* Quisque suos, sua, se, pro Christi spernat amore. [1]

ANACHORITA

31* Nomen, causa, locus in quo claudatur et a quo/ [2]
32* Includunt homines amor ac imitatio Christi/ [2]

QVALITER DOMINVS APPARVIT HELYE

33* Spiritus et motus ignis, post sibilus aure/ [2]

(24v)

ABSOLVTIO

34* Absoluunt animas defunctorum ospes et Ely. [1]

ABLVTIO

35* In uerbis, precibus, lacrimis, in sanguine, limpha/ [3]

ARMA

36* Virtutes et uerba Dei fletusque precesque/ [3]

DE AQVA BENEDICTA ET ASPERSORIO

37* Lignum, seta rigens, aqua, sal ad uulnera mordens/ [3]

AQVA

38* Est aqua baptismi, scripture, flaminis almi. [1]
39* Est aqua doctrina uel gratia spiritualis/ [6]

(25r)

40* Limpha Dei donum, populus, doctrina, uoluptas/ [6]

AQVE PROPRIETATES

41* Labitur, extinguit, fecundat, et abluit unda/ [3]

ARVNDO

42* Debilis et uacua, leuis et radice lutosa/ [3]

ARS

43* Ars uitium nescit, uitiosus abutitur arte. [1]

AVDIRE
44*   Non te pretereat narratio presbiterorum/ [2]

AVRVM
45*   Auro sunt signata fides, amor, atque sophia/ [3]

ARCHA
46*   Est homo uel Christus, mens, ecclesie, domus archa/ [2]

ADEPS
47*   Dant adipem triplicem: cor, epar, renunculus extis/ [3]

                                                              (25v)

AMBVLARE
48*   Qui gradiuntur ubi, uel quo duce, quomodo, quando/ [3]

AGER
49*   Plantas et segetes produc et gramina flores/ [5]

ANIMALIA IN EZECHIELE
50*   Sis uitulus te sacrificans, homo sis ratione/ [4]

ANIMALIA IMMVNDA
51*   Sunt immunda lepus, cirogrillus, susque camelus. [1]

ANIMALIA ET AVES
52*   Nasciscuntur enim fera siluas, bestia campos/ [4]

ARIES
53*   Est ab ares dictus aries, mactatur ad aram/ [4]

ASINVS
54   Est asinus stolidus, immundus, hebesque Manasses/ [4]

                                                              (26r)

AVIS
55*   Corpore sicut aues, sic mente superna petamus. [1]
56*   Angelus et Christus, sanctus, demonque superbus/ [2]

ARIDITAS
57*   Auris, ocellus, et os, cor, pes, manus, arida fiunt. [1]

ANATHEMA
58   Corpus, culpa, sathana, mundus, tibi sint anathema/ [3]

AVARVS
59*   Naufragus ut retinet manibus si forte quid hesit/ [2]

AVARITIA
60* Ydrops et dipsas, species, bitumen, irudo/ [10]

AMBITIO
61 Magnum querit honus, magnum qui querit honorem. [1]

ADVLATIO
62 Oscula ficta Ioab, pestis blandumque uenenum/ [6]

(26v)

62a A petra resilit quamuis sit acuta sagitta/ [2]

ATTENVATIO
63* Attenuant hominem studium, ieiunia, pallor/ [2]

AMBIGENA
64 Hec sunt ambigena natura dispare nata/ [5]

AN OMNIS ACTIO SIT A DEO
65 Est longinqua Deus non causa propinqua malorum/ [3]

ADVERSITAS
66 Iustus in aduersis non spernitur immo probatur. [1]

ACETVM
67 Materies, sapor et species pensentur aceti. [1]

ARANEA
68 Egerit, irretit, tabet, suspenditur, aret/ [2]

BEATITVDO CELESTIS
69* Hec bona sunt patrie: dulcedo, uita beata/ [4]

(27r)

BAPTISMVS
70* Primum fons et crux intranti sancta patescunt/ [5]
71* Flatus, crux, et sal, sputum cum crismate, uestis/ [3]
71a* Sponsor baptismi uotum dissoluere noli. [1]

BENEFICIA DEI
72* Tot Dominus nobis et tanta dedit bona quod non/ [3]

BONVS HOMO
73* Que bona sunt bonus in lingua uel pectore tractat/ [6]

BONA
74* Que secum non ferre potest hominis bona non sunt/ [2]
75* Temporis hec bona sunt non effectu licet usu. [1]

QVOT MODIS DICATVR BONVM

76   Affectu care luneue resigno uel ex spe/ [2]

(27v)

BENEDICERE

77*   Cui uel ubi, quando, qui, quomodo, cur benedicant/ [2]

BLANDITIE

78*   Inuiscos uolucres cogit cum cantibus auceps/ [2]

BIBERE

79*   Dum bibis et rebibis componitur unde peribis/ [2]

BOS

80*   Bos, demon, stolidus, Iudeus, sollicitusque/ [4]
81*   Bos mactatur, arat, lactat, pascit, corium dat. [1]

BACVLVS PASTORIS

82*   Curua trahit quos uirga regit, pars ultima pungit. [1]
83*   Curua trahit mites, pars pungit acuta rebelles. [1]
84*   Recte uiue, feri, flexus propera misereri. [1]
85*   Attrahe per primum, medio rege, punge per imum/ [3]

BACVLVS

86*   Percutit, irritat, sustentat, protegit, ornat/ [2]

(28r)

BELLVM

87   Aduersus Christum legitur comittere bellum/ [2]
88*   Ad bellum doctus, armatus, fortis et audax/ [3]

BREVITAS VITE

89*   Apocopant infelices sibi tempora uite/ [20]

BREVITAS RERVM

90*   Vita, salus, requies, substantia, doxa, uoluptas/ [3]

(28v)

BEATITVDO

91   In patria requies sanctis erit et stola duplex/ [11]

BENEDICERE

92   Confert, augmentat, conseruat, denique firmat/ [6]

BASAN

93   Basan turpe sonat, siccum, confusio, bruchus/ [2]

BRACHIVM DOMINI
94   Cum tibi diuinus scriptura promitur armus/ [2]

SANCTVS BENEDICTVS
95*   A puero spreuit Benedictus florida mundi/ [2]

CORPVS CHRISTI
96*   Egris et sanis est sana refectio panis/ [6]

(*29r*)

CARITAS
97*   Fons, radix et adeps amor est et forma, caracter/ [7]

(*29v*)

98*   Fons, gluten, bernix, amor est alatus et ignis/ [4]
99*   Alligat atque legit amor, et coniungit et unit/ [4]
100* Quis sit amandus, quomodo, quantum, curque uideto. [1]
101* Quomodo, cur, quantum, Dominus sit amandus et a quo. [1]
102* In bello fortis instar dilectio mortis/ [2]
103* Arche ligna lita non soluunt uentus et unda/ [2]
103a Cedrus odore suo fugat angues, sic amor almus/ [2]

CASTITAS
104* Baltheus est bissus, iacinctus, gemmaque flos, sal/ [9]

(*30r*)

105* Subtrahe ligna foco si uis extinguere flammam/ [2]

CONCORDIA
106* Timpana, sal, munus, reddit concordia grata. [1]
107* Iustis concorda ne fias dissona corda/ [2]

CONCORDIA MALORVM
108   Pressio squame, lappaque uiscus, nexio praua. [1]

CONCORDIA BONORVM
109   Cementum, gluten, iuncturaque nexio iusta. [1]

CONSTANTIA
110* Tu te non alius celis auferre ualebis/ [2]

CVSTODIA
111   Serues sollicitus carnis cum sensibus artus/ [2]
112* Vt te ipsum serues, non expergisceris/ [5]
113   Conseruant castum labor et fuga, sobrietasque/ [5]

(*30v*)

CONTEMPLATIVVS
114*   Si mundo moreris moriendo non morieris. [1]

CAVE
115*   Inspice cui uel cur, attendas qualiter, a quo/ [2]

CAVTELA
116   Lapsus malorum fiat cautela minorum. [1]
117*   Quod leo non tetigit dum mordet aranea ledit/ [2]
118*   Felix quem faciunt aliena pericula cautum. [1]
119*   Prouideas, campus oculos habet et nemus aures. [1]
120*   Non detur sathane locus aut membris sathaninis/ [4]
121*   Vehementi occurrite morbo/ [4]

CONSILIVM
122*   Subtrahe consilio dilectum quem petit hostis. [1]

COGITA CHRISTVM
123*   In Christo lapide submissa mente recumbe. [1]

REMEDIVM CONTRA MALAS COGITATIONES
124*   Hec muscas abigunt: ramus, contunsio, clauus. [1]

CONVERSIO
125*   Qui conuertentur, quando, cur, qualiter, unde. [1]
126   Sit cita, discreta, conuersio plena, fidelis. [1]

(31r)

127*   Vnde et quo, qualis conuersio, quomodo, quare/ [3]
128   Conuerti dant ista: fides contritio cordis/ [6]

CONFESSIO
129*   Peniteas plene, si uere peniteat te/ [5]
130*   Est fidei, fraudis, ueri, confessio laudis/ [4]
131   Sint comites Iude pudor et submissio spesque. [1]

(31v)

CASTELLVM
142*   Fossa, latex, collis ac murus celsaque turris/ [2]

CENA DOMINI
143   Villa, boues, uxor, cenam clausere uocatis/ [2]
144*   Ara, pes, et missa, pax ecclesiastica, crisma/ [2]

CANDELABRVM
145*   Christus et ecclesia, doctor scripturaque iustus/ [2]

CONFIDENTIA
146* In quo, cur, qualis sit confidentia nobis. [1]
147* Omnis in hoc mundo fidens est sicut arundo/ [2]

COMMVNICATIO
148* Veste, loco, uase, cultu potuque ciboque/ [2]

CVRIA
149* Currere, pascere, parcere, querere curia prestat/ [3]

(32r)

COLVMPNA
150* Denotat antiquam benedicta columpna columpnam/ [3]

CORPVS
151* Terra, lutum, uestis, uas, fascis, seruus, et hostis/ [4]

CORPVS HOMINIS
152* Est aurum purum regis diadema futurum/ [3]

CARO
153* Vilior est humana caro quam pellis ouina/ [4]
154   Quid tam curate nutritur inutilis a te/ [2]
155* Spirituique uiro mulier caro sepe repugnat/ [2]

(32v)

155a* Candidus et mundus lauat et sanat cinis ignis/ [2]

CAPTIVITAS
156* Dulcis in hostili patrie memoratio terra. [1]

CARCER
157* Vinctos educit Dominus de carcere ceco/ [4]
158* Sunt timor et tenebre, uermes, in carcere fetor/ [2]

CVRA
159* Cura uigil macerat, sollicitatque timor. [1]

CLAMOR
160* Ad quem quis clamet, cur, quomodo, quando, quid, unde. [1]
161* Sanguinis et fletus, operis quoque cordis et oris/ [2]
162* Clamant sanguis, opus, uirtus, et spiritus, os, cor. [1]

CONTINVATIO
163* Expedit, infigit, rude continuatio tollit/ [3]

CONSVETVDO
164* Assuetudo mali fetet ad ora Dei. [1]

165*   Quod noua testa capit, inueterata sapit/ [2]
166*   Mollibus assuetus clipeum bene non gerit armus/ [2]

(*33r*)

CIRCVITVS
167*   Circueas scripta, mentem, loca, tempora, membra/ [3]

CRVX ET PASSIO CHRISTI
168   Dat tibi spontanei crux, mors seu passio Christi/ [4]

CONSCIENTIA
169*   Nil conscire sibi, nulla pallescere culpa. [1]

COLVMPNA
170   Christus et ecclesia, doctor nubisque columpna/ [2]

COMPASSIO ET CONGRATVLATIO
171   Si bona uicinis dentur congratulor illis/ [2]

CAPVD
172*   Initium capud est, mens, Christus, dux aliorum. [1]

CAPILLVS
173   Spissus uel rarus, tenuisque leuisque capillus/ [4]

<CRINIS>
174*   Est crinis capitis gracilis uariique coloris/ [2]

CASVS
175   Gratia, natura dant casum, pena scelusque/ [2]

CARACTER
176   Est tiphus reprobi titulus signumque caracter. [1]

CIBVS
177   Vsus et ara, liber et gratia, gloria, culpa/ [3]

CENA MAGNA
178   Ad mensam socius fuerit quicumque uocatus/ [2]

CVRRVS
179   Currus prelatus est; quatuor iste rote sunt/ [5]

CINIS
180   Puluis siue cinis Abraham fertur Iob et Adam/ [2]
181   Imposito cinere capiti subeant tibi quinque/ [3]

CECITAS
182   Talpa, canis, Naas, coruus Samsonque Thobias/ [3]

CATVS
183 Accipiendo seu quasi cautum dicito catum. [1]

CIBVS DIABOLI
184 Delicie silique fenumque fauillaque ficus/ [2]

QVANDO CLAVDETVR IANVA CELI
185 In sero mundi claudetur ianua regni/ [4]

COREA
186 Ducentes gratas, iocunda mente, choreas/ [5]

CEDRVS
187 Cedrus odorifera serpentibus est inimica/ [2]

QVOMODO COR PATET
188* In facie legitur hominum secreta uoluntas/ [4]

CIRCVMSTANTIE
189* Mos, modus et causa, tempus, persona locusque/ [2]

(33v)

190* Aggrauat ordo, locus, peccata, scientia, tempus/ [2]

CIRCVMSTANTIE IN CONFESSIONE
191* Quis, quid, ubi, quibus auxiliis, cur, quomodo, quando/ [2]

CRVX
192* Crux est muscipula, baculus, torcular, et ara/ [8]
193* En epigrama crucis Christum regem manifestat/ [4]
194* Salue crux, hoc est, sis nobis causa salutis. [1]
195* Christus quadrifidi concendit robora ligni/ [2]
196* Lingua Latina potens, Hebreaque religiosa/ [4]

(34r)

197 In ligno limphe Marath indulcantur amare/ [8]

CALIX
198* Dant calicem nobis lex, gratia, gloria, culpa/ [2]

CELI
199* Celi sunt sancti qui celant mistica prauis/ [3]

CLAVES REGNI CELORVM
200* Quis liget aut soluat, ubi, quem, cur, quomodo, quando. [1]

(34v)

CANTVS
201* Quis, quid, cui cantet, ubi, quando, quomodo, quare. [1]
202* Corde pio ac opere Domino cantemus et ore/ [2]

CITHARA
203* In cithara lignum cordeque cauillaque plectrum/ [2]

CONTENTIO BONA
204* Cursus, martirium, contendere donat et artum/ [2]

CVRRERE
205* Quis cursus, quis currat, ubi, quibus auxiliis, quo/ [2]

CVRRVS
206* Currus amor, gemineque rote dilectio duplex/ [3]

CADERE
207* Qui cadit in faciem quo decidat aspicit ipse/ [2]

CONSOLATIO
208* Solatur scriptura, Deus pius, actaque pena. [1]

CVLTVS
209* Obsequio cole patronum, pietate parentem/ [2]

CIBVS
210* Dum uacat os mense ferat ad celestia mens se. [1]

CENA
211* Post cenam standum, uel passus mille uagandum. [1]

(35r)

CONGREGATIO
212* Quis, quo, quos, unde, cur, quomodo congregat, ad quid. [1]

CAVSA
213* Efficiens causa Deus est, formalis ydea/ [2]

QVE SE CELARE NON POSSVNT
214* Dicitur et uere nequeunt hec quinque latere/ [2]

CONTRARIA
215* Gratificat flores spinetum, coruus olores. [1]

CECVS
216* Quis uidet agnoscens quid credendum, quid agendum/ [5]

CALCIAMENTVM
217* Sumas exemplum quod tanquam calceus aptus/ [2]

COLLIRIA
218* Que bona sunt oculis cordis colliria si uis/ [2]

CRASSVS

219* Telluris loca Tigris obit, qua sorbuit aurum/ [2]

CVPIDVS

220* Est cupidus Pharius mersus, Crassus, canis, orchus/ [2]

(35v)

221* Quid lucra terrea uos male ferrea corda gerentes/ [2]
222* Eris seruus eris si te species trahit eris. [1]
223* Attrahit, absorbet naues pontina uorago/ [2]

CVPIDITAS

224* Spongia, ianua, uiscus et ignis, rete, uorago/ [2]

QVE DESTRVVNT CVPIDITATEM

225* Radicem prauam, mens leti, falco necabit/ [2]

CVPIDO

226* Pingitur alatus ueterum ratione Cupido/ [2]

CRVDELITAS

227* Sanguine non uesci, mel non offerre iuberis/ [2]

CONQVESTIO CLERICORVM SVSPENSORVM

228* Nobis suspensis Christi suspenditur ensis/ [2]

CLERICI

229* Non discunt quicumque scolas ubicumque frequentant/ [2]

CANIS

230* Inuidet, immundus, redit ad uomitum canis atque/ [2]

(36r)

PROPRIETAS CERVI

231 Apotoy keraton, hoc est a cornibus apte/ [8]

CAPRA

232* Balatu querulo subiens sublimia sepe/ [2]

COLVMBA

233* Est socialis auis cui nidus petra, columba/ [7]

(36v)

CORVVS

234* Pasco, Caym, macro, clamosus, cras, niger, imbre. [1]

CIBVS DIABOLI

235 Serpentis cibus est fenum puluisque fauilla/ [2]

Cognitio Dei
236*   Resplendet sole paries pelui mediante/ [2]

Carnalia desideria
237*   Hec terrena teras: carnem cum fomite motum. [1]

Qualiter Dominvs compescat malos
238   Compescit prauos Dominus reprimens furiosos/ [2]

Cavsa
239   Causa super causas Domini ualor atque uoluntas/ [2]

Caritas
240   Si desit panis est mensa et inops et inanis/ [2]

Caritas et patientia
241   Dant calor ac humor flores et gramina, fructus/ [3]

(37r)

Devs
242*   En Deus excelsus nulli dabit esse secundum. [1]
243*   Est Deus excelsus pariter metuendus amandus/ [3]
244*   Desinit esse modo quod numquam desinit esse. [1]
245*   Vt rota principio uel fine carere uidetur/ [2]
246*   Nobis blanditur Deus et quandoque minatur/ [2]
247*   Quales nos illi, talis nobis Deus extat/ [2]
248*   In Domino gaude simul expergiscere et aude/ [2]
249*   Omnia discernit, trutinat Deus, omnia cernit/ [2]
250*   Omne bonum nostrum referamus ad omnipotentem/ [3]
251*   Concipiens mundum ratio diuina secundum/ [3]
252*   Ad benedicendum uel agendum suspice celum. [1]
253*   Cuncta uidet, curat, mala uindicat et bona reddit/ [2]
254*   Tu Deus adiutor, medicus, dux, rex, mihi pastor/ [5]
255*   Cetera sunt cure, Deus est obliuio solus. [1]
256*   Quem ter ter[re]nus apex diuini numinis index/ [2]
257*   Pectus eum uoluit, uox protulit, actio prompsit/ [2]

(37v)

258*   Principium rerum, fons lucis, origo bonorum/ [3]
259*   Summe Pater uerbi, perimentis iura superbi. [1]

Devs Trinitas
260*   Qui uoluit uerbum de se sine tempore natum/ [5]
261*   Mens, sol, fons, candela, manus, trinus Deus unus. [1]

Devs creator
262* Viuens eternum Deus omnia condidit una/ [2]

Devs rector
263* Ne mors trina premat, cor et os rege factaque uestra. [1]
264* Per nec, perque pie, scitur solus Deus esse. [1]

Velle Dei
265* Precipit et prohibit, permittit, consulit, implet/ [2]
266* Vellet, si uellent, Deus omnes saluificari. [1]
267* Consulit, hortatur, iubet, omnes saluificari. [1]

Beneficivm Dei
268* Expectat, uocat, et bona dat Deus, hic sceleratis/ [2]

Patientia Dei et beneficivm
269* Multa diu patitur, pulsans Deus et bona prestat. [1]

Devs trahit
270* Sol trahit ardore nebulas, nos Christus amore/ [2]

Devs svos exaltat
271* Summus ab extremis nebulas leuat opiliones/ [2]

Largitas Dei
272* Munificus Deus est dans omnibus omnia dona/ [2]

(38r)

273* Quod plusquam tollat, promittat siue petatur/ [3]

Dona Dei
274* Magna mihi sunt dona Dei, pro dantis amore/ [2]
275* Dat Dominus posse, meritum producere nosse/ [3]
276* Dat Deus hic quedam nobis in pignus et arram/ [4]

Qve nvmeret Devs
277* Tempora cum stellis numerat Deus utile, carum/ [4]

<Devs verax>
278* Omnibus uerbis uerax Deus atque fidelis/ [2]

Dvlcedo Dei
279* Hic mundus sit uas quoddam dulcedine plenum/ [2]

Stare Dei
280* Stat Dominus stabilis, prouidus atque uiuans. [1]

Sedes Dei
281*   Sedes firma Dei, lenis subiectaque mollis/ [7]

(38v)

Devs ivdex
282*   Est iudex iustus, districtus, terribilisque/ [2]
283   Hec attendantur in summo iudice, quantum/ [2]

Ivdicivm Dei
284*   Iudicis aduentus seu iudex, iudiciumue/ [5]

(39r)

285*   Vt proruperunt quondam cathaclismus et ignis/ [3]
286*   Premunit gentes Christus ac premonet omnes. [1]

(39v)

287*   Ignis, uox, et uentilabrum, fera uisio, signum/ [3]
288*   Iudicium metuo quod timet omnis homo/ [3]
289*   Ventilabrum dextra gerit et paleas facit extra/ [2]

Ira Dei
290*   Ira furorue Dei quid nisi pena rei. [1]

Cvr Devs flagellat
291*   Vt domet, ut dampnet, ut purget et ut mereatur/ [2]

Qvatvor flagella Dei
292*   Esuries, ensis perimunt, mala bestia, pestis. [1]

Devs penitet
293   Penitet et mutat aliquid Deus, istud idem sit. [1]

<Dominvs intvetvr cor>
294*   Non ut homo faciem Deus aspicit exteriorem/ [2]

Devs dedvcit
295   Deducit Dominus dum deduci sinit usquam/ [2]

Devs mvtat consilivm
296*   Consilium mutat Dominus, sententia perstat/ [2]

(40r)

Qve debentvr Deo
297*   Debemus Domino nos nostraque tempora, mentem/ [2]

Qve svnt Deo reservanda
298*   Laus et uindicta sunt et promotio nostra/ [2]

Reddite qve svnt Dei Deo
299*   Dentur honos et amor Domino, timor obsequiumque/ [3]

LAVS DEI
300*   Cuncta Deum laudant uel per se uel mediate/ [2]

LOQVI DEO
301*   Cor Domino loquitur, meditatio nostra fatetur/ [3]

DIACONVS
302*   Attendas qualis, cui, quomodo, curque ministres. [1]

DISCRETIO
303*   Sal sacrificii cithare discretio plectrum/ [2]

DISCERE
304*   Dum uiuis discas ad quid uel quomodo uiuas/ [3]

DOCERE
305*   Quod doceas sane tu multo tempore disce/ [4]

                                                            (40v)

DOCTRINA
306*   Doctrine librum nobis assumite mundum/ [2]
307*   Ars, usus, locus et tempus, scriptura, creata/ [3]

DOCTRINA ET GRATIA
308   Sol est doctrina, tenebras pellendo chorusca. [1]
309*   Est imber doctrina Dei, ros gratia Christi/ [2]

QVE NECESSARIA SVNT AD DISCIPLINAM
310*   Mens humilis, studium querendi, uita pudica/ [3]

DISTINCTIO
311*   Personas actusque modos, loca, tempora, causas/ [2]

DETERMINATIO CONTRARIETATEM
312*   Que forsan reputo contraria soluere quero/ [3]

DECALOGVS
313*   Sperne deos, non periures, requies celebretur/ [6]

DEDICATIO ECCLESIE
314*   Octo concurrunt ad templum sanctificandum/ [5]

                                                            (41r)

315*   Cum uino sit aqua, cinis et sal mixtaque sint hec/ [2]

DARE
316*   Si donas tristis et dona et munera perdis/ [2]
317   Vel rem uel uerbum tribuas cuicumque petenti/ [2]

318   Dans Aidanus equum, gladium dans Brigida patris/ [2]
319* Fers aliquid nihil, esto foras, fero, quid nimis, intra. [1]

DIVISIO
320* Tempus, opes et opus, operam quoque diuide recte. [1]

DENARIVS
321* Denarius sit homo regis retinendo rotundus/ [2]

DIVITIE
322* Cum dat sero Deus bona temporis, insinuatur/ [4]
323* Diuitie nullum dare possunt esse beatum/ [2]

                                                                    (41v)

324* Vnde habeas nemo querit set oportet habere. [1]
325* Apparet fantasma uiris, set rursus ab illis/ [4]
326* Spina facultatis suppungit corda, maresque/ [4]
327* Fortune fragilis fiat tibi copia uilis. [1]
328* Pauperibus large tua dum tibi copia sparge. [1]
329* Sunt fluuius, Pharius, maris unde, sarcina, gibbus/ [8]

                                                                    (42r)

DIVES MALVS
330* Vt colatorum locuples, loculusque camelus/ [6]

DECIME
331   Prima Deo decima detur, decimaque secunda/ [3]
332* Quis, cui, cur uel ubi, decimas det, qualiter, ad quid. [1]

DIOGENES
333* Ridens derisit, flens defleuit mala mundi. [1]

SEPTEM DORMIENTES
334* In Celio monte septem dormisse leguntur/ [2]

DOMVS
335* Prima datur nobis uterus domus, altera mundus/ [4]

                                                                    (42v)

DOMVS ORNATVS
336* Virtus exornat mentem, contritio mundat/ [2]

DESERTVM
337* Sunt in deserto serpens, sitis, ardor, harena. [1]
338* Existi liber Pharias fugiendo tenebras/ [4]
339* Scorpius ac dipsas et serpens flatibus urens/ [2]
340   Desertum carnis est mortificatio, uestis/ [8]

DOMINICA OCTODECIM POST PENTECOSTEN
341 Labes, diuitie sancte, detectio Christi/ [4]

(43r)

DOMINICA PALMARVM
342* In ramis agnus ac ebdomadarius, hospes/ [6]

DOLOR
343* Est dolor ingrati, desperati uel auari/ [5]

(43v)

DAMPNVM
344* Temporis ac anime, necnon et uirginitatis/ [2]

DIES MALI
345* Dat bona iustitia tempora, culpa mala. [1]

DERISIO
346* Quam sit uitanda derisio quamque nefanda/ [2]

DENTES
347* Ordine stant dentes albi multisque molentes/ [7]

DETRACTIO
348* Praui solamen iustorum carpere uitam/ [3]

DETRACTOR
349* Est homicida canis, detractor musca uel hircus/ [4]

DESPERATIO
350* Nemo desperet pro quantocumque reatu. [1]

DIABOLVS STELLA
351* Tanquam fax ardens de celo decidit ingens/ [3]

(44r)

DIABOLVS
352* Est canis, est ursus, leo, bos, draco, simia, serpens/ [3]
353* Piscator stigius habet hamum, rete, sagenam/ [2]
354* Sollicite scrutans et lustrans lustra ferarum/ [3]
355* Culpis aut penis nocituris incubat hostis/ [2]
356* Obseruat partum, draco, stans captatque uorandum. [1]

(44v)

357* Transire et capere, simul in coniunge decore/ [2]
358* Est sathan ut fulgur, terret, micat, irruit, urit/ [2]
359* Exerit ut fallat uelum, prestigia, folles/ [10]

(45r)

360* Est Zabulus dipsas, prester, salamandra, phareas/ [3]
361* Est perdix, adamans, sathanas, aquiloque, Golias/ [3]

(45v)

362* Demon deformat, set sanctum pneuma reformat. [1]
363* Sub specie recti fallit temptatio plures. [1]
364* Principio Pharao, medio Ysmael insidiatur/ [2]
365* Terret et illudit per sompnia uana malignus/ [2]
366* Visibus intentis scrutatur ab ethere terram/ [4]
367* Per minimum serpens serpit uetus ille foramen/ [5]
368* Serpens antiquus a quo uix est homo tutus/ [3]
369* Decidit in casses preda petita meos/ [2]
370* Efficiunt fortem beemoth natura, libido/ [2]

QVE FVGANT DIABOLVM

371* Hec exorcismus et crux, aspersio, uirtus/ [3]

(46r)

372* Crux, aqua, munus, opus, oratio, pectoris ictus/ [4]

DECLINATIO

373 Declinant fragilis, ignorans atque superbus. [1]

DIES IVDICII

374 Ventus, caligo, fulmen, tonitrus sonus, imber/ [2]

BENEFICIVM DEI

375 In de, pro signum, causam, noto materiamque/ [2]

DOMINVS PAVPEREM FACIT ET DIVITEM

376 Ditat et apporiat, necat et sic uiuere donat/ [2]

VENIRE AD DEVM

377 Venimus a Domino per quem redeamus ad ipsum/ [2]

QVOMODO DEVS VBIQVE EST

378 Vt uox, lux, anima simul hic ibi, sic Deus extat/ [5]

DOMINVM MAGNIFICARI

379 Dicit scriptura Dominum tunc magnificari/ [2]

QVOMODO DEVS DOCET

380 Instinctu, scriptis, doctoribus atque creatis/ [2]

DEVS TERRET ET MVLCET

381 Consueuit Dominus uulgari more docentis/ [4]

CVR DEVS DET DIVITIAS

382 Vt Deus alliciat, ut dampnet, premia soluat/ [2]

DECIME

383 Cur decime dentur sex hee cause perhibentur/ [4]

DISCAS

384 Discas ut sapias, facias, doceas, merearis/ [4]

DOCTRINA

385 Nos elementa docent elementatisque docemur/ [8]
386 Lectio non modicum, set plus collatio prebet/ [2]
387 Est totum tempus presens quod cepit ab Adam/ [8]

DAVID ET SIBA

388 Fallax Siba, Dauid preceps, hinc peccat uterque. [1]

CVI PLVS DIMITTITVR PLVS DEBET

389 Promissum, comissum, dimissum, meritumque/ [2]

DETRACTOR

390 Alterius bona perpendens qui detrahit ille/ [5]

DIVITIE

391 Amissis habitis dolor attestatur amorque. [1]

QVE SVNT VITIA DIVITVM

392 Isti sunt morbi quibus egrotant opulenti/ [4]

VERMES DIVITVM

393 Diuitis hii uermes: elatio, cura, uoluptas. [1]

DEMONIVM

394 Iustus demonium conculcat et effugat ipsum/ [2]
395 Accedit nobis aduersans callidus hostis/ [3]
396 Bestia censetur sathanas et causa notetur/ [10]

DEMONES

397 Hii post derident qui primum crimina suadent. [1]

VOX DIABOLI

398 Hunc teneo certus meus est errore repertus. [1]
399 Qui dat diuitias tibi si Deus adicit ullas/ [2]
400 Hostes crudeles felicis fallit aragnes. [1]

ECCLESIA

401* Ecclesia est archa, discus, domus, ara, sagena/ [6]

(46v)

402* Dicitur ecclesia Domino famulans, humilisque/ [2]
403* Ecclesie tres sunt partes; pars una laborat/ [4]

404* Ecclesiam subiens ores, discas, doceasue. [1]
405   Vt medicus, rethor, Dominus curare, tueri/ [5]

ECCLESIASTICA EDIFICANT
406* Fons, aqua, sal oculis occurrunt introeuntis/ [4]

(47r)

VT VINVM IN DOLIO SIC MALI HOMINES IN ECCLESIA
407* Ima petunt feces cupidorum terrea mentes/ [2]

EVCHARISTIA
408* Pondus ibi color atque sapor si queritur an sint/ [2]
409* Primum curauit Dominus quos denique pauit. [1]
410* Qui proprie carnis dape corda fidelia ditas/ [2]
411* Hoc sacramentum uas poscit crimine mundum/ [2]
412* Corporis et cordis soluit uel sufficit una/ [2]
413* Constat in altari carnem de pane creari/ [4]

DE ESV AGNI PASCHALIS
414   A quibus et quando comedatur pascha notato/ [2]

EXALTATIO CHRISTI
415   Crux et pascha, fides, ascencio, iudiciumque/ [2]

ETERNVM
416* Dicitur eternum mundi, legis, iubelei/ [3]

(47v)

EWANGELISTE
417* Matheo, Luce, Marco datur atque Iohanni/ [4]

QVE SIT MATERIA EWANGELISTIS
418   Sunt euuangelica nature themata Christi/ [2]

EVANGELIVM
419   Sunt ewangelia paradisi flumina, dragme/ [3]

EPISCOPI
420* Pontifices perimunt caro, curia, pompa, fauorque. [1]
421* Aufers prebendis uerum nomen quia uendis/ [2]
422* Hoc baculo fultus stas, prouidus erige uultus/ [3]

EPIPHANIA
423* Est aurum triplex, thus triplex, mirraque triplex/ [7]

(48r)

ELEMOSINA

424* Sal sacrificii personaque iussio, causa/ [3]
425* Sal, modus in dandis, et circumstantia queuis/ [4]
426* Extinguit munus districti iudicis iras/ [8]

(48v)

427* Floritio, satio, tibi sit largitio doni/ [2]
428* Liberat et mundat donum, redimitque tuetur/ [3]
429* Truncus, pons, glacies, bosilac dans, talpa, columba/ [2]
430* Est pietatis opus oleum, flos, ala, thesaurus. [1]
431* Est Christi pastus aqua, fenus, semen, aroma. [1]
432* Cum trunco tellus, leo, pelta, columba, puella/ [3]

(49r)

433* Da large, lete, sis intendens quoque recte/ [4]

EXEMPLVM

434* Sanctorum uita uiuendi sit tibi forma/ [2]
435* Est uitalis odor ducens ad uiuere uerum/ [3]
436* Sanctorum uita nobis est lectio uiua/ [2]
437* Non petere exemplum set dare dignus eras. [1]

EXAVDIRI

438* Ex meritis exauditur quicumque sacerdos/ [2]

DE ELIGENDIS

439* Sunt preponenda maiora minoribus atque/ [3]

DE EPVLIS

440* Esca Dei uerbo prius et prece sanctificetur/ [9]

(49v)

EMORDISSA

441* Non res in uitium ueniunt set abusio rerum/ [3]

EGRITVDO

442* Ira Dei prauis morbus, miseratio iustis/ [3]

(50r)

SERMO EGROTIS

443* In pape, flaui, labis, puri, Iob, ara, ui/ [2]

EMPLASTRVM

444 Vulneris ardorem lenit, seditque tumorem/ [2]

EXPECTATIO

445* Attendas qualis expectes, qualiter et quid. [1]

(50v)

EICERE

446* Cerne quis eiciat, quid, quem, quo, qualiter, unde. [1]

EDVCERE

447* Quis quos educat, quo, quando, qualiter, unde. [1]

EGRESSVS BONVS

448* Lazarus et Petrus, Moyses, Cananeaque Christus/ [2]
449* Moyses cum Christo, seniores cum Cananea/ [5]

(51r)

EXITVS DE EGYPTO

450* Exeat Egyptum quis, quando, qualiter, ad quid. [1]

EGYPTVS

451* Egyptus tenebre, tribulans, afflictio, meror/ [2]

EGRESSVS MALVS

452* Egressum nobis ostendunt perniciosum/ [3]

EDIFICARE LIGNVM, FENVM, STIPVLA

453* Edificat qui multa diu collecta reseruat/ [3]

EXPROBRATIO

454* Quam texit Dominus culpam non detegat ullus/ [2]

EBRIVS

455* Dum pisces uolucresque cibos capiunt, capiuntur/ [2]

EBRIETAS

456* Est lectus beemoth, bibio, bibulus Gedeonis/ [6]

(51v)

457 De gradibus quinque quartum quintumque relinque/ [4]
458 Erietas furor est, fuge qui bibis ebrietatem/ [2]

ERROR LAICORVM

459* Scito quod a multis laicis erratur in istis/ [7]

EQVVS

460* Cor feruens erexit equum, deiecit asellum/ [2]
461* Corpus equus domitus, nec desint cingula, frenum. [1]

LABOR ECCLESIE

462 In conuertendo, patiendo, timendo, dolendo/ [2]

EFFVSIO

463 Hec dant effundi nunc presens pena iehenna/ [3]

EVGE
464   Detrahit, applaudit, palpareque dicitur euge/ [2]

EDVCTIO PETRI DE CARCERE
465   Luciferi laqueus captus quicumque fidelis/ [2]
466   Est carcer cecus, fetens, artusque profundus/ [4]

EXCLVSIO A REGNO DEI
467   Institor in templo, Iudeus, stultaque uirgo/ [4]

ETATES MVNDI
468   Etates mundi sunt sex et septima currit/ [2]

ECCLESIA SVPRA
469   Fundatur domus, erigitur, munitur et intus/ [2]

EXEMPLA PATRVM
470   Iustus Abel parens Abraham Samuelque benignus/ [6]

EXPROBRATIO
471   Hostes improperant quos fellea uiscera uexant/ [3]

EXALTATIO HVMANE NATVRE
472   Eleuat humanam naturam dum creat ad se/ [2]

EXCLVSIO A REGNO DEI
473   Iudeus, fatua uirgo, Pharius, canis, are/ [2]

EXALTATIO CHRISTI SVPRA
474   Efficitur Christus altissimus, altior, altus/ [2]

FERCVLA PATRIE
475*   Visio, laus, locus et socii, saluatio iusti/ [3]

                                                    (52r)

FIDES
476*   Gratia prima fides, mater, basis et uia, piscis/ [8]
477*   Est deuota fides uite meritoria feruens/ [5]

                                                    (52v)

478*   Crede Deum, credesque Deo, mage credo salubre/ [2]
479*   Vna fides in te faciens subsistere uitam/ [4]
480*   Opprobrium semper Didimus cognomine gestat/ [2]

FACILITAS CREDENDI VEL IRASCENDI
481*   Credula suspicio, mens preceps, impetus ire/ [2]

FAMA

482* Pomum prodit odor, splendor quoque detegit ignem. [1]
483* In nichilum nix alta fluit si desuper imber/ [2]

FESTVM

484* Quod festum, cuius, que sunt adnexa uideto/ [2]
485* A quibus et quando, cur, quomodo sit feriandum. [1]
486* Sunt legis festa cum iugi sabbata festo/ [9]

                                                              (53r)

FRATRES

487* Dat dici natura, fides et adoptio fratres/ [2]

FEMINA

488* Crede ratem uentis, animum ne crede puellis/ [3]
489* Femina nulla bona, set si bona contigit ulla/ [2]
490* Plurima cum soleant mores euertere sacros/ [2]
491* Omnia consumens uitio consumitur omni/ [2]
492   Carduus, urtica, sus, lappa tenax, et yrudo/ [4]

FALLACIA

493* Rara fides, simulatus amor, speciosa supellex/ [2]
494* Nullum decipies nec decipieris ab ullo/ [2]

FVGA

495* Quid fugis ex illo qui claudit cuncta pugillo/ [2]

FVGA IN BONO

496* Moyses et Iacob, Ioseph, Iosue, Mare, Parthus/ [3]
497* Est fuga cautele, tutele, strenuitatis/ [3]

FVGA IN MALO

498* Prodigus et fictus Ionas, iuuenisque Iohannes/ [4]

                                                              (53v)

QVE SVNT FVGIENDA

499   Peccatum, mundus, hostis, sociusque malignus/ [4]

FICVS

500* Est ficus sterilis ypocrita uel balamita/ [2]

FLOS

501* Flos tener et tenuis, lenis, leuis et speciosus/ [6]
502* Est flos cum fructu, flos fructus, flos sine fructu/ [2]

FONS

503* Christus amorque timor, fons est, sapientia, doctor/ [2]

FORTITVDO

504*   Cum niue, cum pluuia, cum grandine uertere capras/ [4]

FABER

505   Fallax folle faber primas exsuflat in igne/ [4]

(54r)

FESTINATIO

506   Nemo nimis propere didicit nocitura cauere/ [2]

FINIS

507*   Non tardes: properat populus, pastor cito currens/ [3]

FENIX

508   Plurima pars celo sustollitur unica fenix/ [2]

FACIES

509*   Humanus uultus os est et littera mentis/ [2]

QVE SVNT CAVSE FAMIS

510*   Fastus et excessus, templi desertio, uerbi/ [2]

FERMENTVM

511*   Acre calens simile pani rumpens zima turget. [1]

FRAGILITAS HOMINIS

512*   Imponit terram capiti qui mente reuoluit/ [2]

FVNDAMENTA

513*   Fundamenta fides, paries dilectio duplex/ [2]

FOMES PECCATI

514*   Paulus ait: Carne peccati seruio legi/ [2]

FVR

515*   Fur Dominus, Dominique dies, mors, hostis iniquus. [1]

FRAVS ET FVRTVM

516   Fraus, dolus, insidie, fallacia, fictio, furtum/ [2]

(54v)

FVRIE

517   Tres Herebi furie sunt ira, cupido, libido. [1]

CAVSA FLETVS

518   Hec nostrum crimen, regni dilatio, culpa/ [2]

FLAGELLVM DEI

519   Non Deus hic parcit ut parcat denique iustis/ [2]

FVNDAMENTVM

520   Fundamentorum fundamentum Iesus ipse. [1]

FVNDA DAVID

521   Sint funes opus atque fides constantia funda/ [6]

FOVEA

522   Sic foueam uici, pene, uirtutis, et orti/ [3]

<FIRMVS>

523   Esto columpna domus postis firmus, non arundo/ [2]

<FLETVS>

524   Fletus causa tibi sunt hec: dilatio regni/ [3]

<FAVOR>

525   Ne fauor inclinat cui sors uaga, blanda proponat/ [2]

<FENERATOR>

526   Est sathane similis et irudo, spongia, perdix/ [3]

GLORIA CELI

527*   Aula celesti sunt semper gaudia festi. [1]
528*   Cognitio cibus est patrie, dilectio potus. [1]
529*   Quamuis perfecti, mortali carne grauati/ [2]
530*   Est stulti, mundi, iusti, pleneque beati/ [2]

GLORIA MVNDI

531*   Est quasi muscipule cibus huius gloria uite/ [2]

GLORIA VANA

532*   Gloria uana quid est? Vmbra est, uesica tumescens/ [2]
533*   Gloria cum reprobo sua non descendet in orchum/ [4]
534*   Vite presentis si comparo gaudia uentis/ [2]

GAVDIVM

535*   Demon, peccator, mundus, contritus, et equi/ [3]

(55r)

GRATIA

536   Culpa reo nox est et iusto gratia lux est/ [2]

GRATIA PRIMA

537   Gratia prima sit ut lux, funis et hospes et imber/ [3]

GRATIARVM ACTIO

538*   In casu quoque grates age, semper ubique/ [2]

GRATISSIMA

539*   Rebus in humanis tria sunt gratissima laude/ [6]

GENELOGIA ANNE

540*   Anna uiros habuit Ioachim, Cleopham, Salomamque/ [6]

GALLVS

541   Est doctor gallus qui noctis discutit horas/ [3]

GALLINA

542*   Est simplex uolucris gallina, domestica, mitis/ [4]

GVSTVS

543*   Querit ut expoliet uenatibus, alite, pisce/ [2]

                                                             (55v)

GVLA

544   Primus ferre moram nequit, immo preuenit horam/ [5]
545*   Ingluuiem uentris sequitur petulantia carnis. [1]

GLADIVS

546*   Terribilis, durus et grandis, semper acutus/ [3]

GVRGVLIO

547*   Gurgulio non est uermis piscisue set ales/ [2]

GAVDIVM

548   Gaudia mundani, contriti, proficientis/ [2]

HVMILITAS

549*   Est ysopus, gluten, primaria filia, nutrix/ [7]

                                                             (56r)

550   Guttas solaris non fluctus attrahit ardor/ [4]
551*   Conseruant humilem si se reputet sibi uilem/ [3]

HONESTAS

552*   Sobrius a mensis, a lecto surge pudicus. [1]

HONOR

553*   Cui decus exhibeas, cur, qualiter, unde uideto. [1]
554*   Est honor humanus breuis et sine pondere fumus. [1]
555*   Dant natura, decus, et gratia, doxa, potestas. [1]

HONOR TERRENVS

556*   Est terrenus honor ut fumus spumaque sompnus. [1]

HOMO

557*   Est homo mendicus, ouis errans, perdita dragma/ [6]

                                                             (56v)

558*   Quomodo uel de quo, qualis uel qualiter, ad quid/ [2]
559*   Nasceris ut uiuas, uiuis moriturus, et unus/ [2]

HOSPES
560*   Verum dixit anus quod piscis olet triduanus/ [2]

HOSTIS
561*   Hostes peccatum, uitium, mundus, caro, demon/ [2]

HOSTES CHRISTI
562*   En saluatoris Iudeus, mors, sathan, orbis/ [2]

                                                                    (57r)

HOMICIDIVM
563*   Mente, manu, uerbo, causa neco denique rendo. [1]

HERODES
564*   Occidit pueros Herodes ascalonita/ [3]

YPOCRISIS
565   Fallit enim uitium specie uirtutis et umbra. [1]

YPOCRITA
566   Miles scaccorum uel simia, canna, sophista/ [5]
567*   Non reputes aurum totum quod splendet ut aurum/ [6]

HISTRIO
568*   Diues eram dudum, me fecerunt tria nudum/ [2]

HYMNI
569*   Noscitur hic series hymnorum sex feriarum/ [7]

                                                                    (57v)

HORE
570   Septem uocales sunt hore totque reales/ [3]

HIRCVS
571   Fetet lasciuus et amaris uescitur hircus/ [2]

HERBA
572   Vtilis est herba succosaque, lenis, amena/ [3]

HAMVS
573*   Est hamus Christus, peccatum, sermo Dei, mors. [1]

HOSTES SECVNDA
574   Nobis bella mouent hii tres: mundus, caro, demon/ [2]

HOSTIA

575 Hostia carnalis operis seu corporis, oris/ [3]

DESCRIPTIO BONI HOMINIS

576 Absque malo plenusque bono prodesse paratus/ [3]

QVE PARIANT HVMILEM

577 Conditio, culpa, transacta pie memorata/ [2]

DVRITIA IVDEORVM

578 Durus Iudeus ad librum, dona, flagella/ [2]

(58r)

IHESVS

579* Testantur Christum Moyses, Pater atque Iohannes/ [2]

QVE TESTANTVR IHESVM ESSE DEVM

580* Scripture uerba, miracula, uita pudica/ [3]

IOHANNES BAPTISTA

581* Forma tibi speculum, turtur, nubesque columpna/ [6]
582* Constans et patiens, castus, baptista Iohannes/ [20]

(58v-59r)

583* Ecclesie lampas radiat baptista Iohannes/ [5]

DE SANCTO IACOBO ET FRATRE EIVS

584* Linque ratem, rete, mare, patrem, quatuor hec sunt/ [2]

IMMOLATIO ISAACH

585* Cum strue lignorum ponas Ysaac super altum/ [2]

IOSEPH

586* Non potuit Ioseph animo set ueste teneri. [1]

IVSTITIA

587* Est uaga communis uirtus astrea peragrans/ [2]

IVSTVS

588* Nulla tui meriti perturbent nubila lucem/ [3]

IVDEX

589* Regula fabrilis est hec terrena potestas/ [2]
590* Blandus erit iustis iudex, districtus iniquis/ [2]

(59v)

IVDICIVM

591 Iudico, discerno, dampno, delicta reuelo/ [2]
592* Decernat quis, que uideas, et qualiter, unde/ [3]

593*   Non ius iudicii clementia flectere debet/ [3]
594*   Qui mandit non mandentem non spernat inique/ [2]
595*   Non manducantem manducans spernere uitet/ [2]

IVRAMENTVM
596*   Si male iurandi species sit cura notandi/ [2]
597*   Pax et fama, fides, reuerentia, cautio dampni/ [2]

INTENTIO
598*   Est oculus cordis thesaurus in arbore radix/ [6]

IVGVM DOMINI
599*   Hec dicit Dominus: uos lene iugum, leue pondus/ [2]

                                                        (60r)

IEIVNIVM
600*   Abstinet infirmus, patiens fastidia, iustus/ [2]
601   In facie memora quod sunt ieiunia plura. [1]

INVOCATIO
602   Confugii turris Domini fortissima nomen/ [2]

INTERROGATIONES ET RESPONSIONES MORALES
603*   Quis, quid, ubi, quando, quo, qualiter, ad quod et unde/ [2]

IVNIPERVS
604*   Hispida iuniperus humilis, uilis, sterilisque/ [3]

INDVMENTVM
605*   Est in ueste triplex excessus, si nimis ampla/ [2]

INTRARE
606*   Quis, quo, cur, quando, uideas, et qualiter intret. [1]

                                                        (60v)

IRE
607*   Infirmus, claudus, pede uinctus non bene uadunt. [1]

IMAGINATIO
608*   Est moriens musca, uolucris mordens abigenda/ [2]

IVMENTVM
609*   Iumentum reputatur homo, fedus, fatuusque/ [2]

IVDEVS
610*   Ista locus, tempus, habitus, caro, cultus et esus/ [2]
611*   Iudeis signa, Grecis sapientia grata/ [3]

QVOT MODIS VTIMVR IMPERATIVO MODO
612* Imperat, hortatur, permittit, precinit, orat/ [3]

INFRVNITVM
613* Hec infrunitum nobis exponere posse/ [2]

IDRA
614 Excedra multorum capitum draco dicitur ydra/ [2]

(61r)

IGNIS
615* Lucet, consumit, ascendit, dequoquit ignis/ [7]
616* Lex ignis celi, rogus, orchus, feruor auari/ [7]

(61v)

617* Ignis auaritie zelique libidinis, ire/ [3]
618 Ignis amor, Deus ipse, rubor, tribulatio, pena. [1]
619* Est ignis liuor set et ira, libido, cupido. [1]
620* Ignis diuinus Pater est, natusque, rubaque/ [3]
621 Suscipiunt ignem sanctum bonus atque beatus/ [3]
622 A culpis ignis altum purgabit et imum. [1]

IGNORANTIA
623* Non scit, non sentit, non experiendo, probando/ [4]

IMPETVS
624* Nil subito faciat qui sensu tardior extat. [1]

(62r)

IRA
625* Ira furor trabs est, aries, turbatio et ignis/ [3]

INVIDIA
626 Non aliud nisi se ualet ardens Ethna cremare/ [7]
627* Bestia, fel, uirus, tinea est rosaria, liuor/ [4]

INCONSTANTIA
628* Inconstans Balaam modicam compunctus ad horam/ [3]
629* Lepra uolans, Canaan, lunaticus, instabilis Nod/ [5]

(62v)

INGRATITVDO
630* Ne ferias ipsum donato fuste datorem/ [3]
631 Ingratus sibi uel meritis propriis sua donat/ [3]
632* Cum bona donantur nisi grates hinc referantur/ [2]

IDOLATRIA
633* Hoc illi Deus est quod quis cupit et ueneratur. [1]

INFERNVS
634*   Est locus indignis quo non extinguitur ignis/ [4]

QVE DESTRVIT IOSVE
635   Hec sunt que Iosue tipico uelamine uastat/ [5]

(63r)

<IMAGO>
636   Extat ymago triplex: formans, formata, reformans/ [2]

INVITATIO
637   Inuitat Christus, impellit et ad bona mundus/ [2]

INTENTIO
638   Munda sit et pura simplex intentio nostra. [1]

<YDROPS>
639   Ydropi languet male luxuriosus, auarus/ [2]

<IMAGO REGIS>
640   Innato nummo speculo limphaque relucet/ [2]

LEX
641   Lex uetus inchoat, ad noua preparat, abdita signat/ [3]
642*   Lex est forma, tipus, signum, uelamen et umbra/ [4]
643*   Lex obscura fuit set Christus clarificauit/ [5]

LIBER SCRIPTVS INTVS ET FORIS
644*   Mentis in excessu liber est datus Ezechieli/ [5]

LIBER
645   Est scriptura sacra prelati preuia uita/ [2]

LECTIO
646*   Est Domini lingua, recreatio, lectio sacra/ [4]

(63v)

LVX
647*   Letificat tenebrasque fugat lux atque decorat/ [2]

QVE NOS ILLVMINANT
648   Lux primitiua, superaddita sidera clara/ [6]

LINGVA LOQVI
649*   Eucharis est lingua que tum bona tum bene profert/ [7]
650   Ex se Gad, Moyses, Ionas, Paulusque loquuntur/ [3]

(64r)

LAVS DEI

651 Res modice, magne Domini magnalia monstrant/ [4]
652* Nescio nec ualeo nec sufficio tibi laudum/ [2]

QVALIS LAVS DEI

653* Sit laus discreta, concors et uiuida, leta/ [2]
654* Voce Deum laudes: Vt lingua Deo famuletur/ [3]

QVE IMPEDIVNT LAVDEM DEI

655 Impietas praui, rerum subtractio mundi/ [4]

QVE SVNT AD DEVM LEVANDA

656* Cum pedibus genibusque capud tollamus in altum/ [3]

LACRIME

657* Contriti lacrime salse, clare, calideque/ [5]

LIBAMINA

658* Granum, sal, simila, thus sunt libamina sicca/ [2]

(64v)

LARGITAS

659* Et prelarga Tithi dextera spargit opes. [1]

LIBERARE

660* Expedit et curat, absoluit, liberat hec dat. [1]

LETITIA MVNDI

661* Non bene letatur cui flendi causa paratur/ [2]

LVCTVS

662* Est perfectorum luctus, lusus puerorum. [1]

LABOR

663* Quis labor et quantum uel quomodo quisque laborat/ [5]

LABAN

664 Iacob ditari meruit, Laban apporiari. [1]

LATRO

665* Non qui clam sumit, set clam uult sumere fur est. [1]

LAQVEVS

666* Est laqueus triplex, Zabuli suggestio, uite/ [4]

LABARVM

667* Signabat labarum clipeorum insignia Christus/ [2]

LICHNVS

668   Ast alii tenebras et opacam uincere noctem/ [2]

LVNA

669*   Est uaga, mendica, mutabilis et maculosa/ [5]
670*   Terris uicina mutabilis et uaga luna/ [3]

LVNATICVS

671*   Parua fides aut nulla fides aut eiciendi/ [2]

(65r)

LEO IN BONO

672*   Est leo rex, audax et largus, pectore fortis/ [7]

LEO IN MALO

673*   Est leo crudelis, immundus terribilisque/ [4]

LVPVS

674   Insidians ouibus lupus est et seuus, ouile/ [4]

(65v)

LOCALITAS

675   Esse locale facit quoduis dimensio corpus/ [2]

LIQVEFACTIO

676*   Eloquio, uento, res sole, calore liquescunt. [1]

LEPRA

677*   In quot consistat, qualis sit lepra uideto/ [4]
678*   Lepra fit in ueste, tumor in uirtute, set illam/ [10]

LIS

679*   Impatiens litis defecit flumine mersa/ [2]

LIBIDINOSVS

680*   Est asinus, porcus, prunis in corpore tactus/ [2]
681*   A ueneris sorde uirgo mundissima uere/ [2]

LIBIDO

682*   Est auidis Cipris uersans male corda uenenis/ [4]

(66r)

683*   Spurcus homo porcus est, mergendus, scabiosus/ [6]

LVXVRIA ET CVPIDITAS

684   Pratum talpa fodit, conculcat et inquinat illud/ [5]

EFFECTVS LVXVRIE

685*   Est ulcus carnis, in carneque lurida lepra/ [6]

(66v)

686* Tollit opes, animam, sensum cum nomine famam/ [2]
687 Scorpius, eruca, Venus, ignis, uirus, yrudo/ [7]

QVE PERIMANT LIBIDINEM
688 In lare, flare, fuge, set et oc, uenerem necat in te. [1]

<LEPROSVS>
689 Fedus et eiectus, turpis, fetens male, raucus/ [2]

<LVX>
690 Lux Deus et ratio, scripturaque gratia, uerbum. [1]

<LABOR>
691 Obsunt non prosunt, uitanda superflua uerba/ [4]

LVMINARIA
692 Cursum continuant sublimia sidera fulgent/ [4]

LIGNA
693 In campis ligna dat et ortus, uinea, silua. [1]

LEGALIA
694 Disparent umbre legis ueteresque figure/ [2]

LEGATI AD CHRISTVM MITTENDI
695 Legati sunt dona manus, ieiunia, fletus/ [4]

MARIA VIRGO
696* Virgo Dei genitrix, rosa, lilia, fons, paradisus/ [6]

(67r)

697* Ancillans, dominans, regnans est femina fortis/ [5]
698* Femina peccauit, peccatum femina lauit/ [2]

(67v)

699* Protulit humano tellus sine semine panem/ [2]
700* Terra, solum uel humus uirgo est, glis, arida, tellus. [1]
701* Credit et assentit, optat, mox concipit alma/ [2]
702* Stella maris, regina poli, miseratio mundi/ [6]
703* Tu fons signatus, tu clausula, clausaque porta/ [4]
704* Extat stella Iacob et matutina Maria/ [4]
705* Mater uirgo pia nobis succurre Maria. [1]
706 Fons in scriptura uelud Hester, uirgo Maria/ [4]
707 Transit preclara nubes, fecunda, leuata/ [11]
708 Dicitur ancilla Domini pia uirgo Maria/ [6]

MAGDALENA
709 Actus solamen, amor et compassio cordis/ [2]
710* Non dum regna poli petii me tangere noli/ [2]

Maria Magdalene
711   Martha quod irritat uel prouocat aut dominatur/ [2]
712   Stella Maria maris, uel amarum sit mare dicta/ [5]

(68r)

Melchisedech
713* Absque parentela Salem rex atque sacerdos/ [11]

Mansio Abrae
714* Inter Sur, Cades, Abraham posuit sibi sedes/ [4]

Martialis
715* Vxorem quare locupletem ducere nolim/ [2]

Misericordia Dei
716* Extat longanimis Domini clementia larga/ [2]

Magnalia Dei
717* In minimis etiam Domini magnalia clarent. [1]

Misericordia
718* Est pietas, oleum, pretium, uiror, ydria, fenus/ [6]

(68v)

Opera misericordie
719* Vestio, poto, cibo, tectum do, uisito, soluo/ [2]
720* Commodo, compatior, conuerto, dono, remitto/ [2]
721   Sunt porte uite clementia iudiciumque/ [2]

Modvs
722* Imponit finem sapiens et rebus honestis/ [4]

(69r)

Mensvra
723* Pro modulo finis tandem tibi de bene gestis/ [2]
724* Metitur Christus attendens omnia nostra/ [2]

Martires
725* Feruens ad pugnam, properans ad premia martir/ [4]

Martirivm
726* Letificant testes, patientia, causaque merces/ [4]

Privilegivm martirii
727* Martirium dans aureolam non transit in ignem/ [2]
728* Martirium faciunt legis defensio ueri/ [2]

MONACHVS

729*   Culpam magnificant monachis tot corporis arma/ [10]

(69v)

730*   Ingrediens heremum puerum dimisit Helyas/ [3]
731*   Ordo labor grandis, res aspera, dura probandis/ [3]
732   Ad formam morum prestat nomen monachorum/ [2]

MONIALIS

733*   Est uirgo prudens, sol, sidus, filia Chore/ [3]
734*   Celebs et terra, mons, fons, pomum, fauus, archa/ [4]

(70r)

735*   Ortus conclusus, bis sancta, soror mea, sponsa/ [3]

(70v)

736*   Sunt sponse Christi uel amice, lumina mundi/ [6]

MONIALES INFESTANT

737   Sollicitudo, uenus, discordia, murmur et ira/ [2]

MERITVM

738*   Auget amor meritum, maior meliorque uoluntas/ [6]
739*   Tempus sudoris breue, mercedis prope iusto/ [2]
740*   Attendas quis, quid, quo uel quando mereatur/ [2]
741   Martirium, sacramentum, tribulatio, sermo/ [2]
742*   Est meritum prauum signum, uia, causa gehenne/ [2]

VARIATIO MERITORVM

743*   Hec uariant meritum: tempus celesteque donum/ [2]
744*   Tempore uel genere, numero, pretio, minus affert/ [2]

MISTERIA

745*   Ecclesie sacra sacro sunt tegmine tecta. [1]

(71r)

MINISTRARE

746*   Quomodo, cui, qualis, in quo, cur, quando ministret. [1]

MEMBRA

747*   Si gaudet membrum congaudent omnia membra/ [2]
748*   Adiutor manus est, oculus prouisor et est pes/ [2]

MVLIER

749*   Est adamas mulier, pix, rampnus, carduus asper/ [2]
750*   Sunt tria grandia: laus, sapientia, gloria rerum/ [2]

Matrimonivm

751* Coniugium mundat, mutat, fecundat et unit/ [2]
752* In quibus articulis liceat non reddere sponsis/ [8]

(71v)

Qvalis debeat esse vxor

753* Casta, fidelis, amans, humilis, subiecta, ministrans/ [2]
754* Pluribus adiunctos seu coniugibus sociatos/ [2]
755   Coniugium quasi lex ligat et munit, monet, unit/ [3]

Vnde dicitvr vxor

756   Fertur ab ungendo dici uelud unxior uxor/ [3]

Meretrix

757* Scorpius et laqueus, uestis, stercus, poliandrum/ [2]
758   Est peccatoris laqueus meretricis ocellus. [1]

(72r)

Mvndatio

759* Gratia, uerba, preces, lacrime quoque sanguis et unda/ [2]

Mvndvs

760* Vertitur, opprimit, atterit, eicit ut mola mundus/ [4]
761* Ista senem circumueniunt incomoda mundum/ [3]
762* Terre curuatur, amat hanc, finemque minatur/ [3]

Mvndana

763* Mundi tollit opes scintilla aut bestia parua. [1]

Mandata temporalia

764* Nunc alii mores, alii pro tempore leges. [1]

Merces temporalis

765   Vesicam loculo preponens stultus habetur/ [2]

Manna

766* Man cum nocturno descendit rore minutum/ [7]

(72v)

Mvnitio

767* Regi paret eques, uerbis munitus et armis/ [2]

Secvndvm qve mvtatvr aliqvid

768   Agnoscas quod res uariant diuersaque mutant/ [4]

Primvs motvs

769   Paruulus est primus, et uulpes paruula motus/ [4]

METALLVM

770*   Argentum seruat dum purificatur in igne/ [3]

(73r)

MVSICA INSTRVMENTA

771*   Est in uoce chorus, lira pulsu, tibia flatu. [1]

MENS

772*   Nauis et archa, capud, tectum presepeque mens est/ [2]

MEMORIALIA

773*   Stent in mente Dei uerbum Dominique flagellum/ [6]

MEMORIA PECCATI

774   Vt plus committat culpe memor impius extat/ [2]

MEMORIA MORTIS

775*   In mentem tempus obitus immittere possunt/ [3]

(73v)

776*   Nuntius, umbra, sopor, capud et pictura, uetustas/ [5]
777*   En monumenta monent, mente mortis reminisci/ [2]

MORS

778*   Atropos, atra nimis, pernicibus aduolat alis/ [3]
779*   Incisor burse, fur, falx et ianua, limen/ [2]
780*   Mors falcem gestat meritis, ac felle molestat/ [4]

(74r)

781*   Mortis causa, modus, locus et tempus latitant nos. [1]
782*   Ecce premunt, circumdant, uilificat quoque rodit/ [3]
783   Porta, foramen acus, mors est et terminus, hamus. [1]
784*   Mutari nequeunt post obitum merita. [1]
785*   Mors cunctis dura, cunctos trahit in sua iura/ [2]
786*   De toto regno superest post fata sepulcrum/ [2]
787*   Cui putredo pater, uermis soror, arrida mater/ [4]
788*   Incedo gressum non promittendo regressum/ [2]
789*   Premeditans mortem parat hosti reddere sortem/ [2]
790*   Qui sumus addicti pro nostro crimine morti/ [2]
791*   Est Domino carum quod nobis uile uidetur. [1]
792*   Mane, techel, phares, uigili si mente notares/ [2]
793*   Non appellandi locus hic, non calculus iste/ [2]
794*   Quid fueris, quid sis, quid eris, circumspice, si te/ [2]
795*   Fac mihi forte suum prestet fortuna fauorem/ [2]
796*   Delicias et opes rapit inclementia mortis. [1]
797   Mors duplex anime, duplex et corporis est mors/ [5]

(74v)

798   Est mors nature, mors culpe, morsque gehenne/ [6]
799*   Mortuus expallet, liuet, fetetque liquatur/ [11]

MORS SANCTORVM
800*   Sancti nascuntur cum migrantes moriuntur/ [7]
801   Cum sis ipse cinis, memor esto per omnia finis/ [2]

MORTIFICATIO CARNIS
802*   Pessimus est hostis qui cum benefeceris illi/ [4]
803   Carnem mortificat qui carnis pernecat actus/ [2]

MARATH
804*   Felleus amnis erat, per lignum melleus extat. [1]

MIRRA
805*   Mirraque de cuius lacrimis in corpora functa/ [2]

MARE
806*   Est mare diffusum, feruens, salsumque profundum/ [3]

(75r)

807   Fluctiuagum fluuidum, salsum, tumidumque profundum/ [3]

MERSIO
808   Merguntur Pharius, ferrum, plumbum, mola, porcus. [1]

MONS
809*   Mons celum, Sathael, Deus est elatio sancti/ [3]

MILVVS
810   Miluus auis mollis est uiribus atque uolatu/ [9]

MVS
811*   Ventris ob ingluuiem mus nulla pericula uitat. [1]

MOLESTA IN DOMO
812   Cum requiem uolumus, uxor mala, stillaque fumus/ [2]

(75v)

EFFECTVS MEDICINE
813*   Aufert et confert, dehinc augmentat medicina/ [2]

MALVM
814*   Est auctor demon, homo uel Deus ipse malorum/ [4]

MALITIA
815*   Serpentem innocuum faciunt deserta locorum/ [2]

MALVS HOMO
816*   Mente, manu, lingua, mala qui malus est operatur/ [2]

MENDATIVM

817* Nec uolo mentiri nec debeo prodere quemquam. [1]

MALEDICTIO

818* Imprecor aut nudo uel detraho uel manifesto/ [4]

VIRGO MARIA

819 Fons in scriptura uelud Hester, uirgo Maria/ [14]

(76r-v)

MITTERE

820* Quis, quales et quos, quot, quomodo, quando, uel
ad quos/ [2]

SECVNDA MVLIER

821 Cor leue, uox lenis atque fidelitas in muliere/ [4]

SECVNDA MENDACIVM

822 Qui fuerit mendax et amans mendacia fallax/ [7]

(77r)

NATIVITAS CHRISTI

823* Sancta Maria, Ioseph, panni, presepeque fenum/ [11]

(77v)

824 Set postremus Adam, natus de uirgine quadam/ [2]

NEGATIO PETRI

825 Ter Dominum Petrus funesta uoce negauit/ [2]

NEMVS ABRAHE

826 Hic qui uult Abraham fieri, fiat prius Abram/ [5]

NEGLIGENTIA SACERDOTVM

827* Ara, locus, cura, doctrina, liber, sacramenta/ [2]

NOBILITAS

828 Hunc genus extollit, set si fastigia penses/ [2]

QVE SVNT IN NVPTIIS

829* Sub tecto nupte sunt plurima, uestis honesta/ [3]

(78r)

NARRATIO

830* Narrabo primum mea iam commissa fatendo/ [4]

NVBES

831* Ex imis terre diuina sorte leuate/ [4]

NEGOTIATIO

832*   Arguo mercandi non officium set abusum/ [2]

                                                                    (78v)

NVMERATIO POPVLI

833*   Qui numerantur, ubi, quotiens et quando uel ad quid. [1]

QVI NVMERANTVR AD BELLVM

834*   Non puer aut mulier, seruus, Pharius numerantur/ [2]

NOX

835*   Est uobis nota nox longa, pauendaque sancta/ [4]

NOCIVA

836   Ledunt, inficiunt scabies, zima, fel sibi iuncta. [1]

NOVISSIMA HOMINIS

837   Prudens prouideas humana nouissima que sunt/ [2]

SECVNDA NVBES

838   Est nubes Christus, caro Christi, Virgo beata/ [3]

                                                                    (79r)

NOMEN BONVM

839   Diuitiis multis nomen prepollet honestum/ [2]

NIMIETAS

840   Lucis, aque nimium prius obtundit tibi uisum/ [3]

SANCTVS OSWALDVS

841*   Rex sacer Oswaldus seuas acies feriturus/ [6]

ORATIO

842*   Est medicamentum sanans oratio, scutum/ [2]
843*   Orat pro nobis chorus ecclesie generalis/ [2]

                                                                    (79v)

844*   Audax, assidua sit nostra precatio iusta/ [8]
845*   Dant precibus spatium dolor et submissio, donum. [1]
846*   Carnis munditia caste, ieiunia sancta/ [13]

                                                                    (80r)

OPVS

847*   Quid sit agendum, quomodo, quando, curque uideto. [1]
848*   Quid, cui uel quantum, cur, qualiter est operandum/ [2]
849*   Sola reuiuiscunt que quondam uiua fuerunt/ [3]
850*   Quid pariat uentura dies nescis, celer esto/ [2]
851*   Quos informat amor actus, deuotio condit. [1]

852* Curre miser dum currendi concessa potestas/ [2]
853   Sunt pulcri flores, set fructus utiliores. [1]

                                                              (80v)

854* Crede, fidelis age de cunctis, elige, sperne/ [5]
855* Exemplum nobis operis dant ista fidelis/ [7]

                                                              (81r)

856   Quid, cui uel quantum, cur, qualiter est operandum/ [2]

QVINQVE NECCESARIA IN OPERE
857* Affectus purus, discretio, finis et ordo/ [2]

QVE DESTRVVNT OPERA BONA
858* Damien, impurum, casti, declinat omissum. [1]

                                                              (81v)

OBLATIO
859* Quis, quid, ubi, quando, cur offerat intueamur/ [2]
860* Aspice quis, quid, ubi uel qualiter offerat, ex quo. [1]
861   Corporis ac operis est hostia cordis et oris. [1]
862* Offer tu uitulum Christum credens memoransque/ [2]
863   Quod scio, quod ualeo, totum simul offero Christo/ [11]

OBLATIO IN PASCHA
864   Sunt hec in Pascha: uituli duo, sunt simul agni/ [3]

                                                              (82r)

OBLATIO IN PENTECOSTEN
865* In Pentecoste legis textu referente/ [5]

OBSEQVIVM
866* Affectus, sensus, mores, meditatio, motus/ [4]

OBEDIENTIA
867* Te parere docent Bethania, sidera, uenti/ [4]

OLEVM
868* Est oleum pingue, calidum, nitidum recreansque/ [2]

                                                              (82v)

OS
869* Os nequam mulce; nequid sapiat nisi dulce. [1]

OS
870* Os siccum, durum, rigidum uacuumque medulla/ [2]

ORTVS
871* Ortum pomiferum cuius sunt poma fideles/ [6]

OVIS

872*   Molle pecus lanis, animo placidum set inherme/ [3]

OLOR

873*   At solus qui sentit olor, discrimine quanto/ [2]

OCCASIO IVSTA

874   Nulli mirentur non hinc aliqui moueantur/ [2]

ONVS

875   Est onus infirmi, peccati, legis et actus/ [3]

(83r)

OBSCVRATIO OCVLORVM

876   Obscurant oculos tenebre, lux, fumus et ignis/ [2]

OS DOMINI

877   Os Domini Christus, facundia, scripta, propheta. [1]

OS

878   Verbum, sputamen, hec egrediuntur ab ore/ [4]

OPERA DEI

879   Fac tu fasciculos operum Domini tibi binos. [1]

OPERA

880   Vt prohibent aliqui bona sunt tantum uia, signum/ [4]

OBSEQVIVM

881   Obsequio famulus deuitandus uel amandus. [1]

<OPERARE>

882   Tu sapiens, instans, mundus, constans et amans sis/ [7]

(83v)

PETRVS

883*   Est Simon Petrus missorum bar-iona primus/ [8]

PAVLVS

884*   Est liber, seruus, pius, omnibus omnia factus/ [11]

(84r)

PETRVS ET PAVLVS

885*   Dat tibi contentum Petri Pauli documentum/ [5]

PETRVS ET ANDREAS

886*   Ad fratrem uictum nichil est a patre relictum/ [2]

PRELATVS

887*   Pastor, prelatus, nox, seclum grexque, popellus/ [2]
888*   At post flagra patris, pietas dabit ubera matris/ [2]
889*   Vitam pastoris perdit commissio plebis/ [2]
890*   Vitam maiorum disponit uita minorum/ [2]
891*   Fiat prelatus sapiens, facundus, honestus. [1]
892*   Vertat pre silo presbiter officio. [1]
893*   Cum sub prelatis qui sensus lumina perdunt/ [2]
894*   Officium, lingua, meritum, sapientia, uita/ [5]
895*   In naui rector non sorte set arte legendus. [1]

                                                      (84v)

896*   Angelus, athleta, miles, medicusque magister/ [8]

                                                      (85r)

PRELATI MALI

897*   Eden procurant, nec dampna gregis mala curant/ [4]

DESIDERIVM PRELATIONIS

898   Cum zelo fragrat animus tibi proficiendi/ [2]

PRINCEPS ET PRELATVS

899*   Ara prophanata, fatuum sal, cesaque uitis/ [3]

ABSENTIA PRELATI

900   Si timor abscedat Domini pastorque recedat/ [4]

QVALIS DEBEAT ESSE PRELATVS

901*   Prelatus mitis, affabilis atque benignus/ [32]

                                                      (85v)

PATER FAMILIAS

902*   Est Domini facies, famulus, speculumque magistri/ [4]

PATER

903   Demon, patrinus, pater est Deus, angelus, Adam/ [2]

PASTOR

904   Helyas uiduam pascit qua pascitur ipse. [1]

                                                      (86r)

905*   Dirigit et pascit, seruat, cogitque requirit/ [2]
906*   Conuocat ad granum pullos gallina repertum/ [5]

PREDICATOR

907*   Reddat se populumque fide factisque disertum/ [7]

QVALIS DEBEAT ESSE PREDICATOR

908*   Sit testamenti ueterisque nouique peritus/ [6]

PREDICATIO

909 Sermo diuinus acus est dissuta retexens/ [2]

910* Non tolerabit equus eius cum tangitur ulcus/ [2]
911* Est humilis, prudens, constans, instans Ieremias/ [2]
912* Non minus est dulcis de paruo fonte recepta/ [7]
913* Est aqua baptismi lix uiaque, cerea, fax, es. [1]

PREDICATOR MALVS

914* Doctor, peccator, crux, petrinusque canalis/ [11]
915* Mi, fa, sol, carus est sermo commaculosus/ [3]

PREDICATIO

916* Arguit, abscidit, monet et iubet, instruit, ungit/ [3]

QVID SIT PREDICANDVM

917* Virtutes, uitia, quid credendum, quid agendum/ [4]

QVE DETINEANT AD TEMPVS PREDICATIONEM

918* Os hominis, locus et tempus, persona, reatus/ [2]

PASSIO CHRISTI

919* Agnus, ouis, Christus, humilis, mitis, taciturnus/ [2]
920* Fossa dabit tellus optato tempore fructus/ [2]
921 ede memor narraque fatens, uenerans imitansque/ [2]

<PAX>

922* Nos elementorum doceat connexio pacem/ [3]

PATIENTIA

923* Est fornax conflans firmamentumque columpna/ [6]

924* Absint o patiens consensus, talio, murmur/ [3]

PATIENTIA DEI

925* Fortior est feriente ferens, nec secula pulcrum/ [10]
926* Copia mercedis, ueteris purgatio culpe/ [2]
927* Fortius excidit magis acta securis in altum/ [6]

PROVIDENTIA

928 Prouideas, campus oculos habet et nemus aures. [1]

PERSEVERANTIA

929* Est pars longa crucis, constantia, lancea, finis/ [3]
930* Continuat cursum sol inter sidera sursum/ [2]

931   Vt sambucus eris plebs israelitica, tigris/ [2]

(88r)

PROPHETIA
932*   Dico prophetiam rem, uerbum, munus et actum. [1]
933*   Sit tibi presagus, presignans, pseudo propheta/ [4]

PASCHA
934   Tristes ac humiles Dominum sancte mulieres/ [6]

PENTECOSTE
935*   Scriptura teste sunt in legis datione/ [2]

(88v)

936   Cerne locum uentumque situs ignemque loquelas/ [3]

PANIS
937*   Corporis esca, Dei uerbum, contritio cordis/ [3]
938   Panis peccatum, peccator, passio pascens/ [3]

DE SEPTEM PANIBVS ET DVOBVS PISCIBVS
939*   Sunt septem panes enarrans sermo saluber/ [5]

QVINQVE PANES ET DVO PISCES
940*   Panes quinque dolor, uerbum, deitas, caro Christi/ [4]
941*   Corripias, moneas, promittas atque mineris/ [3]

PANIS, PISCIS, OVVM
942*   Panis amor piscisque fides, spes dicitur ouum/ [3]

PISCIS
943   Est uagus atque uorax piscis, silet, amne moratur/ [2]

(89r)

PISCINA
944*   Mota piscina periit uetus illa ruina/ [2]

POTVS CELESTIS
945   Est diuinus amor dulcis super omnia potus. [1]

PARADISVS
946   Est locus, ecclesia, paradisus, Virgo beata/ [2]

PASCVA
947*   Pascua scriptura, caro Christi, uita beata. [1]

PROCESSIO
948*   Profectum sanctum signat processio nostra/ [3]

Ex omnibvs profice
949*   Sensus corporei fiant tibi causa merendi/ [2]

Prevenire
950*   Preueniunt Iacob, Iudas Petrusque Iohannes/ [2]

Palma
951   Alta uirens uictrix cui radix aspera palma/ [2]

(89v)

Premivm
952   Premia iustorum pendent de fine laborum/ [3]

Prosperitas
953*   Otia, pax et delicie Dauid superabant/ [7]

Prosperitas et adversitas
954   Sorte nocent equa stultis aduersa, secunda/ [3]

Pavpertas
955*   Paupertas uera est contemptus diuitiarum. [1]

Qve sint vitia pavpervm
956   Sunt inopum uitia murmur, detractio, liuor/ [2]

Proprietates pveri
957*   Credulus, incultus, simplex, humilis patiensque/ [3]

Primogenitvra
958*   Sunt primogenita uestis benedictio dupla/ [5]

(90r)

Qvid parens proli debeat
959   Educo, corripio, doceo natam michi prolem. [1]

Qvid proles parenti
960   Exhibeo, ueneror, illi parendo parentem. [1]

Promissio
961*   Nuda uelud pactum reddit promissio tutum/ [2]

Qvaliter aliqvid probandvm
962*   Exemplum, simile, factum, uerbum ratioque/ [2]

Posse
963*   Posse quidem rebus dant ius, natura, facultas/ [2]

Pes
964*   Pes est affectus Domino per cuncta placendi/ [4]

(90v)

PRINCIPIVM

965 Principium Pater et natus spiransque creator/ [2]

PROPRIVM

966* Tu nisi peccatum nil reputes proprium/ [3]

PAVCI ELECTI

967* Plurima stultorum messis, set rara bonorum. [1]

PORTARE

968* Hec portant Christum: Virgo, Symeon et asellus/ [4]

PORTA

969 Iustitie porta Christus doctrinaque, mors est/ [2]

PACTVM

970 Que bona sunt per se, pactio praua facit. [1]

PVLLI

971* Pasce columbinos pullos, etate nouellos/ [3]

(91r)

PASSER

972 Instabilis, pugnans, petulans auis, alta requirens/ [4]

PAPAVER

973 Plana soporatum terra papauer habet. [1]

PLVVIA

974 Gratia, pena, Deus doctrinaque dicitur imber. [1]

PARALITICVS

975* Christo curandum presentant quatuor egrum/ [3]

PECCATOR

976* Stulte quid egisti, cur non miser extimuisti/ [3]
977 Est uere stultus qui ius discretus adultus/ [3]
978 Hostis fit peccans sponsi sponseque suique. [1]
979 Nascitur ut fimo scarabo, sic sordibus hostis/ [2]
980* Es, ferrum, plumbum, stagnum reputatur iniquus/ [2]
981 Dans sathane uires, reus hosti reddidit arma. [1]
982 Sus de sorde leuat, saltem dum colligit escam/ [2]
983* Qui uitiis mille se tradit, consecrat ille/ [2]

DENIGRATIO PECCATORIS

984* Cum male ludentis facies mendosa paratur/ [4]

Presvmptio
985* Errant qui sperant se sibi sufficere/ [8]

(91v)

Pompa
986 Sunt pompe mundi tanquam fantasmata noctis. [1]

Pollvtio
987 Ne macules animam quam Christus mundificauit/ [6]

Peccatvm
988* Sunt peccata fores inferni, scoria, feces/ [5]
989 Est uitium seu peccatum pestis simulacrum/ [2]
990 Carduus est motus radix fomes tibi culpe/ [3]
991 Nubes, sartago, paries murusque chaosque/ [2]
992 Inruha cum fertur non solui culpa, nocentur/ [2]
993 Presbiteri culpa cumulatur et ordine pena. [1]
994 Ordo sacerdotum cumulat scelus et cruciatum. [1]
995 Non culpas proprias defendas aut alienas. [1]
996* Tunc stulti cernit ratio, scelus horret et odit/ [2]

(92r)

997* Sepius unius in plures culpa redundat/ [10]
998* Morbi principia sunt hec: gula, luxus et ira/ [5]
999* Non oleum, non thus, pro culpa sacrificatur/ [2]
1000* Splendorem meriti sceleris caligine fuscant/ [11]
1001* Conflatus uitulus Ihericoque anathema cremandum/ [4]
1002* Statim post culpam dolet et rubet et pauet Adam/ [4]

(92v)

1003* Est anime uitiis subici confusio grandis/ [3]

Peccatvm veniale
1004 Vim tu caute caue, retinens moderamina lingue. [1]
1005* Gutta cadens igni subseruit noxque diei/ [4]

Qve peccata magis pericvlosa
1006* Canon deflorans, heres, proles, lupa, perplex/ [2]

Circvmstantie aggravant peccatvm
1007* Aggrauat ordo, locus, peccata, scientia, tempus/ [3]

Cvr peccatvm vitandvm
1008* Vitet homo culpam ne seruus damnificetur/ [8]

(93r)

De corporalibvs et spiritvalibvs peccatis
1009* Corporis ut maculas anime sic crimina pandas/ [8]

EFFECTVS PECCATI
1010*   Aggrauat et fedat peccatum uilificatque/ [7]

(93v)

PECCATVM
1011*   Est peccatorum saccus, uelum pariesque/ [3]

AFFECTVS PECCATI
1012*   Fallit peccatum falsa dulcedine stultum/ [9]
1013   Peccatum parit exilium dampnumque ruborem/ [2]

(94r)

REMISSIO PECCATI
1014*   Hec baptisma, fides, pietas, contritio, Christi/ [3]
1015*   Dimittit Dominus solus peccata, sacerdos/ [2]

PENITENS
1016*   Contritus doleat, rubeat, fidat metuatque/ [2]
1017   Contritus natum Iacob est deflendo peremptum/ [2]
1018*   Peniteas cito peccator cum sit miserator/ [2]

QVE SVNT NECCESARIA PENITENTI
1019*   Spes uenie, cor contritum, confessio culpe/ [2]

AVSTERITAS PENITENTIS
1020*   Sit tibi potus aqua, cibus aridus, aspera uestis/ [11]

PENITENTIA INFIRMI
1021*   Eger peniteat et crimina confiteatur/ [5]

(94v)

PENITENTIA
1022*   Ex uiridi ligno limphas calor exprimit ignis/ [6]
1023*   Omnia peccata lustret contritio nostra/ [13]
1024   Contrito formam dant Iob Ionasque columba/ [3]

PLANCTVS PECCATORIS
1025*   Plango quod amisi, quod commisi, quod omissi/ [5]

(95r)

1026*   Fons, fluuius, mare, diluuium piscinaque labrum/ [8]

(95v)

1027*   Accelerent nos conuerti, deflere reatus/ [5]
1028*   Attendas cur peniteas et quomodo, quando/ [5]

(96r)

1029*   Baptizat, sanat, mutat, contritio uelat/ [11]

(96v)

1030* Plango quod offendi, lesi, nocui, male caui/ [2]
1031* Canon deflorat, heres, proles, lupa, perplex/ [13]
1032* Sunt extrema crucis contriti quatuor ista/ [2]

(97r)

1033* Sunt persepe simul solaris fulgor et imber/ [21]

(97v)

CVR ACCELERANDA PENITENTIA
1034 Ad Dominum festinandi sint hee tibi cause/ [3]

DIGNVS FRVCTVS PENITENTIE
1035* Vt pariat dignos homini contritio fructus/ [2]

SATISFACTIO PENITENTIALIS
1036* Vt dimittaris, aliis peccata remitte/ [5]

PLANCTVS
1037 Plango parum meriti, flens otia temporis acti. [1]

PVNITIO
1038 Hebrei, Pharii, peruerse, luxuriosi/ [3]

(98r)

1039* Cur homo torquetur: Vt ei meritum cumuletur (Iob)/ [5]

PENA
1040* Presentes pene sunt seue signa gehenne/ [8]
1041* Celestis medicus non parcens hic secat, urit/ [2]
1042 In culpis minus est, in penis plus reperitur/ [2]

PENA SIMILIS CVLPE
1043* Qui teneros pueros mergunt merguntur et ipsi/ [2]

PENA PRECEDIT GLORIAM
1044* Da si ditari, ieiuna si satiari/ [2]

PENA PECVNIARIA
1045* Sepe crumena tumens, emuncta cohercet auarum/ [2]

PLAGE EGYPTI
1046 Sanguis, rana, culex, musce, pecus, ulcera, grando/ [7]

(98v)

PENE INFERNI
1047* Vt reprobi penas uigilanti corde reuoluas/ [2]

POTESTAS SATHANE
1048 Est sathane triplex scriptura teste potestas/ [4]

PRECEPTA DEI
1049* Custodi precepta Dei, cuius placitum fac/ [2]

(99r)

PRECEPTVM
1050* Quis, quid, ubi, cui precipiat, cur, quomodo, quando/ [2]

PRELATI
1051 Orbem continue lustrant sol, sidera, Phebe/ [2]

PREDICATIO
1052 Doctrinis, donis, uirtutibus allice gentes/ [4]

PREDICATOR
1053 Est nubes doctor, fulmen, doctrina, mineque/ [4]

VOX MINORIS PREDICATORIS
1054 Riuulus et medici puer exto, fistula plumbi/ [4]

(99v)

PRESBITER
1055 Presbiteris caste sint uxores et amice/ [2]

VIOLENTE SVNT PRECES MAGNATVM
1056 In prece prelati uis est nonnulla iubendi/ [2]

PERSECVTOR
1057 Qui iustos uexant, merito tandem cruciantur/ [2]

QVE PERIMANT PECCATA
1058 Est lac doctrine mores quod sopit equinos/ [4]

PENA REPROBORVM
1059 Quis dormire facit concentus carmina celi/ [2]

(100r)

PREDICATOR
1060 Quod dicis facto doctor complere memento/ [2]

PREDICATIO
1061 Aures pascuntur ubi tantum uerba loquntur/ [2]

PAX
1062 Ficta, reconcilians, pax est tranquilla, beata/ [2]

PROPHETA
1063 Sit tibi presagus, presignans, pseudo propheta/ [5]

(100v)

QVERERE

1064*   Quis Dominum querat, ubi, quando, quomodo, quare/ [2]

QVADRAGESIMA

1065*   Pugnat et impugnat solito nunc seuius hostis/ [2]

QVINQVAGESIMA

1066*   Per quinquagenum numerum sunt significata/ [2]

QVONIAM

1067   Adiunctum, signum, causam, uerum, quoniam dat. [1]

QVADRAGENA

1068   Tempestas, tenebra, seruire, parasceue, limpha/ [3]

                                                                    (101r)

REDDITE QVE SVNT DEI DEO

1069*   Rem templi, uotum, laudem, grates et honorem/ [2]

QVE SVNT DEO REDDENDA

1070*   Laus et uindicta sunt et promotio nostra/ [2]

RESPONDERE DEO

1071*   Respondere Deo quid sit si querimus, hoc est/ [2]

RESPICERE CHRISTVM

1072*   Sit mens in Christo, cor defigatur in ipso/ [2]

REDIMERE

1073   Personam redimas, res et loca, tempora, causas/ [2]

RELIQVIE SANCTORVM

1074*   Sanctorum nos reliquias quasi pignus habemus/ [2]

REVERSIO

1075*   Quomodo, quo, quando, cur, unde reuersio fiat. [1]

RENVNTIATIO

1076   Denariis, rebus uel amore renuntio sponte. [1]

RENOVATIO

1077*   Serpens, ceruus, auis, arbor, sol lunaque tellus/ [2]

RELIGIO

1078*   In uestimentis non est meditatio mentis/ [3]

REGVLA

1079*   Obseruant motum sibi celitus astra statutum/ [2]

ROMA

1080   Roma manus rodit, quos rodere non ualet odit. [1]

VITIA RELIGIOSORVM

1081*   Religiosorum sunt hee species uitiorum/ [4]

(101v)

REMISSIO

1082*   Quis, quid uel quantum, cui, quomodo, quando remittat/ [2]

REQVIES

1083*   Hic requies sanctis breuis et longus labor extat. [1]

REX

1084*   Si bene membra regis es dignus nomine regis/ [4]

RECTOR

1085   Dedecet ut uite iudex fiat aliene. [1]

REGERE

1086*   Exemplo, uerbo, nos subsidio, precibusque/ [2]

RATIO ET SENSVALITAS

1087*   Suggerit in primis serpens, deliberat Eua/ [10]
1088*   Vir rationis apex, mulier pars ima uocatur/ [6]

(102r)

RIGOR

1089   Quadrupedes adaquare nequis dum percutis illos/ [2]

ROS

1090   Ros est ipse Deus et copia, gratia, uerbum. [1]
1091   Ros in scriptura Deus est et gratia, uerbum/ [2]

RECIDIVATIO

1092   Caute deuitet contritus ne recidiuet/ [4]

RVINA

1093*   In laqueum uolucris et cesa solotenus arbor/ [3]

RESVRRECTIO

1094*   Vt sompnolentes, sementis, et archa resurgit/ [2]
1095   A triplici morte presenti tempore surge/ [4]

(102v)

RESVRRECTIO MORTVORVM

1096*   Corpora quod surgent declarant uerba, figure/ [6]
1097*   Carbo reaccensus, ustus fenix rediuiuus/ [2]

RETE

1098 Verbi rete, doli, peccati, iudiciique/ [4]

RVBVS

1099 Est rubus ecclesia, Iacob, et crux, uirgaque doctor. [1]

RAMPNVS

1100 Ruscus inhorrescens et eisdem rampnus in armis/ [2]

REPVGNANTIA

1101 Quando repugnatur, calcari bis stimulatur. [1]

(103r)

REPROBI

1102 Sunt palee reprobi, sunt purgamenta metalli/ [4]

REMVNERATIO

1103 Hic obstetrices, rex Iehu, rex Babel, Achab/ [2]

RECIDIVATIO

1104 Respiciens retro, collum uelud Orpha reflectens/ [3]

RECORDATIO PATRIE

1105 In terra hostili patrie memoratio dulcis. [1]

RINOCEROS

1106* Vno rinoceros cornu pugnans, elephantem/ [18]

(103v)

SPIRITVS SANCTVS

1107* Est uirtus, donum, digitusque Dei, calor, ignis/ [16]

(104r-v)

1108* Spiritus est ignis precellens atque columba. [1]

SEPTEM DONA

1109* Hec intellectus, pietas, sapientia, robur/ [2]

SAPIENTIA

1110* Annus et annus abit, semper sapientia stabit. [1]
1111* Si probus es tepet hoc, formosus abit, locuplex es/ [2]

SCIENTIA

1112* Qui uitant falsa, ueniunt ad uera scienda/ [3]

SPES

1113* Spes mola, pes, cedrus, altum crucis, anchora, tectum/ [3]
1114* Spes est pes nobis ad Christum progrediendi/ [4]

1115   Dant Magdalena, spine, tibi, limus, asellus/ [2]
1116   Confidas nec diffidas lapsus, crucifixus/ [2]

SOBRIETAS
1117*   Sobrietas uires uitiorum comprimit omnes/ [3]

STABILITAS
1118   Sunt adamantina nostri non cerea corda. [1]

DE SANCTIS, ANGELIS, ET CHRISTO
1119*   Hec animal, firmamentum, tronus, et super hunc uir/ [5]
                                                    (105r)

SANCTVM
1120   Sanctificans alios, sanctus proprie Deus in se/ [13]

SANCTVS
1121*   Sis mundus, firmus, agyos, Dominoque dicatus/ [2]

SANCTI
1122*   Terra argillosa, uirgeque Iacob tibi sancti/ [3]

STEPHANVS
1123*   Disputat atque docet Stephanus confessus et orat. [1]

QVE DEBEMVS SANCTIS
1124*   Vt dominis plenus honor, obsequiumque fidele/ [2]
                                                    (105v)

SACERDOTIVM AARON
1125*   Emulus exustus, oratio, uirgaque florens/ [2]
1126*   Sta stabilis, firmus, pugnans et prouidus altus/ [2]

SACERDOS
1127*   Presbiter est pastor, sal, lux, miles, medicusque/ [4]
1128*   Si quis ad altare malus accedit celebrare/ [4]
1129*   Dux sacer ad sacrum te duc dans sacra sacerdos/ [5]
1130   Est cophinus sordis fragmentorumque sacerdos/ [2]
                                                    (106r)

SACRIFICIVM
1131*   Quis, cui, quando litet quid, ubi, cur intueamur. [1]
1132*   Corporis et cordis, operis simul offer et oris/ [2]

SYNA
1133   Amphora mensura mea si iungatur utrique/ [2]

STARE
1134   Quadraginta dies pia per ieiunia complens/ [4]

SERVIRE DEO
1135* Quis Domino seruit inductus amore metuue/ [2]

SERVVS
1136 Aspice quis, quando, cuius, quomodo seruiat et cur. [1]
1137 Pascens seruus arans, rediens, dominoque ministrans/ [3]
1138 Seruus seruatur ut seruiat inde uocatur. [1]

(106v)

1139 Vendere cum possis captiuum occidere noli. [1]

SAPIENS
1140* A Phebo Phebe lumen capit; a sapiente/ [2]

SAPIENS ET ELOQVENS
1141 Facundus sapiens argentum fertur et aurum. [1]

SERVVS NEQVAM
1142* Non recolit seruus collata sibi bona prauus/ [6]

NEMO POTEST DVOBVS DOMINIS SERVIRE
1143* Nullaque sunt pacis federa cum uitiis. [1]

SECVRITAS
1144* Tutior in terra locus est quam turribus altis/ [2]

SALVARE
1145 Vnde Ihesus saluet, quos, quando, quomodo, quare. [1]

SCRIPTVRA
1146 Sunt nobis uarie scripture sicut et esce. [1]

SCRIPTVRA MARE
1147* Est mare terribile magnumque uoraxque, profundum/ [3]

QVE SIGNIFICENT IN SACRA SCRIPTVRA
1148* Res, persona, locus, gestum, tempus, numerusque/ [3]

(107r)

SERMO DEI. QVID SIT SERMO
1149* Est sermo ratione quidem subnixa loquela/ [2]

SEMEN
1150 Quis, quid, ubi, quando serat, ad quid, quomodo,
     quantum/ [2]
1151* Vita breuis, casusque leuis, nec spes remeandi/ [4]

SAL
1152* Conficit ignis, aqua, sal quod post infatuatur/ [4]

SAGITTA
1153* Pennis ornata, uelox penitransque sagitta/ [3]

(107v)

SPECVLVM
1154* Est speculum Christus, ratio, scriptura, creata. [1]
1155   Sunt speculum quo conspicitur Deus ista creata/ [2]

SYLOE
1156* Paruaque set felix Syloe uisura, prophetam/ [2]

SOLATIVM CONTEMPLATIVORVM
1157* Exemplum ueterum diuersaque causa piorum/ [2]

SACRAMENTA
1158* Ordo, lingua, Dei corpus, thorus, unda, bis ungi. [1]
1159* Preparat et firmat, reparat Deus, abluit, armat/ [2]
1160* Ista requiruntur: intentio, forma, potestas/ [2]

SIGNA
1161   Signa futurorum sunt hec presentia queuis/ [6]

(108r)

SCALA IACOB
1162* Mens capud est, Christus lapis est, iacobita uiator/ [3]

ALIQVIS SECVLARIS PREFERTVR CLAVSTRALI, ET PENITENS INNOCENTI
1163   Fruge uigent ualles, algent de frigore montes/ [4]

QVALITER PSALLENDVM
1164   Psallite discrete, constanter, cordis amore/ [2]

DE SERVVLO PARALITICO
1165* Et laus celestis et odor tibi seruule seruit/ [2]

SENECTVS
1166* Affectus non effectus habet egra senectus. [1]

SENEX
1167* Vespere gallina scandit pro uulpibus alta/ [3]
1168* Culpe sit finis cum uite sit prope finis/ [6]

(108v)

SENEX FATVVS
1169* Post annos centum puer alphesibeus adhuc est/ [4]
1170* Bos semel est uitulus, semel et canis ipse catellus/ [4]
1171* Olla recens fracta ualet ex facili reperari/ [2]

SEMINIFLVVS
1172*   Garrulus est uir, spermaticus uel prodigus omnis. [1]

SVCCESSORES ALEXANDRI
1173   Est orientalis Babilon subiecto Seleuco/ [4]

SOLLICITVDO
1174*   In quid sollicitus sis, quantum, quomodo, quando/ [3]

SIMILITVDO
1175   Dat similem dici rem, gratia, gloria, culpa/ [3]

(109r)

SVSTENTATIO
1176*   Ille natat leuiter cui mentum sustinet alter. [1]

SORS
1177*   Que sors et qualis, quando quibusue datur/ [3]

SOL
1178*   Sol ueluti solus lucens est orbicularis/ [2]
1179*   Solus prelucens, exsiccans, letificansque/ [8]

(109v)

1180   Siccat et indurat sol presens, lucet et ardet/ [3]

QVATVOR EQVI SOLIS
1181*   Vt ficte narratur, equi sunt bis duo Phebi/ [4]

STELLA
1182*   Stella fides, Christus, sancta exhortatio, sermo est/ [3]

(110r)

SALIX
1183*   Alta salix, sterilis et amica paludis, amara/ [2]

SINAPIS
1184*   Sinapis granum, calidum, siccum, modicumque/ [10]

(110v)

STIPVLA
1185*   Est fragilis stipula, terre radicitus herens/ [2]

(111r)

STVPPA
1186   Accendi facilis, uilis, leuis, aspera stuppa/ [3]

STRAMEN
1187*   Fecundat, tegit et signat, sustentat et ornat. [1]
1188*   Stramen fedatur, calcatur, et igne crematur. [1]

SPELVNCA
1189*   Est spelunca caro uel mundus siue sepulcrum. [1]

SACCVS
1190   Est saccus sathane teter, gemine quoque pene/ [2]
1191*   Vsus, homo, culpa, cordis contritio, pena/ [2]

STATERA
1192*   Sit distincta crucis, distincta statera sit oris/ [2]

SICLVS
1193*   Argenti quinque redimenda pro sibi prole/ [3]

(111v)

SENSVALITAS
1194   Rampnus, apis, Ioab, mulier, pars infima siche/ [2]

SERPENS
1195   Est heresis, demon, peccatum pseudoque serpens/ [6]

(112r)

SVPERBIA
1196*   Morphosis et mater, nutrix, uredo et origo/ [11]
1197*   Quatuor hiis fastus speciebus fit manifestus/ [4]

(112v)

QVE PERIMANT SVPERBIAM
1198*   Depede, prefati, rumor, fit ruptio tifi. [1]

SYMONIA
1199   Qui uendunt uel emunt res quaslibet ecclesiales/ [4]

SECTA
1200   Falsa Saduceis astrea dedit, Phariseis/ [2]

SOCIETAS
1201*   Fragrantes uicina rosas urtica perurit/ [2]

SOCIETAS MALORVM
1202*   Inter peruersos iusti Loth et Ezechiel, Iob/ [2]

SCANDALVM
1203*   Scandalon equiuocant obex, impactio, casus/ [2]

QVATVOR CAVSE SVBVERSIONIS SODOME
1204*   Subuertunt Sodomam tumor, otia, copia panis/ [2]

NVSQVAM SECVRITAS
1205*   Tutus uir quis, quoque statu, cur, quomodo, quando. [1]

SEPVLCRVM

1206*   Sunt bustum, domus, infernus, corpus, monumentum. [1]

(113r)

1207   Culpa, gehenna, solum dant gratia, gloria bustum. [1]

SECVNDA SERMO DEI

1208   Sermo Dei lux est, si diligis hunc tibi dux est/ [2]
1209   Sermo Dei sanat, seruat, corroborat, armat. [1]

SECVNDA SIMILITVDO

1210   Esse Deo similem si uis per scripta doceri/ [2]

SVBIECTIO

1211   Corpus spiritui, sensus subsit rationi/ [2]

SICVT

1212   Dat minus aut maius uel par uel ratione sicut. [1]

SECVLVM

1213   Est ut hiemps seclum presens, nox longa diesque/ [3]

(113v)

QVINQVE SENSVS

1214   Ad noctis tenebras, ad fulgura claude fenestras/ [4]

TANGIT DEVS

1215   Curans, inspirans, compungens atque flagellans/ [2]

DEVS TRADIT HOMINEM DIABOLO

1216   Cur Dominus sathane quemquam tradat, tibi cause/ [2]

TEMPLVM CHRISTI

1217*   Nos sibi munus, nos sibi templum querit amenum/ [2]

THESAVRVS VIRTVTVM

1218*   Etsi deest aurum, non deest thesaurus honesti/ [2]

TIMOR ET SPES

1219*   Non prodest sine spe timor, aut spes absque timore/ [2]

TIMOR

1220*   Qui timet ille sibi cauet et reueretur et horret. [1]
1221*   Culpam cum pena Dominumque timere uideris/ [5]
1222*   Terreat hos pena quos non inuitat amena/ [2]

SERVILIS TIMOR

1223*   Seruilis bonus est timor ac effectus et usus/ [2]

(114r)

1224*   Fassio, notitia, grates, honor atque sequela/ [3]

TIMOR IN BONO
1225*   Heth pauor est, hic est semen, uia uitaque compes/ [9]

(114v)

TIMOR IN MALO
1226*   Porta sathan timor est, febris horrida, pallida lepra/ [2]

THOMAS
1227*   Est Didimus geminus, set Thomas fertur abissus/ [3]

TESTIS
1228*   Stephanus et Christus mulierque pudica Susanna/ [2]

TRIBVLATIO
1229*   Nos homo, mens, culpa tribulant, Zabulus, caro, mundus/ [2]
1230*   Quod fornax auro, quod ferro lima, flagellum/ [2]
1231*   Fullo, faber, miles, genitor, medicusque sacerdos/ [3]
1232*   Sunt mala mixta bonis humane conditionis/ [2]
1233*   Cum furit aura foris premit auram feruor amoris/ [2]
1234*   Propter doctrinam nostram, solatia, culpam/ [3]

EFFECTVS TRIBVLATIONIS
1235*   Signat, submittit, purgat, conseruat et auget/ [6]

(115r)

TVRBATIO
1236*   Iudicii baratrique metus, presentia culpe/ [5]

TVRBO
1237*   Irruit, inuoluit turbo, paleas rapit, aufert. [1]

TEMPESTAS
1238*   Tempestas uento, tonitru fit, fulgure, nimbo. [1]

TRISTITIA
1239   Tristitiam culpa, dampnum, contritio, pena/ [5]

(115v)

TORPOR
1240*   Tedia torpentem faciunt, labor atque secunda. [1]

TACITVRNITAS
1241*   Laus male, sermo Dei, correptio, culpa tacetur/ [2]

TEMPTATIO
1242*   Dat tria temptare: seducere, scire, probare. [1]

1243* Temptant nos homines, Deus et demon, caro nostra/ [3]
1244* Quando temptaris, Christi mala si meditaris/ [2]
1245 Pulsat nec frangit, impellit ne mouet, auget/ [4]

TEMPTARE DEVM
1246 In puteum uero temptans Dominum cadit Hero/ [2]

ABSCONDERE TALENTVM
1247* Non minus hic peccat qui censum condit in agro/ [2]

TERRA
1248* Tellus sustentat, induit atque cibat. [1]

TERRE CVLTVRA
1249 Tellus purgetur, scindatur, deinde seratur/ [2]

TEMPVS
1250* Tempora cum ueniunt abeunt, sic tempora fiunt/ [2]
1251* Mensis qui caret R. sompnis solet esse saluber/ [2]

(116r)

OBSERVA TEMPVS
1252* Obserua tempus in dicendis et agendis/ [7]

TRANSIT HOMO
1253* Mundus abit tanquam lanugo, spuma, sagitta/ [6]

TECTVM
1254 Protegit et munit, transcendit, suscipit imbrem/ [3]

(116v)

VECTES TABERNACVLI
1255* Vt tabulas uectes, sic iustos ista tenebunt/ [2]

THVRIBVLVM
1256* Mistica sunt uas, thus, ignis, quia uase notatur/ [2]

TVBA
1257* Conuocat Hebreos legis tuba, clangit et ipsa/ [2]

TVRTVR
1258* Turtur, soliuaga uolucris, gemebunda, pudica/ [4]

TROPVS
1259* Rem uariant tempus, locus, etas, causa modusque/ [3]

TRIBVLATIO SECVNDA
1260 Exurit paleas ignis, propurgat et aurum. [1]

TEMPTATIO SECVNDA
1261   Excitat, excercet Zabuli temptatio iustum/ [6]

(117r)

TIMOR SERVILIS SECVNDA
1262   Dum tu seruilem credis saluare timorem/ [2]

VIRTVS
1263*   Spes triplex triplexque fides, dilectio triplex/ [2]
1264*   Virtus res simplex, nec crescere nec minui scit/ [7]

VIRGINITAS
1265*   Tardior in nobis set et ictibus apta ferendis/ [8]

VIRTVTES ET VITIA
1266*   Lente uenit uirtus, uitium ruit impetuose. [1]
1267*   Prepropero uitium lentoque uenit pede uirtus. [1]
1268*   Accidiam generant iteratio, copia, morbus. [1]

VERBVM
1269*   De uacuo uerbo ratio reddetur, acerbo/ [2]
1270*   Vtilis ut sermo sit et ut uideatur honestus/ [2]

(117v)

VERBVM DEI
1271*   Sermo diuinus est aduersarius, ignis/ [6]
1272*   Collige frumentum sit ut id cibus esurientum/ [2]

(118r)

VIS
1273   Vis est in uerbis, gemmis, oculis, et in herbis. [1]

<VERBVM DEI>
1274*   Sermo Dei uiuus ueraxque per omnia, castus/ [10]

(118v)

1275*   Sacre scripture succendunt crimina prune. [1]

VIDERE
1276   Nos uideat Ihesus semper uideamus ut ipsum. [1]

VVLT
1277*   Sustinet atque probat, placet et proponit et optat/ [2]

VIA
1278*   Ampla uia est uere que ducit ad atra gehenne/ [3]
1279   Est error cordis, praue credendo, putando/ [4]

1280*   En callem Samye monstrat pars dextra figure/ [2]
1281*   Nec iaceas neque stes, set eas in tramite recto/ [3]

VIA VEL PROFECTVS
1282*   Recte progrediens, oblitus posteriora/ [2]
1283   Angustant iter hec: mundus, caro, demon et usus/ [2]

VIATORES
1284*   Omnibus est optanda salus, saluentur ut omnes/ [2]
1285   Subsidium, cautela, Dei clementia, gressus/ [2]

VITA
1286   Degeneri uita, uitam corrumpere uita/ [4]

                                                              (119r)

1287*   Viuere natura dat, gratia, gloria, culpa. [1]

VITA ET MORS
1288   Non sibi set Domino uiuat quis uel moriatur/ [2]

VITA PRESENS
1289*   Vite labentis et in arto tempore mortis/ [8]

VENIRE AD DEVM
1290*   Qui uenient, ad quem, quando uel qualiter, unde. [1]

VIGILARE
1291*   Vt naute uigiles, pastores, angelus, ales/ [7]

VIRGA
1292*   Virga Dei rectos regit et contundit iniquos/ [2]
1293   Percutitur uirga Moysi puluis, mare, petra. [1]

VIRGA AARON
1294*   Est florens uirga qui penitet alma Maria/ [2]

                                                              (119v)

VIVERE
1295   Viuere natura dat, gratia, gloria, culpa. [1]

VINEA
1296*   Prudens et fidus instans operarius extet/ [2]
1297*   Falx, ignis, nexus, paxillus, fletus et uua/ [2]
1298*   Vinea uallatur, complantatur foditurque/ [6]

                                                              (120r)

1299*   Mane dedit uiti cultores, tertia, sexta/ [4]
1300*   Vinea culta fuit, cultores premia querunt/ [4]

VINVM

1301* Est uinum cum letitia, dilectio, sensus/ [3]
1302   Est uinum luxus, fallax mordaxque furoris/ [2]

VINVM EST HOMO IVSTVS

1303* Res pretiosa merum, potu, libamine dignum/ [5]

(120v)

VRIAS

1304   Coniuge pro pulcra metuat iam quisque sepulcra. [1]

CVR PLVRES VXORES ANTIQVORVM

1305* Pluribus adiunctos seu coniugibus sociatos/ [2]

VXOR

1306   Est uxor sensus et sollicitudo, uoluptas. [1]

VELVM

1307* Quatuor in uelo designant ista colores/ [5]
1308* In uelo uarii signant diuersa colores/ [7]

VECTES

1309* Spes, amor, exemplum sunt et meditatio mortis/ [2]

VESTES

1310   Vestitur tellus gramine, fronde nemus/ [10]

(121r)

VITVLVS

1311* Est uitulus mundus, mitis, lactens, nouus, insons/ [4]

(121v)

VICTORIA

1312* Nolumus a sociis uinci qui uincimur ira/ [2]

VIS

1313   Non uinolentus regnum rapit, at uiolentus/ [2]

VRBS

1314   Vrbes munitas uastat bonus aut malus ignis. [1]

VINCVLA

1315   Est uinculum culpe, pene legisque superne/ [4]

VINCVLA PECCATI

1316* Affectu tentus reus est porcus pede uinctus. [1]

(122r)

1317*   Mundi, nature, culpe, peneque gehenne/ [2]
1318   Extant in culpa mortali uincula plura/ [3]

VVLPES
1319   Tramitis amfractus, fraus cordis, fetor et oris/ [2]

VENTVS
1320   Est uentus uelox, siccat, mouet, obruit ignem/ [7]

(*122v*)

VLTIO
1321*   Vermis corrodens, subtractio gratuitorum/ [3]
1322   Rosio, ruptio, demptio, pressio, temporis huius/ [2]

VASA
1323   Aurea uasa bonus amor et sapientia prestat/ [4]

(*123r*)

VETVSTAS ET NOVITAS
1324   Iudei ueteres sunt crimine, tempore, lege/ [2]
1325   Est culpe pene non ignorata uetustas/ [2]

VERMES
1326*   Sunt qui cum clauso putrefacta est spina sepulcro/ [5]

VMBRA
1327*   Commemora culpam, tempus mortemque per umbram/ [4]

VANA
1328*   Dicimus hoc uanum quod transit, inutile, falsum/ [2]

VITIA
1329*   Maiorum tumor in iussu, formido minorum/ [2]

(*123v*)

1330*   Esuries, ensis perimunt, mala bestia, pestis. [1]

SEPTEM VITIA CAPITALIA
1331*   Culparum fontes sunt fastus, liuor et ira/ [2]

VITIA CANONICA
1332   Gorgias timor est, Vsias cupit, atque Nichanor/ [4]

VENVS
1333*   Qua specie Martis cedit uictoria Parthis/ [2]

VSVRA
1334   Dicitur usura sors, siue quod accidit illi/ [4]

VENDITIO

1335 Ex quouis pacto, uel quouis mutuo nacto/ [2]

VALLIS

1336 Est uallis floris, fontis, farris, terebinti/ [2]

EQVALITAS VEL INEQVALITAS VIRTVTVM

1337 Prestant equales uirtutes enea nobis/ [2]

VOLVPTAS

1338 Est tibi carnalis, suauis, mel dulce, uoluptas/ [2]

VITA HOMINIS

1339 Est mihi militia modo seu temptatio uita/ [2]

(124r)

VANA

1340 Gloria, prosperitas et uita, potentia uana. [1]

VITA PRESENS

1341 Quem rapit atque leuat fluctus uite trahit huius. [1]

VVLNVS

1342 Est actu, culpe, rupture uulnus inique/ [2]

VIRTVS ET VITIVM

1343 De uitiis uitia, nimirum cernimus orta/ [4]

XPC

1344* Christus acus, capud est, dux, pastor, stella, columpna /[2]
1345* Ecclesie fundamentum, fundator et idem/ [3]

(124v)

1346* Christus fons uiuus, mons summus, pons tibi factus/ [30]
1347* Rex sedet in solio, mala dissipat aspiciendo. [1]
1348 Christus et ecclesia duo sunt, set carne sub una/ [2]
1349* Non Deus est nec homo presens quam cernis ymago/ [2]

MATER ET VIRGO

1350* Virgo Deum peperit, set si quis quomodo querit/ [4]
1351 Cedens uiuificat, lapides transponit, inaltat/ [6]

CHRISTVS VERBVM

1352* Est uerbum Christus lumenque lucernaque nobis/ [5]

(125v)

SOL IN VIRGINE

1353* Incircumscriptus sol est in Virgine Christus. [1]

Domvs Christi
1354* Virgo, presepe, crux tumbaque mundus, olimpus/ [7]

Qve portant Christvm
1355* Portitor ipsius portatur uirgine clausus. [1]
1356* Nauis, iumentum, crux, uirgo senexque sepulcrum/ [2]

Vita et doctrina Christi
1357* Exemplar, forma speculique nitor, uia, norma/ [8]

Christvs sponsvs
1358   Virgo tibi sponsus sit is est cui grata iuuentus/ [2]

(126r)

Christvs medicvs
1359   In celis residens terris medicamina prestat/ [3]

Vestis Christi
1360   Purpura cum clamide rubicunda, candida uestis/ [2]

Meritvm Christi
1361   Si Christus meruit, cui, quando, qualiter et quid/ [2]

Passio Christi
1362* Est sanguis cordis signum cordalis amoris/ [8]
1363* Cum moritur uita nobis est reddita uita/ [2]
1364* Cur Dominus passus, ubi, quot uel quomodo, quando/ [4]

(126v)

1365* A pomo quod primus homo gustauit, acetum/ [2]

Corpvs Christi
1366* Saluator cibus et uitis, lux atque leuamen/ [2]

Resvrrectio Christi
1367* Forma, fides, causa, nobis surrectio Christi/ [5]
1368* Quis uel ubi surgat, cur, quando, qualiter, unde. [1]

Victoria Christi
1369* Mors cum Iudeo, mundus cum demone uicti/ [2]

Stare Christi
1370   Christus se monstrans stat, et auxilians stabilisque. [1]

Christvs fvr
1371   Est Christus latro, fur in mundo uel auerno/ [2]

Testes Christi
1372* Sunt Pater et Verbum Christi cum Pneumate testes/ [3]

SEQVI CHRISTVM

1373*   Morbus, signa, cibus, blasphemia, dogma, fuere/ [2]

QVE ATTESTETVR CHRISTO

1374   Sanguis, opus, testes dant Christum uera locutum. [1]

MIRACVLA CHRISTI

1375   Firmant et fulgent, Christi miracula terrent. [1]

II.13

De septem sacramentis ecclesie

These questions on the Church's sacraments reflect William's teaching at Paris in the 1180's or at Lincoln Cathedral during the last decades of the twelfth century. They address a mixture of speculative and practical issues, and evince a familiarity with the teachings of the canon lawyers as well as the theologians. Although called a "treatise" (*tractatus*) in some of the manuscripts, the *De septem sacramentis*, at least in its present form, is a rather unsystematic collection of *quaestiones* on the sacraments. It seems to have developed out of William's actual classroom teaching, and to address the questions that were raised in his school.

One of the most important inventions of twelfth-century scholasticism was the doctrine of the seven sacraments. Great energy was devoted, by theologians and canonists alike, to differentiating "sacraments" from "sacramentals" and to defining the nature and operation of the seven ecclesiastical sacraments.[1] Gratian's canonical textbook, the *Decretum* (c. 1140), came to include inchoate discussions of the sacraments in the two sections *De penitentia* and *De consecratione*, but scholars are still uncertain as to the genesis and intention of these seemingly imperfect additions to the end of the *Decretum*.[2] In the 1160's Peter Lombard was able to devote the bulk of the fourth book of his *Sentences* to the seven sacraments and thus give evidence of a growing body of scholastic teaching on the topic.

---

[1] See Damien Van den Eynde, *Les définitions des sacrements pendant la première période de la théologie scolastique (1050-1240)* (Rome: Antonianum, 1950); Nikolaus Häring, "The Interaction between Canon Law and Sacramental Theology in the 12th Century," *Proceedings of the Fourth International Congress of Medieval Canon Law* (Vatican City: Biblioteca Apostolica Vaticana, 1976), pp. 483-493. For a general bibliographical orientation see Josef Finkenzeller, *Die Lehre von den Sakramenten im allgemeinen: Von der Schrift bis zur Scholastik* (Freiburg im Br.: Herder, 1980), pp. 1 and 78.

[2] See John H. van Engen, "Observations on the *De consecratione*," *Proceedings of the Sixth International Congress of Medieval Canon Law* (Vatican City: Biblioteca Apostolica Vaticana, 1985), pp. 309-320, and the literature cited there.

Sacramental theology in the schools, however, was not relegated to the last place in the curriculum that might be suggested by its situation at the very end of the two great textbooks of theology and canon law. The novelty of the subject matter and its importance for both speculative theology and day-to-day practice in the churches insured that it would be discussed frequently in the schools. The academic setting of such discussions is unclear, but from the 1160's onward there is abundant evidence that the seven sacraments were a subject for detailed comment and dispute in their own right.[3] By the end of the century, discussions of the sacraments had come to have a respected place in the theology curriculum, often in conjunction with the school exercise of disputed questions.[4] William's *De septem sacramentis ecclesie* contributes to our understanding of the early development of sacramental doctrine in the schools. He draws on both the canonical materials in the *Decretum* and Lombard's theological *summa*, but adds significant elements from his own teaching and, presumably, from other Parisian masters of the period between 1170 and 1185. That scribes continued to copy these *quaestiones* well into the fifteenth century indicates the perspicacity that William brought to his task.

The two versions of this work that can be identified in the extant copies seem to reflect two *reportationes* of the (original) questions. Neither version represents the original in its entirety, and both preserve elements that have been excised or rearranged in the other. A critical edition of all the manuscript witnesses will be necessary to establish a reliable text; such an edition would provide valuable insight into sacramental teaching and practice during this formative period.

AUTHENTICITY AND DATE

Unlike William's other writings, which survive in numerous manuscript copies from the first half of the thirteenth century, the earliest extant copies of the *De septem sacramentis* date from the end of the thirteenth century and are unascribed. Two late manuscripts (nos. 8 and 9), copied in 1375 and 1423 respectively, ascribe the work to William. Since his fame was shortlived outside of thirteenth-century England, these un-

---

[3] See Raymond M. Martin, "Pierre le Mangeur De sacramentis: Texte inédit," appendix to Henri Weisweiler, *Maitre Simon et son groupe De sacramentis: Textes inédits* (Louvain: Spicilegium sacrum, 1937).

[4] The most famous example is that of Peter the Chanter at Paris, whose *Summa de sacramentis et animae consiliis* is a collection of questions on the sacraments disputed in his school; cf. Baldwin, *Masters*, 1: 13-14.

ambiguous attributions in manuscripts copied in Germany more than 150 years after his death could hardly have originated with their scribes; they must reflect an earlier manuscript tradition. Likewise, the excerpts of this work preserved in a Trinity College, Cambridge, manuscript of the fifteenth century (MS B.15.20 [356]) and incorrectly attributed to Robert Grosseteste (bishop of Lincoln 1235-1253) probably point to an earlier tradition that ascribed the work to William de Montibus, chancellor of Lincoln.[5]

Arguments for William's authorship based on internal evidence must await a collation of all the manuscripts and the establishment of a reliable text, but many similarities between doctrines and expressions in the *De septem sacramentis ecclesie* and William's other writings strengthen the case for the authenticity of this work.[6]

In style and content the work is typical of the twelfth century rather than the thirteenth. Arguments for dating the questions on the eucharist to the 1170's or 1180's have been presented elsewhere.[7] The references to the "character" impressed on the soul by baptism and confirmation confirm this dating. Nikolaus Häring has demonstrated that the notion of a sacramental character entered the theological vocabulary in the Parisian schools about the years 1175-1180.[8] An earlier usage of the term "character" understood it not as a substantial element of the sacrament but as a sign by which the baptized (or confirmed) would be discerned from the unbaptized (or unconfirmed) in the Last Judgement.[9] Both the old and the new usage are present together in the

[5] See Goering, "*Diffinicio eucaristie*," p. 95, where it is suggested that the false attribution to Robert Grosseteste (*alias* "Lincolniensis") most probably reflects the tendency of later scribes to subsume references to less well-known Lincoln writers under the name of the famous bishop.

[6] Examples are given by Goering, ibid., p. 94. One of William's favorite similitudes — the twin dangers of Scylla and Charybdis — is employed in the discussion of whether one should rather commit fornication than masturbate. William replies that fornication is the lesser evil, but that one should not avoid Scylla to enter into the whirlpool Charybdis (William, or the scribe, has transposed these two classical loci): "Item queritur de illis qui ducendo et reducendo tractant uirgam et dicuntur molles, utrum peccant mortaliter, quod non est dubium, set queritur utrum potius debeant fornicari. Respondeo quod minus malum est fornicari, set non debet uitare Cariddam ut intret Cillam," Aberdeen, University Library MS 240, fol. 197ra.

[7] Goering, "*Diffinicio eucaristie*," pp. 92-94.

[8] "The Augustinian Axiom: *Nulli Sacramento Injuria Facienda Est*," *Mediaeval Studies* 16 (1954) 114.

[9] See Nikolaus Häring, "Character, Signum, und Signaculum: Die Einführung in die sacramentalischen Theologie des 12. Jahrhunderts," *Scholastik* 31 (1956) 182-212; cf. Van den Eynde, *Définitions des sacrements*; Henri Weisweiler, "Das Sakrament der Firmung in den systematischen Werken der ersten Frühscholastik," *Scholastik* 7 (1933) 481-523.

De septem sacramentis, suggesting that they were composed during the transitional period between 1175 and 1190. The existence of many copies of this text in continental libraries and the relative paucity of copies in English collections might suggest that they were composed during William's Parisian career, before c. 1186.

SOURCES

The sources used in this text are typical for the period. William appears to draw many of his authorities — Ambrose, Augustine, Isidore, Jerome, Pope Pius I, Pope Urban I — from Gratian's *Decretum*, although many of them are also found in Lombard's *Sentences*. The *Decretum* itself is cited once. Biblical citations, of course, are adduced throughout, and occasional references are made to the authority of the Church's liturgy.

The questions treated here are those that were current in the schools during the 1170's and 1180's where no sharp distinction was drawn between the purview of the canonists and the theologians. One question on penance is prefaced by the remark: "Questio est inter theologos,"[10] but most are pertinent to students in both disciplines. Many of the questions posed are of a general and theoretical nature, but some reflect current events. For example, after defining marriage as involving the consent (*in eadem uoluntate*) of a man and a woman, William introduces a question arising from a recent case ("unde queritur de quodam casu qui in temporibus nostris accidit") where two nobles decided to make peace with each other by joining their children in matrimony. The daughter was unwilling to marry and took a solemn vow of chastity to foil her father's plan. Upon learning of this he beat her and threatened to put her in the stocks, whereupon she decided that the humiliation planned for her would be worse than marriage, and acceded to her father's wish. To the question of whether this was a legitimate marriage William responds that it was not because it was forced and made without free consent.[11]

---

[10] "Questio est inter theologos utrum peccata reuiuiscant, quidam dicunt quod non. Solutio: Sed nos dicimus quod reuiuiscunt ... ," Baltimore, Walters MS W.131, fol. 155v.

[11] "Vnde queritur de quodam casu qui in temporibus nostris accidit. Discordia erat inter duos principes; uoluerunt ergo terminare discordiam per filiam unius eorum, quam uoluit alter eorum copulare filio alterius principis ut ita pax fieret et concordia. Set illa puella uouerat Deo castitatem et illa sic discordabat a proposito patris sui. Tunc pater iratus prostrauit eam et dixit ei quod in patibulo statueret eam. Vnde

MANUSCRIPTS

1. *A* = Aberdeen, University Library MS 240, fols. 194vb-198ra. Late 13th century.

> Title: (*Tractatus de vii sacramentis ecclesie*).
> Inc. Prol.: *Septem sunt sacramenta ecclesiastica.*
> Inc. Txt.: *Primo tractandum est de baptismo.*
> Expl.: (*De coniugio*) ... . *Secunda est fornicacionis remedium.*

Excerpts of this text are printed below as "Version A."

2. *B* = Baltimore, Walters Art Gallery MS W.131, fols. 133r-174v. Late 13th century.

> Title: (*De septem sacrementis ecclesie*).
> Inc. Prol.: *Septem sunt sacramenta.*
> Inc. Txt.: (*De baptismo*) *Primo agendum est de baptismo.*
> Expl. Txt.: (*De extrema unctione*) ... *et ideo debet esse uel fieri in forma deprecatiua.*

Excerpts of this text are printed below as "Version B." The initial letter of each chapter is replaced with an illuminated miniature portraying the dispensation of the sacrament in question.

3. Budapest, Egyetemi Könyvtár (University Library) MS 39, fols. 90r-94r. 14th/15th century.

> Title: (*Sequitur de septem sacramentis matris sancte ecclesie*).
> Inc. Prol.: *Septem sunt sacamenta que nominantur in his verbis.*
> Expl.: *Et hec dicta sufficiant de septem sacramentis sancte ecclesie.*
> Colophon: *Expliciunt septem sacramenta que multum sunt necessaria ad salutem animarum fidelium et cetera.*

The description is taken from Ladislaus Mezey, *Codices latini Medii Aeui Bibliothecae Universitatis Budapestinensis* (Budapest: Akadémiai Kiado, 1961), pp. 55-57.

4. Cambridge, Gonville and Caius College MS 61/155, fols. 149va-176rb. Late 13th century.

> Title: *Incipit tractatus de vii sacramentis*
> Inc. Prol.: (*De baptismo.*) *Septem sunt sacramenta.*
> Inc. Txt.: *Primo agendum est de baptismo.*
> Expl. Txt.: (*De sacris ordinibus*) ... *officium sacerdotis perfecit.*

This copy represents Version B, although the wording and word-order differs somewhat from that in the other manuscripts of this version.

---

ipsa uidens pudorem nimium sibi innuere nupsit iuxta uelle patris sui filio principis. Queritur ergo utrum legitimum fuerit matrimonium. Solutio: Respondemus quod non quia coacta, et non fecit hec spontanea uoluntate," ibid., fol. 166v.

It omits the seventh sacrament, extreme unction, and the section on holy orders omits the introductory remarks and the discussion of the first six orders; it begins with the seventh: *Sequitur ordo presbiterorum ... .*

5. Cambridge, Gonville and Caius College MS 380/600, fols. 17va-19vb. Late 13th century.

> Inc. Prol.: *Septem sunt sacramenta ecclesiastica.*
> Inc. Txt.: *Quia ergo baptismus est magis necessarium sacramentum.*
> Expl. Txt. (imperfect in *penitentia*): *Item queritur de prauo sacerdote et indiscreto ... dummodo diuites sint.*

This copy is idiosyncratic, combining elements of both Version A and B, but generally following the outline of Version B. It includes the first five sacraments, ending in mid sentence of a question on penance; the rest of folio 19v is blank.

6. Leipzig, Universitätsbibliothek MS 423, pp. 308-313. 15th century.

> Inc.: *Bos vt erat petulans cernentibus obice cursum.*
> Expl.: *error non separat eos.*

The description is taken from Rudolf Helssig, *Katalog der lateinischen und deutschen Handschriften der Universitäts-Bibliothek zu Leipzig,* 1/1 (Leipzig: S. Hirzel, 1926-1935), pp. 653-657.

7. Mainz, Stadtbibliothek MS I.117, fols. 19ff. This manuscript could not be microfilmed and has not been examined. It is cited by M. Bloomfield, *Incipits,* p. 470, no. 5461.

8. Munich, Bayerische Staatsbibliothek MS Clm 8885, fols. 270ra-274rb, 274vb-ra. AD 1375.

> Title: (*De septem sacramentis ecclesie. Primo de baptismo*).
> Inc.: *Septem sunt sacramenta.*
> Expl.: (*De ordinibus*) ... *officium sacerdotis inplet et perficit Christi. Abluo firmo cibo penitet vngit et ordinat vxor.*
> Colophon: *Explicit summa magistri Wilhelmi de montibus super septem sacramenta gloriose compylata ex vno versiculo.*

This copy contains the first six sacraments as in Version B. The scribe apparently mistook the end of section 5, *De coniugio,* for the end of the treatise. The section ends on the bottom of fol. 274rb, and the scribe writes: *Anno Domini mº cccº lxxvº. Conpletus est liber iste per manus Nicolai in die sancti Ruperti.* He then began copying a sermon on fol. 274va, (inc.: *Sapiencia edificauit sibi domum ... . Legitur quod Salomon sapientissimus construxit templum*). After copying only one column, he returns abruptly to William's text and copies section 6, *De ordinibus,* on fols. 274vb-275ra.

9. Munich, Bayerische Staatsbibliothek MS Clm 8961, fols. 163r-173r. AD 1423.

> Inc. Prol.: *Septem sunt sacramenta.*
> Inc. Txt.: *Primo est agendo de baptissimo.*
> Expl. Txt.: (*De sacris ordinibus*) ... *officium sacerdotis implet et perfecit Christi. Abluo firmo cibo penitet ungit et ordinat uxor.*
> Colophon: *Explicit summa magistri Willhelmi de montibus super septem sacramenta gloriose complete ex uno uersiculo. Anno <Domini> m° cccc° 23° frater Symon.*

Text of Version B, sections 1-6. Like Clm 8885, sections 5 and 6 are separated by the same extraneous sermon fragment, copied here on fol. 172r-v.

10. Munich, Bayerische Staatsbibliothek MS Clm 14706, fols. 11r-18v. AD 1380.

> Inc. Prol.: *Septem sunt sacramenta.*
> Inc. Txt.: *Primum querendum est de baptismo tamquam de digniori.*
> Expl. Txt.: *si forte fuerit consanguinea sua, licet ambo baptizantur, debet eam dimittere.*

This copy contains Version A of the first five sacraments. Section 3, *De eucaristia*, is incomplete, omitting the last 26 questions. Sections 4 and 5 omit some of the materials in *A* and supply others found in *B*. The text is followed immediately by the treatise *Qui uult uere confiteri ad salutem anime sue* attributed to Robert of Sorbon in other manuscripts. The scribe concludes on fol. 22r: *Explicit libellus septem sacramentorum questionibus ... . Deo gloria et honor, conpletus sub anno Domini 1380 in proximo tertia feria post festum natiuitatis Marie, ab Henrico locato.* An incomplete and unascribed copy of William de Montibus's *Peniteas cito peccator* is found on fols. 27r-28v.

11. Oxford, Balliol College MS 228, fols. 220rb-225rb. Early 14th century.

> Title: (*Questiones de sacramentis ecclesie*)
> Inc. Prol.: *Septem sunt sacramenta.*
> Inc. Txt.: *Primo agendum est de baptismo. Queritur autem baptismus.*
> Expl. Txt.: (*De coniugio*) ... *quia illi sunt de una progenie.*

This copy contains sections 1-5 of Version B.

12. Tours, Bibliothèque Municipale MS 473, fols. 196r-198v, 202r-207v, 216v, 217r. 14th century.

> Inc.: *Septem sunt sacramenta.*
> Expl. (in *Coniugio*): ... *quia coacta hoc fecit et non sponte.*

The description is taken from M. Collon, *Catalogue général des manuscrits des bibliothèques publiques de France* (Paris, 1900), 37: 375-378.

13. Troyes, Bibliothèque Municipale MS 1514, fols. 90va-96va. 15th century.

> Inc.: *Septem sacramenta que notantur in isto versiculo.*

The description is taken from Jacques Guy Bougerol, *Les manuscrits franciscains de la Bibliothèque de Troyes* (Rome: Collegii S. Bonaventurae, 1982), p. 203.

14. Utrecht, Bibliotheek der Universiteit MS 387, fols. 50r-52v.

> Inc.: *<B>os ut erat peculans cernentibus obice cursum. Nota quod per hunc versum.*
>
> Ends in *Coniugio.*

The catalogue description by P.A. Tiele, *Catalogus codicum manu scriptorum bibliothecae Universitatis Rheno-Trajectinae* (Utrecht, 1887), 1: 132-133, fails to note that another work has been appended on fols. 53r-59v. This is a work on confession beginning: *Confessio est legitima peccatorum coram proprio sacerdote ... .* The scribe notes correctly on fol. 59v: *Explicit liber de sacramentis ac liber penitenciarum.*

15. Worcester, Cathedral Library MS Q.27, fols. 226v-234v. 14th century.

> Inc.: *Septem sunt sacramenta, que nominantur hoc versiculo.*

The description is from John Kestell Floyer, *Catalogue of Manuscripts Preserved in the Chapter Library of Worcester Cathedral*, ed. and rev. S.G. Hamilton (Oxford: J. Parker, 1906), pp. 121-123.

Excerpts from section 3 are preserved in Cambridge, Trinity College MS B.15.20 (356), a fifteenth-century codex, where they are ascribed to Robert Grosseteste: *Diffinicio eucaristie secundum sanctum Robertum Episcopum Lincolniensem.*[12] A treatise in Vatican Library MS Reg. lat. 440 begins with the same unusual verse that introduces the *De septem sacramentis*: *Bos ut erat petulans cernentibus obice cursum.* In his catalogue of the Vatican manuscripts, Wilmart identified this treatise as the work ascribed to William de Montibus in MS no. 8, above, but it is a quite different work and seems to have no direct relationship to William's authentic writings.[13]

All of the manuscript copies of this treatise preserve late and rather corrupt redactions of the text. Two clear recensions have been pre-

---

[12] See Goering, "*Diffinicio eucaristie*," pp. 91-104.
[13] *Codices Reginenses Latini*, ed. Wilmart, 2: 561-563; cf. Goering, "*Diffinicio eucaristie*," p. 96. The suggestion made in that study that the Vatican treatise might also belong in the canon of William's writings has not been borne out by further study of the texts.

served, probably reflecting the work of two different "reporters" of the original questions. The two versions are represented here by manuscript *A* = Aberdeen, University Library MS 240 (Version A) and manuscript *B* = Baltimore, Walters Art Gallery MS W.131 (Version B).

The prologue and the first section, *De baptismo*, are printed in their entirety. Version A is edited from MS *A*, with emendations from Munich, Bayerische Staatsbibliothek MS Clm 14706 enclosed in angle-brackets < >. Version B is edited from MS *B*, with emendations from Munich, Bayerische Staatsbibliothek MS Clm 8885. Sections 2 to 7 are represented by a numbered list of the questions in each, edited from MSS *A* and *B*, with variant readings given in the footnotes.

De septem sacramentis ecclesie

[Version A]	[Version B]
Aberdeen, University Library MS 240, fols. 194vb-195vb:	Baltimore, Walters Art Gallery MS W.131, fols. 133r-137r:

TRACTATVS DE VII SACRAMENTIS ECCLESIE	DE SEPTEM SACRAMENTIS ECCLESIE

Septem sunt sacramenta ecclesiastica que notantur hoc uersu:

> Bos, ut, erat, petulans, cernentibus, obice, cursum.

Per hanc dictionem *bos* notatur baptismus, per *ut* unctio, per *erat* eucaristia, per *petulans* penitentia siue confessio, per *cernentibus* confirmatio, per *obice* ordo, per *cursum* coniugium.

Septem sunt sacramenta que notantur isto uersiculo:

> Bos, ut, erat, petulans, cernentibus, obice, cursum.

Per hanc dictionem *bos* notatur baptismus; per *ut* unctio, per *erat* eucaristia, per *petulans* penitentia siue confessio, per *cernentibus* confirmatio, per *obice* ordo, per *cursum* coniugium.

<BAPTISMVS>

Primo tractandum est de baptismo tanquam de digniori. Baptismus est caracter impressus anime quo

DE BAPTISMO

Primo agendum est de baptismo.

discernuntur baptizati a non baptizatis.

[1] Queritur in primis quid conferat baptismus. Respondemus
quod delet mortale peccatum quod
contraximus ab Adam.

Set uidetur posse probari quod
nichil confert baptismus, quia nullum sacramentum ualet sine fide,
et puer non habet fidem, ergo
nescit articulos fidei, ergo non
ualet baptismus. Respondemus
quod ualet habitu et non actu. Et
sicut puer habet instrumentum uidendi et palpandi et non potest eis
uti, ita habet fidem et non potest
ea uti.

[2] Sct queritur in qua fide puer
baptizatur <cum non habeat fidem maturam.

Respondemus quod baptizatur in
fide patrinorum. Et si patrini infideles sint, baptizatur> in fide
ecclesie. Et si ibi nullus sit in
mundo christianus, baptizatur in
fide Apostolorum qui precesse-
runt.

Vnde Augustinus: Est fides sementiua et fides germinans et fides
matura. Sementiua, quando puer
defertur ad baptismum, quia cum
baptizatur in eo est fides sementiua
a Spiritu sancto. Fides germinans
est quando puer est quinquennis
uel septennis. Fides matura est

Queritur utrum baptismus conferat gratiam quia delet originale
peccatum, ergo confert gratiam.
Contra: Sine fide non potest aliquis placere Deo, et puer non
habet fidem quia nescit articulos
fidei, ergo baptismus ille non
placet Deo.

Solvtio Respondemus quod confert gratiam illi puero habitu et
non actu. Et sicut puer habet
instrumenta eundi et palpandi et
tamen non potest eis uti, <habet
enim facultatem nondum matu-
ram> sed iuuenculam, similiter
non habet fidem operatiuam, sed
adhuc iuuenculam.

Qvestio Item queritur in qua fide
puer baptizetur, quia non habet
fidem et nulla sacramenta ualent
sine fide, ergo istud non ualet.
Solvtio Dicimus quod baptizatur
sed in fide patrinorum, et si patrini
sunt infideles, dicimus quod in fide
ecclesie. Et si in mundo nullus
christianus in qua fide baptizatur?
Dicimus quod in fide Apostolorum.

Et est fides sementiua, ut in
puero quando baptizatur, germinans quando est quinquennis,
herba quando est septennis, matura quando peruenit ad annos
discretionis.

quando uenit ad annos discretos et scit discernere bonum a malo et econuerso.

[3] Vnde oritur questio: Ponatur quod duo sint pueri quorum unus sit baptizatus alter non, et nescitur utrum istorum sit baptizatus. Queritur utrum debeant baptizari an non. Probatur quod non, quia oporteret quod alter rebaptizetur, et nemo debet rebaptizari.

QVESTIO Item de duobus pueris quorum alter est baptizatus et alter non, sed nescitur quis, queritur utrum ambo debeant rebaptizari. Probatur quod non quia nemo debet rebaptizari. Vnus baptizatus est, ergo oporteret quod rebaptizaretur. Contra: Alter illorum non baptizatus est, ergo baptizari deberet, sed nescitur quis, ergo ambo debent baptizari.

Respondemus: Debent ambo baptizari propter ambiguitatem remouendam.

SOLVTIO Respondemus quod ambo debent baptizari ad remouendum incertitudinem.

[4] QVESTIO Item de puero qui raptus est a paganis uel a iudeis et querit baptismum, et non est qui baptizet, et habet uoluntatem baptizandi, queritur utrum saluetur. SOLVTIO Respondemus quod baptizatus est spiritu; habet enim bonam uoluntatem et bona uoluntas pro facto reputatur.

[5] Item, Ambrosius dicit quod qui male sentit de Trinitate non baptizat, sed malus male sentit de Trinitate, ergo non baptizat. Dicimus quod non baptizat quantum in ipso est, id est quantum ad fidem suam, sed in fide ecclesie. Vnde semper debemus confugere ad bonum sacerdotem.

[6] Queritur utrum baptismum factum a bono sacerdote melior sit

QVESTIO Item queritur utrum magis ualeat baptismus a bono

quam a malo. Respondemus quod sacramenta non possunt deteriorari uel meliorari nec per bonum nec per malum, set tutius est a bono quam a malo.

sacerdote quam a malo. SOLVTIO Respondemus quod sacramenta non possunt deteriorari uel meliorari per bonum sacerdotem uel per malum,[1] sed melius et tutius a bono, et necessitate potest baptizari a malo.

[7] Item queritur si necessitate cogente laycus baptizet proferendo uerba corrupta sic dicendo: "In nomine Patrias et Filias" et cetera. Probatur quod non, quia non sunt uerba sacramenti immo corrupta, ergo non faciunt sacramentum, ergo non baptizat, ergo puer non baptizatur, quod non est uerum. Respondemus sic: Laycus non baptizat set uerba secundum intentionem, quia Deus nouit abscondita cordis.

QVESTIO Item queritur si aliquis baptizet puerum in nomine Patrias et Filias et Spiritusanctias, ita corrupte, utrum baptizet. Si dicatur ita, contra: Iste non facit sacramentum quia non dicit uerba sacrata sed corrupta.

SOLVTIO Dicimus quod baptizat quia habet fidem et intentionem, et Deus nouit abscondita cordium.

[8] Item probatur quod quilibet sacerdos facit maius miraculum quam Petrus uel alius sanctus, quia dicente scriptura "magis est corpus Christi conficere quam mortuum suscitare."

QVESTIO Item uidetur posse probari quod quilibet sacerdos facit maius miraculum quam Petrus quia maius est conficere corpus Christi quam suscitare hominem, et quilibet sacerdos potest conficere uel consecrare corpus Christi, ergo magis facit quam Petrus. SOLVTIO Dicimus quod sacerdos non consecrat, sed uerba consecrata.

Respondemus quod debemus deferre Petro et aliis sanctis, et sacerdos non consecrat set uerba consecrata consecrant.

[9] Item inuenitur in Euangelio [Io 3:5]: "Nisi quis renatus fuerit ex aqua et Spiritu sancto non potest intrare in regnum Dei." Set

ARGVMENTVM Item dicitur in Euuangelio [Io 3:5]: "Nisi quis renatus fuerit ex aqua et Spiritu sancto non potest introire in reg-

---

1 malum] et habet enim facultatem nondum inacutam per malum *add. B*

innocentes non fuerunt renati ex
aqua et Spiritu sancto, ergo non
intrabunt in regnum celorum. Respondemus quod fuerunt baptizati
in sanguine suo, quia uero inuenitur <in legendo sua>: "Non
loquendo set moriendo confessi
sunt," et ita baptizati sunt.[2]

[10] Item queritur de Maria que
nunquam baptizata fuit in aqua
nec in sanguine, ergo non intrabit
in regnum celorum. Solutio: Dicimus quod multiplex est baptismus. Est enim baptismus necessitatis qui fit in patella, et emun-
dationis ut Marie que obumbra-
tione Spiritus sancti baptizata est.
Et est baptismus innocentium qui
fit in sanguine. Et est baptismus
usitatus qui fit in sacris fontibus.

num Dei." Contra: Innocentes non
fuerunt baptizati, ergo non intrabunt in regnum Dei.

SOLVTIO Dicimus quod multiplex
est baptismus — baptismus sanguinis ut innocentium, baptismus
aque ut baptismus usitatus, et est
baptismus necessitatis qui fit in
patella, et est baptismus emunda-
tionis ut Marie, que diuinitus
obumbrata in terris interius et exterius baptizata fuit, quia ipsa est
sedes totius Trinitatis.

[11] ARGVMENTVM Item: "Nisi
quis renatus fuerit" et cetera. Sed
confessio abluit peccata et delet
quo<d>libet peccatum. SOLVTIO
Dicimus quod confessio est actualis et ideo delet quodlibet actuale,
sed non originale quod deletur in
baptismo.

[12] QVESTIO Sed queritur quid
confert confessio ex quo baptismus
delet peccatum. SOLVTIO Dicimus
quod homo, quando est baptizatus, est quasi in archa et euasit
diluuium cum Noe, sed adhuc non
habet nuntium salutis scilicet co-

---

2 *Collecta*, 28 Dec.

lumbam, que defert florem in ore; sed quando confessus est tunc per columbam (id est per confessionem) flos (id est gratia sancti Spiritus) ei confertur.

[13] Item ponatur quod aliqua uilla obsideatur nec possit haberi aqua, et tunc deferatur puer ad sacros fontes, quomodo potest baptizari. Respondemus quod sacra uerba sacerdotis prolata ualebunt cum ceteris usitatis consuetudinibus, et quam cito remoueatur obsidio deferatur ad ecclesiam ut insinuetur ei fides et mergatur in aqua <ter>.

QVESTIO Queritur utrum quis possit baptizari sine aqua, posito quod <obsidiatur in aliquo castro> et ibi non sit aqua nec possit aqua inueniri ut possit baptizari nec baptizatur. SOLVTIO Dicimus quod baptizatur per inuocationem Trinitatis et per sacra uerba ibi memorata, et excusat necessitas[3] quod ibi <deest> ad supplendum misterium.

[14] QVESTIO Item pastores et multi alii faciunt baptismum sine presbitero et episcopo, et baptizant et dicunt in nomine Patris et Filii et Spiritus sancti, Amen. Queritur si ille baptismus ualet. SOLVTIO Dicimus quod ualet, sed insinuanda est fides sancte Trinitatis ei cum tres immersiones sint.

[15] Item queritur quare tres immersiones fiant in baptismo, et utrum baptismus fiat in prima immersione, uel in secunda, uel in tertia. Respondemus sicut cum dico "homo est animal" modo perfecta locutio, et ita nec in prima nec in secunda fit baptismus, set in tertia.

QVESTIO Queritur utrum baptismus fiat immersione prima, uel in secunda, aut in tertia; si in secunda eadem ratione in tertia. SOLVTIO Dicimus quod fit in tertia, sicut cum dico "homo" non dico uerum uel falsum, "est animal" non dico uerum uel falsum, "homo est animal" modo est perfecta oratio et perfectum sensum generat; ita nec in prima nec in secunda sed in tertia perficitur baptismus.

3 necessitas] necessitatis *B*

[16] Item si contingat negligentia sacerdotis quod non fiat nisi una immersio uel bina, queritur si ualeat. Respondemus quod ualet quantum ad puerum non quantum ad sacerdotem.

[17] Item queritur si baptizati ab hereticis debeant rebaptizari. Probatur quod sic. Dicit beatus Gregorius: "Qui male sentit de Trinitate non baptizat," ergo iste non baptizat, ergo baptizati ab hereticis debent rebaptizari.
Contra: Dicit Augustinus:[4] "Baptizatos ab hereticis malis esse rebaptizatos. Set ignauissimum scelus baptizatos a legitimis est rebaptizari." Dicimus tamen quod baptizati ab hereticis non debent rebaptizari, set cum uenerint ad annos discretionis uenire debent ad ecclesiam ut insinuetur eis fides catholica a bono sacerdote.

QVESTIO Queritur utrum baptizatos ab hereticis liceat rebaptizari. Quod probatur: "Qui male sentit de Trinitate non baptizat," ergo hereticus non baptizat, ergo puer debet baptizari.

Contra dicit Augustinus: "Ab infidelibus baptizatos malum est rebaptizari, si a fidelibus baptizatos immanissimum scelus est rebaptizari."

Item probatur quod bonum est baptizatos ab hereticis rebaptizari sicut contingit de confessione. Licet enim bis confiteri si confessio sit insufficiens.
Solutio: Non est simile de confessione et baptismo. Baptismus est caracter impressus anime quo discernuntur baptizati a non baptizatis.

Item licet bis confiteri peccata si confessio insufficiens habeatur, ergo a simili debet fieri de baptismo.

SOLVTIO Dicimus quod non debet rebaptizari, et non est similitudo de confessione, quia in baptismo imprimitur quidam caracter anime quo discernentur in die iudicii baptizati a non baptizatis, set in confessione non.

---

4 Cf. *De cons* D.4 c.108

[18] Queritur quo tempore inuentus fuit baptismus. Respondemus quod eo tempore quo Dominus dixit discipulis [Mt 28:19]: "Ite et docete omnes gentes baptizantes eos in nomine Patris" et cetera.

QVESTIO Queritur quando fuit inuentus primo baptismus. SOLVTIO Dicimus tunc quando Dominus dixit [Mt 28:19]: "Ite, baptizantes eos in nomine Patris et Filii et Spiritus sancti."

[19] Item queritur quare baptismus non habet suum officium sicut missa et euangelium, quia dicitur missa illius et euangelium illius, quare non baptismus illius.

QVESTIO Item queritur utrum baptismus suum proprium habeat sicut euuangelium et sicut missa. Dicitur enim missa illius et euuangelium illius scilicet hominis, et sic de aliis, a simili debet dici baptismus illius.

Respondemus quod non est simile. Missa enim et euangelium constant in prolatione uerborum, baptismus uero in caractere.

SOLVTIO Dicimus quod baptismus non habet suum proprium, et non est similitudo de baptismo et de missa. Missa enim et euuangelium in prolatione uerborum se habent uel consistunt, baptismus autem est impressus caracter anime.

Item puer inundatus aqua non debet iterum mergi, sed tantum inungi crismate.

[20] Item ponatur quod aliquis baptizet puerum et dicat: "In nomine Patris" et statim hoc dicto cadat in extasim et moriatur, et dicat alter: "et Filii et Spiritus sancti." Et tunc queritur utrum ille puer sit baptizatus an non. Si concedatur, contra: Baptizatur ergo ab aliquo uel ab aliquibus, non ab aliquo ergo ab aliquibus, ergo ab illo et ab illo, ergo bis baptizatur. Solutio: Dicimus quod ab istis baptizatur coniunctim, et est ibi compositio dictionis.

QVESTIO Item si contingat quod aliquis sacerdos teneat puerum et dicat: "In nomine Patris," et statim decidat in estasim et moriatur et ueniens alter inueniat eum dicens: "et Filii" et sequentia. Queritur utrum baptizatus sit, et si concedatur, contra: Iste baptizatur, ergo ab aliquo uel aliquibus, non nisi ab aliquibus et non nisi ab istis, ergo ab isto uel ab illo. SOLVTIO Dicimus quod ab istis communiter baptizatur ita quod nec ab isto nec ab illo diuisum uel diuisim.

De confirmatione
(*A* = fol. 195vb; *B* = fols. 137v-138v)

Confirmatio est sacramentum, et iuste[5] dicitur sacramentum quia sacrat mentem. ...

[1] Queritur ergo utrum confirmatio deleat originale peccatum sicut baptismus, uel aliud aliquod peccatum patens. Et certum est quod non delet, ergo uidetur esse superfluum hoc sacramentum.[6]

[2] Item queritur utrum liceat reconfirmare puerum.[7]

[3] Item posito quod sint quatuor pueri quorum duo confirmentur et duo non, set nescitur qui, queritur utrum sint confirmandi aut non.[8]

[4] Item queritur quare non liceat sacerdotibus confirmare sicut baptizare cum baptismus sit dignior confirmatione.

[5] Item quando puer baptizatur imprimitur caracter, set caracter qui est in confirmatione datur in baptismo, unde duo caracteres imprimitur in baptismo.[9]

De evcaristia
(*A* = fols. 195rb-197rb; *B* = fols. 138v-151v)

Eucaristia est tertium sacramentum et dicitur ab "eu" quod est bonum, et "carisma"[10] quod est gratia, quasi bona gratia ... . Eucaristia dicitur angelorum panis ... . Et dicitur manna ... .

[1] Vnde huic sacramento opponunt heretici: Ille panis est corpus Christi, set ille panis incepit esse quando materia data est ex farina et aqua, ergo corpus Christi incipit tunc esse.[11]

[2] Set queritur utrum sit panis qui consecratur an non.[12]

---

5 iuste] iure *B*
6 Queritur ... sacramentum] Set queritur quid confert ex quo in baptismo deletur originale peccatum, in confirmatione(!) uero actuale *A*
7 Item ... puerum *om. A*
8 Item ... non *om. A*
9 Item ... baptismo *om. B*
10 carisma] caristia *A*
11 Vnde ... esse *om. A*
12 Set ... non *om. B*

[3] Queritur si sit corpus Christi an non.[13]

[4] Item uidetur quod tunc incepit esse quando assumpsit humanam carnem,[14] ergo corpus Christi conficitur ex duplici materia.[15]

[5] Queritur de cibo quem Deus comedit post resurrectionem quando comedit partem piscis assati et fauum mellis, quomodo usus est talibus cibariis ex quo corpus Christi erat glorificatum.[16]

[6] Set queritur ab aliquibus quando datum fuit hoc sacramentum.[17]

[7] Set queritur utrum habuerit duo corpora quando eleuatis oculis in celum post agnum misticum panem benedixit dicens, "hoc est corpus meum," et ipse Christus; et corpus Christi passibile esset, et illud corruptibile quod tenebat.[18]

[8] Item ponatur quod aliquis laboret in extremis et accipiat corpus Christi et statim euomat; queritur utrum euomit id quod comedit uel quod non comedit.[19]

[9] Queritur utrum prauus sacerdos inuitandus sit ad celebranda diuina; habes penes te sacerdotem non aptum, est autem longe positus sacerdos castus et adest ebrius.[20]

[10] Item queritur utrum tantum ualeat missa celebrata[21] a malo sacerdote quantum[22] a bono.

[11] Item queritur quomodo conficitur[23] corpus Christi.

[12] Item opponitur de hoc quod dicit Dominus ante passionem in cena discipulis, "hoc est corpus meum," demonstrans panem; ergo habuit duo corpora, unum quod traxit de uirgine et aliud quod erat in pane.[24]

[13] Item queritur quomodo mutatur panis ille in corpus Christi.

---

13 Queritur ... non *om. B*
14 quando ... carnem] quando ipse assumpsit carnem in uentre matris *B*
15 ergo ... materia] ergo fiunt de diuersis materiis *B*
16 Queritur ... glorificatum *om. A*
17 Sed ... sacramentum *om. A*
18 Set ... tenebat *om. A*
19 Item ... comedit *om. B*
20 Queritur ... ebrius *om. A*
21 celebrata] cantata *B*
22 quantum] quam *A*
23 conficitur] per uerba *add. A*
24 Item ... pane *om. A*

[14] Item uidetur quod habeat diuersa corpora, quia in ista ecclesia est et in illa, totum huc et totum illuc.

[15] Item queritur utrum sine aqua liceat missam celebrare[25] causa necessitatis, posito quod aliqua uilla obsidiatur et non habeat aquam.

[16] Item queritur quare iusti et perfecti singulis dominicis accipiunt[26] eucaristiam.

[17] Queritur a quibusdam quare aqua benedicta precedat crucem.[27]

[18] Item queritur si corpus Christi cotidie immolatur.

[19] Item queritur utrum liceat presbitero bis cantare missam in die, sicut ter uel quater baptizare.

[20] Item queritur si corpus Christi frangitur.

[21] Item queritur quid significent tres partes quarum una intingitur uino, due uero remanent in manu sacerdotis.[28]

[22] Item queritur si ex[29] pane fit corpus Christi. Si concedatur, contra: Ergo panis est corpus Christi, set panis non potest esse corpus Christi.

[23] Item queritur si hereticus consecret corpus Christi.

[24] Item queritur utrum sit bonum iusto sumere cotidie eucaristiam, et utrum sit bonum sacerdoti cotidie celebrare missam.

[25] Item queritur de sacerdote uel monacho[30] qui peccat et scit se non posse abstinere a peccato, utrum debeat celebrare missam.

[26] Item queritur utrum sacerdos debeat dare eucaristiam feneratori in die Pasche, et si sciat illum non dimittere peccatum, et querit eucaristiam.

[27] Item queritur de sacerdote suspenso[31] ab episcopo et uadit in alium episcopatum et ibi cantat missam. Consecrat?

---

25 celebrare] cantare *B*
26 accipiunt] accipiant *B*
27 Queritur ... crucem *om. A*
28 Item ... sacerdotis *om. A*
29 ex] in *A*
30 uel monacho] symoniaco *B*
31 suspenso] qui excommunicatus est *B*

[28] Item queritur de scismaticis et hereticis quibus dixit Dominus, "maledicam benedictionibus uestris," et eadem ratione maledictionibus eorum benedicet, ergo uidetur quod uerba eorum habeant efficaciam aliquam, et potius uerba consecrata,[32] ergo uidetur quod possunt consecrare.[33]

[29] Item queritur de feneratore, utrum possit saluari.

[30] Item queritur de meretrice utrum possit facere elemosinam[34] de rebus adquisitis fornicando.

[31] Item queritur de nocturna pollutione, utrum liceat sacerdoti in crastino missam celebrare.

[32] Item queritur utrum nocturna illusio[35] auferat a casto castitatem suam si contingat eum se uidere mulierem formosam[36] et ita[37] ebulliat eius[38] caro.

[33] Item queritur de illis qui ducendo et reducendo tractant uirgam et dicuntur molles, utrum potius debeant fornicari.[39]

[34] Item questio est etiam inter theologos utrum peccata reuiuiscant.[40]

[35] Item dictum est superius quod bonum est iusto cotidie sumere eucaristiam, set dicit Augustinus, "Sumere cotidie eucaristiam nec laudo nec uitupero." Et Augustinus hoc non approbat, ergo non uidetur esse bonum.

[36] Item queritur de mure qui corrodit eucaristiam utrum comedat corpus Christi.[41]

[37] Item queritur si gutta uini sacrata cadat in dolium plenum uino, utrum totum efficiatur sanguis Christi.

[38] Item si musca uel[42] aranea uel aliquid aliud[43] cadat in calicem utrum sit accipienda.

---

32 consecrata] sacramenta *A*
33 consecrare] sacrare *B*
34 facere elemosinam] elemosina prosit meretrici quam facit *A*
35 illusio] pollutio *A*
36 formosam] aliquam *B*
37 ita] intra *B*
38 eius] ei *B*
39 potius ... fornicari] mortaliter peccant *B*
40 Item queritur de feneratore ... reuiuiscant *qq. 30-35 infra, De penitentia, B*
41 utrum ... Christi *om. A*
42 musca uel *om. A*
43 uel aliquid aliud *om. A*

[39] Item queritur quid debeat fieri de corporali si gutta sanguinis[44] cadat super illud.

[40] Item queritur quare dicitur missa.[45]

[41] Item, ob hoc quod dictum est quod nemo debet cantare missam nisi semel in die, opponitur quod in die natiuitatis Domini ter missa celebratur, ergo falsum est quod dictum est superius.

[42] Queritur de aspersione eucaristie,[46] si uinum illud quod funditur in calicem post consecrationem fit eucaristia.

[43] Item queritur utrum frangat ieiunium uel non, posito quod sacerdos uouerit non bibere uinum, quia ibi nulla[47] est transubstantio cum non[48] transit in corpus.

[44] Item queritur utrum aqua que exiuit de latere Christi cum sanguine[49] sit sacramentum.

[45] Item queritur de pane ordeaceo utrum possit consecrari in eucaristiam causa necessitatis.

[46] Item queritur si ibi sint tria grana frumenti et quatuor ordei et ex illis fiat eucaristia si transubstantio sit ex illa parte et non ex uel in alia.[50]

[47] Item queritur utrum de frumento[51] uel de uino cui admiscetur species aromatica uel[52] herbe, utrum liceat inde facere[53] sacramentum.

DE PENITENTIA
(A = fols. 197rb-198vb; B = fols. 151v-165v)

Penitentia est maximum sacramentum et necessarium. Ait enim Ieronimus, "Penitentia est secunda tabula post naufragium" ... .

[1]   Set queritur quare potius datur septennis penitentia quam alia.

---

44 sanguinis] uini B
45 Item ... missa om. B
46 de aspersione eucaristie om. A
47 nulla om. A
48 cum non] nec B
49 latere ... sanguine] corpore Christi A
50 Item ... alia om. A
51 frumento] pigmento B
52 aromatica uel om. A
53 inde facere] fieri B

[2]   Item queritur si aliquis habeat rem cum uxore fratris sui utrum debeat dimittere[54] uxorem suam.

[3]   Item queritur de sacerdote feneratore, quid debeat fieri de eo, et quomodo possit sanari.[55]

[4]   Quidam dicunt quod confessio cordis sufficit ad salutem anime, et hoc probant per istas auctoritates ... .

[5]   Item queritur utrum confessio oris ualeat, posito quod aliquis accedat ficte ad sacerdotem.

[6]   Item queritur utrum confessio cordis saluet hominem, posito quod sit in articulo mortis et non possit habere sacerdotem.

[7]   Item queritur utrum aliquis possit esse saluus sola confessione sine baptismo.

[8]   Item dictum est superius quod pena decennalis debet iniungi presbitero[56] pro sola fornicatione siue usura. Set queritur si fecerit tres fornicationes triginta anni debeant ei iniungi.

[9]   Item queritur quid confert illa confessio que fit ante missam et ad primam in quibusdam ecclesiis.

[10]   Item queritur de elemosina que fit in mortali peccato. Dicitur superius quod non ualet.

[11]   Item queritur de confessione que fit in articulo mortis; probo quod non ualet.

[12]   Item uidetur posse probari quod sit Deus iniustus quia pro sola fornicatione, licet in tota uita sancte et[57] iuste uixerit, dampnat hominem[58] eternaliter.

[13]   Item queritur de prauo sacerdote et indiscreto utrum possit dare penitentiam.

[14]   Item queritur de illo cui iniuncta est penitentia et non peracto termino moritur utrum residuum peragat in alio seculo, qui adhuc si uiueret peniteret, ergo preuentus mortis uidetur eum excusare.[59]

---

54 dimittere] desinere *B*
55 sanari] saluari *A*
56 debet ... presbitero] debetur *A*
57 sancte et] sua *A*
58 dampnat hominem] dampnetur *A*
59 Item ... excusare *om. A*

[15] Item queritur si ei qui moritur debeat dari[60] penitentia.

[16] Item queritur utrum fornicatio cuiusdam sapientis sit maius peccatum quam adulterium rudis.[61]

[17] Item queritur utrum peccatum quod fecit aliquis iustus[62] qui numquam peccauit sit maius[63] illo peccato quod aliquis iterat post confessionem.

[18] Item queritur utrum pro excommunicato sit orandum, posito quod eat ad ecclesiam ut absoluatur et post moriatur; et si illius elemosina debeat accipi.

DE CONIVGIO

A = fols. 198vb-199ra; B = fols. 165v-171r)

Cum baptismus dignum sit sacramentum et eucaristia, tamen coniugium dignissimum dicitur quia prius[64] inuentum fuit. ...

[1]   Vnde queritur de quodam casu qui in temporibus nostris accidit.[65] Discordia erat inter duos principes; uoluerunt ergo terminare discordiam[66] per filiam unius eorum quam uoluit alter eorum copulare filio alterius principis ut pax fieret et concordia.[67] Set puella uouerat Deo castitatem et illa sic discordabat a proposito patris sui.[68] Tunc pater iratus prostrauit eam et dixit ei quod in patibulo statueret eam, unde ipsa uidens pudorem nimium sibi munere nupsit iuxta uelle patris sui filio principis.[69] Queritur utrum legitimum fuerit matrimonium.

[2]   Queritur ergo utrum diuortium possit celebrari.

[3]   Vltimo queritur quare[70] coniugium sit indissolubile.

---

60 dari] septennis *add. B*

61 Item ... rudis] Item, quanto enim aliquis magis sapiens et prudens est tanto maius est peccatum illius, unde grauius peccant archiepiscopi quam episcopi et sic de aliis secundum ordinem. Vnde soluitur questio que solet fieri de Adam, quomodo ex solo morsu pomi tam grauiter peccauit *A*

62 aliquis iustus] rusticus *B*

63 sit maius] si iniustus *A*

64 prius] primo *B*

65 de ... accidit] hoc quod contingit *A*

66 terminare discordiam] pacificari *A*

67 per ... concordia] coniungendo filium unius filie alterius in coniugio *A*

68 illa ... sui] non fauebat patri *A*

69 Tunc ... principis] Set patre minas inferente tandem adquieuit ei *A*

70 quare] utrum *A*

[4]   Item queritur si contingat quod aliquis rex habeat duas filias et
      promittat maiorem alio regi et det ei minorem natu, utrum possit
      eam dimittere.[71] Certum est quod licet ei dimittere eam quia ipse
      non assensit ei et non est matrimonium nisi ibi sit assensus
      utriusque,[72] set queritur utrum possit aliam ducere in uxorem.

[5]   Item queritur de eo qui habuit rem cum sorore uxoris sue[73] utrum
      debeat rem habere cum uxore sua deinceps.

[6]   Item queritur de illis quorum unus dixit alii, sine iuramento, se
      nubere insimul, postea unus eorum uult resilire a primo proposito;
      queritur utrum liceat resilire.[74]

[7]   Item difficilior est questio utrum ille qui promiserit, interposita
      religione sacramenti, debeat tenere; et queritur utrum illud sit
      coniugium et utrum possit stare quia uerba sunt de futuro.[75]

[8]   Item queritur de illo qui ficte[76] iurat alicui se nupturum utrum
      coniugium sit tenendum.

[*explicit A*]

[9]   Set queritur si pater alicuius puelle cogat filiam suam ad nubendum
      alicui uiro, illa quantum potest respuit, utrum coniugium istud
      sit tenendum.

[10] Queritur ergo si aliquis accipiat uxorem de causis approbatis
      utrum sit coniugium legitimum.

[11] Item queritur de Ioseph et Maria, quia ibi non fuit spes sobolis
      nec remedium fornicationis.

[12] Item queritur utrum liceat alicui ducere concubinam, etiam illam
      quam polluit adulterio.

[13] Item queritur utrum liceat alicui ducere seruam; uel si ipse duxerit
      eam queritur utrum disiungi liceat.

[14] Item queritur si coniugium possit celebrari inter infideles.

[15] Set queritur utrum fidelis possit accipere infidelem putans eam
      esse fidelem.

71 dimittere] relinquere *A*
72 Certum ... utriusque] certum est quod non consensit ei *A*
73 sorore ... sue] uxore fratris sui *A*
74 Item ... resilire *om. A*
75 Item ... futuro *om. A*
76 ficte] stricte *A*

[16] Item queritur de iudeo et iudea utrum possit dimittere quia uult baptizari.

[17] Notande sunt cause quare prohibuit lex quod aliquis non capiat consanguineam suam.

DE ORDINIBVS
(*om. A*; *B* = fols. 171r-174r)

Vltimum sacramentum est de septem ordinibus qui sunt septem gradus per quos clericus efficitur: hostiarius, lector, exorcista, acolitus, sub-diaconus, diaconus, sacerdos. Primus gradus est hostiarius cuius est discernere quos ab ecclesia iuste repellat et quos digne recipiat ... [*sine quaestionibus*].

DE EXTREMA VNCTIONE
(*om. A*; *B* = fols. 174r-174v)

Queritur de sacramento extreme unctionis, et dicitur hoc sacramentum morientium.

[1]   Queritur ad quid est.

[2]   Item queritur quid sit materia huius sacramenti et que forma.

[3]   Item queritur utrum istud sacramentum sit iterabile.

[4]   Set queritur a quibus confertur hoc sacramentum.

[5]   Item queritur quare fit in forma deprecatiua. Respondeo quia in hoc sacramento fit remissio peccatorum per orationem et ideo debet esse uel fieri in forma deprecatiua.

II.14

Super Psalmos

William seems to have published none of his own lectures on the Bible. We infer from his thorough knowledge of the Bible and its various glosses that lectures on Scripture were a staple of his school, but it is only in this student *reportatio* that evidence of these lectures has survived. The student reporter, Samuel Priest (*Presbyter*), also recorded a number of scholastic exercises from William's school; these are described in the next chapter (*Collecta*). Here he gives us a valuable glimpse of William's classroom lectures on the Bible, and reveals something of the qualities that made him a famous and respected teacher.

These lectures are important not only because they provide a glimpse into William's actual classroom teaching, but also because they represent a type of commentary that, although soon to fall out of favour, was widespread around the beginning of the thirteenth century. More than a simple gloss or exposition (*postilla*) of the biblical texts, these lectures comprise a kind of theological *summa*. By elaborating in distinction-form the various meanings that a word in the Psalms might bear in theological discourse, William introduces the major concepts of medieval theology. (See the *distinctiones* on the words *resurrectio, consilio/concilio, iudicium*, and *noscere*, and on the similitudes or metaphors *puluis*, and *terra*, below).

William takes care to expound the historical and "mystical" context of each Psalm, and to interpret the literal meaning of the verses. Here he has frequent recourse to the principles developed in his *Tropi*. For example he explains that Psalm 16:1, *Exaudi Domine*, is a figure of speech: "Similis tropus loquendi est ibi: Ihesus proficiebat sapientia, id est uidebatur proficere" (fol. 23ra). But he is seldom constrained by the Psalm text itself, and discourses at length on such theological and pastoral topics as: the limits of philosophical knowledge (11ra), the causes of the incarnation (18rb), the nature of the preaching office (29ra-30ra), the eucharist (33ra), grace and free choice (37va-b), the relation of logical and theological truth (55va, etc.), the nature of the virtues (82rb), and the question of whether one can merit salvation (88vb).[1]

Occasionally topics for later classroom disputation are identified, as in the exposition on the Last Judgement in Psalm 1: "Dubitant an uerbo proferetur sententia, an in conscientiis fiet manifesta absque uerbo." Often such questions are taken up immediately, as in Psalm 26, in a discussion of sacramental unction: "Potest hic queri quare Dauid post primam inunctionem iterum inunctus fuerit, quia uidetur quod iniuria facta fuerit priori sacramentali unctioni; et queri potest si plenius collata est spiritualis gratia per secundam unctionem. Queri etiam potest si sacerdos in ueteri testamento debet iterum inungi sicut sacerdos in nouo testamento ..." (39vb).

It is perhaps misleading to consider these lectures in the context of biblical exegesis as represented by Andrew of St. Victor, Stephen Langton, and the thirteenth-century Friars.[2] William's commentary is at once less orderly and more wide ranging. It resembles most nearly in style and content the *Distinctiones* on the Psalms by Peter of Poitiers,[3] and the *Summa super Psalterium* of Praepositinus,[4] both written at the end of the twelfth century. The writings of Peter Comestor and Peter the Chanter on the Psalms have yet to receive careful attention, but Smalley's general remarks concerning them are appropriate for William's lectures as well: "The Comestor and the Chanter represent an earlier and less differentiated state .... . They do not limit themselves to questions relevant to the text and the *Gloss*, as Langton does, but discuss much more general topics."[5] A careful investigation of the commentaries written between 1170 and 1230 may well reveal that this "less differentiated" state of affairs continued well into the thirteenth century,[6] and that William's lectures are representative of a general attempt to find a suitable vehicle for systematizing theological teaching. By the mid thirteenth century clear distinctions would be

---

[1] This last discussion contains the observation: "Magister Gilebertus dixit quod nullus meretur uitam eternam, et dixit mala merita esse signum et uiam et causam ad dampnationem, et bona merita esse signum et uiam non causam ad uitam eternam, nisi accipiatur 'causa' pro 'causa sine qua non.'" The reference apparently is to Gilbert of Poitiers.

[2] This context is portrayed brilliantly by Beryl Smalley, *Study of the Bible*, chapters Five and Six.

[3] See Moore, *Works of Peter of Poitiers*.

[4] See Lacombe, *La vie et les oeuvres de Prévostin*.

[5] Smalley, *Study of the Bible*, p. 212.

[6] See Smalley's brief comments on the "uncharted territory" between 1206 and 1230, ibid., pp. 264-268.

drawn between lecturing on the books of the Bible and lecturing, systematically, on theology. In the absence of a consensus, in the twelfth and early thirteenth century, on the best way to summarize and systematize theological knowledge, biblical commentaries like this one served both as a gloss and as a rudimentary *summa theologiae*.

AUTHENTICITY AND DATE

The inscription of the work in the only surviving manuscript, "Hec collecta sunt ex auditis super Psalmos in scola magistri Willelmi de Montibus," is unusually informative. It suggests that this commentary on the Psalms comes from William's actual classroom lectures. A study of the contents of the lectures reveals many similarities to William's other authentic works, especially the *Distinctiones*, the *Similitudinarium*, and the *Tropi*.

Although the student-collector fails to identify himself in this part of the manuscript and in the collection "ex diversis auditis in scola magistri Willelmi de Montibus" that follows immediately (fols. 94r-107v; see below, *Collecta*), a third collection, on fols. 108r-206v, bears his name. It begins, like the two preceding texts: "Hec collecta sunt ad habendam memoriam quorundam utilium in sacra scriptura, et eorum quedam sumpta sunt a uerbis expositionum ewangeliorum, et quedam ab ipsis uerbis ewangelicis, et quedam ab aliis uerbis neccesariis ad salutem anime; et hec composita sunt post dicessum a scola." This collection ends on fol. 206v with the words "Expliciunt collecta Samuelis Presbiteri." Unfortunately this Samuel, a student in William's school, eludes further identification.[7] His extant writings were originally preserved in the library of Bury St. Edmunds in England.[8] The surname "Presbyter" or "Priest," although unusual, is found with some frequency in the city of Lincoln (see above, Chapter One), so it may be postulated that Samuel attended William's lectures in Lincoln rather than in Paris. A casual reference in the text to the British Isles and the British language helps to confirm this assumption.[9] No evidence suggests a particular

---

[7] See Russell, *Dictionary of Writers of Thirteenth Century England*, p. 147, under "Samuel Presbyter."

[8] Ibid.

[9] "Patet quod loquitur ecclesia quia quis posset clamare a finibus terre [Ps 60:3] ut ecclesia que est diffusa per orbem terrarum set clamat ab extremis terre et ab insulis. Vnde dicit super hunc locum: Iam lingua britanie que nihil nouit nisi barbarum fremitum, resonat Hebreum alfabetum," fol. 59rb.

date within the period c. 1186-1213, when these lectures on the Psalms were delivered.

SOURCES

In addition to the Bible and to both the Hebrew and the Roman versions of the Psalms, explicit references are made to Ambrose, Anselm, Aristotle, Augustine, Boethius, Cassiodorus, Claudius, Gregory, Isidore, Jerome, Lucan, Methodius, Origen, Ovid (*Poeta*), Plato, Seneca (*Philosophus*), Tyconius, Virgil, and masters Peter Lombard and Gilbert. The *legenda* of Sts. Agatha, Agnes, Katherine, and Martin are also invoked, as are various hymns and other liturgical sources. The *Glossa ordinaria* is never cited as such, although some of the authorities listed above are quoted from it.

MANUSCRIPT

Oxford, Bodleian Library MS Bodley 860 (sc 2723), fols. 9ra-93vb. Early 13th century (above top line).

    Title: *Hec collecta sunt ex auditis super Psalmos in scola magistri Willelmi de Montibus.*
    Inc.: "*Non sic impii.*" *Dicendo bis non sic.*
    Expl.: *Ecclesia semper est.*

The text is incomplete at beginning and end. It begins with Psalm 1:4, omitting what may have been an introductory sermon or lecture on the first three verses of the Psalm. It breaks off in the commentary on Psalm 87:16, at the end of a gathering. The catchwords *inter malleum et incudem*, at the bottom of fol 93v, indicate that the text originally continued on one or more quires. On folio 53ra, the text breaks off in the commentary on Psalm 33:10. The remainder of fol. 53 is blank, and the text resumes on fol. 54ra with Psalm 55. A partial index to this work, in a fourteenth-century hand, is found on fols. 207-208.

    The transcription that follows, from fol. 9ra-b of the unique manuscript, displays the salient characteristics of the commentary. A full and accurate summary is impossible here; the text deserves to be studied in its entirety.

Super Psalmos

Hec collecta sunt ex auditis super Psalmos in scola magistri Willelmi de Montibus.

<PSALMVS 1:4-6>

Non sic impii. Dicendo bis non sic duo superius attributa beato, scilicet esse immunem ab omni malo, plenum omni bono, remouet ab impio; tertium non remouet — esse utilem proximo — quia impius uiuit iusto. Quod fornax auro, quod lima ferro, quod flamma tibi, hoc tribulatio iusto.

Set tanquam puluis, scilicet aridi, carentes humore gratie. Puluis quandoque notat ariditatem, ut hic; quandoque ueniale peccatum: Excutite puluerem de pedibus uestris [Mt 10:14]; quandoque humilitatem: Ego qui pulvis sim et cinis clamo ad te [cf. Gen 18:27].

Quem proicit uentus, id est sugestio diaboli, uel superbia, *a facie terre*. Terra dicitur elementum siue elementatum. Vnde dicitur solum quasi solidum, et dicitur: Terra stat in eternum [Eccl 1:4], scilicet quoad substantiam, non quoad formam; et dicitur: Transiet sicut celum, [cf. Mt 25:35], scilicet quoad formam, non quoad substantiam.

Et dicitur terra ecclesia militans: Ce. a. t. li.

Et dicitur ecclesia triumphans: Credo uidere bona Domini in terra uiuentium [Ps 26:13].

Proiciuntur impii a presentia stabilitatis quia instabiles sunt, et a presentia ecclesie militantis, et a presentia stabilitatis eterne, scilicet eterne beatitudinis.

Ideo non resurgent. Est resurrectio anime a morte, scilicet a mortali peccato. Vnde dicitur: Surge a mortuis qui dormis, et illuminabit te Christus [Eph 5:14].

Est resurrectio generalis, scilicet corporum in die iudicii. Vnde dicitur: Omnes quidem resurgemus [1 Cor 15:51].

Non resurgent impii in iudicio. Vnde iudicent se, et ita actiue legitur iudicio. Boni iudicant se. Vnde Paulus: Quod si nos iudicaremus non utique diiudicaremur [1 Cor 11:31].

Neque peccatores in consilio iustorum, id est in iudicio, quod dicitur consilium, quia discrete et consulte fit.

Vel sic, consilium iustorum est non consentire proprie uoluntati set uoluntati Christi. Vnde Dominus dixit Petro: Vade retro sathana [Mc 8:33], id est noli consentire proprie uoluntati. In tali consilio non resurgunt peccatores, quia consentiunt propriis uoluntatibus.

Vel potest dici *in concilio iustorum,* id est in concordi multitudine iustorum. Constituunt differentiam inter impios et peccatores dicentes impios aduersantes pietati, scilicet diuino cultui, et in compositione est aduersatiua. Peccata dicunt falsos christianos qui recesserunt a fide. Infideles non resurgent die nouissimo. In iudicio scilicet <non> iudicentur, quia iam iudicati sunt. Vnde Dominus ait: Qui non crediderit iam iudicatus est [Io 3:18].

Quidam iudicabunt et non iudicabuntur, ut sancti electi.

Quidam nec iudicabunt nec iudicabuntur, ut infideles.

Eorum qui iudicabuntur: Quidam iudicabuntur et saluabuntur, ut mediocriter boni. Quidam iudicabuntur et dampnabuntur, ut mali christiani.

Est iudicium auctoritatis, quod conuenit toti Trinitati.

Est iudicium amministrationis, quod conuenit soli Filio. Vnde illud: Omne iudicium dedit Filio [Io 5:22], quia persona Filii apparebit in die iudicii et proferet sententiam: Esuriui etc. [Mt 25:35, 42]. (Dubitant an verbo proferetur sententia, an in conscientiis fiet manifesta absque uerbo.)

Est iudicium confirmationis, quod conueniet sanctis. Sancti iudicabunt altiori sessione. Vnde illud: Sedebitis super sedes duodecim, etc. [Mt 19:28]. Iudicabunt maiori cause cognitione, quia magis aliis cognoscent quare unus ad uitam predestinatus fuerit, alter ad mortem prescitus. Et iudicabunt sentente confirmatione, unde illud: Vt faciant in eis iudicium conscriptum, etc. Qui conscribunt post datam sententiam quodammodo confirmant. Sancti confirmabunt sententiam quia assessorum est confirmare sententiam iudicis. Quidam etiam iudicabunt die iudicii comparatione minoris mali.

Quoniam nouit Dominus. Deus dicitur quandoque noscere uel scire per cognitionem comprehensiuam et plenariam, non per enigmaticam ut nos. Quandoque per experientiam, ut nouit que sunt in homine, scilicet famem et sitim, per experientiam. Quandoque per efficientiam, unde dicit ad Abraham: Nunc cognoui quod timeas Deum [Gen 22:12], id est feci scire. Et alibi de die iudicii: Neque sancti neque angeli sciunt, neque filius scit [Mt 24:36], id est non facit scire, et hoc utiliter.

Quandoque noscere uel scire dicitur approbare, ut hic: *quoniam nouit Dominus uiam iustorum*; et alibi: Nouit qui sunt eius [2 Tim 2:19]; et alibi: Nescio uos [Mt 25:12].

Et iter impiorum peribit, ubi uidentur debere dicere: non nouit uiam impiorum, dicit equipollens, scilicet iter impiorum peribit.

<PSALMVS SECVNDVS>

Quare fremuerunt gentes. Hec distinctio dicitur Psalmus Dauid, et potest legi sub persona Dauid uel persona Christi, quia Christus potest dici Dauid, id est manu fortis, quia uicit forti manu, non armata set clauis confixa, non in equo residens, set in cruce pendens; uel Dauid, id est aspectu desiderabilis, quia ipse est in quem desiderant angeli prospicere, id est desiderabiliter prospiciunt.

Psalmus dicebatur modulatio que fiebat ante arcam federis Domini cum psalterio, et transumitur ad appellandum tractatus qui modulabantur cum psalterio, sicut pertica terre dicitur quia pertica mensuratur, funiculus terre quia funiculo mensuratur.

Hec distinctio monet ad bene operandum pro superna mercede per psalterium. Psalterium resonat tactu manuum, in quo designatur operatio, et resonat a superiori, in quo designatur superna merces. Dauid uel Christus dicit:

Quare fremuerunt gentes, id est gentiles fremuerunt fremitu fremitatis, sicut fere. Est et fremitus pietatis, ut ibi: Ihesus fremuit spiritu [cf. Mc 14:5; Io 11:38].

Et populi, id est multi, uel ciues Ierosolimitani, scilicet Iudei.

Meditati sunt inania, scilicet detinere Christum in morte; uel expectantes Messiam cum asinina tarditate, stolida, sicut duo ministri Abrahe expectabant cum asino, quando Abraham debuit immolare [Gen 22:3] ... .

II.15

Collecta

This collection of "diverse sayings" (*de diuersis auditis*) from William's school, made by Samuel Priest (Presbyter), offers a unique insight into the educational milieu from which it derives. The "sayings" are, in fact, glossed mnemonic verses on many different topics of theological and moral interest. They summarize and repeat many of the doctrines found in William's writings and in the lectures on the Psalms that Samuel reported earlier in this same manuscript. The occasions for these sayings are unspecified, but they would seem to derive from *collationes* or *repetitiones*, possibly held later in the day or in the evenings, that served to reinforce the teachings conveyed in William's more formal lectures and disputations.

Although other *reportationes* of formal lectures by medieval scholastics have survived from the schools of Paris and from the thirteenth-century universities, this is a rare example of the teaching practice at a cathedral school. Even more unusual, this collection of diverse materials from William's school appears to be a report of something other than the formal lectures on the set books of the medieval curriculum. We know from other sources that William lectured on the Psalms,[1] perhaps on the Gospels, and probably on other books of Scripture. He also provided his students with a number of works for extracurricular study. But in this *Collecta* Samuel preserves evidence for a kind of teaching that falls outside the bounds of the scholastic activities as they are usually defined, i.e. lecturing (on set texts), disputing, and preaching.

William himself may provide a clue to the nature of the exercises that are collected here by Samuel Presbyter. Under the rubric DOCTRINA in his *Versarius* William includes the couplet:

Lectio non modicus set plus collatio prebet,
Hiis opus adiungas ut mage proficias.

---

[1] See above, *Super Psalmos*.

He is addressing, here, the students in his school and reminding them that, while the lectures are important, *collationes* offer even more. The nature of such scholastic "collations" is elusive, and the term is used in a number of different contexts by medieval writers, but there can be little doubt that they formed an important part of the curriculum in many medieval schools.[2] It is quite possible that many of the collections of *notulae*, *sententiae*, and other *dicta* that survive in innumerable medieval manuscripts derive from records of informal *collationes* in the schools.[3] That brief mnemonic poems might serve as the basis or "text" for such collations can also be inferred from the twelfth-century evidence. When John of Salisbury wished to praise Bernard of Chartres as an outstanding teacher, he did so by quoting examples of his verse and describing his method of teaching in a way that brings to mind the verses and teachings found in Samuel's *Collecta*.[4]

If these poems and glosses may be understood, at least provisionally, as records of William's scholastic collations, what do they tell us about the form and content of such exercises? First, they make clear the sense in which *collationes* are to be identified with *repetitiones*. Many of the teachings that are expounded in William's lectures on the Psalms are taken up again in this *Collecta*. Since both works are copied together in this codex by William's student, it may be inferred that they are reports of Samuel's work during a single academic term. We might imagine Samuel recording William's formal exposition of the Psalms, and then attending his collations where the master would reiterate, in a less formal way, the same doctrines or others that he feels are of special import to his students.

Second, this record of a classroom exercise built around mnemonic verses helps to provide a meaningful context in which to place the thousands of such poems that were collected by William de Montibus in his *Versarius*, *Peniteas cito*, and *Tractatus metricus*, and that so impressed his students and contemporaries.[5] William, after all, won

---

[2] See G. Paré, et al., *La renaissance du XIIe siècle*, pp. 123-124; Glorieux, "L'enseignement au moyen âge," pp. 120-122, 156-157.

[3] See Beryl Smalley's comments on Hugh of St. Victor's *Notulae*, in *Study of the Bible*, pp. 85-86, 97-106.

[4] *Metalogicon* 1.24, 4.35, ed. Clement C.J. Webb (Oxford: Clarendon Press, 1929), pp. 55-56, 205-206; *Policraticus* 7.13, ed. Webb (Oxford: Clarendon Press, 1909), 2:145. Cf. Paul Edward Dutton, "The Uncovering of the *Glosae super Platonem* of Bernard of Chartres," *Mediaeval Studies* 46 (1984) 192-195.

[5] The most notable being William's student, Richard of Wetheringsett, whose *Summa Qui bene presunt* is filled with such verses.

his fame as a teacher rather than as a literary poet, but no plausible explanation for the usefulness of such verses in teaching has been proposed heretofore.

Finally, the range of topics suggested by the rubrics and the poems indicates clearly the interests of the teacher and, presumably, of the students in a cathedral school around the beginning of the thirteenth century. These topics give concrete expression to the common but indistinct notion of a "biblical-moral school" of theological education that flourished during these years.[6] They range from rather abstract discussions of the relation of grace to free choice (no. 1), sacramental theology (no. 36), and the nature of apostolic poverty (no. 42), to practical questions concerning vows (nos. 7, 18, 54) and marital relations (no. 17). Many take the form of biblical exegesis (e.g. nos. 2-6, all based on the scriptural accounts of Abraham). Nearly all of the expositions touch on the moral qualities of the Christian life as well as on the specific qualities required of the monk (no. 21), the preacher (nos. 23, 38), the confessor (nos. 5, 12), and the priest (nos. 2, 4, 16).

Although Samuel has collected here a mere fragment of William's teachings, he provides us with a unique opportunity to put William's literary compositions into their proper context — the theological classroom. Because teaching is an ephemeral art it is understandable that historians should tend to judge medieval scholastics as authors rather than as teachers; as authors they leave discernable traces in their books. In this record of William's teaching, however, we can see how his major literary productions, the *Versarius*, *Distinctiones*, *Similitudinarium*, and others, were composed in the service of the classroom. One might well be puzzled by their (lack of) form or their seeming incoherence when studied in their own right, but from the perspective of William's classroom teaching the practical usefulness of didactic verses — and of the *distinctio*, the *similitudo*, and the proverb as means of explicating them — is readily apparent.

AUTHENTICITY AND DATE

The manuscript containing this work appears to have been written by Samuel himself; it also contains a *reportatio* of William's lectures on the Psalms (see above, *Super Psalmos*), and another collection of

---

[6] See above, Chapter Two.

verses that Samuel composed after leaving the schools.[7] It was suggested above that Samuel attended William's school at Lincoln rather than at Paris, but no further precision concerning the date of this composition is yet possible.

If there were any doubts concerning the veracity of Samuel's inscription — "Hec collecta sunt ex diuersis auditis in scola magistri Willelmi de Montibus" — they are removed by the numerous similarities in style and content to William's other writings. Six of the poems reported here are also found in William's *Versarius*, and the style of commenting on brief mnemonic verses is typical of his writings. Several of the longer glosses of the *Collecta* are nearly verbatim repetitions of texts in William's exposition of the Psalms, reported earlier in the same manuscript.[8] Similarities to other works, especially the *Numerale*, *Distinctiones*, *Tropi*, *Similitudinarium*, *Prouerbia*, and the *Peniteas cito*, also abound in the glosses, although it is difficult to know whether these other collections were already made when Samuel heard William's lectures or whether they were composed later as the fruits of his lecturing.

SOURCES

Other than the Bible, very few authorities are adduced in the *Collecta*. The sources that underlay William's teachings here are the same that inform his more formal treatises, especially the *Numerale*, the *Distinctiones*, and the *Versarius*. None of the poems has been identified as the work of another author. As noted above, six of the poems

---

[7] "Hec collecta sunt ad habendam memoriam quorundam utilium in sacra scriptura, et eorum quedam sumpta sunt a uerbis expositionum ewangeliorum, et quedam ab ipsis uerbis ewangelicis, et quedam ab aliis uerbis necessariis ad salutem anime; et hec composita sunt post dicessum a scola. IN HIS MONEMVR SECTARI HVMILITATEM, ET NON DEDIGNARI PROXIMOS LICET SINT MISERI, SET EIS SVBVENIRE ALIQVA CVRA QVE PROSIT EIS. Leprosum tetigit Christus sic omnia munda/ ... ," fol. 108r.

Another of Samuel's collections is found in MS 115 of Pembroke College, Cambridge: *Collecta Samuelis presbyteri ex speculo Beati Gregorii*; cf. Russell, *Dictionary of Writers of Thirteenth Century England*, p. 147.

[8] The gloss to line 3 of the first poem, printed below, concerning grace and free choice, is based on the exposition of Psalm 24 in the *Super Psalmos*: "Dicit tamen leuaui pro libero arbitrio quod cooperatur gratie. Quedam auctoritates attribuunt totum gratie Dei, et hoc est contra Pelagianos qui dicunt liberum arbitrium sufficere absque gratia. Quedam attribuunt totum libero arbitrio, quod est contra pigros qui reputant gratia conferri bonum absque illorum conamine. Quedam auctoritates partiuntur, et quedam attribuunt gratie Dei, quedam libero arbitrio, unde Paulus ait: 'Non ego set gratia Dei mecum; Dei enim adiutores sumus.' Set licet liberum arbitrium cooperetur gratie, tamen gratia preuenit et in ea est principalitas," MS Bodley 860, fol. 37va-b.

are found in William's *Versarius*; only the first poem is listed by Walther, and it is cited from this manuscript.[9]

MANUSCRIPT

Oxford, Bodleian Library MS Bodley 860, fols. 94r-107v. Early 13th century (above top line).

> Title: *Hec collecta sunt ex diuersis auditis in scola magistri Willelmi de Mont'.*
> Inc. Gloss: *Duo necessaria sunt ad hoc*
> Inc. Txt.: (*In his primis ostenditur quod liberum arbitrium cooperatur ratione*) *Nulli cernentur*
> Expl. Gloss: *fidelitate, acceleratione, caritate*
> Expl. Txt.: *Redditioque notent circum ue ho de mo ca ue fac*

The following extracts are transcribed from the unique manuscript copy. The first topic, *Quod liberum arbitrium cooperatur gratie*, is transcribed in its entirety; it consists of four lines of verse and an interlinear gloss (written above the line of verse being glossed). Subsequent sections are represented by the topical rubric, and by the first line of verse in that section. The number printed within square brackets [ ] after the first line of verse indicates the total number of verses in the "poem." Where the section includes only two verses, both have been printed.

Collecta

Hec collecta sunt ex diuersis auditis in scolis magistri Willelmi de Montibus.

1 IN HIS PRIMIS OSTENDITVR QVOD LIBERVM ARBITRIVM COOPERATVR GRATIE

Nulli cernentur oculis que subicientur
> Duo necessaria sunt ad hoc ut aliquid uideatur usu corporeo: claritas exterior et uisus interior.

---

[9] Hans Walther, *Initia*, no. 12376.

Ni lux exterior assit et interior

> lux interior, id est uisus interior.

Nulli cernentur celestia ni socientur

> Ad hoc quod aliquis uideat spiritualia oportet quod duo concurrant, gratia Dei et bona uoluntas. Vnde in Psalmo [15:1] dicitur: "Conserua me Domine quoniam speraui in te," id est serua me inesse. Per hoc notatur quod liberum arbitrium cooperatur gratie. Etiam notandum quod quedam auctoritates attribuunt totum gratie Dei, et hoc contra Pelagianos qui dicunt liberum arbitrium sufficere absque gratia ad meritum uite eterne. Quedam auctoritates attribuunt totum libero arbitrio, et hoc contra pigros qui reputant gratia conferri bonum absque libero arbitrio et illorum conamine. Quedam auctoritates partiuntur, et attribuunt partem gratie partem libero arbitrio. Vnde Paulus [1 Cor 13:10, 3:9] dicit: "Non ego set gratia Dei mecum. Dei enim adiutores sumus." Set licet liberum arbitrium cooperetur gratie, tamen gratia preuenit et in ea est principalitas. Vnde ait quidam:
>
>> Quicquid habes meriti, preuentrix gratia donat;
>> Nil Deus in nobis preter sua dona coronat.
>
> Etiam in oratione [Dom. vi. post Pentecost.] dicitur: "Gratia tua Domine nos preueniat et sequatur." Gratia preuenit ut homo bonum uelit, sequitur ne frustra uelit. Gratia semper preuenit liberum arbitrium naturali ordine et causa licet non tempore. Infusio gratie causa est quare conuertatur homo ad Deum, set quam cito infunditur gratia et conuertitur homo ad Deum, et ita gratia non preuenit tempore set naturali ordine et causa.

Bina: Dei donum gratia, uelle bonum.

2 HIC NOTANTVR SEX QVORVM OBSERVATIO
NECESSARIA EST SACERDOTI

Absque parentela Salem rex atque sacerdos [11 lines]

3 DE SPIRITVALI OBLATIONE SECVNDVM OBLATIONEM
SACRIFICII ABRAHE

Offerto trimam uaccam, capram quoque trimam [5 lines]

4 HIC MONETVR VT QVI VVLT FIERI RECTOR POPVLI PRIVS PRECELLAT
IN SAPIENTIA ET BONIS MORIBVS

Hic qui uult Abraham fieri fiat prius Abram [5 lines]

5 HIC NOTANTVR DVO QVE NECESSARIA SVNT AD DELENDVM
ET CAVENDVM PECCATA

Inter Sur, Cades, Abraham posuit sibi sedes [4 lines]

6 Hic monetvr in Domino gavdere

Cum strue lignorum ponas Ysaac super altum,
Non perimentur ibi gaudia fixa tibi.

7 De ivramento

Iuramenta Deo reddas, tribus hec revocato [4 lines]

8 De hvmilitate

Te sub maiori, te sub pare siue minori [8 lines]

9 De mansvetvdine

Si tu mitis eris scripturis erudieris,
Applaudent homines, regna superna preces.

10 De lacrimis

Gratia si lacrimis assit solamen habebit,
Non hoc set lacrimis dat mala culpa suis.

11 De esvrie spiritvali

Est grauis illa fames doctrine pane carentes [8 lines]

12 De misericordia

Tu dimitteris, tu premia digna sequeris [8 lines]

13 De mvnditia

Illum conspiciet, si mundum cor tibi fiet,
Quem nisi mundus eris cernere non poteris.

14 De pace

Pax solide mentis non temporis est bona cunctis [4 lines]

15 De patientia

Quandoque nature numquam patientia culpe [4 lines]

16 Hic habetvr instrvctio svmpta ex hoc qvod Christvs in die sabbati svrrexit legere, et in his monemvr aptari his qve legimvs in sacra scriptvra in qvibvs possvmvs

Christus surrexit, sibi tradita scripta reuoluit [10 lines]

17 DE ARTICVLIS IN QVIBVS LICET VIRO NON REDDERE DEBITA SPONSE
In quibus articulis liceat non reddere sponsis
Persoluenda thoro sponsis, per S C I N D E notato.

18 DE FORMIS MALE IVRANDI
Si male iurandi formas sit mens memorandi
Per primas F A T O per I D O N E A commemorato.

19 HINC POTEST SVMI EXEMPLVM
FVGIENDI QVANDOQVE PERSECVTIONEM
Christus in Egyptum fugiens, sic esse fugandum [4 lines]

20 DE DIVISIONE CORPORIS CHRISTI SVPER ALTARE
Diuiditur partes caro Christi pro tribus in tres [4 lines]

21 HIC DOCETVR DISCRETIO FVGIENDI IN HEREMVM
SIVE IN ALIQVOD CLAVSTRVM
Si deserta petis non sit dux aura fauoris,
Huc sis expulsus seu ductus. Quo duce? Christus.

22 HIC NOTATVR QVOD PECCATVM COMMISSVM ALIVD ATTRAHIT
Non scandit montem Loth, habens incredulitatem,
Incestumque specii commisit ob ebrietatem.

23 HIC NOTANTVR QVEDAM QVE PREDICATOREM CONGRVIT OBSERVARE
Strenuus ut Christus, sis utilis atque benignus [3 lines]

24 DE SCANDALO VITANDO
Que mala sunt in eis, que nec mala nec bona sunt his [6 lines]

25 HIC DATVR INTELLIGI QVALITER CHRISTIANVS VERO
CRISMATE DEBET INVNGI
Balsama conficias oleo, te talibus ungas.
Sic aliis redole, sic tibi mente nite.

26 HIC HABETVR QVALITER HOC NOMEN PANIS
IN PLERISQVE SCRIPTVRIS ACCIPIATVR
Diuersos queres a celesti patre panes;
Hoc ex S C O P E D O C E S O dempta concipe panes.

27 HIC DATVR INTELLIGI QVALITER HEC NOMINA,
SINISTRA DEXTERA, SOLENT ACCIPI

Quid fiat dextra non debet scire sinistra?
Prudens in dextra cor habet stultusque sinistra.

28 DE ORATIONE

Non prece deuota phariseus, ypocrita, scriba [5 lines]

29 DE IEIVNIO

Ex F A C I E memora quod sunt ieiunia plura
Quod designat C generale uel est speciale.

30 DE INTENTIONE

Si fuerit simplex intentio, si plica duplex [4 lines]

31 DE SIGNIFICATIONE HORVM NOMINVM: SERAPH, CHERVB,
SERAPHIN, CHERVBIN, SERAPHIM, CHERVBIM

Ordine maiori seraph, et cherub inferiori [4 lines]

32 IN HIS MONEMVR PECCATA CAVERE ET COMISSA CITO RELINQVERE
QVIA MORA IN HIS MAIVS ATTRAHIT PERICVLVM

Propter sex caueas peccata citoque relinquas [4 lines]

33 HIC NOTATVR QVARE DEVS DIFFERAT LIBERARE
ALIQVOS IN AFFLICTIONE LABORANTES

Sepe laboranti differt Deus auxiliari [4 lines]

34 DE COLLIRIIS OCVLORVM CORDIS

Que bona sunt oculis cordis colliria si uis
Noscere, mente F V I T habeas primasque P O P O scit.

35 DE ERVDITIONE DEI

Qualiter erudiat Deus ut tibi notio fiat [4 lines]

36 HIC NOTATVR QVIBVS DIGNE SVMI POSSIT SANCTA EVCHARISTIA

Est humili, miti, caro sancta, Deumque timenti [6 lines]

37 EX HIS POTEST INTELLIGI QVID SIGNIFICET CANDELA BREVIS
IN MEDIO CANDELABRI IN TRIBVS NOCTIBVS ANTE PASCHA,
ET QVID PER CEREVM ERECTVM IN SABBATO PASCHE

Christum signantem post candelam breuiorem [5 lines]

38 Hɪᴄ ɴᴏᴛᴀɴᴛᴠʀ ǫᴠᴇᴅᴀᴍ ǫᴠᴇ sᴠɴᴛ ɴᴇᴄᴇssᴀʀɪᴀ ᴘʀᴇᴅɪᴄᴀᴛᴏʀɪ
Erudiens homines transi prefulgida nubes [11 lines]

39 Dᴇ ʙᴏɴᴏ ᴄɪʀᴄᴠɪᴛᴠ ꜰᴀᴄɪᴇɴᴅᴏ
Scripta, creaturas, exemplaque, premia, penas [5 lines]

40 Iɴ ʜɪs ɴᴏᴛᴀᴛᴠʀ ǫᴠᴏᴅ sᴇx ᴅᴇ ᴄᴀᴠsɪs Dᴇᴠs ᴅɪꜰꜰᴇʀᴀᴛ
ᴅᴀʀᴇ ᴄᴏɴᴠᴇʀsɪs ᴀᴅ sᴇ sᴀɴɪᴛᴀᴛᴇᴍ
Sepe Deus multis differt dare dona salutis [6 lines]

41 Hɪᴄ ɴᴏᴛᴀᴛᴠʀ ǫᴠᴏᴅ sᴇx ᴅᴇ ᴄᴀᴠsɪs ᴘʟᴇʀᴀǫᴠᴇ sᴏʟᴇɴᴛ ᴛᴀᴄᴇʀɪ
Quosdam sex cause quedam fecere tacere.

42 Dᴇ sᴏʟʟɪᴄɪᴛᴠᴅɪɴᴇ
Prouida nature, pastoralis quoque cure [3 lines]

43 Dᴇ ᴘᴇʀᴍɪssɪᴏɴᴇ ᴇᴛ ᴀᴄᴄᴠsᴀᴛɪᴏɴᴇ
Est permissio triplex, accusatio triplex,
Tu distinguendo ᴄɪs atque ᴅɪᴠ memorato.

44 Iɴ ʜɪs ʜᴀʙᴇᴛᴠʀ ǫᴠᴇ ᴘᴏʀᴛᴀᴍ ᴠɪᴛᴇ ʟᴀᴛᴀᴍ ᴇᴛ ǫᴠᴇ ᴀʀᴛᴀᴍ ᴇꜰꜰɪᴄɪᴀɴᴛ
Ingresso portam uite faciunt tria latam [5 lines]

45 Dᴇ ᴛɪᴍᴏʀᴇ
Non naturalem poteris remouere timorem [6 lines]

46 Hɪᴄ ɴᴏᴛᴀᴛᴠʀ ǫᴠᴀɴᴅᴏǫᴠᴇ ᴇxᴄᴇᴘᴛɪᴏɴᴇᴍ ꜰᴀᴄɪᴀᴛ ʜᴇᴄ ᴅɪᴄᴛɪᴏ
"ɴɪsɪ" ɪɴ ǫᴠɪʙᴠsᴅᴀᴍ ᴄᴏɴsᴛʀᴠᴄᴛɪᴏɴɪʙᴠs
Per nisi tollantur que his duo sᴘ ᴀʀ sᴇ notantur.

47 Ex ʜɪs ᴘᴏᴛᴇsᴛ ɪɴᴛᴇʟʟɪɢɪ ǫᴠɪʙᴠs ᴅᴇ ᴄᴀᴠsɪs ꜰʟᴀɢᴇʟʟᴇᴛ
Dᴇᴠs ʜᴏᴍɪɴᴇs
Torquentur uariis homines plerique flagellis [6 lines]

48 Iɴ ʜɪs ᴏsᴛᴇɴᴅɪᴛᴠʀ ᴀᴅ ǫᴠᴇ ᴠᴀʟᴇᴀɴᴛ ᴏᴘᴇʀᴀ ᴍɪsᴇʀɪᴄᴏʀᴅɪᴇ
ꜰᴀᴄᴛᴀ ᴀʙ ᴇᴏ ǫᴠɪ ᴘᴇᴄᴄᴀᴛᴏ ᴍᴏʀᴛᴀʟɪ ᴄᴏɴsᴛʀɪɴɢɪᴛᴠʀ
Culpa mortali dum sis omittere noli [4 lines]

49 Dᴇ ᴄʀᴠᴄᴇ Dᴏᴍɪɴɪ ꜰᴇʀᴇɴᴅᴀ
In cruce tollenda que sunt tibi semper habenda
Hec ʀ sublato per ᴠ ᴇ s ᴄ ᴀ ʀᴠ ᴍ memorato.

50 DE SEPTEM VITIIS CAPITALIBVS SIVE PRINCIPALIBVS
EX QVIBVS ALIA VITIA ORIVNTVR

Crimine manantes sunt tres et bis duo fontes;
Tu per A G I L A I C I qui sunt poteris reminisci.

51 IN HIS DATVR INTELLIGI QVE CONTEMPLATIVE VITE
ET QVE ACTIVE VITE CONVENIANT

Vt grates donet, legat et meditetur et oret [6 lines]

52 DE SVPERBIA CAVENDA

Neue tibi tribuas bona si qua tenes neque credas [5 lines]

53 HIC NOTATVR QVOD NECESSARIA EST CONIVNCTIO SPEI ET TIMORIS

Ex spe prorumpit presumptio si timor absit [4 lines]

54 DE VOTO

Quoddam discrete quoddam uotum fit inepte [5 lines]

II.16

Sermones

Preaching was an integral part of William de Montibus's activities as a teacher and as chancellor of Lincoln Cathedral. In addition to the many references to preaching and preachers in his other writings, 149 sermons can be attributed to William with some confidence. They are listed below in four groups. The first seventy-three sermons represent an early collection of William's sermons in the schools and the cathedral at Lincoln. A second group of sermons (nos. 74-115) is addressed to an unnamed acquaintance whom, in two rather acerbic letters, William urges to take up the preaching office that he has neglected. To this end William supplies his friend with forty-two brief and simple sermons to serve as models for learning the art of preaching. A third group of fifteen miscellaneous sermons (nos. 116-130) is comprised of individual works that circulated in the manuscripts alongside the sermons in collections One and Two, but form an integral part of neither group. A final collection of nineteen sermons (nos. 131-149), found in a unique manuscript copy, would seem to represent William's preaching at Lincoln towards the end of his career.

The sermons ascribed to William in MS *C* (nos. 1-73, below) are addressed primarily to a clerical audience of priests and students in the schools. No overall plan of organization according to the liturgical year is evident in this collection. Indeed, it contains no sermons at all for the seasons of Advent, Christmastide, or Epiphany. Of the sermons whose occasions are clearly specified, ten are Lenten sermons, one is for Easter, eight for the feast of the Ascension, ten for Pentecost, two for Holy Trinity, and one each for the feasts of St. Peter and of All Angels. The inclusion of many sermons for the same feast suggests that this collection was not the work of a single "auditor"; perhaps it derives from a sermon-collection made by William himself.

The original form and extent of such a collection cannot now be guessed at, but the purpose of the sermons in MS *C* can scarcely have been to serve as a practical aide to preachers. The absence of a liturgical ordering of the sermons, the imbalance of sermons (too many or too few) for specific feasts, and the lack of any indication of a liturgical context for many of the sermons, make it less than ideal for the practising preacher. An alternative is to understand the collection, at least in part, as an aide in the education of students in the schools. That William conceived of his sermons as serving such a purpose is clear from references to them in his *Numerale*.[1]

Many of the sermons collected here seem to have been addressed to students. These sermons are characterized by the copiousness of the scriptural citations, the introduction of alternative readings to the scriptural texts, the explication of the "mystical" sense of texts, the use of technical vocabulary concerning tropes and figures of speech, frequent use of *distinctiones*, and pointed references to the special responsibilities of the learned in christian society. Such academic preaching embodies the twofold purpose of moral and intellectual education that William intended for his theologians. A detailed study of these sermons would help to specify the ways preaching extended and, indeed, consummated the academic exercises of the theological teacher.

If this first group of sermons is primarily academic, the purpose of the second collection (sermons 74-115) is rigorously practical. William designated his audience as those who are learned and capable of memorizing written sermons and preaching them to their flock, but who are too lazy or negligent to undertake the task. For one such acquaintance William composed these sermons. "Desiring by the goad of artificial brevity," William writes, "to motivate you to the task of preaching, I have composed short and easy sermons, so that this simple collection of them might rouse your delicate spirit, which can be deterred from the labour of memorization by the length or difficulty of other sermons, to that same work."[2]

The sermons are, indeed, masterpieces of brevity and clarity. It would be difficult to find a more accessible collection in all of the Middle Ages. Nevertheless William feared that the first batch of these simple sermons might fail to achieve their purpose. In the introduction to a second series (nos. 98-115) he comments: "I sent the promised work to you as one sowing seed in the field of your heart ... . That field,

---

[1] See above, p. 56. One reference in the *Numerale* is to a sermon that is found in none of the collections above: "Homicidiorum autem duodecim genera distinximus in sermone qui sic incipit: Misit Herodes rex manus, etc.," *Numerale*, 10.1. A sermon with this incipit is noted by R.W. Hunt, *The Schools and the Cloister*, p. 153, no. 130, among sermons attributed to Alexander Neckam.

[2] See below, p. 545, preceding sermon no. 74.

however, remains sterile and uncultivated, thus far neither producing nor promising fruit." William expresses his hope that this second series will leave the recipient with no excuse for continued silence in the pulpit. He concludes:

> If this brevity seems to you wordy, this simplicity onerous, this usefulness bitter, I will toil no longer in this intractable field, but leave you to your own fate as one hopeless and incurable, afflicted by sorrow and sloth. If, however, roused by my chastisement and inspired by God's grace, you are led to open your lips to preach the word of God, you will bring joy and gladness to my ears.[3]

Manuscript *L* provides our best guide to the original contents of these two series of sermons. The first series in that manuscript begins with twelve sermons from the temporal cycle of the liturgy, beginning with Christmas and ending with Pentecost. A sermon for Advent (no. 96) has, perhaps, been misplaced from the beginning of the series to near the end. These are followed by eleven sermons from the sanctoral cycle, beginning with the Nativity of John the Baptist (24 June) and ending with St. Nicholas (6 December). The second series follows the same format. It begins with ten temporal sermons (Christmas to Pentecost), and is followed by seven sanctoral sermons (Nativity of John the Baptist to All Saints).

Although these sermons surely represent something of William's own preaching at Lincoln Cathedral, they have been tailored specifically to the needs and experience of the addressee. Sermon number 76, on Epiphany, begins with a *captatio benevolentiae* that would be inappropriate for William but seems to suit the preacher to whom he addressed these collections: "As I am no expert in the more subtle arts, I will lay before you not subtle but simple things, not mysteries but common knowledge, not doctrines but admonitions. You know that today the Wise Men brought gifts ... ."

In a sermon on the Presentation of Jesus in the Temple (no. 101) William puts in the mouth of his preacher an even more embarrassing admission: "Since a 'pastor' receives his name from pasturing, he is wrongly called 'pastor' who never feeds his flock. What plea, therefore, have I, who have the name of pastor and do not feed my flock? How will I answer to the Great Shepherd? What excuse can I make? If I am able to feed them and do not I am guilty of negligence ... . Hence, fearful and trembling, will I strive today to speak, lest I be convicted

---

[3] See below, p. 557, following sermon no. 115.

of persistent silence. Today Jesus's parents brought him into the temple ... ."

Other sermons in these collections add to our knowledge of their recipient and of his audience. Sermons to the laity and to *claustrales* both are found here. The emphasis on St. Augustine's teachings in sermon 91, for example, might suggest that the *claustrales* were Augustinian canons. The remarkable sermon on St. Andrew (no. 95) makes it clear that the recipient is a preacher in a monastery dedicated to St. Andrew, and that the parochial churches in the city all pertain to the monastery. It begins: "This is the day on which, and this is the place in which, we ought to pay special honor to St. Andrew ... . This is one of his principal churches in England; this is his splendid citadel, his holy cloister. Here is his distinguished army — this venerable congregation of monks ... who are able to defend this citadel and this city from the devil's fiery missiles." The sermon goes on to describe St. Andrew's city: "This city is under St. Andrew's special care; all its churches are assigned to his monastery, and thus are all the inhabitants of this city, as it were, his parishioners."

William obviously had a particular setting in mind when he composed this sermon. Although the city and church are unnamed, there are few important monasteries dedicated to St. Andrew in England, and even fewer where all the churches of the town are assigned to the monastery, and where the monks or canons follow the rule of St. Augustine. The monastic cathedral at Rochester is dedicated to St. Andrew, but it is a Benedictine foundation. The monastery in the important Lincolnshire town of Northampton is also dedicated to St. Andrew and had possession of all the other churches in the city, but it is an alien monastery dependent on Cluny and following the rule of St. Benedict. St. Andrew's Cathedral in Scotland, served by Augustinian canons, fits all the criteria. William is known to have spent time in Scotland and even to have died there, but he would scarcely have described that church as "in England" (*in Anglia*). The Augustinian houses dedicated to St. Andrew in England — Hexham (Northumberland), Owsten (Leicestershire), and Barnwell (Cambridgeshire, dedicated to both St. Andrew and St. Giles) — might possibly fit the description in this sermon.

A final and intriguing possibility is that the sermons were written for a canon of the Gilbertine house at Sempringham. The monastery at Sempringham, dedicated to St. Andrew and St. Mary, was the mother house of the Gilbertine Order. The rule of St. Augustine served as one of the bases for the Gilbertine rule. William was closely associated with the order throughout his life, and might well have composed such works for the use of the prior or one of the canons. On the other hand, it is less than clear that the monastery at Sempringham could be considered one of St. Andrew's "principal churches in England." Nor does the sermon's reference to the "city" with "all its churches" seem particularly descriptive of the village of Sempringham.

The third group of sermons (Collection Three, nos. 116-130) are a mixed lot only because we can place them neither in Collection One nor Collection Two on the basis of the extant manuscripts. If we had access to William's original collection of his own sermons or to the original versions of his epistolary treatises on preaching, many of these sermons would certainly be found therein.

The sermons in the final group (nos. 131-149) are found only in MS R. They follow the liturgical year, from Advent to Pentecost, and end with three Marian sermons. They were probably preached in the schools, and the cross-references to the *Versarius* indicate their didactic purpose. These sermons represent William's mature preaching, at the end of a long career as chancellor of Lincoln Cathedral and master of theology in the Lincoln schools.

AUTHENTICITY AND DATE

A consideration of the authenticity of the 149 sermons listed below raises a number of problems. The secure attribution of medieval sermons is a notoriously difficult task. We can, perhaps, achieve only verisimilitude and not certainty in following the clues left in the extant manuscript copies. In compiling the list of sermons I have been guided by the internal evidence of the sermons themselves and by the external evidence of the manuscript traditions.

The earliest surviving sermons seem to be those in MS C (nos. 1-73, below). They are explicitly ascribed to William in the manuscript, they contain many echoes of his teachings and his style as witnessed in other authentic works, and several of them are also found in MS O (nos. 2, 17-19, 29, 52, 55, 60 [twice], and 63), a manuscript containing many ascribed and unascribed excerpts from William's writings.

An early date for these sermons in MS C is suggested by several factors. Sermon no. 3 includes a reference to William's masters: "Secundum enim assertionem magistrorum nostrorum ... ." The opinion voiced in this sermon is found, substantially verbatim, in the *Historia*

Scholastica of Peter Comestor, whom we suspect to have been one of William's teachers in Paris. William seldom refers to his own teachers in his later writings, and this reference would seem to date the sermon to the early years of his regency in Lincoln, or even earlier. Sermon no. 16 contains a reference to Saladin's recent conquest of Jerusalem (1187): "Iam Saladinus ... uineam illam Ierosolimitanam ... depascus est, conculcauit, et exterminauit." This sermon may have been preached during the enthusiasm accompanying the Third Crusade (1189-1192); it would have lost much of its force not long thereafter. Finally, the bulk of the sermons in MS *C* seem to be addressed to clerics in the schools. Only sermon no. 14, addressed to the people in Pentecostal procession, can be positively associated with William's preaching responsibilities as chancellor of Lincoln Cathedral. In itself this is no argument for an early date of these sermons, but taken with the two unmistakably early references above, we might presume that William's earlier preaching concentrated on the students in his schools, and that only gradually did he begin to collect and distribute his sermons preached *ad populum*.

The sermons numbered 74 to 115, above, are found variously distributed among MSS *E, F, L,* and *O.* The original form of this collection is suggested by MS *L,* where forty-two sermons are included in two epistolary treatises on the art of preaching. The treatises are anonymous in *L,* but nineteen of their sermons are among those ascribed to William de Montibus in MS *E.* The first of the two treatises in *L* is introduced by the preface: "Inter omnia opera misericordie ... ."[4] This preface also is found in MS *E,* where it has been edited so as to serve as a part of the general introduction to the sermons ascribed to William in that codex. In MS *L,* we find not only the original form of the preface, but the entire work that it introduced, as well as a companion piece by the same author (Collection Two A and B, below). These two treatises were written by a single author for an identifiable purpose — the education of a lazy colleague. Although anonymous in MS *L,* the presence of nearly half of the sermons in these two treatises among the ascribed sermons in MS *E,* which also preserves a form of the preface to *L*'s first treatise, allows us to suggest that all forty-two sermons are attributable to William de Montibus.

The unascribed sermons in MS *F* add no direct support to the hypothesis of William de Montibus's authorship, but they confirm the impression that the sermons in *E* and *L* are by the same author. Of

---

[4] See below, p. 544, at sermon no. 74.

the twenty-five sermons in *F*, twenty-four are identical in content and in order to the sermons in *L*'s first treatise.

If the scribe of MS *F* was copying his sermons primarily from those contained in the first treatise on preaching in MS *L*, the early thirteenth-century scribe of MS *O* had before him the sermons of the second treatise, as well as a number of William de Montibus's other sermons and writings. At various places throughout his codex he inserted copies of all but three of the eighteen sermons in *L*'s second treatise, along with nine of the other sermons ascribed to William in MS *E*. These sermons are all anonymous in MS *O*, but when taken with the evidently high regard in which its scribe held William de Montibus, and his familiarity with William's sermons and other writings, this manuscript, too, can be seen to add support to the argument for William's authorship of the sermons in question.

No internal references reveal the date of the sermons collected in the two epistolary treatises, but the tone of the collections is magisterial and authoritative. They must have been composed after William was well established as a teacher and preacher. The sermons themselves evince long practice in addressing popular audiences outside of the schools, a practice that William would have gained in fulfilling his duties as chancellor of Lincoln Cathedral. A date of composition in the thirteenth century (1200 x 1213) is likely.

The third group of sermons listed here, nos. 116-130, comprises those sermons in MSS *E*, *L*, and *F* that were not included in *L*'s two epistolary treatises on preaching. Nine of the fifteen sermons in this group are found only in MS *E*, where they are among the sermons ascribed to William. Two sermons in *E* (nos. 121 and 128) are also found in MS *C*, at the end of group of sermons ascribed to Alexander of Ashby; both attributions — to William and to Alexander — are plausible. Another sermon in *E* (no. 117) is preserved also in MS *L*. Sermon 116 follows immediately after the second epistolary treatise in *L*, and is also found in MS *O*. The final sermon in this third group is found only in MS *F*, but it is the first sermon in the codex and is followed immediately by twenty-four of William's authentic sermons.

The final group of William's sermons listed here occur in a discrete block in MS *R*. This manuscript, from Bardney Abbey in Lincolnshire, contains a copy of William's *Distinctiones* (fols. 1ra-115ra), and a number of other theological works from the early thirteenth century. On fols. 205ra to 211va one finds an interesting set of questions disputed in the schools that include a reference (fol. 208vb) to William's teachings: "Vnde dicit magister W. de monte ... ." The sermons on fols.

142ra-149va bear no ascription to William, but three references to *uersibus nostris* in sermon nos. 132 and 139 reveal his authorship. These are precise and accurate references to William's *Versarius*.[5] The other sermons in this group are written in the same style, and should probably be assigned to William as well.

No doubt refinements will be made to this list of 149 sermons; some will prove to be inauthentic, and more sermons remain to be identified. William, himself, seems to have made a collection of sermons for use in the schools that is yet to be discovered.[6] But one interesting sermon collection that has long been associated with William's name should probably be removed from the canon of his writings.

The *Filius matris* collection, a series of sermons from the late twelfth century expounding the gospel readings for Sundays and the greater festivals, seems first to have been attributed to William de Montibus by Henry of Kirkestead (whose *Catalogus scriptorum ecclesie*, formerly attributed to Boston of Bury, is from the mid fourteenth century).[7] None of the extant manuscripts copies of the *Filius matris* sermons is ascribed to William de Montibus.[8] In the prologue the anonymous author dedicates his exposition to a Lord William, dispenser of the church at Lewes, whom he asks to read it critically, correct its errors, and, if it is found suitable, to publish it.[9] Other than this William of Lewes, obviously the recipient and not the author of the sermons, there is nothing in the text to associate it with a "William," let alone William de Montibus. Neither do the content, language, and style of the sermons themselves bear more than a superficial resemblance to William's authentic sermons or to his other writings.

---

[5] Sermon 132: "Deus inquid Dominus timendus, et illuxit nobis multiplici luce. Quere in uersibus nostris, L: 'Lux'" = *Versarius*, nos. 647, 648; Sermon 139: "'Asinus utilis ac humilis' et cetera. Quere in uersibus nostris, A: 'Asinus'" = *Versarius*, no. 54; ibid., "Huius autem opera quere in uersibus, O: 'Opera misericordie'" = *Versarius*, nos. 718-721.

[6] William refers the readers of his *Numerale* to such a collection; see above, note 1.

[7] See Helen L. Spencer, "Vernacular and Latin Versions of a Sermon for Lent: 'A Lost Penitential Homily' Found," *Mediaeval Studies* 44 (1982) 271-305, at 274, n. 17; cf. idem, "A Fifteenth-Century Translation of a Late Twelfth-Century Sermon Collection," *Review of English Studies*, n.s. 28 (1977) 257-267.

[8] On the manuscript copies see Spencer, "Lost Penitential Homily," p. 280, and n. 32; idem, "Translation," pp. 259, n. 3.

[9] "Viro bone fame uitaque celeberimo, Domino Willelmo Dei gratia Latisaquensis ecclesie dispensatori fidelissimo, Filius matris sue ... . Ea maxime de causa, uir totius prudentie, ut ueste serenitatis et discretionis censura eiusdem codicilli superflua deleat, uitiosa corrigat, minus dicta suppleat, tolerabilia commendet, et ad laudem nominis Christi si sic uobis placuerit in lucem proferat," Cambridge, Pembroke College MS 116, fol. 69r.

The attribution of the *Filius matris* sermons to William de Montibus probably rests on a confusion in the manuscript tradition such as could easily arise, for example, from a careless or cursory interpretation of the information in MS *E* above. This manuscript includes two sermon collections, the first explicitly ascribed to William de Montibus, and the second — the *Filius matris* collection — without ascription. A scribe has provided for both collections an alphabetical subject index, and two separate "catalogues" of the sermon themes in the two collections. In a table of contents he ascribes the first set of sermons to William de Montibus: *Sermones Guilelmi de monte de tempore*, but he leaves a blank for the author of the second collection: *Sermones* [lac.] *de tempore*." A casual reader might understandably extend the first ascription to the second set of sermons, and conclude that William was the author of both.

The only bit of evidence that might suggest William's authorship of the *Filius matris* sermons is an oblique reference in an epitaph composed by Matthew of Rievaulx.[10] One of Matthew's four epitaphs for William de Montibus begins with a word-play calling to mind his *Numerale*: "In libro vite numeretur, qui Numerale/ Fecit ... ." Another begins with the words: "Filius in matris utero merito sepelitur." It is possible that Matthew intended these words, too, as a reference to one of William de Montibus's writings. But this is a rather slender thread on which to hang an argument for William's composition of the *Filius matris* sermons. Further study of this interesting and important sermon-collection may clarify the question of authorship, but for the present we find no compelling arguments for including it among the authentic works of William de Montibus.

MANUSCRIPTS

Incipits and explicits are given in the numbered list of sermons below. The manuscript descriptions here discuss that part of each codex in which William's sermons are to be found.

1. *C* = Cambridge, University Library MS Ii.I.24, fols. 77ra-103vb, 179ra-181rb. Mid 13th century (above top line).
    Title (77ra): (*Sermones magistri Guillelmi de Montibus*)
    Fols. 77ra-103vb = sermon nos. 1-73 (Collection One, below).
    Fols. 179-181 = sermon nos. 121 and 128 (at the end of a collection of sermons ascribed in this MS to Alexander of Ashby.)

---

[10] See above, Chapter One, p. 26.

This early manuscript contains a number of important works from the twelfth- and early-thirteenth-century schools, including sermons ascribed to Hilduin (the chancellor of the Parisian schools, c. 1178-1190), Alexander Neckam, and Alexander of Ashby, as well as copies of Alan of Lille's *De arte predicandi*, Alexander of Ashby's *De artificioso modo predicandi*, and Peter the Chanter's *De tropis loquendi*.

2. *E* = Cambridge University Library MS Dd.IV.27, fols. 1ra-137vb. 14th century.

> Title (5va): (*Incipiunt sermones magistri Willelmi de monte Cancellarii Lincolniensis. De aduentu Domini*).
>
> Fols. 5va-13vb = sermon nos. 96, 117, 74, 98, 75, 99, 118, 76, 100. (A sermon on fols. 8ra-9va, ascribed to "Hildewin" in MS *C*, is excluded from this list).
>
> Fols. 37rb-49rb = sermon nos. 119-122, 82, 123.
>
> Fols. 115ra-137vb = sermon nos. 80, 124, 81, 105, 83, 106, 125, 84, 107, 126-128, 85, 108, 129. (One sermon on fol. 116vb-121ra is omitted here; it is attributed to Stephen of Tournai by Schneyer).

A table of contents on the verso of the last flyleaf (= fol. iiiiv) reads: *Contenta*:

> Introductio ad artem concionandi fol. 1
> Sermones Guilelmi de monte de tempore fol. 5b
> Catalogus thematum et locorum eorundem fol. 138
> Item index alphabeticus in eosdem supra ad "A" [= flyleaf i]
> Sermones [*lac.*] de tempore fol. 143
> Catalogus thematum et locorum eorundem fol. 139b
> Item Index alphabeticus in eosdem supra ad "D" [= flyleaf ii]

The item referred to as *Introductio ad artem concionandi*, on fols. 1r to 5r, consists of three brief works, unascribed in this manuscript. The first is an abbreviation of Richard of Thetford's mid-thirteenth-century *Summa de modo predicandi*. It begins on fol. 1ra with the title *Quibus modis themata diuidi possunt*, and the text *Primo per qualemcumque termini positionem*.[11] This work ends incomplete on fol. 1vb: *Rogemus igitur illum in principio in quo sunt omnes*, and is followed by nineteen blank lines.

---

[11] Another copy of this abbreviation of Thetford's *Summa* is found in Oxford, Bodleian Library MS Bodley 631 (sc 1954), and is printed by Fritz Kemmler, *"Exempla" in Context*, pp. 200-201. The entire *summa* has been printed as Part Three of an opusculum entitled *Ars concionandi* in *S. Bonaventurae Opera omnia* (Quaracchi: Typographia Collegii S. Bonaventurae, 1901), 9: 8-21; see Thomas Charland, "Les auteurs d'"artes predicandi' au XIIIe siècle d'apres les manuscrits," *Etudes d'histoire littéraire et doctrinale du XIIIe siècle* 1 (1932) 41-60, at 50-51.

The second part of the so-called *ars concionandi* in MS *E* is a copy of William de Montibus's first letter on preaching, printed below, preceding sermon no. 74. The copy of this letter in MS *E* (fol. 2ra-2va) has been revised so as to remove references to the actual recipient and to give it a wider applicability as an introduction to the preaching office. Only the first portion of the letter is preserved in this manuscript. It is followed immediately by an unascribed copy of Alexander of Ashby's early-thirteenth-century *De artificioso modo predicandi* on fols. 2va-5rb.[12]

Although the title on fol. 5va and the *Contenta* on the flyleaf ascribe all the sermons from fol. 5v to fol. 137v to William de Montibus, not all are his. Most of the sermons on fols. 14ra-37rb (two gatherings) and on fols. 49rb-114vb (five and one-half gatherings) have been attributed by Schneyer[13] to other authors, primarily John of la Rochelle, and the remainder (nos. 76-94 and nos. 101-102 in Schneyer's list of William's sermons) are dissimilar to William's authentic works. The sixty-five sermons in these eight gatherings share a number of common characteristics that distinguish them from William's: They use "Langton numbers" or modern chapter divisions in their citations of Scripture, they are accompanied by marginal distinctions, and they share a common style and organization that is different from William's. None is found in other collections of William's sermons. That these "intrusive" sermons are all found in discrete blocks, helps to confirm that they were copied from other sermon-collections and should not be conflated with the de Montibus sermons in this codex.

The sermons on fols. 143 to 239 comprise a very popular collection known as *Filius matris* from the first words of the prologue. They have often been attributed to William de Montibus, but reasons for rejecting them have been given above in the discussion of authenticity and dates.

An alphabetical index to all the sermons in the codex has been added on the flyleaves i-iiii, which are designated "A" to "H" by the scribe of the index. A catalogue of the *themata* of William's sermons, written by the same scribe, is found on fols. 138r-139r, and another, of the *themata* of the *Filius matris* sermons, is on fols. 139v-140r.

---

[12] On Alexander's preaching manual see Kemmler, *"Exempla" in Context*, pp. 69-76; Russell, *Dictionary of Writers of Thirteenth Century England*, p. 12.

[13] Johannes B. Schneyer, *Repertorium der lateinischen Sermones des Mittelalters*, Beiträge zur Geschichte der Philosophie und Theologie des Mittelalters, 43/2 (Münster: Aschendorff, 1970), pp. 509-524, at p. 524.

3. *F* = Cambridge, University Library MS Dd.IV.50, fols. 1r-24v. 15th century.

> Fols. 1r-24v = sermon nos. 130, 74-97.

Sermon no. 97 ends imperfectly, at the end of a gathering; the catch-words *oculi quibus* are found in the bottom margin of fol. 24v, but not on fol. 25r where a new sermon begins.

Four of the sermons in this manuscript, attributed by Schneyer to William de Montibus (his nos. 130-133), are found in the gathering that begins on fol. 25. This gathering is written in a double-column format unlike the single-column or "long lines" of fols. 1-24. The sermons in this gathering are probably not by William, and two of them (nos. 131-132 in Schneyer) are plausibly ascribed to Alexander of Ashby in MS *E*, fols. 172-173.

4. *L* = Laon, Bibliothèque Municipale MS 309, fols. 41r-52v; 82v-89v. 13th century.

> Fols. 41r-52v = sermon nos. 74-97, (Collection Two A, below).
> Fols. 82v-87r = sermon nos. 98-115, (Collection Two B, below).
> Fols. 87v-89v = sermon nos. 116 and 117.

5. *O* = Oxford, Bodleian Library MS Lyell 8, *passim*. Early 13th century (above top line).

In addition to a number of excerpts from William's other writings, this miscellaneous collection includes the following sermons: nos. 96, 98, 63, 99, 102-104, 113, 105, 29, 52, 60, 55, 2, 109, 18, 110, 19, 111-112, 114-115, 116, 17, 60 (a second copy).

Another of William's "sermons" in this manuscript is edited above (II.6) as the *Epistola ad moniales*.

6. *R* = London, British Library MS Royal 10.A.vii, fols. 142ra-149vb. Early 13th century (above top line).

> Fols. 142ra-149vb = sermon nos. 131-149 (Collection Four, below).

A number has been assigned to each sermon for ease of reference. The number of each sermon in Schneyer's *Repertorium* follows, enclosed in round brackets; (n.l.) indicates that the sermon is not listed by Schneyer in his entry for William de Montibus. The incipit and explicit of each sermon are printed here along with any internal indications of the occasion or the audience of the sermon. The "theme" or scriptural text is italicized (and sometimes abbreviated). Each entry is followed by notices, in round brackets, of the sermon's occasion and its original audience, where these can be determined or deduced from internal evidence, and by a list of the manuscripts known to contain copies of the sermon.

Sermones

COLLECTION ONE: SERMONS FROM MS *C*

1 (134) *Constituit Dominus populum suum super excelsam terram* [Deut 32:13] Alia translatio habet "de petra firma." Hebraica ueritas habet "perduxit eos in uirtute terre." ... Sanctus Dei propheta Moyses plenus Spiritu sancto de Deo et ecclesia, de Christo et Spiritu sancto in hunc modum locutus est: Constituit Deus, etc. ... quod ipse nobis tribuat, conseruet nec subtrahat, qui uiuit et regnat
(Pentecost?) *(C 77ra)*

2 (135) *Ego sum Deus Abraham* [Mt 22:32] Competenter expleta celebritate Pentecostes e uestigio sequitur sollempnitas in ueneratione sancte Trinitatis ... . In hac sancte Trinitatis sollempnitate post Pascha nouem recitamus lectiones ... . Monachi etiam propter Trinitatem lectionum superaddunt ternarium, set et hoc idem faciunt quasi supererogando, ad insinuandum maiorem eorum perfectionem ... ut ad beatam illam sancte atque indiuidue Trinitatis uisionem peruenire ualeamus, quod ipse nobis prestet qui uiuit et regnat
(Holy Trinity; to clerics in the schools?) *(C 77vb; O 99va)*

3 (136) *Homo quidam diues* [Luc 16:19] Homo iste a quibusdam dictus est Tantalus siue Tartarus, a quo locus supplicii gehennalis Tartarus censetur ... . Serus diues iste magister incipit esse, cum iam nec discendi tempus habet nec docendi. "Si quis," inquit, "ex mortuis" etc. Qui uerba Dei despexerat, hec audire non posse suos sequaces existimat. Vos itaque in carne degentes oportebit audire. Neque de cetero ad predicandum nobis prophete uel apostoli descendent de celis aut resurgent ex mortuis. Et nota quia hec lectio euuangelica magis uidetur narratio quam parabola. Secundum enim assertionem magistrorum nostrorum non fuit hec parabola, set in re ipsa quod perpendi potest, quia mendici ibi nomen ponitur, Lazarus scilicet. Ex hoc etiam quod diues de fratribus audiuit, "habent Moysen et prophetas," conicit quod Iudeus fuerat, pro quo et ipse Abraham patrem uocat et ille eum filium non quidem adoptione non imitatione set tantum carne.
(to clerics in the schools?) *(C 78rb)*

4 (137) *Homo quidam erat diues* [Luc 16:19] quasi ignotus et alienus apud Deum, nomine non designatur. "Ego," inquit Dominus, "cognosco oues meas." Dominus autem milites suos signo et uexillo proprio designauit, oues suas caractere impresso discernendo ab edis diaboli distinguit ... . Pauper quidem humilis per approbationem ex nomine scitur et proprio nomine designatur ... . Set et de Lazaro quem suscitauerat Iesus a mortuis cogitauerunt ut eum interficerent quia multi post illum abibant ex Iudeis et credebant in Iesum.
(to clerics in the schools?)   (*C 79ra*)

5 (138) Dixit Iesus Phariseis *Homo quidam erat diues et induebatur purpura et bisso* ... usque illud *Neque si quis ex mortuis resurrexerit credunt* [Luc 16:19-31] "Homo quidam," inquit, "erat diues." Diuitie quidem non sunt ex cupiditate immoderate affectande, non sunt ex tenacitate reseruande. Non enim in habitis opibus confidendum nec ex eisdem amissis excessu tristitie dolendum ... . Diuitias spirituales assimulare studeamus, quibus regnum celorum emere nobis ualeamus, quod nobis prestet qui uiuit et regnat
                                                               (*C 79vb*)

6 (139) *Non est Deus alius ut Deus rectissimi* [Deut 33:26-27] Moyses Spiritu sancto plenus locutus est de Christo. Vnde et Dominus Iudeis in euuangelio [Io 5:46]: "Si crederetis," inquit, "Moysi, crederetis forsitan et mihi." ... contritum numquam eleuabit in nos ad compungendum.
                                                               (*C 80va*)

7 (140) *Educens nubes ab extremo terre, fulgura in pluuiam fecit* [Ps 134:7] Nubes sunt predicatores. Vnde: "Mandabo nubibus meis ne pluant" [Is 5:6] ... . Hic est angelus cuius aspectus ut fulgur est, uestimentum ut nix.
                                                               (*C 81ra*)

8 (141) *Dominus memor fuit nostri et benedixit nobis* [Ps 113:12] Deus memor est miserorum, ad eis subueniendum ... . Memor est etiam Dominus meritorum malorum ad puniendum, memor esto Domine filiorum Edom in die Ierusalem.
                                                               (*C 81va*)

9 (142) *Ecce quam bonum et quam iocundum* [Ps 132:1] Hac tuba Spiritus sancti excitati fortes et bellatores incliti sacramentali militie

astricti indicentes bellum uitiis, diabolo, carni, mundo. In domo
iuramenti ministrant saluatori, militant summo regi. Et quia iam
cessauit aqua contradictionis in nostro habitationis loco excogitauerunt
spirituali martirium subire in monasterio ... . Porro unum est necessario
qui adheret uni uiuet de communi.
(To monks or canons)   (*C 81vb*)

10 (143) *Vado ad eum qui misit me* [Io 16:5] Pauperi elemosinam
petenti dici solet, "Vade ad Deum," hoc est recurre ad Dei suffragium
cum penes nos non reperias subsidium. De fideli etiam discedente
consueuimus pronuntiare quia uadit ad Deum, hoc autem est Dei
fruitionem ... . Solet enim poni presens pro eminenti futuro, ut et ibi:
"Ascendo ad Patrem meum." ... Sic studeamus preparari ut in aduentu
sancti neumatis Paracliti, tanti doni tanti dantis, nam et se una cum
Patre et Filio dat, immittit, infundit, diffundit, accepti habeamur grati
et idonei, quod et ipse nobis prestet qui uiuit et regnat
(Ascension; to clerics in the schools?)   (*C 81vb*)

11 (144) *Et cantent in uiis Domini, quia magna est gloria Domini*
[Ps 137:5] Videndum qui, cui, quid, de quo, cur, quando, ubi, qualiter,
ad quid cantare debeant. Qui, docti: "Eructabunt labia mea ymnum
cum docueris me iustificationes tuas" [Ps 118:171] ... . Alioquin
obicietur exprobationis inuectiua: "Cecinimus uobis et non saltastis"
[Mt 11:17].
(to clerics in the schools?)   (*C 82rb*)

12 (145) *Apparuerunt illis lingue dispertite* [Act 2:3] Sollempnitas
hodierna uenerabiliter et gloriose celebranda Spiritus sancti aduentui
rite est dedicata ... . De aduentu itaque Spiritus sancti prosequemur:
Quis ueniat uideas, quando uel qualiter ... ut a Spiritu sancto ualeamus
inhabitari, quod nobis prestet qui uiuit et regnat
(Pentecost)   (*C 82vb*)

13 (146) *Sic Deus dilexit mundum ut Filium suum unigenitum daret*
[Io 3:6] Ostenditur hic salutis humane causa scilicet dilectio diuina.
O inestimabilis dilectio, proprio Filio non pepercit Deus set pro nobis
omnibus tradidit illum; ut seruum redimeret Filium tradidit ... set suum
dedit autem in Pentecoste Spiritum ad amplius illuminandum et
roborandum ... . Secundo quidem ueniet iudicare et secundum opera
retribuere, ad cuius aduentum hoc modico uite nostre tempore nos

preparare studeamus ut ei parati et prompti et leti occurramus, quod
nobis prestet qui uiuit et regnat
(Pentecost; to clerics in the schools?)   *(C 83va)*

14 (147) *Dum implerentur dies Pentecostes erantque pariter in eodem
loco* [Act 2:1] Rationabilis est consuetudo nostre congregationis etsi
particularis, cum non possit esse nunc uniuersalis; a ueteri namque
lege traducta est hec institutio ubi ter in anno, in uere scilicet estate
et autumpno, hoc est in Pascha, in Pentecoste, cenofagia, iussi sunt
Israelite apparere in conspectu Domini. Et subiunctum est non
apparebit ante Dominum uacuus set offeret unusquisque secundum
quod habuerit iuxta benedictionem Domini Dei sui quam dedit ei. Ad
nos etiam ab Apostolis hoc emanauit et a reliquis discipulis qui
completis diebus, idest quinquagene illius que iam a Domini resurrectione effluxerat, erant omnes pariter in eodem loco in cenaculo
scilicet in Ierusalem ... . Iam igitur fratres ad sinum matris ecclesie
confluxistis de diuersis partibus ... occursu consonantie de habitaculis
uestris per turmas secundum signa, uexilla, quasi in castris contra hostes
spirituales ordinate processistis ... ab illa itaque reproborum turbida
congerie nos defendat et ad cetum sanctorum feliciter perducet qui
uiuit et regnat
(Pentecost; to the people in procession)   *(C 83vb)*

15 (148) *Nescitis quod hii qui in stadio currunt* [1 Cor 9:24] Totus
mundus liber est sapientis. Apostolus ad nostram eruditionem ago-
nistarum proponit similitudinem. Attendendum igitur quia in cursu
stadii sex sunt ... . Sic currite non scilicet in inuio set in uia recta et
arta ducente ad uitam, in hilaritate mentis — liberi, ueloces, sudentes
— ut in unanimitate socialitatis comprehendatis brauium eterne
notionis (brauium Grece, corona uel palma Latine). Ad hoc itaque
ipse dux uie Christus nos perducat qui uiuit et regnat
(to clerics in the schools?)   *(C 84rb)*

16 (149) *Sex annis seres agrum tuum* [Lev 25:3-4] Vinea in qua
Christus uitis et sui palmites est ecclesia siue uita euuangelica que sex
annis excolenda est, idest toto tempore presentis uite que senario
completur etatum ... . Si enim Deus naturalibus ramis non pepercit
ne forte nec tibi parcat. Iam Saladinus quasi singularis ferus uineam
illam Ierosolimitanam meritis eius malis exigentibus depastus est,
conculcauit, et exterminauit. Prouideat nobis Deus ne similia patia-
mur ... . Obsunt autem huic uinee ledentes aquilo, grando, gelu, pluuia,

hec est diaboli suggestio, principum persecutio, algor aduersitatis, et affluentia mundane felicitatis.

(*C 84vb*)

17 (150) *Inspice et fac secundum exemplar quod tibi in monte monstratum est* [Ex 25:40] Moysi cum Domino in monte Sina philosophanti ait idem Dominus agens de constructione tabernaculi et distinctione ministerii leuitici ... . "Officium leuitarum dispone secundum exemplar angelice conuersationis quod ostendo tibi in monte" [cf. Hebr 8:5], idest in celsitudine contempla ... . Hiis itaque uirtutibus precingamur ministraturi, et ut non uituperetur ministerium nostrum bene ministremus ut gaudium nobis bonum in profectu et promotione, meliorem in meriti augmentatione, optimum in premii cumulatione, quod nobis prestet
(to clerics at ordination)   (*C 85va; O 180vb; BL Royal 4.B.viii 180ra*)

18 (151) *Venite post me, faciam uos fieri piscatores hominum* [Mt 4:19] Venit Deus ad hominem ut ad se Deum traheret hominem. Venit in mundum ut uiam patefaceret ueniendi ad Deum ... . Septimum et ultimum erit inuitarium: "Venite benedicti Patris mei percipite regnum," etc. [Mt 25:34].
(The Apostles?; to clerics in the schools?)
(*C 85vb; O 118ra; BL Royal 4.B.viii 184ra*)

19 (152) *Circumdabo domum meam ex his qui militant mihi* [Zach 9:8] Verba Dei sunt in Zacharia propheta. "Circumdabo," inquit, "domum meam" etc. Huic consonat illud in Canticis [3:7-8], "En lectulum Salomonis," idest humilem ecclesiam Christi, "quadraginta fortes ambiunt," scilicet doctores et prelati ecclesiastici perfecte decalogum implentes, "ex fortissimis Israel, omnes tenentes gladios," uerborum diuinorum, "et ad bella doctissimi." Leuite quidem excubant circa tabernaculum. Nos autem ueri leuite laicos muniamus infirmos uerbo sancte predicationis, suffragio pie orationis, et exemplo honeste conuersationis ... . Set "ecce nunc tempus acceptabile" [2 Cor 6:2], presertim in tempore gratie, "uidens uidit Dominus afflictionem populi sui" [Act 7:34].
(to prelates and clerics in the schools)   (*C 86ra; O 136rb*)

20 (153) *Vinea mea coram me est* [Cant 8:12] Ex hodierna euuangelii lectione [cf. Mt 20:1-16] comprehendimus quia paterfamilias horis diei uariis in uineam operarios inducit. Vocatosque in sero munerat singulos

singulis pro conuentione denariis. Hec est similitudo proposita et hec est eius intelligentia: Deus diuersis tum mundi tum hominis etatibus ecclesie aggregat ... . Quintus annus est longanimis perseuerantia ex qua ut ita dicam presumendum est, hoc est confidendum.
(to clerics in the schools?)   (*C 86va*)

21 (154) *Fac tibi archam de lignis leuigatis* [Gen 6:14] Ex serie libri Geneseos conicimus quod cathaclismi cause fuere libido clerorum, ubertas uictualium, et inde natum ut recreare otium ... . Quinque ergo mansionibus <archa> distincta fuit. Prima idest inferior fuit stercoraria quo stercora defluebant ne que erant in archa fetore lederentur. Secunda, apotecaria ... . In apotecaria, omnibus escis que mandi possunt referta, sunt scolares ... . Ingrediuntur igitur seorsum uiri, seorsum femine, quia ab amplexu abstinendum est in afflictione. Set qui disiuncti intrauerant coniuncti exeunt, scilicet uiri et femine, quia iam tunc opus erat amplexu et generis humani multiplicatione. Salomon ait [Eccl 3:1,5], "Omnia tempus habent, tempus amplexandi et tempus longe fieri ab amplexibus."
(to clerics in the schools?)   (*C 86vb*)

22 (155) *Nolite thesaurizare uobis thesauros in terra* [Mt 6:19-21] Thesaurus est substantia non uilis ut stagnea uel plumbea, non modica ut duo nummuli siue tres oboli, nec ad tempus breue collecta, ad horam confecta, neque palam posita in publico scilicet, set in abscondito ... . Sic sit thesaurus tuus in occulto ut condatur in tuto. In tuto condit qui in manu Christi reponit. Ipse enim sibi commendatum ultra loca periculosa raptoribus plena deferens absque detrimento restituet tibi totum ex integro.
                                                                            (*C 87va*)

23 (156) *Beatus est*, et erit, *uir qui timet Dominum* [Ps 111:1-2]
Deum iudicem iustum, qui postquam occiderit potest mittere in gehennam et *qui in mandatis eius uolet* uel cupit *nimis* uel multum. Hic qui uoluntate intensa Dei desiderat implere mandata, *potens in terra erit semen eius*. Semen est opus misericordie ut elemosina ... . Sic igitur omnes semper et ubique elemosinis insistamus, ut ad bona premissa attingere ualeamus, quod nobis prestet qui uiuit et regnat
(to clerics in the schools?)   (*C 88ra*)

24 (157) *Facite uobis amicos de mammona* [Luc 16:9] Mammona lingua Syrorum diuitie nuncupantur, et mammon demon, qui opibus seducit ... . Sic igitur in hilaritate misereamur, in simplicitate elemosinis tradamus, ut per has ad iam dictam beatitudinis celestis mensuram perueniamus.

(to clerics in the schools?)   (*C 88rb*)

25 (158) *Facite uobis amicos de mammona ut cum defeceritis recipiant uos in eterna tabernacula* [Luc 16:9] Diuitie iniquitatis uenialis scilicet non mortalis sunt que cum minori equitate adquiruntur, ut est in negotiatione ubi non omnimoda puritas, non prorsus sincera ueritas ... . Eterna tabernacula dicit mansiones in domo patris, ad quas nos perducat qui uiuit et regnat

(*C 88va*)

26 (159) *Erraui sicut ouis que periit* [Ps 118:176] Iustus et in principio et in fine accusator est sui ... . Scribe etiam in tabulis capacis intelligentie et tenacis memorie commemorationem quidem peccati ac mortis ... ut ouis erronea gregi suo apponatur, dragma decima in erarium summi regis inseratur, et filius prodigus qui perierat inueniatur ac in gratiam patris admittatur.

(to clerics in the schools?)   (*C 88vb*)

27 (160) *Stelle manentes in ordine suo et cursu* [Iud 2:20] Apostolus ait fidelibus [Phil 2:15]: "In medio huius nationis praue et peruerse lucetis sicut luminaria in mundo." Sunt ita lumina celi fideles et iusti presertim ministri ecclesiastici puta clerici ... . Qui bene ministrat gradum sibi adquirit bonum; aduersus Siseram pugnauerunt. Hodie iurati in Christi sacramenta tyrones contra fortem armatum proceditis ad bellum ... ut de hoste triumphum reportantes, mereamur accipere coronam uite, quam nobis conferat, qui uiuit et regnat

(to clerics at ordination)   (*C 89ra*)

28 (161) *Sacerdotes qui ad Dominum accedunt sanctificentur, ne percutiat eos* [Ex 19:22] Sacerdos dicitur quasi sacrum dans siue sacer dux. Sacra sunt sacramenta ecclesiastica que de iure impretiabilia sunt, dari debent non uendi ... . Sacerdos in altari manus expandit in modum crucifixi, quod dicit: crucifixum credo, predico, represento, uicem eius gero ... . Laici toto tempore quadragesimali se preparantes ac salutem suam operantes, cum metu et tremore ad sacramentum altaris inuitati ueniunt in sollempni die Pasche. Quid dicendum de sacerdote existente in mortali qui irreuerenter se ingerit cotidie? ... . Sanctificamini ergo hodie, et estote parati in diem obitus in quo, cum uenerit Dominus,

inueniat uos uigilantes et paratos, ad celestes introducat nuptias, ad quas nos perducat qui uiuit et regnat
(to priests)   (*C 89va*)

29 (162) *Exaltare super celos Deus* [Ps 107:6] Dauid Spiritu sancto plenus interioribus oculis preuidens Dei aduentum ... . Plures legimus Christi exaltationes, prima fuit in cruce, secunda in resurrectione, tertia in ascensione, quarta hodie in gentium conuersione et fide, quinta apparebit in extremo agmine ... . Sane hodie manipulum Ioseph adorant circumstantes manipuli fratrum facientium uoluntatem Patris qui in celis est, adoraturi sunt etiam Iudei in fine conuertendi. Verum Ioseph iam adorant sol idest excellentia sanctorum, et luna idest claritas ecclesie, et stelle idest numerositas populorum. Iam lapillus creuit in montem, et potentum, sapientum, religiosorum in orbis nostri circumstantia regi Christo submittuntur colla ... ad Christi igitur capitis exemplum nos membra sic humiliemur ut cum eo in futuro sublimemur. (Pentecost; "in Ascensione Domini" *O*)   (*C 90ra; O 80ra*)

30 (163) *Videte quomodo caute ambuletis* [Eph 5:15] Verba Apostoli sunt. Viatores sumus nondum comprehensores, in uia sumus non in patria, militantes non triumphantes ... . Hic est draco qui in his rogationibus duobus primis diebus antecedit ... . Sic itaque satagamus in uia Dei caute gradi, immo in stadio currere ad brauium festinantes, ingredi in requiem ut deuitatis periculis ope Dei cursum feliciter consumemus, et strenui post laborem, uinctam pugnam, de omnibus hostibus triumphum gloriose reportemus, quod nobis prestet qui uiuit et regnat
(Rogationtide)   (*C 90rb*)

31 (164) *In conspectu angelorum psallam tibi* [Ps 137:1] Psallere est in psalterio musico instrumento modulari. Psallere etiam dicitur psalmodiam proferre, psalmos scilicet canere. Psallere mistice est bene operare scilicet pro superna mercede ... . Angelici spiritus nobis adesse credendi sunt maxime cum diuinis mancipamur obsequiis, idest cum ecclesiam ingressi uel lectionibus sacris aurem accommodamus uel psalmodie operam damus uel orationi incumbimus, uel missarum sollempnia celebramus ... . Sequitur [Ps 137:2]: "Confitebor nomini tuo," corde scilicet, ore, et opere. Laudabo et in laude magnificabo.
(to clerics in the schools?)   (*C 90vb*)

32 (165) Cananea in oratione perstat et instat [cf. Mt 15:22], cui consonat et illud de Iacob [Gen 32:26]: "Non dimittam te nisi benedixeris mihi." ... Et nobis quidem nocte huius seculi lucta restat post baptismum, non solum cum diabolo, mundo, carne, uerum et cum Deo ... . Tunc Iacob, idest luctator, prius in uia uere dicetur Israel, idest directus uel rectus Dei, princeps cum Deo et uir uidens Deum in patria.
(Second Sunday in Lent?)   (*C 91rb*)

33 (166) *Audiui orationem tuam et uidi lacrimam tuam* [4 Reg 20:5] Instantia Cananee flagitantis in Euuangelio hodierno [cf. Mt 15:21-28] tribuit nobis exemplum et scemam orationis ... . Exemplum autem elemosine habemus in uidua Sareptana, de qua Regum libro tertio.
(Second Sunday in Lent)   (*C 91rb*)

34 (167) *Erat Iesus eiciens demonium* [Luc 11:14] Congruit huic tempori loqui nos de ieiunio, oratione, penitentia, eleemosina, et in hiis quidem laboriosis habunda patientia, ut et anima nostra superne Ierusalem promereatur ingressum, et corpus gloriosam optineat resurrectionem. Hunc quidem tam dictorum ordinem declarant nobis euuangelia dominicarum in quadrigesima ... . Siquidem euuangelica lectio prime dominice quadrigesimalis mentionem facit de ieiunio indicans quia cum ieiunasset Dominus quadragintis diebus et quadragintis noctibus temptatus est a sathana. Sequentis dominice euuangelium proponit nobis orationem mulieris Cananee ... . Tertie uero dominice hoc est diei hodierne euuangelium tangit id quod spectat ad penitentiam ... gloriosam resurrectionem consequamur, quod nobis prestet qui uiuit et regnat
(Third Sunday in Lent)   (*C 91va*)

35 (168) *Estote imitatores Dei sicut filii karissimi* [Eph 5:1] Serui inutiles sumus, filii tamen nominamur ... . Exemplum quidem strenue agendi dant nobis formice, apes, aues, et agricole. Fortius quidem in spiritualibus quam in carnalibus excitare debemus, et diligentius anima excolenda quam ager uel uinea.
(Third Sunday in Lent?)   (*C 91vb*)

36 (169) *Abiit Iesus trans mare Galilee* [Io 6:2] De operibus misericordie exercendis hodierna euuangelii lectione erudimur ... . Set Christus miraculose et multiplici ciborum et potuum uarietate, nec solum corporalis substantie set et esca multiplici spiritualis alimonie.
(Fourth Sunday in Lent)   (*C 92ra*)

37 (170) *Mulier que dampnauit saluauit*, et "sicut per inobedientiam unius hominis peccatores constituti sunt multi, ita per unius obedientiam iusti constituti sunt multi" [Rom 5:19] ... . Ad hec etiam facit quia in hoc quadragesimali tempore dominica una legitur quod "erat Iesus eiciens demonium, et illud erat mutum" [Lc 11:14], et proxima dominica in sequenti legitur euuangelium de edulio panum quinque [Io 6:1-15]. Set et ibi etiam ante refectionem premittit euuangelista infirmorum curationem, presertim lectio de hoc eodem agens conuiuio predicans in hunc modum: "Turbe secute sunt eum et excepit illos et loquebatur illis de regno Dei, et eos qui cura indigebant, sanabat" etc. [Lc 9:11]. Nemo reuera digne Christi cibum accepit nisi antea sanatus fuerit, quia post remissionem peccatorum attribuitur allimonia celestis
(Fourth Sunday in Lent?)   (*C 92ra*)

38 (171) *Meror in corde iusti humiliabit eum, et sermone bono letificabitur* [Prov 12:25] Meror in cordibus antiquorum, gemitus compeditorum, desiderium pauperum humiliauit eos cum cogitarent dies antiquos, et annos eternos in mente haberent, recolentes quantum boni amiserint et quantum mali incurrerint ... . Demum quidem sermone bono letificati sunt cum annuntiatione angelica [Lc 1:28]. De redemptione certificati sunt. "Ave," inquit angelus, "gratia plena," etc. ... . Set etiam in hoc tempore quadragesimali meror penitentialis saluber humiliat, et post per iudicium sacerdotis datum reconciliationis sermo letificat. Sic Dauid cui dictum est [2 Reg 12:13]: "Transtulit Dominus a te peccatum tuum," et Magdalenam de qua "dimissa sunt ei peccata multa quia dilexit multum" [Lc 7:47].
(Annunciation, during Lent)   (*C 92va*)

39 (172) *Dilectus meus candidus et rubicundus* [Cant 5:10] Salomon Christi et ecclesie coniunctionem in Spiritu cernens introducit ecclesiam tanquam sponsa de sponso Christo ita loquentem ... . Hinc eius uicarius hodiernus, scilicet sacerdos, et alba sacerdotali induitur et casula rubea ... . Cinis quippe memoria mortis est. Vnde: Memento hec quia cinis es siue puluis [cf. Gen 18:27]. Hoc est memorare nouissima tua. Et Dominus ait: "Hoc facite in meam commemorationem" [Lc 22:19]. Sponso igitur sponsa studeat assimilari in candore castitatis et rubore karitatis. Vnde: "Sint lumbi uestri precincti et lucerne uestre ardentes," etc. [Lc 12:35].
(To priests?)   (*C 92vb*)

40 (173) *Ascendet sicut uirgultum et sicut radix de terra sitienti* [Is 53:2] Hec dixit Ysaias quando uidit et humilitatem et gloriam Christi ... . Ita et Christus homini humilimus, quod patuit in hodierna pedum ablutione ubi seruis plusquam seruus seruiuit ... . "Sine me," inquit, "nichil potestis facere" [Io 15:5]. Ipse etiam arboris totalitatem sustentat portans omnia uerbo uirtutis sue.
(Maundy Thursday; to clerics in the schools?) *(C 93ra)*

41 (174) *Scrutemur uias nostras* [Lam 3:40-41] Verba sunt Ieremie prophete. "Scrutemur," inquit, "uias nostras," idest actiones. Sicut enim uia uehit ad locum bonum uel malum, ita et actio ducit ad requiem uel penam ... . Perscrutemur et rimemur in confessione nostra in hoc tempore quadragesimali genera peccatorum nostrorum cum circum-stantiis eorum ... ut bona que agimus ad Deum referamus et intuitu superne mercedem non quidem terrene faciamus.
(Lent) *(C 93va)*

42 (175) *Surrexit Dominus sicut predixit*, Mattheo xvii [= Mt 28:6] Exinde cepit Iesus ostendere discipulis suis quia oportet eum ire Ierosolimam, et multa pati a senioribus et scribis et principibus sacerdotum, et occidi, et tertia die resurgere ... . Probat enim et proclamat resurrectionem mortuorum generalis doctrina prophetarum et apostolorum omniumque sanctorum predecessorum necnon et prelatorum ecclesiasticorum magistrorumque omnium modernorum auctenticorum et omnium ortodoxorum. Set et uniuersaliter hoc protestatur fides tum Iudeorum tum Saracenorum ... . Possunt et ad hoc induci similitudines mundiales ... sicque iterum de cineribus suis <fenix> resurgit.
(Resurrection; to clerics in the schools?) *(C 93vb)*

43 (176) *Vado parare uobis locum* [Io 14:2] Verba Domini sunt in cena ante passionem discipulis proposita. "Vado," inquit, quasi per portam mortis, transeo, abeo, recedo ... . Set nota quia accipit homo Deum et Deus hominem. Suscipimus quidem Deum per commercium nature, et societatem scilicet et fraternitatem ... et per edulium sancte eucharistie ... et per participium gratie ... . Vnde et Psalmus intitulatur ita: Psalmus cantici in dedicatione domus Dauid [Ps 29:1], hoc est letitie habite pro dedicatione, idest confirmatione, ecclesie in gloria.
(Ascension?; to clerics in the schools?) *(C 94ra)*

44 (177) *Vado ad eum qui me misit* [Io 16:5] Euuangelia que hiis diebus dominicis leguntur post octauam Pasche usque in ipsum diem Pentecostes ... . Mors autem porta uite est que ad uisionem Dei transmittit claudens oculos quibus homines uidebuntur et mundus, et interiores oculos aperiens ut uideatur Christus.
(Pentecost)   (*C 94va*)

45 (178) *Hic Iesus qui assumptus est a uobis* [Act 1:11] Quis, quotus ascendat, quare uel quomodo, quando. Quis: aquila singularis ... sic ueniet manifeste in aere ipse idem in corpore presentibus angelis et hominibus.
(Ascension)   (*C 95ra*)

46 (179) Vnde Iesus scandat, uel quo, uel ubi uideamus ... hec erunt in medio terre, in medio populorum.
(Ascension)   (*C 95ra*)

47 (180) *Passer* [Ps 83:4], hec auis Christus. Ysaia cxxxvi [= 46:11]: "Vocans ab oriente," idest Iudea, "auem" Christum, "et de terra longinqua," idest mundo qui longe a celo, "uirum uoluntatis mee," Filium in quo mihi complacui, *inuenit sibi domum*. In domum Domini ibimus ... sicut turtur nidum, fidei quietem, ubi reponat pullos suos
(Ascension?)   (*C 95rb*)

48 (181) *Beatus uir cuius auxilium est abs te*, etc. [Ps 83:6] Est ascensus electionis, Ysaia xliii [= 14:14]: "Ascendam super altudinem nubium et similis ero altissimo." Est ascensus discretionis ... . Ascensionis gradus sunt meriti inchoatio, augmentum, alternatio, continuatio, et perseue-rantia, et consecutio premii, cum scilicet salit ascensor in paradisum.
(Ascension; to clerics in the schools?)   (*C 95rb*)

49 (182) *Ex Egipto uocaui Filium meum* [Os 11:1] In infantia, contra Herodes et complices eius; et in passione, de Egipto idest de mundo uocatus ... . Tunc absorbebitur in uictoria mors cum omni familia sua, idest defectionibus et penalitatibus presentis status. Auctor etiam mortis occidetur et sepelietur, Ysa. lxxi [= 27:1]: "Dominus occidet cetum qui in mari est."
(Ascension?)   (*C 95va*)

50 (183) Figura dominice ascensionis fuit ante legem translatio Enoch, et in lege subuectio Helie. Item quadraginta mansio est Hely ... . Si tamen gustastis quoniam dulcis est Dominus.
(Ascension)   (*C 95va*)

51 (184) *Cum uenerit paraclitus* [Io 15:26] Quis ueniat uideas, quando uel qualiter, ad quos, in quibus et maneat. Quis, paraclitus idest consolator uel aduocatus et spiritus ueritatis ... . Ita et quinquagensima die a die Resurrexionis dominice hoc est cum complerentur dies Pentecostes ... datus est Spiritus sanctus ... . In columba enim quando apparuit Spiritus sanctus, et auis ista celica plures ramiculos attemptans sessionem morosam non facit nisi in fronde firma.
(Pentecost; to clerics in the schools?)   (*C 95va*)

52 (185) *Cum complerentur dies Pentecostes* [Act 2:1] Pentecostes dicitur hic non sollempnitas illa septem diebus protelata, set quinquagena dierum que fluxit a die Resurrexionis dominice usque ad aduentum Spiritus sancti, quibus completis ultimus dies dicebatur Pentecostes ... . Non enim uos estis qui loquimini, set Spiritus Patris uestri qui loquitur in uobis.
(Pentecost; to clerics)   (*C 95vb; O 87ara*)

53 (186) Quis ueniat, quid agat, in quos, ubi, quomodo, quando. Quis ueniat, Spiritus sanctus qui est arca future beatitudinis cum Christo, et uinum profluens a uite uera Christo ... . Hoc inebriati sunt Apostoli, exhilarati, diserti effecti ... . In spirituali iubileo rei soluuntur, debita dimittuntur, exules in patriam remittuntur, hereditas amissa redditur, serui idest homines peccato uenundati quolibet a iugo seruitutis liberantur.
(Pentecost; to clerics in the schools?)   (*C 96va*)

54 (n.l.) *Ignem ueni mittere in terram* [Lc 12:49] Venit autem Dominus per aquam et sanguinem [1 Io 5:6]: aquam scilicet baptismatis et sanguinem redemptionis, per que Dominus saluat sicut econtra diabolus enecat ... . Ignem etiam idest Spiritum sanctum misit Dominus in Pentecoste ... et facta sunt tonitrua, idest miracula, et terremotus magnus, quibusdam ad bonum, quibusdam ad malum.
(Pentecost)   (*C 96vb*)

55 (187) *Beati mundo corde* [Mt 5:8] Congrue sollempnitatem Pentecostes e uestigio sequitur festum sancte Trinitatis, eo quod Apostoli

in Pentecoste roborati Spiritu sancto fidem sancte Trinitatis predicabant, et in nomine Patris et Filii et Spiritus sancti baptizabant ... . Ne aduertas faciem tuam a me.
(Holy Trinity)   (*C 97ra; O 96ra*)

56 (188) *Honora patrem et matrem* [Ex 20:12] Honora parentes carnales, eis impendens duplici honore ... in gremium suum admittendo, in sinum reponendo.

(*C 97va*)

57 (189) *Homo quidam erat diues* [Luc 16:19] In diuite isto quattuor detestanda reperiuntur scilicet inanis gloria induitur purpura et bisso ... attendendum etiam quia si inhibetur et dampnatur tenacitas.

(*C 97va*)

58 (190) *Vos estis sal terre* [Mt 5:13-14] Verba Domini sunt ad Apostolos. Ipsi nos salliunt doctrina, illuminant uita ... . Nos igitur Petrum et alios sanctos imitemur in sanctitate ut in futuro eis sociemur in beatitudine, quod nobis prestet qui uiuit et regnat
(St. Peter)   (*C 97vb*)

59 (191) *Omnia facite sine murmurationibus* [Phil 2:14-15] Verba sunt Apostoli. Omnia inquit facite sine murmure, uigilias, orationes, ieiunia, elemosinas ... . Magdalena quidem exemplar est penitentie ... hanc igitur nos imitari concedat, qui uiuit et regnat

(*C 98ra*)

60 (192) *Nisi conuersi fueritis* ... usque *angeli semper uident faciem Patris mei* [Mt 18:3-10] Quis putas maior est idest sublimior et uenerabilior in regno celorum, in collegio iustorum? Et aduocans Iesus paruulum, statuit eum in medio eorum, et secundum Marcum, complexus est eum [9:35] ... . Quilibet igitur caueat ne in oculis angeli sui et etiam in conspectu Dei turpia committat. Angelis igitur in dilectione, munditia, obedientia, et laude diuina, hic in uia assimilemur ut postmodum in patria eis associemur, quod nobis prestet qui uiuit et regnat
(All Angels?; to clerics in the schools?)
(*C 98vb; O 94ra, 181ra;* ʙʟ *Royal 4.B.viii, 190rb*)

61 (193) *Nudus egressus sum de utero matris mee* [Iob 1:21] Tria intelligenda sunt et memoriter tenenda: Ingressus hominis in mundum, progressus per mundum, et egressus a mundo ... . Vade et tu fac similiter: felici commercio pro modicis uniuersa, pro terrenis celestia, pro perituris mansura commutemus, ut ad eternam beatitudinem pertingere mereamur, quod nobis prestet qui uiuit et regnat

(*C 99rb*)

62 (194) *Lapidem quem reprobauerunt edificantes* [Ps 117:22], uel sicut Ebreus habet, "Lapis, quem reprobauerunt edificantes," *hic factus est in caput anguli.* Lapis iste Christus est qui in euuangelio dicit Iudeis [Mt 21:42]: Nunquam legistis in scripturis ... abiciat amor Dei.
(to clerics in the schools) (*C 100ra*)

63 (195) *Domine dilexi decorem domus tue* [Ps 25:8] Dei plures sunt domus, habitacula et mansiones. Christus Dei Filius propter nos non dedignatur habere reclinatorium angustum, paupercule et questuarie uirginis uterum ... . Ecclesia etiam in Christi nomine constructa et dedicata domus Dei est de qua scriptum est [Is 56:7, Lc 19:46], "Domus mea domus orationis uocabitur."
(to clerics in the schools?) (*C 100va; O 23rb*)

64 (196) *State succincti lumbos uestros in ueritate* [Eph 6:14-15] O quam uenerabile, quam gloriosum, quam insigne fuit apud antiquos nomen sacerdotii, set hodie ... equis passibus ambulat cum artibus mechanicis, immo inspecta rei ueritate longe uilius est eis, quia ut satyrice loquamur sicut expedit quandoque ex cognitione cause ad arguendum uitia que hodie in ecclesia pullulant prostat, et in questu quasi pro meretrice sedet. Huius autem tam digni nominis abiectio unde habet esse nisi ex indiscreta ministrorum promotione? Proh dolor. Hodie in ecclesiasticis gradibus, ubi summa debet haberi diligentia, nulla adhibetur industria. Multo cautius hodie agitur in secularibus ... . Vtraque ergo manu, O sacerdos, si uis placere Domino, tam otio contemplationis quam opere actionis; modo uaca uigiliis et orationibus ut gregem tibi commissum doceas exemplo, modo insta predicationi ut eum reficias sacro eloquio, modo ministra sacramentum ut esuriens spiritualis spirituale suscipiat alimentum. Oportet te esse ualde circumspectum quia teneris reficere ecclesiam tuam triplici edulio, uerbo scilicet, exemplo, et sacramento ... ut ex miseria huius mundi transeatis ad gloriam, ex luctu triplici ad eternam pacem, quam nobis conferre dignetur Deus, et dilectionis etc.
(to priests) (*C 100vb*)

65 (197) *Ignem ardentem extinguit aqua et elemosina resistit peccatis* [Eccli 3:33] Facienda est quidem larga elemosinarum profusio, ut ualeant elemosine ad potiorem satisfactionem post penitentiam, ad pleniorem reconciliationem post offensam, ad completiorem recompensationem, et ad cumulatiorem remunerationem ... . Idem sapientia dicitur [cf. Prov 3:16]: "In dextera eius anni uite, et in sinistra eius diuitie et honor."

(*C 101vb*)

66 (198) *Beati misericordes quoniam ipsi misericordiam consequentur* [Mt 5:7] Misericordes sunt qui opera misericordie faciunt, que sunt compati, dimittere, dare, et commendare. Opera misericordie sunt elemosine ... . Qui enim perseuerauerit saluabitur

(*C 102ra*)

67 (199) *Honora patrem tuum et matrem tuam ut sis longeuus super terram* [Ex 20:12] siue ut longo uiuas tempore, et bene sit in terra, *quam Dominus Deus dabit tibi.* Hoc est maximum et primum mandatum in altera tabula Moysi, primum septem mandatorum que pertinent ad proximum ... . Est enim pater spiritualis qui dicitur Patris summi uicarius, qui te ecclesiasticorum semine sacramentorum ministerio regenerauit. Hic est sacerdos, hunc igitur uice Christi honora qui talibus ait [Lc 10:16]: "Qui uos audit me audit, et qui uos spernit me spernit." Mater etiam spiritualis ecclesia est que conciperit, de fidei rudimentis instruit, alit enim proficere facit, per baptismum in lucem edit, simplici doctrina lactat, ulnis gestat, de bonis moribus informat, ad mensam mittit dum ad solidioris cibum doctrine idoneum accedere facit, infirmis sacramenta medicinalia dispensat, mortuorum corpora gremio atrii sui confouens resurrectionem gloriose reseruat. Huic igitur tam pie matri et sollicitudine sedula diligenti in honorificentia debita uicem condignam recompendamus, ut iuxta diuinam pollicitationem bene longeui esse mereamur et uitam eternam consequamur in terra uiuentium, quod nobis prestet qui
(to clerics in the schools?)   (*C 102rb*)

68 (200) *Vendite que possidetis et date elemosinam* [Luc 12:33-34] Elemosina debet esse preambula, excisiua, pretiosa, ac in tuto loco reposita ... . Thesaurus enim substantia pretiosa est et celum locus tutissimus. In hoc igitur summi regis erarium substantiam multam inferamus, ut Christi commendata manibus in extrema necessitate repperiamus, quod nobis prestet qui uiuit et regnat

(*C 102va*)

69 (201) *Fili si habes benefac tecum* [Eccli 14:11-15] "Fili," inquit, "si habes." Si enim, ut ait Apostolus, uoluntas prompta est dando, scilicet quod habet accepta est [cf. 1 Cor 4:7]. Qui autem non habet exteriorem facultatem, habeat interius piam uoluntatem ... . Nos autem similiter plures Deo offeramus oblationes in sustentionem sacerdotum, in fabricam ecclesiarum, in necessitates pauperum, et huiusmodi ... . Elemosina quidem purgat peccata et liberat a morte tum corporis tum anime tum a morte gehenne, et ipsa facit filios olim uiros soliditatis. Elemosinarios loquor in extrema necessitate uitam eternam inuenire, ad quam nos perducat.
(to clerics in the schools?) *(C 102va)*

70 (202) *Nisi Dominus edificauerit domum* [Ps 126:1] Attendenda sunt in edificando loco soliditas, expensarum sumptuositas, congruitas etiam materie et idoneitas sceme. De primo habetur ibi [Mt 16:18]: "Super hanc petram edificabo ecclesiam meam." ... Magister igitur immo minister ecclesiasticus, qui in se turrim prelationis construit, sedens computet sumptus qui necessarii sunt ad perficiendum, ne querat fieri iudex cum non ualeat uirtute irrumpere iniquitates ... . Nunc nauigat, nunc arat, nunc fabricat, sculpit, pingit, format; sine huiusmodi non edificatur ciuitas. Exigitur etiam in edificio apta materies lapidum seu lignorum, fit eruderatio lapidum et latomorum industria; fit incisio, politio, et celatio. Succiduntur ligna, planantur, componuntur, exponuntur ne peccetur in materia et in forma. Et iusti quidem constantia stabiles, fide fortes, spe firmi, caritate robusti ... suisque aptantur locis per manus artificis, disponuntur permansuri sacris edificiis ... . Est autem anima Dei domus, thalamus, templum, ortus, ager, uinea diligenter excolenda. In uanum laborauerunt qui edificant eam, quia "neque qui plantat neque qui rigat est aliquid, set qui incrementum dat, Deus" [1 Cor 3:7].
(C 102vb)

71 (203) *Nisi Dominus custodit ciuitatem* [Ps 126:1] Statum ciuitatis turbant ciuis, ignis, et hostis. Mos est ciues ciuibus inuidere. Ciues se inuicem accusant, impugnant, maiores etiam minoribus molestiam multipliciter inferunt. Hostis manifestus est ut depredator, occultus ut fur. Ad custodiam igitur ciuitatis necessaria est ciuium unanimitas in bono et amicabilis confederatio ... . Est autem ciuitas Dei ecclesia Christi siue conscientia iusti ... si tamen homo bene custodiatur Deo totum tribuatur, quia nisi Deus etc.
(C 103ra)

72 (204) *Ad uesperum demorabitur fletus et ad matutinum letitia* [Ps 29:6] Iam uespera mundi est. Iam nouissima hora est. Nos enim sumus in quos fines seculorum deuenerunt, et iudicium illud finale iam in ianuis est ... . Dum tempus habemus operemur bonum ... . Exaltabunt enim sancti in gloria, letabuntur in cubilibus suis, ad quam letitiam nos perducat qui uiuit et regnat

(C 103rb)

73 (205) *Omne datum optimum et omne donum perfectum desursum est* [Iac 1:17] Quasi dicit: Quo datum melius eo collatum a Deo magis agnoscamus. Dona Dei necesse est ... . Datur quidem Spiritus ad sanctificandum sicut datus est a Domino in insufflatione; datur ad roborandum, ut in Pentecoste. Verbo enim Domini celi firmati sunt et spiritu oris eius omnis uirtus eorum [Ps 32:6], datur ad beatificandum ut ad fruitionem.

(C 103va)

COLLECTION TWO: SERMONS FROM MS *L*

II.A [Sermons numbered 74 to 97 are prefaced by the following introduction, found in both MSS *E* and *L*. The text is printed here from *L*; the copy in *E* has been changed from second-person singular to third-person plural throughout].

Inter omnia opera misericordie excellentissimum opus est diuini uerbi predicatio qua errantes possint ab inuio in uiam reuocari, et in uia positi ne deficiant refici. Quantum sit hoc opus saluatori nostro acceptum et nobis necessarium, ipse innuit hiis uerbis: "Messis quidem multa, operarii autem pauci. Rogate ergo dominum messis ut mittat operarios in messem suam" [Lc 10:2]. Vnde beatus Gregorius super eundem locum de tam necessarii operis omissione conqueritur dicens: "Ecce mundus iste plenus est sacerdotibus, et tamen ualde rarus inuenitur in messe Dei operator. Nam etsi sint qui bona audiant, desunt qui dicant." Pauci sacerdotes uerbum Dei predicant, multi tacent, alii ex ignorantia, alii ex negligentia. Set nec isti nec illi poterunt in conspectu Dei de culpa taciturnitatis excusari, cum nec isti preesse debeant qui predicare nesciunt, nec illi tacere qui predicare sciunt.

Quantum periculosa sit predicatorum ignorantia patet ex eo quod ait Veritas: "Si cecus ceco ducatum prestet ambo in foueam cadunt" [Mt 15:14]. Quam nociua sit negligentia innotescere ex illa Salomonis sententia: "Piger propter frigus arare noluit, mendicabit ergo estate, et non dabitur ei" [Prov 20:4]. Quidam autem ex negligentibus licet literature subtiliori expertes sint, tamen, quia capax habent ingenium et linguam intelligunt Latinam, possent saltem sermones scriptos addiscere et sub eadem uerborum serie uel sub leui quadam trans-mutatione subiectis suis exponere, sicque animas suas aliquatenus liberare ab ira illius qui ait: "Si non annuntiaueris populo meo scelera eorum, sanguinem eorum de manu tua requiram" [Ez 3:18]. Set multi illorum tam pigri tam delicati sunt ut, quia sermones scripti uidentur eis aut difficiles aut prolixi, laborem recordationis sustinere non curent.

Quia ergo tibi amice huiusmodi negligentiam inesse perpendi, cupiens te quodam artificiose breuitatis stimulo ad opus predicationis excitare, sermones breues et leues composui, ut animum tuum delicatum quem in aliis sermonibus aut difficultas aut prolixitas a labore recordationis deterrere potuit, horum facile compendium ad eundem laborem prouocaret. Hiis sermonibus si uti consueueris tam magnum pariet tibi consuetudo profectum, ut quandoque iuxta horum exemplar alios eque bonos et forte meliores proprio possis ingenio formare, quibus sonorus incedas et precepta sapientie predices ne legis censura moriaris set cum elucidantibus sapientiam uita perfrui merearis eterna.

(*L 41r; E 2ra-va*)

74 (69) *Christus hodie natus est, gaudeamus* Ne argui possim nihil doctrine uobis impendisse quibus omnia debeo, propono Deo donante aliquid hodie loqui quod spectet ad uenerationem hodierne festiuitatis, ad profectum religionis, ad edificationem animarum. Ecce euuangelizo uobis gaudium magnum: Christus hodie natus est, gaudeamus. Tres sunt natiuitates ... nec in cor hominis ascendit, quam promittis dili-gentibus te, saluator mundi
(Nativity of Jesus)   (*L 41r; E 9va; F 2v*)

75 (71) *In nouissimis diebus circumcides cor tuum* [Is 2:2] Dies ista, quia diem iudicii significat, tam magnum timorem et honorem mihi incutit ut tacere non possim, et loqui me oporteat de circumcisione que tunc plenarie fiet. Tres circumcisiones, prima est carnalis, secunda spiritualis, tertia est corporalis ... . O Domine Iesu Christe rex glorie qui dignatus es hodie pro nostra utilitate circumcidi in teneris membris uulnera ferens dura, fac nos in presenti uita circumcidi, idest purgari ab omni peccato ut mereamur in die iudicii ab omni corruptione circumcidi et in templum superne Ierusalem cum hostiis bonorum operum transferri et tecum ibi uiuere et regnare
(Circumcision of Jesus)   (*L 41v; E 10va; F 3v*)

76 (74) *Obtulerunt Magi Domino aurum, thus, et mirram* [Mt. 2:11] Quia non cognoui litteraturam subtiliorem ideo non propono uobis subtilia set simplicia, non incognita set nota, non doctrinam set admonitionem. Scitis quod hodie obtulerunt magi Domino munera ut, quod corde de eo credebant, muneribus testarentur ... . Imitemur eos offerendo nos et spiritualia munera nostra Deo. Offeramus ei aurum sapienter uiuendo, thus deuote orando, mirram discrete nos mortificando, ut mereamur in die nouissimo nos illi offerre in illa superna Bethlem ... qui omnes electos satiabit et sanabit, ut in eternum uiuant et gaudeant gaudio ineffabili. Quod nobis prestare dignetur
(Epiphany)   (*L 41v; E 13ra; F 4r*)

77 (117) Nam et Maria et Ioseph et Symeon et Anna hodie uenerabilem processionem fecerunt et puerum Iesum in templum presentauerunt. Suscipiens Symeon puerum in manibus, benedixit Dominum dicens, *Nunc dimittis seruum tuum Domine* [Luc 2:29]. Hodie beata Virgo filium suum ad templum detulit. Sicut illi duo portauerunt hodie Christum in manibus suis corporaliter, sic eundem debemus in manibus nostris portare spiritualiter, scilicet per uirtutem sacramenti ... . Offeramus et nos candelas nostras manibus sacerdotis per ipsum pro nobis Deo offerendas ... et lumen illuminans nos uirtutibus, et gloria glorificans nos premiis uite eterne et perpetue beatitudinis, in qua ipse uiuis et regnas
(Presentation in the Temple; to the laity)   (*L 42r; F 4v*)

78 (118) *Sacrificium Deo spiritus tribulatus* [Ps 50:19] Tria sunt sacrificia spiritualia scilicet sacrificium penitentie, sacrificium iustitie, sacrificium laudis ... . Hodie inchoamus quadragesimale ieiunium ... hodie cineres per sacerdotum manus capitibus nostris imponi ... ut in die resurrectionis ualeamus sacramentum corporis et sanguinis tui tam digne suscipere ut non sit nobis reatus ad penam set intercessio salutaris ad ueniam, purgatio peccati, augmentum meriti, profectus uirtutis, et causa salutis, quam salutem nobis concedere digneris
(Ash Wednesday; to the laity)   (*L 42r; F 5r*)

79 (119) *Cum appropinquaret Iesus Ierusalem uidens ciuitatem fleuit* [Lc 19:41-42] Quatuor processiones fecit Iesus in terra. Primam fecit hodierna die quando, appropinquante tempore passionis sue, loco passionis sue approprinquare uolens, eo modo uenit quo eum uenturum propheta predixit, scilicet sedendo super asinam ... ubi erit uisio pacis,

splendor lucis perpetue, et dulcedo ineffabilis glorie, quam dulcedinem nobis prestare digneris saluator mundi, qui cum Patre
(Palm Sunday, in procession; to the laity) (*L 42v; F 5v*)

80 (103) *Absit mihi gloriari nisi in cruce* [Gal 6:14] Imitemur Apostolum et gloriemur in Domino pro nobis crucifixo gratias ei agentes et uestigia eius quantum possumus sequentes ... . Hodie serui Christi erimus per obedientiam si, sacre institutioni ecclesie obedientes, inclinato capite, flexis genibus, fusis lacrimis, corde contrito et humiliato crucem eius adoremus deosculando et gratias ei agendo quod pro nobis in cruce hodierna die mortem pati dignatus ... . Concede Domine ut per plagas tuas et per mortem quam pro nobis pati hodie dignatus es, mereamur a plagis peccati, a penis inferni, et a morte eterna liberari, et ad regnum tuum transferri, Domine Iesu Christe rex glorie, fons pietatis, misericordie, et dulcedinis.
("De cruce" *E* = Good Friday)
(*L 43r; E 115ra; F 7r; Oxford, Bodley 230, 138r*)

81 (105) *Si consurrexistis cum Christo* [Col 3:1] Duplex est resurrectio sicut duplex mors. Est mors corporis, est mors anime ... . Ad eum de quo locuti sumus predicando conuertamus uerba orando: Domine Iesu Christe rex glorie qui hodierna die pro nobis a mortuis resurrexisti fac nos in presenti resurgere de peccato ad iustitiam et in futuro de morte ad uitam, de corruptione ad incorruptionem, de dolore ad gaudium interminabile quod commune erit omnibus electis suis saluator mundi, qui cum Patre
(Easter Sunday) (*L 43v; E 121ra; F 7v; Reims* MS *582, f. 38v*)

82 (99) *Lauamini mundi estote* [Is 1:16] In hiis uerbis Ysaie prophete notari possunt due uirtutes, scilicet penitentia et perseuerantia ... . Ecce fratres mei in hac sacra quadragesima nuper preterita per ueram penitentiam et opera bona purgata fuit conscientia uestra, hospitio cordis uestri mundato Dominum nostrum in die paschali digne suscepistis ... . Perseuerate ergo in illa munditia ne Dominum uestrum digne susceptum indigne expellatis et ad iracundiam prouocetis, ne polluatis hospitium eius sicut polluit olim populus Romanus et graui ultione percussus est, scilicet peste inguinaria, pro cuius remotione instituta fuit Rome hodierna letania que dicitur letania maior ... . Ut ipse per Romanorum processionem et preces et ieiunium placatus eos a peste inguinaria hodierna die liberauit, ita per eadem a nobis placatus nos ab omnibus peccatis et periculis liberet et in preceptis suis faciat

pacem usque ad finem uite perseuerare et post finem in ipsos sine fine uiuere et regnare, qui cum Patre
(Major Litanies)   (*L 44r; E 46vb; F 8v*)

83 (107) *Bona est oratio cum ieiunio et elemosina* [Tob 12:8] Hiis uerbis commendauit Raphael Tobie et filio eius et nobis in eis orationem, ieiunium, et elemosinam quasi tria sacrificia quibus possimus iram Dei placare et amicitiam nobis restituere ... . Unde emanauit ieiunium horum dierum trium qui dicuntur dies rogationum ... et inde institutum est ieiunium illius diei qui dicitur Letania maior ... . Si ergo uolumus ut processio nostra Deo placeat sicut processio illorum placuit, offeramus Deo illa tria sacrificia ... . Scimus Domine quod bona est oratio cum ieiunio et elemosina, pro quibus tecum uiuimus et regnamus, qui cum Patre
(Major Litanies, in procession; to the laity?)   (*L 44r; E 122ra; F 9v*)

84 (110) *Ascendens Christus in altum captiuam duxit captiuitatem* [Eph 4:8] Quatuor sunt ascenciones Domini. Prima facta fuit in capite et paucis membris; secunda et tertia sunt solis membris; quarta fiet in capite et in omnibus. Prima fuit hodie, secunda et tertia cotidie, quarta fit in nouissimo die ... . Studeamus sic per secundam ascencionem proficere ambulantes de uirtute in uirtutem, ut anime nostre per tertiam ascencionem ad uidendum Deum deorum in Syon quamcito fuerint a corporibus separate, et nos omnes in die nouissimo simul cum animabus et corporibus glorificatis per quartam ascencionem perueniamus ad celestem patriam ubi erit perfectio quietis et eternitas beatitudinis, quam nobis prestare digneris saluator mundi, qui cum Patre
("In Ascensione Domini" *E*)   (*L 45r; E 126rb; F 12r*)

85 (114) *Si quis diligit me sermonem meum seruabit* [Io 14:23] Hiis uerbis inuitat nos Dominus ad dilectionem suam ostendens eius effectus ... . Ad hoc dicimus quod ualde necessarium esset omnibus scire quot et que sint criminalium peccatorum genera. Set horum distinctionem usque in alium sermonem differemus, ne presens sermo promisse breuitatis metas excedit. Deprecemur modo Spiritum sanctum qui est uerus et omnipotens Deus cum Patre et Filio ut sicut hodie corda apostolorum plena scientia illuminauit et perfecta caritate accendit, ita nos illuminet et accendat ut hinc sciamus et inde uelimus mala uitare et bona facere quibus mereamur ad celestem patriam

transferri et eterna beatitudine perfrui in eodem Spiritu sancto, qui cum Patre
(Pentecost) (*L 45v; E 133ra; F 12v*)

86 (120) Ait angelus de beato Iohanne: *Multi in natiuitate eius gaudebunt* [Luc 1:14-15] Magnum est testimonium angeli de magnitudine Iohannis, sed maius est testimonium Dei, qui ait: Inter natos mulierum ... . Gaudeamus hodie in natiuitate eius, suplicantes ut intercedat pro nobis ad Dominum et nobis impetret eius gratiam qua sic imitemur beatum Iohannem ... ut mereamur peruenire ad consortium eius et magni esse cum eo coram Domino et angelis eius et omnibus electis in eterna beatitudine, quod nobis prestare dignetur
(Nativity of John Baptist) (*L 46r; F 13v*)

87 (121) *Qui sunt isti qui ut nubes uolant* [Is 60:8] Isayas propheta sancti Spiritus reuelatione edoctus preuidit quales et quam preclari futuri erant Apostoli ... . Imploramus ergo Apostolos omnes et maxime Petrum et Paulum quos hodie specialiter ueneramur, ut sicut nos hodie de illis loquimur in terris, ita illi pro nobis loquantur in celo et nos Deo reconcilient, ut mereamur ad eorum consortium peruenire, et cum eis in eternum uiuere et regnare
(Peter and Paul) (*L 46v; F 14v*)

88 (122) *Dilectissimi emendemus nos ab omni inquinamento carnis et spiritus* [2 Cor 7:1] Cum nec possim nec sciam omnia in presenti exponere que uobis necessaria sunt, propono illa saltem explicare que scire est utilius et nescire periculosius. Nichil autem est ut arbitror utilius scire quam mala quibus, et bona sine quibus, salus esse non potest ... . Mala enim sunt criminalia peccata ... hec septem sunt illa septem demonia que Dominus eiecit de beata Maria Magdalena cuius hodie festiuitatem colimus ... . Deprecemur eam ut ipsa pro nobis intercedat ad Dominum quatinus sicut ipse eiecit ab illa septem demonia, ita eiciat a nobis omnia uitia, et emundet ab omni inquinamento carnis ac spiritus, et emundatos transferat ad regnum suum.
(Mary Magdalene) (*L 47r; F 15v*)

89 (123) *Dispersit dedit pauperibus* [Ps 111:9] Quattuor in hoc uersu possunt notari que faciunt elemosinam magni meriti, scilicet larga uoluntas, discreta intentio, prudens humilitas, et pia hilaritas ... . Hec quatuor egregie compleuit beatus Laurentius cuius hodie martirium celebri deuotione ueneramur ... . Obsecremus ergo beatum Laurentium

ut nobis a Domino impetret gratiam qua mereamur dona nobis
commissa sic dispergere et dare pauperibus, ut iustitia nostra maneat
in seculum seculi, et cornu nostrum exaltetur in gloria sempiterna, quod
ipse prestare dignetur
(St. Laurence)					(*L 48r; F 16v*)

90 (124) *Multe filie congregauerunt diuitias* [Prov 31:29] Sermo iste
dirigitur ad mulierem fortem et dirigi potest ad tria, scilicet ad ecclesiam,
ad fidelem animam, ad beatam Virginem ... . Set omissis aliis ad presens
loquimur de Virgine singulari cuius assumptionem hodie singulari
ueneratione celebrare debemus ... Quas diuitias et delicias nobis prestare
dignetur per merita et intercessionem eius Filius qui cum Patre
(Assumption of the Virgin)					(*L 48v; F 17v*)

91 (125) *Ecce sacerdos magnus, pater multitudinis gentium et non
inuentus similis illi in gloria* [Eccli 44:20] Hec sunt uerba prophetie
commendantis beatum Augustinum, scilicet ab officio, a probitate, a
lucro ... . Pater erat, est, multarum gentium, idest multarum congre-
gationum tripliciter scilicet in canonicis regularibus, in theologis
secularibus, in populis conuersis ... . Imitemur eum in hiis tribus pro
modulo nostro, ut simus sacerdotes in oblationem hostie uiue, magni
ex merito uite, patres multitudinis gentium et in lucro animarum quas
possimus Deo presentare, et cum eis et pro eis uiuere et regnare, quod
nobis prestare dignetur per merita et per intercessionem beati Augustini
(St. Augustine; to the clergy)					(*L 49r; F 18v*)

92 (n.l.) *Gaudeamus omnes in Domino diem festum celebrantes sub
honore Marie uirginis de cuius natiuitate gaudent angeli* Merito debent
homines hodie gaudere in terra unde angeli gaudent in celo, scilicet
de natiuitate beate Virginis ... . O beata Virgo que nata es hodie, adiuua
nos cotidie, salua nos in nouissimo die, ut mereamur ad consortium
tuum peruenire, prestante filio tuo.
(Nativity of the Virgin)					(*L 49r; F 19r*)

93 (126) Cum summa deuotione celebranda est beati Michaelis festiuitas
quia ipse est, scriptura testante, princeps celestis militie, prepositus
paradisi, susceptor animarum ... . Diximus breuiter quid sit angelus,
quot sunt ordines angelorum, que officia, et que nomina. Videamus
modo quomodo ad eorum consortium peruenire possimus ... quatinus
mereamur eis sociari in luce et regere in gaudio et gloria, in qua ipse
uiuit et regnat
(St. Michael and all Angels; to the laity?)					(*L 49r; F 19v*)

94 (127) *Beati pauperes spiritu quoniam ipsorum est regnum celorum* [Mt 5:3] Hoc euuangelium pulcherrime congruit hodierne festiuitati in qua sub una celebritate ueneramur omnes sanctos, qui per septem uirtutes que in hoc euuangelio enumerantur ad serenitatem peruenerunt ... . Studeamus ergo predictas uirtutes habere ut mereamur ad tam magna premia peruenire, et per experientiam scire quam beati sunt pauperes spiritu quoniam ipsorum est regnum celorum. Quod nobis prestare dignetur per merita et intercessionem omnium sanctorum, saluator mundi
(All Saints; to the laity?) (*L 50r; F 20r*)

95 (128) *Dilexit Andream Dominus in odorem suauitatis* Hec est dies in qua, hic locus in quo, speciali deuotione uenerari debemus beatum Andream. Ideo in hac die specialius quam in aliis honorandus est a nobis beatus Andreas, quia ipse in hac die specialius et excellentius obsequium Deo exhibuit, offerendo se illi in ara crucis ... . Hic est una ex principalibus ecclesiis eius quas habet in Anglia. Hic est preclarum castellum eius, scilicet hoc sacrum cenobium. Hic est insignis excercitus eius, scilicet uenerabilis congregatio monachorum, pulcra et decora tamquam filia celestis Ierusalem, terribilis ut castrorum acies ordinata, que in hoc castello se et ciuitatem hanc ab igneis telis diaboli potenter defendit. Hec ciuitas est specialiter patrimonio beati Andree subiecta, quia omnes ecclesie in ea constitute huic cenobio sunt assignate, et ita omnes habitatores huius ciuitatis sunt beato Andree tamquam parochiani subiecti sui ... . Quarum beatitudinem nobis prestare dignetur per merita et intercessionem beati Andree saluator mundi.
(St. Andrew; to the canons, clergy, and people) (*L 50v; F 21v*)

96 (67) *Qui sedes super cherubin manifestare* [Ps 79:2] Tres sunt aduentus Domini de quibus cantamus et legimus in hoc tempore, unus in spiritu, duo in carne. Aduentus Domini spiritualis est quando uenit per gratiam ad peccatorem uel ad iustum ... gaudio magno et multiplici et interminabili. Quod nobis prestare dignetur saluator mundi, qui cum Patre et Spiritu sancto uiuit et regnat per omnia secula seculorum.
(Advent) (*L 51r; F 23r; E 5va; O 9brb*)

97 (129) *In lapide uno septem oculi sunt* [Zach 3:4] Hiis uerbis ostendit propheta quam utilis sit nobis Christus. Ipse enim est lapis in fundamento ecclesie positus ... . Hec septem dona que plenissime in Christo erant ipso donante manifeste refulserunt in beato Nicholao,

cuius solempnitatem hodie celebramus ... quam dulcedinem nobis
prestare dignetur saluator mundi
(St. Nicholas)   (*L 52r; F 24r*)

Habes amice quod promisi, sermones scilicet compendiosos, quibus
si uti uolueris, tibi et aliis plurimum prodesse poteris. Vt autem utilitati
tue et honori propensius inuigilem, plures adhuc sermones tibi com-
ponam eodem ordine in illis processurus quo in istis processi.

                                                       (*L 52v*)

II.B [Sermons numbered 98 to 115 are prefaced by the following
introduction, found only in ms *L*, fol. 83r]

Promisi me tibi amice in Christo dilecte scripturus sermones quibus
te ad predicationis operam compendiose instruere<m> et artificiose
excitarem. Promissum tibi opus transmisi tanquam semen agro cordis
tui comittendum ut quod modicum erat in semine, multiplicaretur in
messe. Ager tamen ille quasi sterilis et incultus permanens, adhuc nec
fructum nec spem fructus pretendit. Quid de tante utilitatis omissione
dicam? Qua differs fronte tam necessario operi operam dare? Quid
specialius pertinet ad pastorem quam pascere gregem? Quid ergo de
te dicam nisi quod uerissimum est, scilicet quod te ab excellentissimo
opere officii tui perniciose auertunt aut ludi, aut labores, aut pocula
Lethes? Set quia fortasse desidiam tuam aut negligentiam excusando
obicis quod a compendio promissi operis in doctrina mea sermo in
dispendium declinauerit, aut a metodo plana in salebras saltum dederit,
icirco tibi iterato sermonem dirigo, tam breuiter et tam leuiter loquens,
ut nulla occurat difficultas in sermone, nulla excusatio de taciturnitate.

98 (70) *Hodie descendit lux magna super terram* Triplex est lux de
qua loquitur sacra scriptura, scilicet lux mundi, lux Dei, lux Deus ... .
Descendit hodie super terram quia hodie natus est Christus de beata
Virgine. Deprecemur eum ut per lucem gratie sue faciat nos lucere
per iustitiam et per uite munditiam, et sic mereri lucem perpetuam
et requiem sempiternam
(Nativity of Jesus)   (*E 10rb; L 83r; O 16ra*)

99 (72) *Renouabitur ut aquile iuuentus tua* [Ps 102:5] Duplex est
renouatio, scilicet una anime, altera corporis. Prima fit cotidie, secunda
in nouissimo die ... . Aquila enim non renouatur ad immortalitatem,
set data est similitudo de aquila quanta potest esse de re mortali ad

immortalem. Hanc circumcisionem et renouationem conferat nobis
saluator mundi
("In circumcisione Domini" *E*) (*E 11ra; L 83r; O 29ra*)

100 (75) *Surge illuminare Ierusalem quia uenit lumen tuum* [Is. 60:1]
Hodierna festiuitas uocatur epiphania, idest manifestatio, triplici ratione,
scilicet quia Christus hodie erat tripliciter manifestatus. Set quibus, ubi
et quando? Hodie fuit Christus manifestatus tribus magis in Bethleem
ductu noui sideris. Hodie fuit ipse manifestatus Iohanni in Iordane
Patris uoce. Hodie fuit ipse manifestatus discipulis suis in Chana Galilee
aque in uinum conuersione. Ecce iste tres manifestationes erant facte
uno et eodem die, set non in eodem anno ... . Hodie et cotidie ita
illuminet ut uideamus eum in presenti per fidem et in futuro per speciem
in illa superna Bethleem ubi ipse uiuit et regnat
("In epiphania Domini" *E*) (*E 13va; L 83v; O 29ra*)

101 (n.l.) *Tulerunt Iesum in Ierusalem* [Luc 2:22] Cum pastor a
pascendo nomen acceperit, iniuste uocatur pastor qui gregem sibi
commissum nunquam pascit. Quid igitur dicam ego miser, qui pastoris
nomen habeo et gregem meum non pasco? Quid summo pastori
respondebo? Qua ratione me excusabo? Si scio pascere et non pasco,
manifesta est negligentia. Si nescio, aperta presumptio. Qua enim
temeritate presumpsi quod nesciui? Hinc timens et tremens nitor hodie
loqui ne semper tacuisse conuincar. Hodie tulerunt parentes Iesum
ipsum in templum cum hostiis legalibus Deo Patri offerendum. Vnde
nos ad imitationem illorum et memoriam illius gloriose oblationis hodie
in manibus nostris portamus candelas accensas ... . Ipse Christus nos
portabit usque in templum celestis patrie ubi cum eo sine fine uiuemus
et regnabimus, quod ipse patrare dignetur.
(Presentation of Jesus in the Temple) (*L 83v*)

102 (n.l.) *Penitentiam agite, appropinquabit enim regnum celorum*
[Mt 3:2] Inuitat nos beatus Iohannes ad penitentiam ostendendo
quantus sit fructus penitentie ... ad ueram penitentiam inuitat nos hodie
impositio cinerum. Ideo namque imponuntur cineres capitibus nostris
ut memores simus quod sumus cineres, idest fragiles et mortales, ut
ita memoria mortalitatis et mortis pariat nobis timorem, et timor
confessionem et satisfactionem, et sic sit in nobis uera penitentia, per
quam appropinquet ad nos regnum celorum.
(Ash Wednesday) (*L 84r; O 53ra*)

103 (n.l.) *Aue Maria gratia plena* [Luc 1:28] Eisdem uerbis quibus salutauit angelus beatam Virginem hodie salutemus eam cotidie ut ipsa nobis subueniat modo et maxime in nouissimo die. Maria interpretatur maris stella ... per merita et intercessionem beate Virginis conferat nobis Filius eius.
(Annunciation)   (*L 84r; O 53ra*)

104 (n.l.) *Egredere de terra tua* [Gen 12:1] Per hec uerba que Dominus dixit ad Abraham inuitat ipse quemlibet peccatorem ad spiritualem processionem ... . Ad hanc spiritualem processionem inuitat nos corporalis processio quam hodie facimus et corporalis processio quam hodie fecit Dominus ueniens in Ierusalem. Ierusalem interpretatur uisio pacis et signat celestem patriam ubi eterna pax uidetur et possidetur, ad quam nos perducat saluator mundi.
(Palm Sunday, in procession?)   (*L 84r; O 53ra*)

105 (106) *Beatus qui habet partem in resurrectione prima* [Apoc 20:6] Duplex est resurrectio scilicet resurrectio anime et resurrectio corporis. Prima est resurrectio anime qua resurgit de morte peccati ad uitam iustitie ... . Christus qui hodie surrexit et in nobis fidem et spem resurrectionis confirmauit, ipse faciat nos partem habere in resurrectione prima et in secunda immortalitatis gloriam et perhennis uite beatitudinem, in qua ipse cum Patre
(Easter Sunday)   (*E 121va; L 84v; O 67ra*)

106 (108) *Bona est oratio cum ieiunio et elemosina* [Tob 12:8] Memini me dixisse in capite ieiunii quod uera penitentia exigit tria scilicet contritionem, confessionem, satisfactionem. Set quia non ostendi quot et que sint necessaria de quolibet istorum, ideo quod tunc minus dixi modo subplebo ... . Iccirco institutum est ut hiis diebus qui dicuntur dies rogationum ieiuniemus et elemosinas faciamus ut oratio nostra ieiunio et elemosina quasi duabus alis subuecta celum penetret et celesti Domino nobis impetret in presenti prosperitatem et pacem et in futuro gloriam et honorem. Hec omnia nobis patrare dignetur saluator mundi qui cum Patre
(Major Litanies)   (*E 123rb; L 84v*)

107 (111) *Ascendit Deus in iubilo et Dominus in uoce tube* [Ps 46:5] Hoc uersu predixit propheta ascencionem Domini et duplex testimonium ipsius ascencionis, scilicet unum in Apostolis et alterum in angelis ... . Christus autem qui hodie ascendit in celum corpore, faciat nos per predictos gradus ascendere in celum in presenti corde et in futuro cum anima et corpore, et ibi cum eo uiuere et regnare, qui cum Patre

(Ascension) (*E 126vb; L 85r*)

108 (115) *Si quis diligit me sermonem meum seruabit* [Io 14:23] Dilectio alia carnalis, alia spiritualis, alia naturalis. Carnalis erat dilectio qua populus Israel carnalis et rudis Deo seruiebat pro temporalibus ... . Qui uere Deum ex uera caritate diligit omnibus preceptis eius obedit et nullum contempnit. Hanc dilectionem infudit hodie cordibus Apostolorum Spiritus sanctus. Eandem infundat cordibus nostris idem Spiritus sanctus, qui cum Patre

(Pentecost) (*E 134ra; L 85v; O 87brb*)

109 (n.l.) *Iustus ut palma florebit* [Ps 91:13] Palma in inferiori parte et radice habet amaritudinem et asperitatem, set in summo habet florem pulcherimum et fructum suauissimum. Set tarde profert florem et fructum, scilicet in fine anni; sic iustus in imo presentis uite in hac ualle miserie habet laboris asperitatem et doloris amaritudinem, set in summo, idest in superna patria habebit florem pulcritudinis in corpore et anima, et fructum dulcedinis, idest eterne iocunditatis, set tarde, idest post finem huius uite. Iniustus autem non floret sicut palma ... . Ille autem cuius hodie natiuitatem celebramus non floruit sicut fenum set sicut palma ... et per intercessionem beati Iohannis nobis conferre dignetur saluator mundi, qui cum Patre

(Nativity of John Baptist) (*L 85v; O 106ra*)

110 (n.l.) *Domine tu omnia scis* [Io 21:17] Tertio interrogauit Dominus Petrum utrum diligeret eum, ut qui eundem ter negauerat ter se amare confiteretur, et trine confessionis merito trine negationis aboleret infamiam. Ideo etiam facta est trina de Dei dilectione interrogatio, quia tribus modis diligendus est Deus, scilicet ex toto corde, et ex tota anima, et ex tota uirtute, uel ex toto intellectu, et ex toto affectu, et ex toto effectu ... . Imitemur ergo Petrum unusquisque nostrum diligendo Deum ex toto corde ... . Ad cuius gloriam per martirii palmam transtulisti hodie Petrum et Paulum per merita et intercessionem eorum ad societatem ipsorum nos perducere digneris domine Iesu Christe rex glorie, qui cum Patre

(Peter and Paul) (*L 85v; O 118vb*)

111 (n.l.) *Magnificat anima mea Dominum* [Luc 1:46] Beata Virgo de beneficiis ineffabilis gratie ei collatis gratias egit Deo tripliciter,

scilicet ore, opere, et corde ... . Si studeamus eum sic laudare, ascendemus quo beata Virgo hodie ascendit ... ad societatem huius Virginis per merita et intercessionem ipsius perducat nos Filius eius saluator noster, qui cum Patre
(Assumption of the Virgin)   (*L 86r; O 140ra*)

112 (n.l.) *Respexit humilitatem ancille sue* [Luc 1:48] Hiis uerbis beate Virginis exprimitur causa quare magnificauit Deum et exultauerit in eo, quasi dicit, "Ideo magnifico Deum et exulto in eo quia ipse respexit humilitatem mei ancille sue." ... Hec Virgo nata est hodie ut per humilitatem sol fieret et solem conciperet ... . Sic humiliari et sic exaltari per intercessionem beate Virginis faciat nos Filius eius, qui cum Patre
(Nativity of the Virgin)   (*L 86v; O 140ra*)

113 (n.l.) *Cum exaltatus fuero a terra, omnia traham ad me ipsum* [Io 12:32] Triplex est utilitas crucis, quia per passionem eius redempti sumus, per fidem eius roboramur, per signum eius munimur ... . Saluator noster qui pro nobis uoluit in cruce exaltari, per quem hodie in Ierusalem fuit crux exaltata. Ipse nos per uirtutem crucis perducat ad gaudia lucis, qui cum Patre
(Exaltation of the Cross)   (*L 86v; O 53rb*)

114 (n.l.) *Precepit Dominus Moisi ut faceret tabernaculum iuxta exemplar tabernaculi quod ei monstrauerat in monte* [cf. Ex 25:40] Moraliter per hoc significatur quod unicuique nostrum percipitur ut in se construat tabernaculum uirtutum ad similitudinem angelice societatis que nobis monstratur in monte, idest in sacra scriptura que dicitur mons propter celsitudinem misteriorum que in ea continentur. Tria sunt in quibus debemus imitari angelos, scilicet pietas, puritas, caritas ... . Beatum ergo Michaelem et omnes angelos imitemur in tribus uirtutibus predictis, ut imitatione uirtutum perueniamus ad societatem eorum, quod nobis prestare dignetur qui
(St. Michael and all Angels)   (*L 87r; O 178ra*)

115 (n.l.) *Dilectus meus candidus et rubicundus* [Cant 5:10] Hiis uerbis ecclesia dilectum suum scilicet Christum commendat a duplici decore quam habet et in se et in membris suis. Ipse enim est candidus in natiuitate in qua peccatum non habuit, et rubicundus in passione qua nos a peccatis lauit ... . Ita sunt due uie per quas ipsi ad regnum peruenerunt, scilicet uia rubea, et uia lactea. Via rubea est uia martirum, uia lactea aliorum sanctorum. Per alteram uiarum istarum oportet nos

imitari sanctos quorum celebramus hodie festiuitatem si uolumus ad eorum peruenire societatem, ad quam per merita et intercessionem eorum perducat nos saluator mundi, qui cum Patre
(All Saints) (*L 87r; O 178rb*)

[This conclusion is found only in *L*, fol. 87r:]

Ecce habes amice, Deo propitio, ex labore meo sermonum breuitatem, leuem et utilem. Si autem uisa fuerit desidie tue hec breuitas prolixa, hec leuitas ho<ne>rosa, hec utilitas amara, non curabo ulterius egro inobedienti manum apponere, set te tibi tamquam desperatum et incurabilem tristitia et tedio affectus relinquam. Si uero ammonitionis mee stimulo excitatus, diuina gratia inspirante, ad uerbum Dei proferendum labia tua aperire dignum duxeris, auditui meo dabis gaudium et letitiam.

COLLECTION THREE: ADDITIONAL SERMONS FROM *E*, *F*, and *L*

116 (n.l.) *Gustate et uidete quoniam suauis est Dominus* [Ps 33:9] In solemnitatibus sanctorum celebrandis, quanto fuerit nostra deuotio feruentior tanto erit ipsa nobis celebratio fructuosior ... . Copiose autem gustauit dulcedinem Dei et uidit beata Katerina, cuius hodie passionem colimus et uirtutes predicamus ... . Ecce bipartitus est sermo noster, primo enim docuimus quod tria sunt que conferunt beatitudinem, scilicet gustare suauitatem Dei, et uidere et sperare in eo; et de singulis tractauimus ostendendo quod triplex est gustus, triplex uisio, triplex spes. Secundo demonstrauimus quomodo hec tria erant in beata Katerina. Imitando ergo beatam Katerinam gustemus ... . Ut ergo, fratres mei, cauemus huiusmodi confusionis et dapnationis amaritudinem, gustemus dulcedinem Dei in corde, ore, et opere ... . Ipse faciat nos secum beate uiuere et regnare, qui cum Patre
(St. Catherine) (*L 87v; O 178rb*)

117 (68) *Descendit sicut pluuia in uellus* [Ps 71:6] Ad sacratissimam dominice natiuitatis sollempnitatem deuote celebrandam preparanda sunt corda nostra excitanda deuotio ... . Mihi autem querenti uerba ad huiusmodi preparationem idonea et prefate sollempnitati cognata, occurrebant ista: "Descendit sicut pluuia in uellus." Satis nostis, fratres mei et domini mei, quod hiis uerbis propheta pulcherima utens similitudine predixit Christi incarnationem et natiuitatem ... et tecum beatitudinem eternam possidere Domine Iesu Christe rex glorie
("In uigilia natalis Domini" *E*; to bishops and clergy?) (*E 6va; L 89r*)

118 (73) *Cum natus esset Iesus in Bethlehem* [Mt 2:1] De gaudiis ad gaudia transeamus, et exigentibus hodierne festiuitatis auspiciis in conspectu Domini Dei nostri iocundiores appareamus. Huius enim ratio sollempnitatis ab apparitione nomen accepit; Epiphania quippe "apparitio" dicitur Latine. Videamus igitur quis apparuit, et ubi, et quando apparuit, qualiter etiam et quare, uel quibus ... per obedientiam et humilitatem ad eandem reuertamur
(Epiphany; in the schools)   (*E 11va*)

119 (95) Karitas in dilectione Dei et proximi constat. Seruat autem in se dilectionem Dei qui a caritate non diuiditur proximi. Qui a fraterna societate secernitur, a diuine caritatis participatione priuatur; nec poterit Deum diligere qui noscitur proximi delectione errare ... . Teneamus ergo eam fratres uirtute quia possumus ut nobiscum sit, nobiscum maneat, nobiscum surgat, nobiscum pergat, nobiscum letetur et coniuuetur. Decet enim in fratrum congregatione tam regiam iugiter inesse uirtutem.
                                                                       (*E 37rb*)

120 (96) Duo sunt genera dilectionem proximi conseruanda, unum ne malum quis inferat, alterum ut bonum impendat ... . Set hec omnia probauerunt senes magni, et inuenerunt quia bonum est cotidie manducare, parum sibi subtrahentes, et ostenderunt nobis uiam hanc regalem, quia leuior est et facilis.
                                                                       (*E 38va*)

121 (97) Uigili cura, mente sollicita, summo conatu et sollicitudine continua decet nos inquirere et addiscere quomodo et qua uia possimus infernale supplicium uitare et celeste gaudium adquirere, cum nec illud supplicium uitari nec illud gaudium adquiri possit nisi uia cognita qua illud est uitandum et istud adquirendum ... . Fac nos sequi uiam caritatis que ducit ad celestam gloriam. Fac nos ibi in decore tuo delectari, dulcedine tua refici, et bona illa uidere que nec oculus uidit nec auris audiuit nec in cor hominis ascendit, que preparasti diligentibus te. Qui cum Patre
                        (*C 179ra, ascribed to Alexander of Ashby; E 39va*)

122 (98) *Lauamini mundi estote, auferte malum cogitationum uestrarum* [Is 1:16] Ysayas propheta hiis uerbis nobis tria commendat, idest ablutionis munditiam, munditie perseuerantiam, et perseuerandi causam ... . Multa possent utiliter dici de hiis tribus capitulis que, si prosequeremur, fortasse prolixior sermonis nostri contextus in tedium uobis

uerteretur. Iustum est quod caritati uestre breuiorem conteximus telam ex uno filo, scilicet ex eo quod propheta intendit docere per hoc unum uerbum: "Lauamini." ... Tripartitus est sermo iste, primo namque breuiter exposuimus uerba prophete ... secundo diffusius de primo tractauimus dicentes que sint immunditie, a quibus mundari debemus, scilicet peccata, que diximus in duo genera scilicet in uenialia et criminalia. Criminalia autem distinximus in septem genera et de singulis latius tractauimus ostendendo quam nociua sunt et quomodo ualeant uitari per uirtutes illis contrarias. Tertio uero ostendimus quo lauacro mundari possint ... . Ad illud regnum nos perducere digneris Domine Iesu Christe rex glorie, fons pietatis, miserie et dulcedinis, qui cum Patre
(in the schools) (*E 42rb*)

123 (100) *Declina a malo et fac bonum* [Ps 36:27] Hiis uerbis commendat propheta uitam honestam et premium eius ... . Fratres mei in hoc sermone potestis addiscere ea quorum notitia uobis ualde neccesaria est ... . Contra gulam et cetera uitia predicta dedit beatus Augustinus cuius hodie festiuitatem celebramus optima documenta. Contra gulam in regula canonicorum ait ... . Contra reliqua uitia que sequntur possent similiter beati Augustini documenta assignari que causa breuitatis omittimus festinantes ostendere quam magnum sit honeste uite premium, scilicet inhabitare in seculum seculi ... . Quam iocunditatem nobis per merita et intercessionem sancti Augustini prestare dignetur saluator mundi, qui uiuit et regnat
(St. Augustine; to Augustinian canons?) (*E 47va*)

124 (104) *Beati qui audiunt uerbum Dei et custodiunt illud* [Lc 11:28] Consuetudo est sancte ecclesie ut in hac die ueniant ad primam pueri, puelle, pastores, seruientes qui pro seruitio dominorum suorum ad ecclesiam in aliis diebus uenire non possunt. Ideo debetis scire causam. Scitote ergo quod iccirco uenitis ad ecclesiam in hac festiuitate que maior est et sanctior omnibus aliis festiuitatibus per annum ut accipiatis lumen et uiaticum, scilicet lumen quo possitis uidere uiam salutis, et uiaticum idest cibum uie quo possitis sustentari in uia ne deficiatis. Illud lumen est doctrina sacre doctrine ... . Viaticum autem est quod accipere debetis, sacratissimum corpus Christi quod est digne accipientibus ad uitam ... et per illam susceptionem peccata et pericula uitare et hostes nostros, scilicet diabolum, carnem, et mundum, sic expugnare ut mereamur coronam glorie et honoris sempiterni percipere ab eo qui cum Patre
(Easter Sunday; to the laity) (*E 115vb*)

125 (109) *Qui crediderit et baptizatus fuerit, saluus erit* [Mc 16:16]
Ea que aliquis a sua recedens extremo eis dicit mentibus eorum artius
imprimuntur. Inde est quod Dominus et saluator noster sermonem,
quem discipulis suis et omnibus credentibus utiliorem et magis necessarium fore nouit, usque ad hodiernum diem quo erat in celum
ascensurus reseruauit, ut extremo eis dictus eorum memorie firmius
inhereret ... . Domine Iesu Christe qui in celum ascendisti hodie, trahe
nos post te, infunde nobis fidem quam docuisti, et confer nobis salutem
quam credentibus promisisti. Fac nos tecum habitare in celestibus,
modo mente, in futuro mente in corpore, qui uiuis et regnas
("In Ascensione Domini")   (*E 123vb*)

126 (112) *Sedete in ciuitate quoadusque induamini uirtute ex alto* [Lc
24:49] Hiis uerbis precepit Dominus Apostolis suis ut corporaliter
manerent in ciuitate Ierusalem quoadusque induerentur uirtute ex alto.
Per eadem uerba precipit nobis omnibus ut spiritualiter sedeamus in
spirituali ciuitate si uelimus induere uirtute. Oportet ergo in presenti
sermone ut tria dicamus, scilicet quid sit spiritualiter sedere, que sit
ciuitas illa in qua sedendum est, et quid sit indui uirtute ex alto ... .
Studeamus ergo sedere sicut supra docuimus in ciuitate presentis
ecclesie ut mereamur indui uirtute ex alto in presenti et stola glorie
in futuro, quod nobis prestare dignetur per merita intercessione beate
Virginis Marie et sanctorum Apostolorum Spiritus sanctus qui eis
hodierna die datus est, qui cum Patre et Filio
(Pentecost; to the clergy)   (*E 127va*)

127 (113) *Qui habet mandata mea et seruat ea, ille est qui diligit me*
[Io 14:21] Fratres mei dilectissimi qui laici estis intendite diligenter hiis
quibus saluator noster ostendit que sint necessaria ad ueram caritatem
habendam, et quod sit uere caritatis premium ... . Frequentate ergo
libenter ecclesiam, audire attentius uerba predicationis, et addicite
diligentius mandata Dei. ... Si non potestis, fratres mei, esse cum uiris
religiosis mente simul et corpore, sitis cum eis mente, sitis cum eis
beneficii exhibitione, uel saltem bona uoluntate ... . Si ex uera caritate
diligimus Deum, hoc erit premium nostrum quod a Patre et Filio et
Spiritu sancto diligemur, quod Filius se nobis manifestabit ut eum cum
Patre et Spiritu sancto uideamus et de illa uisione eternaliter et
ineffabiliter gaudeamus, quod nobis prestare dignetur idem Dominus
noster Iesus Christus qui cum Patre
(Pentecost; to the laity)   (*E 130ra*)

128 (n.l.) Tota religiosorum debet intentio circa hoc uersari et ad hoc niti ut possint in hac uita prouehi ad illam perfectam caritatem que foras mittit timorem ... . Set omnipotens et pius est Spiritus sanctus per quem hodierna die cordibus Apostolorum infusa et diffusa est perfecta illa caritas ... . Set potius cupiamus dissolui et esse cum Christo, et cum ipse ad hostium pulsauerit ei confestim aperiamus semper uicturi cum Christo, qui cum Patre
(Pentecost; to religious)

(C 180vb, ascribed to Alexander of Ashby; E 132ra)

129 (116) In hac sacra sollemnitate que sancte Trinitati assignatur in materiam sermonis nobis assumimus simbolum Apostolorum quod fidem Trinitatis immo tantam fidem catholicam breuiter comprehendit. Et primo traditum est Christianis ut eo cotidie omnes tam clerici quam laici fidem profitentur. Omnibus ergo expedit et maxime clericis hoc simbolum intelligere, quia clerici non solum fidem que in eo continetur debent tenere set etiam tueri, et iuxta doctrinam beati Petri, semper esse parati satisfacere poscenti rationem de ea que in eis est [cf. 1 Petr 3:15]. Fide et spe hoc simbolum exponere, immo expositiones theologorum inde nobis recitare uolentes, dicemus hec quatuor scilicet quare dicatur simbolum, quare simbolum Apostolorum, et quot habeat partes, et quid in singulis partibus contineatur ... . Studeamus ergo fidem catholicam que in hoc simbolo continetur firmiter tenere, et ad hanc fidem infideles conuertere et fideles in ea confirmare ... . Hanc fidem in nobis confirmet et per hanc fidem perducat ad eternam beatitudinem sancta et indiuidua Trinitas cuius hodie festiuitatem celebramus, qui uiuit et regnat Deus unus et trinus per infinita secula seculorum.
(Holy Trinity; in the schools) *(E 134va)*

130 (n.l.) *Ecce Dominus ueniet et omnes sancti eius cum eo, et erit in die illa lux magna* [cf. Zach 14:5] Nisi Dominus reliquisset nobis semen suum, quasi Sodoma et Gomorra essemus ... . Ecce ueniet Dominus et omnes sancti etc. Hodie fratres karissimi ecclesia magna facit gaudium et festum de adventu Christi. ... Item queritur si missa pro uno defuncto celebrata, ei plus ualet quam aliis. Ad hoc dicendum est quod si celebratur missa pro uno defuncto, omnibus prodest lumen istud. Quod in tenebris ostenditur est lucidum corpus Christi quod omnes illuminat, qui dum uincerent illuminari meruerunt. Verumtamen orationes spirituales et deuotio specialis pro uno facto magis prosunt quam alii.
(Advent; in the schools.) *(F 1r)*

COLLECTION FOUR: SERMONS FROM MS *R*

131 (n.l.) *Fasciculus mirre dilectus meus mihi. Inter ubera mea co-morabitur* [Cant 1:12] Verba sponse sunt de sponso loquentis in cantico amoris. Fasciculus quidem est paruulus qui natus est nobis. Christum etiam et martires eius haut incompetenter comparare possumus fasciculis qui de silua ceduntur, ligantur, coaptantur ... et ubi lenis sibilus aure tenuis, ibi Dominus.
(Advent?)   (*R 142ra*)

132 (n.l.) *Benedictus qui uenit in nomine Domini. Deus Dominus et illuxit nobis* [Ps 117:26, 27] Benedictus sit, laudatus corde, ore, opere, qui uenit. Ad nos uenit per Virginem ... . At quis uenit? Deus. ... Deus inquid Dominus timendus, et illuxit nobis multiplici luce. Quere in uersibus nostris, L: "Lux" ... . Hinc et in ortu solis iustitie claritas Dei pastores circumfulsit, et stellam splendidam et matutinam quam maris stella peperit aeris stella magis indicauit.
(Advent)   (*R 142va*)

133 (n.l.) *Adducet Dominus urentem uentum de deserto ascendentem et siccabit uenas mortis et desolabit fontem eius* [Os 13:15] Tenebrosa aqua in nubibus aeris, idest obscura doctrina in prophetis, ut scilicet diabolo celaretur Christi incarnatio ... . Igitur Osee utrumque Christi aduentum prenuntians, eius incarnationem et natiuitatem insinuans ... . Ex ipso enim hauriunt reprobi mortem corporis et mortem anime, et mortem eternam, idest penam gehenne. Ipse enim auctor potius ex quo mors.
(Advent)   (*R 142vb*)

134 (n.l.) *Offer filium tuum quem diligis Ysaac super unum montium quem monstrauero tibi* [Gen 22:2] Oblatus est in templo masculus paruulus Ihesus pannis inuolutus, et tu offer Domino masculum, idest opus bonum, cui caueas a fluuio Pharaonis, idest luxu seculi, et ab ense Herodis, idest suggestione demonis ... . Et attende quod conceptus est Christus de Spiritu sancto, et tamen ex carne uirginea procreatus. Ita et opus bonum ex gratia Dei prouenit, et libero arbitrio quod tamen ex Deo.
("Sermo in die purificationis sancte Marie")   (*R 143va*)

135 (n.l.) Offer Domino candelam accensam, benedictam, et sancti-ficatam. In hac tria sunt, scilicet cera munda, hec est caro casta qua

offeras secundum illud: "Ne polluatis terram habitationis uestre" [Num 35:33], idest carnem quam inhabitat anima ... . Castitatis quidem exemplum et humilitatis atque caritatis, idest dilectionis, in beata Virgine et eius prole reperimus.
(Purification of the Virgin)   (*R 143va*)

136 (n.l.) *Deus ab austro ueniet* [Hab 3:3], de Bethleem scilicet ad Ierusalem in die purificationis sancte Marie, et tu Deum imitare. Prius sis in austro, ubi maior est splendor solis et calor; hoc est in sapientia et caritate ... et in laudem Dei musica instrumenta, idest iubilus perpetuus.
(Purification of the Virgin)   (*R 143vb*)

137 (n.l.) *Cum optulerit homo sacrificium coctum Domino in clibano de simila, panem scilicet absque fermento, conspersum oleo* [Lev 2:4] Omnia in figura contingebant Hebreis. Clibanus igitur est Virginis uterus siue ipsa Virgo ... . Os autem huius clibani Deus post iudicium opturabit ne panes extrahantur.
("Sermo de annuntiatione sancte Marie")   (*R 143vb*)

138 (n.l.) *Sapientia edificauit sibi domum, excidit columpnas septem, immolauit uictimas suas, miscuit uinum, et proposuit mensam suam* [Prov 9:1-2] Christus Dei uirtus et Dei sapientia, emphatice dictus est sapientia. Ipse enim omnisciens est ... . Domus ista est beata uirgo Maria ... . Peccator quidem fouea uulpis est, cubile demonis. Vnde: "Reuertar in domum meam unde exiui" [Mt 12:44]; Iob xxx, ii [37:8]: "Ingredietur bestia latibulum suum, et in antro suo commorabitur."
("Sermo in annuntiatione sancte Marie")   (*R 144rb*)

139 (n.l.) *Soluite et adducite mihi* [Mt 21:2] Prius iaciatur fundamentum hystorie secundum seriem quatuor Euuangeliorum: Ab aduentu Domini Bethaniam, sabbato scilicet proximo ante dominicam palmarum usque ad eiectionem uendentium et ementium in templo, idest atrio templi. Deinde sic proponatur: Vbi sunt egritudines et uulnera, necessaria est medicina. Spirituales autem egritudines et anime uulnera sunt uitia et peccata. Medicina competens et sanatiua est penitentia, que piscina furum est. In hac fit tum asine tum pulli solutio et eorundem ad Iesum adductio. Vt qui prius fuit asinus stolidus et immundus etc., iam sit Ysachar fortis ut iumentum factus aput Deum [cf. Gen 49:14-15]: "Asinus utilis ac humilis" et cetera. Quere in uersibus nostris, A: "Asinus" ... et fiat dignus fructus penitentie, secundum qualitatem

scilicet et quantitatem culpe. "Oleos" quippe Grece, "misericordia"
Latine. Huius autem opera quere in uersibus, O: "Opera misericordie" ... . Vt deinceps in celesti Ierusalem in templo, idest cetu angelico,
innocentes et puri laudemus ipsum in perpetuum, iuxta illud [Ps 83:5]:
"Beati qui habitant in domo tua, Domine, in secula seculorum
laudabunt te."
("Dominica palmarum")   (*R 144va*)

140 (n.l.) Per montem oliueti tendit Dominus Ierusalem, et per opera
misericordie pro superna mercede facta ad celestem perueniemus
Ierusalem. Bethfage quidem, idest domus bucce, uiculus sacerdotum,
est humilitas in qua maneant sacerdotes ... . In hoc autem humilitatis
uiculo, buccas suas exercent sacerdotes pro se et aliis orando, Deum
laudando, et uerbum Domini populo predicando ... . Bethania igitur
estis si obeditis prepositis uestris. Hospitatur autem Dominus in
Bethania, quia in hiis qui parent eius preceptis habitat, reficitur, et
requiescit ... . Sic itaque Dominum suscipiamus in domum terrestrem
ut post obitum ab ipso suscipiamur in domum celestem. Quod nobis
prestet etc.
("Sermo in dominica palmarum"; to clerics at ordination?)   (*R 145ra*)

141 (n.l.) *Christus humiliauit semetipsum factus obediens usque ad
mortem, mortem autem crucis* [Phil 2:8] Iam passio dominica celebratur.
Redemptori grates agamus, non solum ore set et opere, ne latronibus
assimulemur quorum fertur ingratitudo erga liberatores eorum a
suspendio ... . Specialiter autem quatuor uirtutum nobis relinquit
exemplum; hec autem quatuor sunt humilitas, caritas, obedientia, et
patientia ... . Porro patientia columpna uirtutum est. Nam uidua est
uirtus quam non patientia firmat.
("Dominica in passione")   (*R 145rb*)

142 (n.l.) *Expecta me, dicit Dominus, in die resurrectionis mee* [Soph
3:8] Verba Domini sunt in Sophonia propheta ecclesie proposita.
Fratres non expectetis ad presens leporem politi sermonis, fucati seu
faleris colorum rethoricorum subornati, presertim cum Dominus dicat:
"Non plantabis lucum et omnem arborem iuxta altare Domini Dei
tui" [Deut 16:21]. Luctus, frondibus amenus set minus fructuosus,
secularis est eloquentia ... . Altare dicit mysterium dominice incarnationis, passionis, et resurrectionis. Ad hoc mysterium discutiendum,
non plantabis facundie philosophice lucum ... . Set iam ad rem acce-
damus, hoc est ad sollempnitatem hodiernam. Hodie archa Dei eleuata

est, baculus nuceus exaltatus, cornu salutis erectum, caput exaltatum, cereus magnus in ecclesia erectus ... in huius mundi deserto proficiscentes et proficientes semper in anteriora, nos extendentes et ad terram promissionis desideranter anelantes, ad quam nos perducat qui uiuit et regnat

("Sermo in die Pasche"; to clerics in the schools?)   (*R 145vb*)

143 (n.l.) *Fulcite me floribus, stipate me malis, quia amore langueo* [Cant 2:5] Vox est ecclesie, angelos et homines alloquentis. Flos autem florum Christus est de uirga radicis Iesse ascendens ... . Terra es et in terram ibis. Hec est in uia non suscipiens cultoris uestigia, idest doctoris monita, aratrum doctrine non sustinens, nec uerbi diuini semen admittens ... . Sericum uero, de uisceribus uermium eductum, humilitatem figurabat qua sacerdos, licet ordinis fastigio polleat, se tamen quasi uermem agnoscat ... . Hinc ad beatam Virginem dicimus: "Vt tuis fultum patrociniis ad celeste regnum me perducas"; et "Beati archangeli Michaelis intercessione suffulti supplices te Domine deprecamur ut quos" etc. Sequitur, "stipate me malis." De hiis in sermonibus qui sic incipiunt: "Omnia po. no. et ue."

("Item sermo in Pascha"; to priests)   (*R 147ra*)

144 (n.l.) *Similis factus sum pellicano solitudinis* [Ps 101:7] Hebraica ueritas habet "deserti," Romanum Psalterium "in solitudine." *Factus sum sicut nicticorax in domicilio*, uel in parietinis. *Vigilaui, et factus sum sicut passer solitarius*, uel singularis, uel unicus, *in tecto*, uel super tectum. Verba Christi sunt qui locutus est per os sanctorum prophetarum ... . In qua celsitudine quoad angelos et homines ipse est solitarius. Quia tu solus altissimus Ihesu Christe cum Spiritu sancto in gloria es Dei Patris. Amen.

            (*R 147va*)

145 (n.l.) *Tria sunt difficilia mihi et quartum penitus ignoro: Viam aquile in celo, uiam colubri super terram, uiam nauis in medio mari, uiam uiri in adolescentia sua. Talis est et uia mulieris adultere, que comedit et tergens os suum dicit: Non sum operata malum* [Prov 30:18-20] Salomon in hoc loco Parabolarum mentionem facit de Christo et ecclesia, de diabolo, antichristo, et populo eius ... . Sit igitur unusquisque nostrum non caro, idest carni deditus, quam pungit anguis iste uirosus, set petra que serpentis aculeos non admittit, neque colubri uiam exprimit, ut nichil suum hostis in nobis inueniat. Quod nobis prestet qui uiuit et regnat

            (*R 148ra*)

146 (n.l.) Spiritus sanctus detestatur et odit simultatem. Vnde: *Spiritus sanctus discipline*, suple doctor, *effugiet fictum* [Sap 1:5], qui scilicet aliud dicit et aliud facit. Odit et falsitatem, quia Spiritus ueritatis est [cf. Io 14:17]. Ipse enim tanquam auis ramum stabilem querit, fragilem et deficientem fugit ... . Hii sunt flores qui in ecclesia ab alto iactantur in die Pentecostes ... . Est enim spiritus intelligentie, sanctus, incoinquinatus, et mundus tum in se tum in effectu. Mundos enim facit et diligit; spiritus autem immundus uersatur in immundo sicut scarabeus in fimo.

("Sermo in die Pentecost")   (*R 148va*)

147 (n.l.) *Assumpta est Maria in celum*, etc. Est assumptio hominis ab imo uitiorum in altum gratie et uirtutis ... . Est et finalis assumptio cum unus assumetur et alter relinquetur. Tunc sponsa Christi in thalamum nuptialem plenarie introducetur.

(*R 148vb*)

148 (n.l.) *Sapientia edificauit sibi domum* [Prov 9:1] Maria est domus obumbrationis contra aeris intemperiem ... . Maria ergo, mulier fortis, fortior uino et rege, accinxit fortitudine lumbos suos. In ea Christus et lumen et custos, positus est homo in paradiso ad operandum et custodiendum.

(*R 148vb*)

149 (n.l.) Virgo sapiens desponsata est filio regis summi, epithalamio idest laude nuptiali digna et dulci cantico dragmatis. Quis sponsus eius? Vnigenitus regis qui fecit nuptias filio suo, et ipse filius tanquam sponsus procedens de thalamo scilicet nuptiarum. Thalamus Marie uirginis uterus quo Christus et Ecclesia, coniuncti quondam caritatis copula, facti sunt iam in carne una; et post consensum animorum feliciter subsecuta est coniunctio corporum cum "Verbum caro factum est et habitauit in nobis" [Io 1:14], idest in conformitate siue identitate nature nostre ... . Continens offert commune sacrificium, uirgo holocaustum. Illa fomitem premit, hec perimit.

(*R 149ra*)

Appendix A

Manuscripts containing the writings of
William de Montibus

This list of manuscripts containing copies of William's writings is organized geographically according to the current repositories of the manuscripts. The provenance of each codex, if known, is noted in square brackets following the shelf number. Unless otherwise specified, this information is from Neil R. Ker, *Medieval Libraries of Great Britain: A List of Surviving Books*, 2nd ed. (London: Royal Historical Society, 1964). The term "imperfect" indicates that the work in question was not copied in its entirety; "incomplete" describes a text that is deficient through the loss of leaves or other mutilation of the codex after it was written.

Aberdeen, University Library MS 240 [From St. Paul's Cathedral, London]
    194vb-198ra *De septem sacramentis*

Baltimore, Walters Art Gallery MS W.131
    133r-174v *De septem sacramentis*

Budapest, Egyetemi Könyvtár (University Library) MS 39 [From southern Poland; see Ladislaus Mezey, *Codices latini Medii Aevi Bibliothecae Universitatis Budapestinensis* (Budapest, 1961), p. 56]
    90r-94r *De septem sacramentis*

Bury St. Edmunds, Cathedral MS 4 (B.357) [From the Benedictine abbey, Bury St. Edmunds (Suffolk)]
    88r-95v *Numerale* (incomplete)

Cambridge, University Library MS Dd.iv.27
    1ra-137vb *Sermones*

——, University Library MS Dd.iv.50
    1r-24v *Sermones*

——, University Library MS Ii.i.24
    77ra-103vb, 179ra-181rb *Sermones*

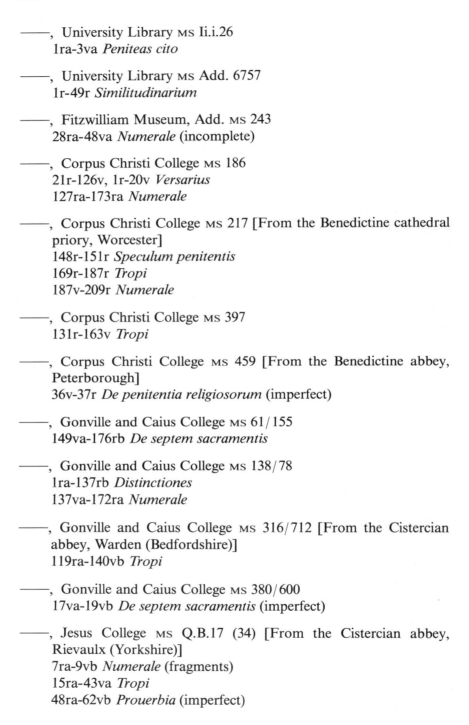

——, University Library MS Ii.i.26
1ra-3va *Peniteas cito*

——, University Library MS Add. 6757
1r-49r *Similitudinarium*

——, Fitzwilliam Museum, Add. MS 243
28ra-48va *Numerale* (incomplete)

——, Corpus Christi College MS 186
21r-126v, 1r-20v *Versarius*
127ra-173ra *Numerale*

——, Corpus Christi College MS 217 [From the Benedictine cathedral priory, Worcester]
148r-151r *Speculum penitentis*
169r-187r *Tropi*
187v-209r *Numerale*

——, Corpus Christi College MS 397
131r-163v *Tropi*

——, Corpus Christi College MS 459 [From the Benedictine abbey, Peterborough]
36v-37r *De penitentia religiosorum* (imperfect)

——, Gonville and Caius College MS 61/155
149va-176rb *De septem sacramentis*

——, Gonville and Caius College MS 138/78
1ra-137rb *Distinctiones*
137va-172ra *Numerale*

——, Gonville and Caius College MS 316/712 [From the Cistercian abbey, Warden (Bedfordshire)]
119ra-140vb *Tropi*

——, Gonville and Caius College MS 380/600
17va-19vb *De septem sacramentis* (imperfect)

——, Jesus College MS Q.B.17 (34) [From the Cistercian abbey, Rievaulx (Yorkshire)]
7ra-9vb *Numerale* (fragments)
15ra-43va *Tropi*
48ra-62vb *Prouerbia* (imperfect)

——, Peterhouse MS 119
31ra-32vb *Speculum penitentis* (incomplete)
33ra-40va *Similitudinarium* (excerpts)

——, Peterhouse MS 255
1r-35r *Numerale*
84r-127r *Similitudinarium*
128ra-133va *Speculum penitentis*
133va-137ra *Errorum eliminatio*

——, St. John's College MS F.4 (141)
1ra-42vb *Numerale*
44ra-47ra *Speculum penitentis* (imperfect)
85ra-88rb *Speculum penitentis*

——, Trinity College MS B.16.18 (392)
1ra-172va *Distinctiones*

——, Trinity Hall MS 24
70r-85vb *Similitudinarium*
86va-101ra *Prouerbia* (incomplete)
102va-107ra *Numerale* (incomplete)
108ra-112rb *Speculum penitentis*

Durham, Cathedral Library MS B.iv.20 [From the Benedictine cathedral priory, Durham]
91a-183b *Numerale*

——, Cathedral Library MS B.iv.26 [From the Benedictine cathedral priory, Durham]
37v-39r *De penitentia religiosorum* (imperfect)

Eton, Eton College MS 82
1r-64r *Numerale*
66r-90v *Similitudinarium*

Heiligenkreuz, Stiftesbibliothek MS 90
1-170 *Distinctiones* (?)

Laon, Bibliothèque Municipale MS 309
41r-52v, 82v-89v *Sermones*

Leiden, Bibliotheek der Rijksuniversiteit MS Vulcanianus 48 (E.173)
195ra-212rb *Tropi*

Leipzig, Universitätsbibliothek MS 423
pp. 308-313 *De septem sacramentis*

Lincoln, Public Record Office MS Ancaster 16/1 [From the Prae-
monstratensian abbey, Newsham (Lincolnshire)]
5vb-45rb *Numerale*
53ra-76ra *Similitudinarium*

London, British Library MS Cotton Vespasian B.xiii [From the
Benedictine abbey, St. Albans (Hertfordshire)]
90va-110va *Similitudinarium*

———, British Library MS Cotton Vespasian D.xiii
60ra-65vb *Speculum penitentis* (incomplete)
114rb-115rb *Peniteas cito*
115rb-118va *Peniteas cito*
118vb-121rb *Speculum penitentis* (imperfect)

———, British Library MS Cotton Vespasian E.x
43v-59v *Tropi* (imperfect)
125v-199r *Numerale*

———, British Library MS Harley 325
38v-82r *Numerale*
87r-94r *Speculum penitentis*

———, British Library MS Royal 6.B.x [From the Benedictine abbey,
Bury St. Edmunds (Suffolk)]
43vb-86vb *Distinctiones* (incomplete)

———, British Library MS Royal 8.C.vii [From the Benedictine abbey,
Tewkesbury (Gloucestershire)]
123v-126r *De penitentia religiosorum*

———, British Library MS Royal 8.D.iv [From the Benedictine abbey,
Pershore (Worcestershire)]
113vb *Similitudinarium* (incomplete)

———, British Library MS Royal 8.G.ii [From the collegiate church,
Tattershall (Lincolnshire)]
2ra-92vb *Distinctiones*

———, British Library MS Royal 9.A.xiv
296ra-298rb *Peniteas cito*

———, British Library MS Royal 10.A.vii [From the Benedictine abbey,
Bardney (Lincolnshire)]
1ra-115ra *Distinctiones*
142ra-149vb *Sermones*

——, British Library MS Royal 11.A.iii
    5ra-34va *Numerale*
    35ra-129vb *Distinctiones*

——, British Library MS Add. 16164 [From the Benedictine abbey, St. Albans (Hertfordshire)]
    15r-58r, 63r-108r *Versarius*

——, Gray's Inn MS 13 [From the Cistercian abbey, Combe (Warwickshire)]
    56ra-101rb *Similitudinarium*

——, Lambeth Palace MS 36
    95v-97v *Peniteas cito*

——, Lambeth Palace MS 122 [From the Augustinian priory, Lanthony (Gloucestershire)]
    178ra-198va *Tropi* (imperfect)

——, Lambeth Palace MS 199
    226ra-248vb *Tropi*

——, Lambeth Palace MS 261 [From the Augustinian priory, Newstead (Nottinghamshire)]
    53r-108v *Numerale*

Mainz, Stadtbibliothek MS I.117
    19ff *De septem sacramentis*

Munich, Bayerische Staatsbibliothek MS Clm 8885
    270ra-274rb, 274vb-ra *De septem sacramentis*

——, Bayerische Staatsbibliothek MS Clm 8961
    163r-173r *De septem sacramentis*

——, Bayerische Staatsbibliothek MS Clm 14706
    11r-18v *De septem sacramentis*

Oxford, Balliol College MS 222
    3ra-27vb *Similitudinarium*
    27vb-48va *Tropi*
    48vb-76vb *Numerale*

——, Balliol College MS 228
    220rb-225rb *De septem sacramentis* (imperfect)

——, Bodleian Library MS Add.C.263 (sc 27646)
    55rb-96va *Numerale*

96vb-113rb *Similitudinarium* (excerpts)
115rb-18ra *Errorum eliminatio*

——, Bodleian Library MS Bodley 419 (sc 2318) [From the collegiate church, Tattershall (Lincolnshire)]
1ra-103rb *Distinctiones* (excerpts)
103va-105rb *Tractatus metricus de septem sacramentis*

——, Bodleian Library MS Bodley 860 (sc 2723) [From the Benedictine abbey, Bury St. Edmunds (Suffolk)]
9ra-93vb *Super Psalmos* (incomplete)
94r-107v *Collecta*

——, Bodleian Library MS Bodley 828 (sc. 2695) [From the Benedictine cathedral priory, Worcester]
225r-226v *De penitentia religiosorum*

——, Bodleian Library MS Bodley 897 (sc. 27888) [From the Franciscan convent, Hereford]
97va-121ra *Numerale*

——, Bodleian Library MS Digby 20 (sc 1602)
92r *Tractatus metricus* (fragment)
103v-104v *De penitentia religiosorum* (incomplete)
158r-161r *Speculum penitentis* (imperfect)

——, Bodleian Library MS Greaves 53 (sc 3825)
55r-106v *Distinctiones* (excerpts)

——, Bodleian Library MS Laud misc. 345 (sc. 1273) [From the Benedictine cathedral priory, Durham]
15ra-18va *Errorum eliminatio*
192rb-206vb *Numerale*

——, Bodleian Library MS Lyell 8 [From the Cistercian abbey, Fountains (Yorkshire)]
56vb-59va, 143rb-va, 169ra-174vb *Numerale* (extracts)
187va-b *Epistola ad moniales*
passim *Sermones*

——, Corpus Christi College MS 43 [From the Augustinian priory, Lanthony (Gloucestershire)]
1ra-12rb, 16ra-46 *Distinctiones* (excerpts)

——, Merton College MS 257
5ra-66ra *Numerale*
68ra-104vb *Similitudinarium*

——, New College MS 98 [From the Benedictine abbey and cathedral priory, Ely]
1ra-32vb *Numerale*
33ra-59rb *Tropi*
59va-123vb *Prouerbia*
123vb-141vb *Similitudinarium*

Paris, Bibliothèque Mazarine MS 730
65rb-67vb *Speculum penitentis*
67v-68r *Errorum eliminatio* (incomplete)

San Marino (California), Henry E. Huntington Library MS HM 19914
159ra-184rb *Numerale*

Tours, Bibliothèque Municipale MS 473
196r-198v, 202r-207v, 216v, 217r *De septem sacramentis*

Troyes, Bibliothèque Municipale MS 1514
90va-96va *De septem sacramentis*

Utrecht, Bibliotheek der Rijksuniversiteit MS 312 [From the Carthusian priory, Utrecht; see P.A. Tiele, *Catalogus codicum manu scriptorum bibliothecae Universitatis Rheno-Trajectinae*, 2 vols. (Utrecht, 1887), 1: 101].
1ra-54vb *Distinctiones* (excerpts)
126vb-142va *Tropi*

——, Bibliotheek der Rijksuniversiteit MS 387
50r-52v *De septem sacramentis* (imperfect)

Worcester, Cathedral Library MS F.61 [From the Benedictine cathedral priory, Worcester]
169ra-180ra *Tropi*

——, Cathedral Library MS Q.27
226v-234v *De septem sacramentis*

Appendix B

Alphabetical listing of the first lines of verse in William's *Versarius*

A culpis ignis altum purgabit et imum. (622)
A petra resilit quamuis sit acuta sagitta (62a)
A Phebo Phebe lumen capit; a sapiente (1140)
A pomo quod primus homo gustauit, acetum (1365)
A puero spreuit Benedictus florida mundi (95)
A quibus et quando comedatur pascha notato (414)
A quibus et quando, cur, quomodo sit feriandum. (485)
A triplici morte presenti tempore surge (1095)
A ueneris sorde uirgo mundissima uere (681)
Abdita propalans, reproborum pectora turbans (5)
Absint o patiens consensus, talio, murmur (924)
Absoluunt animas defunctorum ospes et Ely. (34)
Absque malo plenusque bono prodesse paratus (576)
Absque parentela Salem rex atque sacerdos (713)
Abstinet infirmus, patiens fastidia, iustus (600)
Accedit nobis aduersans callidus hostis (395)
Accelerent nos conuerti, deflere reatus (1027)
Accendi facilis, uilis, leuis, aspera stuppa (1186)
Accidiam generant iteratio, copia, morbus. (1268)
Accipiendo seu quasi cautum dicito catum. (183)
Acre calens simile pani rumpens zima turget. (511)
Actus solamen, amor et compassio cordis (709)
Ad bellum doctus, armatus, fortis et audax (88)
Ad benedicendum uel agendum suspice celum. (252)
Ad Dominum festinandi sint hee tibi cause (1034)
Ad formam morum prestat nomen monachorum (732)
Ad fratrem uictum nichil est a patre relictum (886)
Ad mensam socius fuerit quicumque uocatus (178)
Ad noctis tenebras, ad fulgura claude fenestras (1214)
Ad quem quis clamet, cur, quomodo, quando, quid, unde. (160)
Adiunctum, signum, causam, uerum, quoniam dat. (1067)
Adiutor manus est, oculus prouisor et est pes (748)

Adueniet iudex Christus districtus in ira (6)
Aduersus Christum legitur comittere bellum (87)
Affectu care luneue resigno uel ex spe (76)
Affectu tentus reus est porcus pede uinctus. (1316)
Affectus non effectus habet egra senectus. (1166)
Affectus purus, discretio, finis et ordo (857)
Affectus, sensus, mores, meditatio, motus (866)
Aggrauat et fedat peccatum uilificatque (1010)
Aggrauat ordo, locus, peccata, scientia, tempus (1007)
Aggrauat ordo, locus, peccata, scientia, tempus (190)
Agnoscas quod res uariant diuersaque mutant (768)
Agnus, ouis, Christus, humilis, mitis, taciturnus (919)
Alligat atque legit amor, et coniungit et unit (99)
Alta salix, sterilis et amica paludis, amara (1183)
Alta uirens uictrix cui radix aspera palma (951)
Alterius bona perpendens qui detrahit ille (390)
Amissis habitis dolor attestatur amorque. (391)
Amphora mensura mea si iungatur utrique (1133)
Ampla uia est uere que ducit ad atra gehenne (1278)
Ancillans, dominans, regnans est femina fortis (697)
Angelus, athleta, miles, medicusque magister (896)
Angelus et Christus, sanctus, demonque superbus (56)
Angustant iter hec: mundus, caro, demon et usus (1283)
Anna uiros habuit Ioachim, Cleopham, Salomamque (540)
Annus et annus abit, semper sapientia stabit. (1110)
Antiquuus primum nos suscipit hostis ut ursus (19)
Apocopant infelices sibi tempora uite (89)
Apotoy keraton, hoc est a cornibus apte (231)
Apparet fantasma uiris, set rursus ab illis (325)
Ara, locus, cura, doctrina, liber, sacramenta (827)
Ara, pes, et missa, pax ecclesiastica, crisma (144)
Ara prophanata, fatuum sal, cesaque uitis (899)
Arche ligna lita non soluunt uentus et unda (103)
Argenti quinque redimenda pro sibi prole (1193)
Argentum seruat dum purificatur in igne (770)
Arguit, abscidit, monet et iubet, instruit, ungit (916)
Arguo mercandi non officium set abusum (832)
Ars uitium nescit, uitiosus abutitur arte. (43)
Ars, usus, locus et tempus, scriptura, creata (307)
Ascensus gradus est primus contempnere mundum. (17)
Aspice quis, quando, cuius, quomodo seruiat et cur. (1136)

Aspice quis, quid, ubi uel qualiter offerat, ex quo. (860)
Assuetudo mali fetet ad ora Dei. (164)
Ast alii tenebras et opacam uincere noctem (668)
At post flagra patris, pietas dabit ubera matris (888)
At solus qui sentit olor, discrimine quanto (873)
Atropos, atra nimis, pernicibus aduolat alis (778)
Attendas cur peniteas et quomodo, quando (1028)
Attendas qualis, cui, quomodo, curque ministres. (302)
Attendas qualis expectes, qualiter et quid. (445)
Attendas quis, quid, quo uel quando mereatur (740)
Attenuant hominem studium, ieiunia, pallor (63)
Attrahe per primum, medio rege, punge per imum (85)
Attrahit, absorbet naues pontina uorago (223)
Audax, assidua sit nostra precatio iusta (844)
Aufers prebendis uerum nomen quia uendis (421)
Aufert et confert, dehinc augmentat medicina (813)
Auget amor meritum, maior meliorque uoluntas (738)
Aula celesti sunt semper gaudia festi. (527)
Aurea uasa bonus amor et sapientia prestat (1323)
Aures pascuntur ubi tantum uerba loquntur (1061)
Auris, ocellus, et os, cor, pes, manus, arida fiunt. (57)
Auro sunt signata fides, amor, atque sophia (45)

Balatu querulo subiens sublimia sepe (232)
Baltheus est bissus, iacinctus, gemmaque flos, sal (104)
Baptizat, sanat, mutat, contritio uelat (1029)
Basan turpe sonat, siccum, confusio, bruchus (93)
Bestia censetur sathanas et causa notetur (396)
Bestia, fel, uirus, tinea est rosaria, liuor (627)
Blandus erit iustis iudex, districtus iniquis (590)
Bos, demon, stolidus, Iudeus, sollicitusque (80)
Bos mactatur, arat, lactat, pascit, corium dat. (81)
Bos semel est uitulus, semel et canis ipse catellus (1170)

Candidus et mundus lauat et sanat cinis ignis (155a)
Canon deflorans, heres, proles, lupa, perplex (1006)
Canon deflorat, heres, proles, lupa, perplex (1031)
Carbo reaccensus, ustus fenix rediuiuus (1097)
Carduus est motus radix fomes tibi culpe (990)
Carduus, urtica, sus, lappa tenax, et yrudo (492)
Carnem mortificat qui carnis pernecat actus (803)

Carnis munditia caste, ieiunia sancta (846)
Casta, fidelis, amans, humilis, subiecta, ministrans (753)
Causa super causas Domini ualor atque uoluntas (239)
Caute deuitet contritus ne recidiuet (1092)
Cedens uiuificat, lapides transponit, inaltat (1351)
Cedrus odore suo fugat angues, sic amor almus (103a)
Cedrus odorifera serpentibus est inimica (187)
Celebs et terra, mons, fons, pomum, fauus, archa (734)
Celestis medicus non parcens hic secat, urit (1041)
Celi sunt sancti qui celant mistica prauis (199)
Celicole sunt castra Dei parere parati (12)
Cementum, gluten, iuncturaque nexio iusta. (109)
Cerne locum uentumque situs ignemque loquelas (936)
Cerne quis eiciat, quid, quem, quo, qualiter, unde. (446)
Cetera sunt cure, Deus est obliuio solus. (255)
Christo curandum presentant quatuor egrum (975)
Christus acus, capud est, dux, pastor, stella, columpna (1344)
Christus amorque timor, fons est, sapientia, doctor (503)
Christus et ecclesia, doctor nubisque columpna (170)
Christus et ecclesia, doctor scripturaque iustus (145)
Christus et ecclesia duo sunt, set carne sub una (1348)
Christus fons uiuus, mons summus, pons tibi factus (1346)
Christus quadrifidi concendit robora ligni (195)
Christus se monstrans stat et auxilians stabilisque. (1370)
Circueas scripta, mentem, loca, tempora, membra (167)
Ciues celestes cum parent carne recentis (15)
Clamant sanguis, opus, uirtus, et spiritus, os, cor. (162)
Clarior est solito post maxima nubila Phebus (25)
Cognitio cibus est patrie, dilectio potus. (528)
Collige frumentum sit ut id cibus esurientum (1272)
Colloquii lignis sacer et contrarius ignis (27)
Commemora culpam, tempus mortemque per umbram (1327)
Commodo, compatior, conuerto, dono, remitto (720)
Compescit prauos Dominus reprimens furiosos (238)
Concipiens mundum ratio diuina secundum (251)
Conditio, culpa, transacta pie memorata (577)
Confert, augmentat, conseruat, denique firmat (92)
Conficit ignis, aqua, sal quod post infatuatur (1152)
Confidas nec diffidas lapsus, crucifixus (1116)
Conflatus uitulus Ihericoque anathema cremandum (1001)
Confugii turris Domini fortissima nomen (602)

Coniuge pro pulcra metuat iam quisque sepulcra. (1304)
Coniugium mundat, mutat, fecundat et unit (751)
Coniugium quasi lex ligat et munit, monet, unit (755)
Conseruant castum labor et fuga, sobrietasque (113)
Conseruant humilem si se reputet sibi uilem (551)
Consilium mutat Dominus, sententia perstat (296)
Constans et patiens, castus, baptista Iohannes (582)
Constat in altari carnem de pane creari (413)
Consueuit Dominus uulgari more docentis (381)
Consulit, hortatur, iubet, omnes saluificari. (267)
Continuat cursum sol inter sidera sursum (930)
Contriti lacrime salse, clare, calideque (657)
Contrito formam dant Iob Ionasque columba (1024)
Contritus doleat, rubeat, fidat metuatque (1016)
Contritus natum Iacob est deflendo peremptum (1017)
Conuerti dant ista: fides contritio cordis (128)
Conuocat Hebreos legis tuba, clangit et ipsa (1257)
Conuocat ad granum pullos gallina repertum (906)
Copia mercedis, ueteris purgatio culpe (926)
Cor Domino loquitur, meditatio nostra fatetur (301)
Cor feruens erexit equum, deiecit asellum (460)
Cor leue, uox lenis, atque fidelitas in muliere (821)
Corde pio ac opere Domino cantemus et ore (202)
Corpora quod surgent declarant uerba, figure (1096)
Corpore sicut aues, sic mente superna petamus. (55)
Corporis ac operis est hostia cordis et oris. (861)
Corporis esca, Dei uerbum, contritio cordis (937)
Corporis et cordis, operis simul offer et oris (1132)
Corporis et cordis soluit uel sufficit una (412)
Corporis ut maculas anime sic crimina pandas (1009)
Corpus, culpa, sathana, mundus, tibi sint anathema (58)
Corpus equus domitus, nec desint cingula, frenum. (461)
Corpus spiritui, sensus subsit rationi (1211)
Corripias, moneas, promittas atque mineris (941)
Crede Deum, credesque Deo, mage credo salubre (478)
Crede, fidelis age de cunctis, elige, sperne (854)
Crede memor narraque fatens, uenerans imitansque (921)
Crede ratem uentis, animum ne crede puellis (488)
Credit et assentit, optat, mox concipit alma (701)
Credula suspicio, mens preceps, impetus ire (481)
Credulus, incultus, simplex, humilis patiensque (957)

Crux, aqua, munus, opus, oratio, pectoris ictus (372)
Crux est muscipula, baculus, torcular, et ara (192)
Crux et pascha, fides, ascencio, iudiciumque (415)
Cui decus exhibeas, cur, qualiter, unde uideto. (553)
Cui putredo pater, uermis soror, arrida mater (787)
Cui uel ubi, quando, qui, quomodo, cur benedicant (77)
Culpa, gehenna, solum dant gratia, gloria bustum. (1207)
Culpa reo nox est et iusto gratia lux est (536)
Culpa, salus, meritum, Domini clementia, discum (2)
Culpam cum pena Dominumque timere uideris (1221)
Culpam magnificant monachis tot corporis arma (729)
Culparum fontes sunt fastus, liuor et ira (1331)
Culpe sit finis cum uite sit prope finis (1168)
Culpis aut penis nocituris incubat hostis (355)
Cum bona donantur nisi grates hinc referantur (632)
Cum dat sero Deus bona temporis, insinuatur (322)
Cum furit aura foris premit auram feruor amoris (1233)
Cum male ludentis facies mendosa paratur (984)
Cum moritur uita nobis est reddita uita (1363)
Cum niue, cum pluuia, cum grandine uertere capras (504)
Cum pedibus genibusque capud tollamus in altum (656)
Cum requiem uolumus, uxor mala, stillaque fumus (812)
Cum singillatim mortalia dixeris uni (133)
Cum sis ipse cinis, memor esto per omnia finis (801)
Cum strue lignorum ponas Ysaac super altum (585)
Cum sub prelatis qui sensus lumina perdunt (893)
Cum tibi diuinus scriptura promitur armus (94)
Cum trunco tellus, leo, pelta, columba, puella (432)
Cum uino sit aqua, cinis et sal mixtaque sint hec (315)
Cum zelo fragrat animus tibi proficiendi (898)
Cuncta Deum laudant uel per se uel mediate (300)
Cuncta uidet, curat, mala uindicat et bona reddit (253)
Cur decime dentur sex hee cause perhibentur (383)
Cur Dominus passus, ubi, quot uel quomodo, quando (1364)
Cur Dominus sathane quemquam tradat, tibi cause (1216)
Cur homo torquetur: Vt ei meritum cumuletur (Iob) (1039)
Cura uigil macerat, sollicitatque timor. (159)
Curans, inspirans, compungens atque flagellans (1215)
Curre miser dum currendi concessa potestas (852)
Currere, pascere, parcere, querere curia prestat (149)
Currus amor, gemineque rote dilectio duplex (206)

Currus prelatus est; quatuor iste rote sunt (179)
Cursum continuant sublimia sidera fulgent (692)
Cursus, martirium, contendere donat et artum (204)
Curua trahit mites, pars pungit acuta rebelles. (83)
Curua trahit quos uirga regit, pars ultima pungit. (82)
Custodi precepta Dei, cuius placitum fac (1049)

Da large, lete, sis intendens quoque recte (433)
Da si ditari, ieiuna si satiari (1044)
Damien, impurum, casti, declinat omissum. (858)
Dans Aidanus equum, gladium dans Brigida patris (318)
Dans sathane uires, reus hosti reddidit arma. (981)
Dant adipem triplicem: cor, epar, renunculus extis (47)
Dant calicem nobis lex, gratia, gloria, culpa (198)
Dant calor ac humor flores et gramina, fructus (241)
Dant Magdalena, spine, tibi, limus, asellus (1115)
Dant natura, decus, et gratia, doxa, potestas. (555)
Dant precibus spatium dolor et submissio, donum. (845)
Dat bona iustitia tempora, culpa mala. (345)
Dat Deus hic quedam nobis in pignus et arram (276)
Dat dici natura, fides et adoptio fratres (487)
Dat Dominus posse, meritum producere nosse (275)
Dat minus aut maius uel par uel ratione sicut. (1212)
Dat similem dici rem, gratia, gloria, culpa (1175)
Dat tibi contentum Petri Pauli documentum (885)
Dat tibi spontanei crux, mors seu passio Christi (168)
Dat tria temptare: seducere, scire, probare. (1242)
De gradibus quinque quartum quintumque relinque (457)
De toto regno superest post fata sepulcrum (786)
De uacuo uerbo ratio reddetur, acerbo (1269)
De uitiis uitia, nimirum cernimus orta (1343)
Debemus Domino nos nostraque tempora, mentem (297)
Debilis et uacua, leuis et radice lutosa (42)
Decernat quis, que uideas, et qualiter, unde (592)
Decidit in casses preda petita meos (369)
Declinant fragilis, ignorans atque superbus. (373)
Dedecet ut uite iudex fiat aliene. (1085)
Deducit Dominus dum deduci sinit usquam (295)
Degeneri uita, uitam corrumpere uita (1286)
Delicias et opes rapit inclementia mortis. (796)
Delicie silique fenumque fauillaque ficus (184)

Demon deformat, set sanctum pneuma reformat. (362)
Demon, patrinus, pater est Deus, angelus, Adam (903)
Demon, peccator, mundus, contritus, et equi (535)
Denariis, rebus uel amore renuntio sponte. (1076)
Denarius sit homo regis retinendo rotundus (321)
Denotat antiquam benedicta columpna columpnam (150)
Dentur honos et amor Domino, timor obsequiumque (299)
Depede, prefati, rumor, fit ruptio tifi. (1198)
Desertum carnis est mortificatio, uestis (340)
Desinit esse modo quod numquam desinit esse. (244)
Detrahit, applaudit, palpareque dicitur euge (464)
Dextra, capud, uirgo, latro, sanguis, monumentum (20)
Dic citra factum committere que uoluisti (132)
Dicimus hoc uanum quod transit, inutile, falsum (1328)
Dicit scriptura Dominum tunc magnificari (379)
Dicitur ancilla Domini pia uirgo Maria (708)
Dicitur ecclesia Domino famulans, humilisque (402)
Dicitur et uere nequeunt hec quinque latere (214)
Dicitur eternum mundi, legis, iubelei (416)
Dicitur usura sors, siue quod accidit illi (1334)
Dico prophetiam rem, uerbum, munus et actum. (932)
Dimittit Dominus solus peccata, sacerdos (1015)
Dirigit et pascit, seruat, cogitque requirit (905)
Discas ut sapias, facias, doceas, merearis (384)
Disparent umbre legis ueteresque figure (694)
Disputat atque docet Stephanus confessus et orat. (1123)
Ditat et apporiat, necat et sic uiuere donat (376)
Diues eram dudum, me fecerunt tria nudum (568)
Diuitie nullum dare possunt esse beatum (323)
Diuitiis multis nomen prepollet honestum (839)
Diuitis hii uermes: elatio, cura, uoluptas. (393)
Doctor, peccator, crux, petrinusque canalis (914)
Doctrine librum nobis assumite mundum (306)
Doctrinis, donis, uirtutibus allice gentes (1052)
Ducentes gratas, iocunda mente, choreas (186)
Dulcis in hostili patrie memoratio terra. (156)
Dum bibis et rebibis componitur unde peribis (79)
Dum pisces uolucresque cibos capiunt, capiuntur (455)
Dum tu seruilem credis saluare timorem (1262)
Dum uacat os mense ferat ad celestia mens se. (210)
Dum uiuis discas ad quid uel quomodo uiuas (304)

Durus Iudeus ad librum, dona, flagella (578)
Dux sacer ad sacrum te duc dans sacra sacerdos (1129)

Ebrietas furor est, fuge qui bibis ebrietatem (458)
Ecce premunt, circumdant, uilificat quoque rodit (782)
Ecclesia est archa, discus, domus, ara, sagena (401)
Ecclesiam subiens ores, discas, doceasue. (404)
Ecclesie fundamentum, fundator et idem (1345)
Ecclesie gremium, sanctus locus est fugienti (141)
Ecclesie lampas radiat baptista Iohannes (583)
Ecclesie sacra sacro sunt tegmine tecta. (745)
Ecclesie tres sunt partes; pars una laborat (403)
Eden procurant, nec dampna gregis mala curant (897)
Edificat qui multa diu collecta reseruat (453)
Educo, corripio, doceo natam michi prolem. (959)
Efficiens causa Deus est, formalis ydea (213)
Efficitur Christus altissimus, altior, altus (474)
Efficiunt fortem beemoth natura, libido (370)
Eger peniteat et crimina confiteatur (1021)
Egerit, irretit, tabet, suspenditur, aret (68)
Egressum nobis ostendunt perniciosum (452)
Egris et sanis est sana refectio panis (96)
Egyptus tenebre, tribulans, afflictio, meror (451)
Elatus, fictus, eger, fedusque fatetur (140)
Eleuat humanam naturam dum creat ad se (472)
Eloquio, uento, res sole, calore liquescunt. (676)
Emulus exustus, oratio, uirgaque florens (1125)
En callem Samye monstrat pars dextra figure (1280)
En Deus excelsus nulli dabit esse secundum. (242)
En epigrama crucis Christum regem manifestat (193)
En iam Christus adest quia tempus transuolat omne. (7)
En monumenta monent, mente mortis reminisci (777)
En saluatoris Iudeus, mors, sathan, orbis (562)
Eris seruus eris si te species trahit eris. (222)
Errant qui sperant se sibi sufficere (985)
Es, ferrum, plumbum, stagnum reputatur iniquus (980)
Esca Dei uerbo prius et prece sanctificetur (440)
Esse Deo similem si uis per scripta doceri (1210)
Esse locale facit quoduis dimensio corpus (675)
Est ab ares dictus aries, mactatur ad aram (53)
Est actu, culpe, rupture uulnus inique (1342)

Est adamas mulier, pix, rampnus, carduus asper (749)
Est anime uitiis subici confusio grandis (1003)
Est aqua baptismi lix uiaque, cerea, fax, es. (913)
Est aqua baptismi, scripture, flaminis almi. (38)
Est aqua doctrina uel gratia spiritualis (39)
Est asinus, porcus, prunis in corpore tactus (680)
Est asinus stolidus, immundus, hebesque Manasses (54)
Est auctor demon, homo uel Deus ipse malorum (814)
Est auidis Cipris uersans male corda uenenis (682)
Est aurum purum regis diadema futurum (152)
Est aurum triplex, thus triplex, mirraque triplex (423)
Est canis, est ursus, leo, bos, draco, simia, serpens (352)
Est carcer cecus, fetens, artusque profundus (466)
Est Christi pastus aqua, fenus, semen, aroma. (431)
Est Christus latro, fur in mundo uel auerno (1371)
Est cophinus sordis fragmentorumque sacerdos (1130)
Est crinis capitis gracilis uariique coloris (174)
Est culpe pene non ignorata uetustas (1325)
Est cupidus Pharius mersus, Crassus, canis, orchus (220)
Est deuota fides uite meritoria feruens (477)
Est Deus excelsus pariter metuendus amandus (243)
Est Didimus geminus, set Thomas fertur abissus (1227)
Est diuinus amor dulcis super omnia potus. (945)
Est doctor gallus qui noctis discutit horas (541)
Est dolor ingrati, desperati uel auari (343)
Est Domini facies, famulus, speculumque magistri (902)
Est Domini lingua, recreatio, lectio sacra (646)
Est Domino carum quod nobis uile uidetur. (791)
Est error cordis, praue credendo, putando (1279)
Est ficus sterilis ypocrita uel balamita (500)
Est fidei, fraudis, ueri, confessio laudis (130)
Est florens uirga qui penitet alma Maria (1294)
Est flos cum fructu, flos fructus, flos sine fructu (502)
Est fornax conflans firmamentumque columpna (923)
Est fragilis stipula, terre radicitus herens (1185)
Est fuga cautele, tutele, strenuitatis (497)
Est hamus Christus, peccatum, sermo Dei, mors. (573)
Est heresis, demon, peccatum pseudoque serpens (1195)
Est homicida canis, detractor musca uel hircus (349)
Est homo mendicus, ouis errans, perdita dragma (557)
Est homo uel Christus, mens, ecclesie, domus archa (46)

Est honor humanus breuis et sine pondere fumus. (554)

Est humilis, prudens, constans, instans Ieremias (911)

Est ignis liuor set et ira, libido, cupido. (619)

Est imber doctrina Dei, ros gratia Christi (309)

Est in ueste triplex excessus, si nimis ampla (605)

Est in uoce chorus, lira pulsu, tibia flatu. (771)

Est iudex iustus, districtus, terribilisque (282)

Est lac doctrine mores quod sopit equinos (1058)

Est laqueus triplex, Zabuli suggestio, uite (666)

Est lectus beemoth, bibio, bibulus Gedeonis (456)

Est leo crudelis, immundus terribilisque (673)

Est leo rex, audax et largus, pectore fortis (672)

Est liber, seruus, pius, omnibus omnia factus (884)

Est locus, ecclesia, paradisus, Virgo beata (946)

Est locus indignis quo non extinguitur ignis (634)

Est longinqua Deus non causa propinqua malorum (65)

Est mare diffusum, feruens, salsumque profundum (806)

Est mare terribile magnumque uoraxque, profundum (1147)

Est medicamentum sanans oratio, scutum (842)

Est meritum prauum signum, uia, causa gehenne (742)

Est mihi militia modo seu temptatio uita (1339)

Est moriens musca, uolucris mordens abigenda (608)

Est mors nature, mors culpe, morsque gehenne (798)

Est nubes Christus, caro Christi, Virgo beata (838)

Est nubes doctor, fulmen, doctrina, mineque (1053)

Est oculus cordis thesaurus in arbore radix (598)

Est oleum pingue, calidum, nitidum recreansque (868)

Est onus infirmi, peccati, legis et actus (875)

Est orientalis Babilon subiecto Seleuco (1173)

Est pars longa crucis, constantia, lancea, finis (929)

Est peccatoris laqueus meretricis ocellus. (758)

Est peccatorum saccus, uelum pariesque (1011)

Est perdix, adamans, sathanas, aquiloque, Golias (361)

Est perfectorum luctus, lusus puerorum. (662)

Est pietas, oleum, pretium, uiror, ydria, fenus (718)

Est pietatis opus oleum, flos, ala, thesaurus. (430)

Est quasi muscipule cibus huius gloria uite (531)

Est rubus ecclesia, Iacob et crux, uirgaque doctor. (1099)

Est saccus sathane teter, gemine quoque pene (1190)

Est sanguis cordis signum cordalis amoris (1362)

Est sathan ut fulgur, terret, micat, irruit, urit (358)

Est sathane similis et irudo, spongia, perdix (526)
Est sathane triplex scriptura teste potestas (1048)
Est scriptura sacra prelati preuia uita (645)
Est sermo ratione quidem subnixa loquela (1149)
Est Simon Petrus missorum bar-iona primus (883)
Est simplex uolucris gallina, domestica, mitis (542)
Est socialis auis cui nidus petra, columba (233)
Est speculum Christus, ratio, scriptura, creata. (1154)
Est spelunca caro uel mundus siue sepulcrum. (1189)
Est stulti, mundi, iusti, pleneque beati (530)
Est terrenus honor ut fumus spumaque sompnus. (556)
Est tibi carnalis, suauis, mel dulce, uoluptas (1338)
Est tiphus reprobi titulus signumque caracter. (176)
Est totum tempus presens quod cepit ab Adam (387)
Est uaga communis uirtus astrea peragrans (587)
Est uaga, mendica, mutabilis et maculosa (669)
Est uagus atque uorax piscis, silet, amne moratur (943)
Est uallis floris, fontis, farris, terebinti (1336)
Est uentus uelox, siccat, mouet, obruit ignem (1320)
Est uerbum Christus lumenque lucernaque nobis (1352)
Est uere stultus qui ius discretus adultus (977)
Est uinculum culpe, pene legisque superne (1315)
Est uinum cum letitia, dilectio, sensus (1301)
Est uinum luxus, fallax mordaxque furoris (1302)
Est uirgo prudens, sol, sidus, filia Chore (733)
Est uirtus, donum, digitusque Dei, calor, ignis (1107)
Est uitalis odor ducens ad uiuere uerum (435)
Est uitium seu peccatum pestis simulacrum (989)
Est uitulus mundus, mitis, lactens, nouus, insons (1311)
Est ulcus carnis, in carneque lurida lepra (685)
Est uobis nota nox longa, pauendaque sancta (835)
Est ut hiemps seclum presens, nox longa diesque (1213)
Est uxor sensus et sollicitudo, uoluptas. (1306)
Est ysopus, gluten, primaria filia, nutrix (549)
Est Zabulus dipsas, prester, salamandra, phareas (360)
Esto columpna domus postis firmus, non arundo (523)
Esuries, ensis perimunt, mala bestia, pestis. (292)
Esuries, ensis perimunt, mala bestia, pestis. (1330)
Et laus celestis et odor tibi seruule seruit (1165)
Et prelarga Tithi dextera spargit opes. (659)
Etates mundi sunt sex et septima currit (468)

Etsi deest aurum, non deest thesaurus honesti (1218)
Eucharis est lingua que tum bona tum bene profert (649)
Ex imis terre diuina sorte leuate (831)
Ex meritis exauditur quicumque sacerdos (438)
Ex quouis pacto, uel quouis mutuo nacto (1335)
Ex se Gad, Moyses, Ionas, Paulusque loquuntur (650)
Ex uiridi ligno limphas calor exprimit ignis (1022)
Excedra multorum capitum draco dicitur ydra (614)
Excitat, excercet Zabuli temptatio iustum (1261)
Exeat Egyptum quis, quando, qualiter, ad quid. (450)
Exemplar, forma speculique nitor, uia, norma (1357)
Exemplo, uerbo, nos subsidio, precibusque (1086)
Exemplum nobis operis dant ista fidelis (855)
Exemplum, simile, factum, uerbum ratioque (962)
Exemplum ueterum diuersaque causa piorum (1157)
Exerit ut fallat uelum, prestigia, folles (359)
Exhibeo, ueneror, illi parendo parentem. (960)
Existi liber Pharias fugiendo tenebras (338)
Expectat, uocat, et bona dat Deus, hic sceleratis (268)
Expedit et curat, absoluit, liberat hec dat. (660)
Expedit, infigit, rude continuatio tollit (163)
Extant in culpa mortali uincula plura (1318)
Extat longanimis Domini clementia larga (716)
Extat stella Iacob et matutina Maria (704)
Extat ymago triplex: formans, formata, reformans (636)
Extinguit munus districti iudicis iras (426)
Exurit paleas ignis, propurgat et aurum. (1260)

Fac mihi forte suum prestet fortuna fauorem (795)
Fac tu fasciculos operum Domini tibi binos. (879)
Facundus sapiens argentum fertur et aurum. (1141)
Fallax folle faber primas exsuflat in igne (505)
Fallax Siba, Dauid preceps, hinc peccat uterque. (388)
Fallit enim uitium specie uirtutis et umbra. (565)
Fallit peccatum falsa dulcedine stultum (1012)
Falsa Saduceis astrea dedit, Phariseis (1200)
Falx, ignis, nexus, paxillus, fletus et uua (1297)
Fassio, notitia, grates, honor atque sequela (1224)
Fastus et excessus, templi desertio, uerbi (510)
Fecundat, tegit et signat, sustentat et ornat. (1187)
Fedus et eiectus, turpis, fetens male, raucus (689)

Felix quem faciunt aliena pericula cautum. (118)
Felleus amnis erat, per lignum melleus extat. (804)
Femina nulla bona, set si bona contigit ulla (489)
Femina peccauit, peccatum femina lauit (698)
Fers aliquid nihil, esto foras, fero, quid nimis, intra. (319)
Fertur ab ungendo dici uelud unxior uxor (756)
Feruens ad pugnam, properans ad premia martir (725)
Fetet lasciuus et amaris uescitur hircus (571)
Fiat prelatus sapiens, facundus, honestus. (891)
Ficta, reconcilians, pax est tranquilla, beata (1062)
Firmant et fulgent, Christi miracula terrent. (1375)
Fletus causa tibi sunt hec: dilatio regni (524)
Flatus, crux, et sal, sputum cum crismate uestis (71)
Floritio, satio, tibi sit largitio doni (427)
Flos tener et tenuis, lenis leuis et speciosus (501)
Fluctiuagum fluuidum, salsum, tumidumque profundum (807)
Fons in scriptura uelud Hester, uirgo Maria (819)
Fons in scriptura uelud Hester, uirgo Maria (706)
Fons, aqua, sal oculis occurrunt introeuntis (406)
Fons, fluuius, mare, diluuium piscinaque labrum (1026)
Fons, gluten, bernix, amor est alatus et ignis (98)
Fons, radix et adeps amor est et forma, caracter (97)
Forma, fides, causa, nobis surrectio Christi (1367)
Forma tibi speculum, turtur, nubesque columpna (581)
Fortior est feriente ferens, nec secula pulcrum (925)
Fortius excidit magis acta securis in altum (927)
Fortune fragilis fiat tibi copia uilis. (327)
Fossa dabit tellus optato tempore fructus (920)
Fossa, latex, collis ac murus celsaque turris (142)
Fragrantes uicina rosas urtica perurit (1201)
Fraus, dolus, insidie, fallacia, fictio, furtum (516)
Fruge uigent ualles, algent de frigore montes (1163)
Fullo, faber, miles, genitor, medicusque sacerdos (1231)
Fundamenta fides, paries dilectio duplex (513)
Fundamentorum fundamentum Iesus ipse. (520)
Fundatur domus, erigitur, munitur et intus (469)
Fur Dominus, Dominique dies, mors, hostis iniquus. (515)

Garrulus est uir, spermaticus uel prodigus omnis. (1172)
Gaudia mundani, contriti, proficientis (548)
Gloria cum reprobo sua non descendet in orchum (533)

Gloria, prosperitas et uita, potentia uana. (1340)
Gloria uana quid est? Vmbra est, uesica tumescens (532)
Gorgias timor est, Vsias cupit, atque Nichanor (1332)
Granum, sal, simila, thus sunt libamina sicca (658)
Gratia, natura dant casum, pena scelusque (175)
Gratia, pena, Deus doctrinaque dicitur imber. (974)
Gratia prima fides, mater, basis et uia, piscis (476)
Gratia prima sit ut lux, funis et hospes et imber (537)
Gratia, uerba, preces, lacrime quoque sanguis et unda (759)
Gratificat flores spinetum, coruus olores. (215)
Gurgulio non est uermis piscisue set ales (547)
Gutta cadens igni subseruit noxque diei (1005)
Guttas solaris non fluctus attrahit ardor (550)

Hebrei, Pharii, peruerse, luxuriosi (1038)
Hec animal, firmamentum, tronus, et super hunc uir (1119)
Hec attendantur in summo iudice, quantum (283)
Hec baptisma, fides, pietas, contritio, Christi (1014)
Hec bona sunt patrie: dulcedo, uita beata (69)
Hec dant effundi nunc presens pena iehenna (463)
Hec dicit Dominus: uos lene iugum, leue pondus (599)
Hec exorcismus et crux, aspersio, uirtus (371)
Hec infrunitum nobis exponere posse (613)
Hec intellectus, pietas, sapientia, robur (1109)
Hec mundi finis ac incarnatio, cor, mors (9)
Hec muscas abigunt: ramus, contunsio, clauus. (124)
Hec nostrum crimen, regni dilatio, culpa (518)
Hec portant Christum: Virgo, Symeon et asellus (968)
Hec sunt ambigena natura dispare nata (64)
Hec sunt que Iosue tipico uelamine uastat (635)
Hec terrena teras: carnem cum fomite motum. (237)
Hec uariant meritum: tempus celesteque donum (743)
Helyas uiduam pascit qua pascitur ipse. (904)
Heth pauor est, hic est semen, uia uitaque compes (1225)
Hic mundus sit uas quoddam dulcedine plenum (279)
Hic obstetrices, rex Iehu, rex Babel, Achab (1103)
Hic qui uult Abraham fieri, fiat prius Abram (826)
Hic requies sanctis breuis et longus labor extat. (1083)
Hii post derident qui primum crimina suadent. (397)
Hispida iuniperus humilis, uilis, sterilisque (604)
Hoc baculo fultus stas, prouidus erige uultus (422)

Hoc illi Deus est quod quis cupit et ueneratur. (633)
Hoc sacramentum uas poscit crimine mundum (411)
Hostes crudeles felicis fallit aragnes. (400)
Hostes improperant quos fellea uiscera uexant (471)
Hostes peccatum, uitium, mundus, caro, demon (561)
Hostia carnalis operis seu corporis, oris (575)
Hostis fit peccans sponsi sponseque suique. (978)
Humanus uultus os est et littera mentis (509)
Hunc genus extollit, set si fastigia penses (828)
Hunc teneo certus meus est errore repertus. (398)

Iacob ditari meruit, Laban apporiari. (664)
Ignis amor, Deus ipse, rubor, tribulatio, pena. (618)
Ignis auaritie zelique libidinis, ire (617)
Ignis diuinus Pater est, natusque, rubaque (620)
Ignis, uox, et uentilabrum, fera uisio, signum (287)
Ille natat leuiter cui mentum sustinet alter. (1176)
Ima petunt feces cupidorum terrea mentes (407)
Impatiens litis defecit flumine mersa (679)
Imperat, hortatur, permittit, precinit, orat (612)
Impietas praui, rerum subtractio mundi (655)
Imponit finem sapiens et rebus honestis (722)
Imponit terram capiti qui mente reuoluit (512)
Imposito cinere capiti subeant tibi quinque (181)
Imprecor aut nudo uel detraho uel manifesto (818)
In bello fortis instar dilectio mortis (102)
In campis ligna dat et ortus, uinea, silua. (693)
In casu quoque grates age, semper ubique (538)
In celio monte septem dormisse leguntur (334)
In celis residens terris medicamina prestat (1359)
In Christo lapide submissa mente recumbe. (123)
In cithara lignum cordeque cauillaque plectrum (203)
In conuertendo, patiendo, timendo, dolendo (462)
In culpis minus est, in penis plus reperitur (1042)
In *de, pro* signum, causam, noto materiamque (375)
In Domino gaude simul expergiscere et aude (248)
In facie legitur hominum secreta uoluntas (188)
In facie memora quod sunt ieiunia plura. (601)
In laqueum uolucris et cesa solotenus arbor (1093)
In lare, flare, fuge, set et oc, uenerem necat in te. (688)
In ligno limphe Marath indulcantur amare (197)

In mentem tempus obitus immittere possunt (775)
In minimis etiam Domini magnalia clarent. (717)
In naui rector non sorte set arte legendus. (895)
In nichilum nix alta fluit si desuper imber (483)
In pape, flaui, labis, puri, Iob, ara, ui (443)
In patria requies sanctis erit et stola duplex (91)
In Pentecoste legis textu referente (865)
In prece prelati uis est nonnulla iubendi (1056)
In puteum uero temptans Dominum cadit Hero (1246)
In quibus articulis liceat non reddere sponsis (752)
In quid sollicitus sis, quantum, quomodo, quando (1174)
In quo, cur, qualis sit confidentia nobis (146)
In quot consistat, qualis sit lepra uideto (677)
In ramis agnus ac ebdomadarius, hospes (342)
In sero mundi claudetur ianua regni (185)
In terra hostili patrie memoratio dulcis. (1105)
In uelo uarii signant diuersa colores (1308)
In uerbis, precibus, lacrimis, in sanguine, limpha (35)
In uestimentis non est meditatio mentis (1078)
Incedo gressum non promittendo regressum (788)
Incircumscriptus sol est in uirgine Christus. (1353)
Incisor burse, fur, falx et ianua, limen (779)
Includunt homines amor ac imitatio Christi (32)
Inconstans Balaam modicam compunctus ad horam (628)
Infirmus, claudus, pede uinctus non bene uadunt. (607)
Ingluuiem uentris sequitur petulantia carnis. (545)
Ingratus sibi uel meritis propriis sua donat (631)
Ingrediens heremum puerum dimisit Helyas (730)
Initium capud est, mens, Christus, dux aliorum. (172)
Innato nummo speculo limphaque relucet (640)
Inruha cum fertur non solui culpa, nocentur (992)
Insidians ouibus lupus est et seuus, ouile (674)
Inspice cui uel cur, attendas qualiter, a quo (115)
Inspice cur uel ubi, quis, quo, quem uel quid adoret. (23)
Instabilis, pugnans, petulans auis, alta requirens (972)
Instinctu, scriptis, doctoribus atque creatis (380)
Institor in templo, Iudeus, stultaque uirgo (467)
Integra sit culpe confessio mundaque uera (135)
Inter peruersos iusti Loth et Ezechiel, Iob (1202)
Inter Sur, Cades, Abraham posuit sibi sedes (714)
Inuidet, immundus, redit ad uomitum canis atque (230)

Inuiscos uolucres cogit cum cantibus auceps (78)
Inuitat Christus, impellit et ad bona mundus (637)
Iob tres dilecti non recte recta loquuntur (29)
Ira Dei prauis morbus, miseratio iustis (442)
Ira furor trabs est, aries, turbatio et ignis (625)
Ira furorue Dei quid nisi pena rei. (290)
Iram uenturam recolas, metuas, caueasque. (10)
Irruit, inuoluit turbo, paleas rapit, aufert. (1237)
Ista locus, tempus, habitus, caro, cultus et esus (610)
Ista requiruntur: intentio, forma, potestas (1160)
Ista senem circumueniunt incomoda mundum (761)
Isti sunt morbi quibus egrotant opulenti (392)
Iudei ueteres sunt crimine, tempore, lege (1324)
Iudeis signa, Grecis sapientia grata (611)
Iudeus, fatua uirgo, Pharius, canis, are (473)
Iudicii baratrique metus, presentia culpe (1236)
Iudicio teget extremo confessio culpas (134)
Iudicis aduentus seu iudex, iudiciumue (284)
Iudicium metuo quod timet omnis homo (288)
Iudicium, mors, mens, caro, dant Christum uenientem (8)
Iudico, discerno, dampno, delicta reuelo (591)
Iumentum reputatur homo, fedus, fatuusque (609)
Iustis concorda ne fias dissona corda (107)
Iustitie porta Christus doctrinaque, mors est (969)
Iustus Abel parens Abraham Samuelque benignus (470)
Iustus demonium conculcat et effugat ipsum (394)
Iustus in aduersis non spernitur immo probatur. (66)

Labes, diuitie sancte, detectio Christi (341)
Labitur, extinguit, fecundat, et abluit unda (41)
Lapsus malorum fiat cautela minorum. (116)
Laus et uindicta sunt et promotio nostra (298)
Laus et uindicta sunt et promotio nostra (1070)
Laus male, sermo Dei, correptio, culpa tacetur (1241)
Lazarus et Petrus, Moyses, Cananeaque Christus (448)
Lectio non modicum, set plus collatio prebet (386)
Ledunt, inficiunt scabies, zima, fel sibi iuncta. (836)
Legati sunt dona manus, ieiunia, fletus (695)
Lente uenit uirtus, uitium ruit impetuose. (1266)
Lepra fit in ueste, tumor in uirtute, set illam (678)
Lepra uolans, Canaan, lunaticus, instabilis Nod (629)

Letificant testes, patientia, causaque merces (726)
Letificat tenebrasque fugat lux atque decorat (647)
Lex est forma, tipus, signum, uelamen et umbra (642)
Lex ignis celi, rogus, orchus, feruor auari (616)
Lex obscura fuit set Christus clarificauit (643)
Lex uetus inchoat, ad noua preparat, abdita signat (641)
Liberat et mundat donum, redimitque tuetur (428)
Lignum, seta rigens, aqua, sal ad uulnera mordens (37)
Limpha Dei donum, populus, doctrina, uoluptas (40)
Lingua Latina potens, Hebreaque religiosa (196)
Linque ratem, rete, mare, patrem, quatuor hec sunt (584)
Lucet, consumit, ascendit, dequoquit ignis (615)
Luciferi laqueus captus quicumque fidelis (465)
Lucis, aque nimium prius obtundit tibi uisum (840)
Lux Deus et ratio, scripturaque gratia, uerbum. (690)
Lux primitiua, superaddita sidera clara (648)

Magna mihi sunt dona Dei, pro dantis amore (274)
Magnum querit honus, magnum qui querit honorem. (61)
Maiorum tumor in iussu, formido minorum (1329)
Man cum nocturno descendit rore minutum (766)
Mane dedit uiti cultores, tertia, sexta (1299)
Mane, techel, phares, uigili si mente notares (792)
Martha quod irritat uel prouocat aut dominatur (711)
Martirium dans aureolam non transit in ignem (727)
Martirium faciunt legis defensio ueri (728)
Martirium, sacramentum, tribulatio, sermo (741)
Mater uirgo pia nobis succurre Maria. (705)
Materies, sapor et species pensentur aceti. (67)
Matheo, Luce, Marco datur atque Iohanni (417)
Mens capud est, Christus lapis est, iacobita uiator (1162)
Mens humilis, studium querendi, uita pudica (310)
Mens, sol, fons, candela, manus, trinus Deus unus. (261)
Mensis qui caret R. sompnis solet esse saluber (1251)
Mente, manu, lingua, mala qui malus est operatur (816)
Mente, manu, uerbo, causa neco denique rendo. (563)
Mentis in excessu liber est datus Ezechieli (644)
Merguntur Pharius, ferrum, plumbum, mola, porcus. (808)
Metitur Christus attendens omnia nostra (724)
Mi, fa, sol, carus est sermo commaculosus (915)
Miles scaccorum uel simia, canna, sophista (566)

Miluus auis mollis est uiribus atque uolatu (810)
Mirraque de cuius lacrimis in corpora functa (805)
Mistica sunt uas, thus, ignis, quia uase notatur (1256)
Molle pecus lanis, animo placidum set inherme (872)
Mollibus assuetus clipeum bene non gerit armus (166)
Mons celum, Sathael, Deus est elatio sancti (809)
Morbi principia sunt hec: gula, luxus et ira (998)
Morbus, signa, cibus, blasphemia, dogma, fuere (1373)
Morphosis et mater, nutrix, uredo et origo (1196)
Mors cum Iudeo, mundus cum demone uicti (1369)
Mors cunctis dura, cunctos trahit in sua iura (785)
Mors duplex anime, duplex et corporis est mors (797)
Mors falcem gestat meritis, ac felle molestat (780)
Mortis causa, modus, locus et tempus latitant nos. (781)
Mortuus expallet, liuet, fetetque liquatur (799)
Mos, modus et causa, tempus, persona locusque (189)
Mota piscina periit uetus illa ruina (944)
Moyses cum Christo, seniores cum Cananea (449)
Moyses et Iacob, Ioseph, Iosue, Mare, Parthus (496)
Multa diu patitur, pulsans Deus et bona prestat. (269)
Munda sit et pura simplex intentio nostra. (638)
Mundi, nature, culpe, peneque gehenne (1317)
Mundi tollit opes scintilla aut bestia parua. (763)
Mundus abit tanquam lanugo, spuma, sagitta (1253)
Munificus Deus est dans omnibus omnia dona (272)
Mutari nequeunt post obitum merita. (784)

Narrabo primum mea iam commissa fatendo (830)
Nasceris ut uiuas, uiuis moriturus, et unus (559)
Nasciscuntur enim fera siluas, bestia campos (52)
Nascitur ut fimo scarabo, sic sordibus hostis (979)
Naufragus ut retinet manibus si forte quid hesit (59)
Nauis et archa, capud, tectum presepeque mens est (772)
Nauis, iumentum, crux, uirgo senexque sepulcrum (1356)
Ne fauor inclinat cui sors uaga, blanda proponat (525)
Ne ferias ipsum donato fuste datorem (630)
Ne macules animam quam Christus mundificauit (987)
Ne mors trina premat, cor et os rege factaque uestra. (263)
Nec iaceas neque stes, set eas in tramite recto (1281)
Nec uolo mentiri nec debeo prodere quemquam. (817)
Nemo desperet pro quantocumque reatu. (350)

Nemo nimis propere didicit nocitura cauere (506)
Nescio nec ualeo nec sufficio tibi laudum (652)
Nil conscire sibi, nulla pallescere culpa. (169)
Nil subito faciat qui sensu tardior extat. (624)
Nobis bella mouent hii tres: mundus, caro, demon (574)
Nobis blanditur Deus et quandoque minatur (246)
Nobis suspensis Christi suspenditur ensis (228)
Nolumus a sociis uinci qui uincimur ira (1312)
Nomen, causa, locus in quo claudatur et a quo (31)
Non aliud nisi se ualet ardens Ethna cremare (626)
Non appellandi locus hic, non calculus iste (793)
Non bene letatur cui flendi causa paratur (661)
Non culpas proprias defendas aut alienas. (995)
Non detur sathane locus aut membris sathaninis (120)
Non Deus est nec homo presens quam cernis ymago (1349)
Non Deus hic parcit ut parcat denique iustis (519)
Non discunt quicumque scolas ubicumque frequentant (229)
Non dum regna poli petii me tangere noli (710)
Non ius iudicii clementia flectere debet (593)
Non manducantem manducans spernere uitet (595)
Non minus est dulcis de paruo fonte recepta (912)
Non minus hic peccat qui censum condit in agro (1247)
Non oleum, non thus, pro culpa sacrificatur (999)
Non petere exemplum set dare dignus eras. (437)
Non potuit Ioseph animo set ueste teneri. (586)
Non prodest sine spe timor, aut spes absque timore (1219)
Non puer aut mulier, seruus, Pharius numerantur (834)
Non qui clam sumit, set clam uult sumere fur est. (665)
Non recolit seruus collata sibi bona prauus (1142)
Non reputes aurum totum quod splendet ut aurum (567)
Non res in uitium ueniunt set abusio rerum (441)
Non scit, non sentit, non experiendo, probando (623)
Non sibi set Domino uiuat quis uel moriatur (1288)
Non tardes: properat populus, pastor cito currens (507)
Non te pretereat narratio presbiterorum (44)
Non tolerabit equus eius cum tangitur ulcus (910)
Non uinolentus regnum rapit, at uiolentus (1313)
Non ut homo faciem Deus aspicit exteriorem (294)
Nos elementa docent elementatisque docemur (385)
Nos elementorum doceat connexio pacem (922)
Nos homo, mens, culpa tribulant, Zabulus, caro, mundus (1229)

Nos sibi munus, nos sibi templum querit amenum (1217)
Nos uideat Ihesus semper uideamus ut ipsum. (1276)
Noscitur hic series hymnorum sex feriarum (569)
Nubes, sartago, paries murusque chaosque (991)
Nuda uelud pactum reddit promissio tutum (961)
Nulla tui meriti perturbent nubila lucem (588)
Nullaque sunt pacis federa cum uitiis. (1143)
Nulli mirentur non hinc aliqui moueantur (874)
Nullum decipies nec decipieris ab ullo (494)
Nunc alii mores, alii pro tempore leges. (764)
Nuntius, umbra, sopor, capud et pictura, uetustas (776)
Nutibus et signis internis proditur ignis. (28)

Obscurant oculos tenebre, lux, fumus et ignis (876)
Obsequio cole patronum, pietate parentem (209)
Obsequio famulus deuitandus uel amandus. (881)
Obserua tempus in dicendis et agendis (1252)
Obseruant motum sibi celitus astra statutum (1079)
Obseruat partum, draco, stans captatque uorandum. (356)
Obsunt non prosunt, uitanda superflua uerba (691)
Occidit pueros Herodes ascalonita (564)
Octo concurrunt ad templum sanctificandum (314)
Offer tu uitulum Christum credens memoransque (862)
Officium, lingua, meritum, sapientia, uita (894)
Olla recens fracta ualet ex facili reperari (1171)
Omne bonum nostrum referamus ad omnipotentem (250)
Omnia consumens uitio consumitur omni (491)
Omnia discernit, trutinat Deus, omnia cernit (249)
Omnia peccata lustret contritio nostra (1023)
Omnibus est optanda salus, saluentur ut omnes (1284)
Omnibus uerbis uerax Deus atque fidelis (278)
Omnis in hoc mundo fidens est sicut arundo (147)
Opprobrium semper Didimus cognomine gestat (480)
Orat pro nobis chorus ecclesie generalis (843)
Orbem continue lustrant sol, sidera, Phebe (1051)
Ordine stant dentes albi multisque molentes (347)
Ordo labor grandis, res aspera, dura probandis (731)
Ordo, lingua, Dei corpus, thorus, unda, bis ungi. (1158)
Ordo sacerdotis, intentio conficientis (962)
Ordo sacerdotum cumulat scelus et cruciatum. (994)
Ortum pomiferum cuius sunt poma fideles (871)

Ortus conclusus, bis sancta, soror mea, sponsa (735)
Os Domini Christus, facundia, scripta, propheta. (877)
Os hominis, locus et tempus, persona, reatus (918)
Os nequam mulce; nequid sapiat nisi dulce. (869)
Os siccum, durum, rigidum uacuumque medulla (870)
Oscula ficta Ioab, pestis blandumque uenenum (62)
Otia, pax et delicie Dauid superabant (953)

Panes quinque dolor, uerbum, deitas, caro Christi (940)
Panis amor piscisque fides, spes dicitur ouum (942)
Panis peccatum, peccator, passio pascens (938)
Parua fides aut nulla fides aut eiciendi (671)
Paruaque set felix Syloe uisura, prophetam (1156)
Paruulus est primus, et uulpes paruula motus (769)
Pasce columbinos pullos, etate nouellos (971)
Pascens seruus arans, rediens, dominoque ministrans (1137)
Pasco, Caym, macro, clamosus, cras, niger, imbre. (234)
Pascua scriptura, caro Christi, uita beata. (947)
Passio contriti, cultum petrinus, et herba (139)
Pastor, prelatus, nox, seclum grexque, popellus (887)
Paulus ait: Carne peccati seruio legi (514)
Pauperibus large tua dum tibi copia sparge. (328)
Paupertas uera est contemptus diuitiarum. (955)
Pax et fama, fides, reuerentia, cautio dampni (597)
Peccatum, mundus, hostis, sociusque malignus (499)
Peccatum parit exilium dampnumque ruborem (1013)
Pectus eum uoluit, uox protulit, actio prompsit (257)
Peniteas cito peccator cum sit miserator (1018)
Peniteas plene, si uere peniteat te (129)
Penitet et mutat aliquid Deus, istud idem sit. (293)
Pennis ornata, uelox penitransque sagitta (1153)
Per minimum serpens serpit uetus ille foramen (367)
Per nec, perque pie, scitur solus Deus esse. (264)
Per quinquagenum numerum sunt significata (1066)
Percutit, irritat, sustentat, protegit, ornat (86)
Percutitur uirga Moysi puluis, mare, petra. (1293)
Perdimus anguillas manibus dum stringimus illas (26)
Personam redimas, res et loca, tempora, causas (1073)
Personas actusque modos, loca, tempora, causas (311)
Pes est affectus Domino per cuncta placendi (964)
Pessimus est hostis qui cum benefeceris illi (802)

Pingitur alatus ueterum ratione Cupido (226)
Piscator stigius habet hamum, rete, sagenam (353)
Plana soporatum terra papauer habet. (973)
Plango parum meriti, flens otia temporis acti. (1037)
Plango quod amisi, quod commisi, quod omissi (1025)
Plango quod offendi, lesi, nocui, male caui (1030)
Plantas et segetes produc et gramina flores (49)
Pluribus adiunctos seu coniugibus sociatos (754)
Pluribus adiunctos seu coniugibus sociatos (1305)
Plurima cum soleant mores euertere sacros (490)
Plurima pars celo sustollitur unica fenix (508)
Plurima stultorum messis, set rara bonorum. (967)
Pomum prodit odor, splendor quoque detegit ignem. (482)
Pondus ibi color atque sapor si queritur an sint (408)
Pontifices perimunt caro, curia, pompa, fauorque. (420)
Porta, foramen acus, mors est et terminus, hamus. (783)
Porta sathan timor est, febris horrida, pallida lepra (1226)
Portitor ipsius portatur uirgine clausus. (1355)
Posse quidem rebus dant ius, natura, facultas (963)
Post annos centum puer alphesibeus adhuc est (1169)
Post cenam standum, uel passus mille uagandum. (211)
Pratum talpa fodit, conculcat et inquinat illud (684)
Praui solamen iustorum carpere uitam (348)
Precipit et prohibit, permittit, consulit, implet (265)
Prelatus mitis, affabilis atque benignus (901)
Premeditans mortem parat hosti reddere sortem (789)
Premia iustorum pendent de fine laborum (952)
Premunit gentes Christus ac premonet omnes. (286)
Preparat et firmat, reparat Deus, abluit, armat (1159)
Prepropero uitium lentoque uenit pede uirtus. (1267)
Presbiter est pastor, sal, lux, miles, medicusque (1127)
Presbiteri culpa cumulatur et ordine pena. (993)
Presbiteris caste sint uxores et amice (1055)
Presentes pene sunt seue signa gehenne (1040)
Pressio squame, lappaque uiscus, nexio praua. (108)
Prestant equales uirtutes enea nobis (1337)
Preueniunt Iacob, Iudas Petrusque Iohannes (950)
Prima datur nobis uterus domus, altera mundus (335)
Prima Deo decima detur, decimaque secunda (331)
Primum curauit Dominus quos denique pauit. (409)
Primum fons et crux intranti sancta patescunt (70)

Primus ferre moram nequit, immo preuenit horam (544)
Principio Pharao, medio Ysmael insidiatur (364)
Principium Pater et natus spiransque creator (965)
Principium rerum, fons lucis, origo bonorum (258)
Pro modulo finis tandem tibi de bene gestis (723)
Prodigus et fictus Ionas, iuuenisque Iohannes (498)
Profectum sanctum signat processio nostra (948)
Promissum, comissum, dimissum, meritumque (389)
Propter doctrinam nostram, solatia, culpam (1234)
Protegit et munit, transcendit, suscipit imbrem (1254)
Protulit humano tellus sine semine panem (699)
Prouideas, campus oculos habet et nemus aures. (119)
Prouideas, campus oculos habet et nemus aures. (928)
Prudens et fidus instans operarius extet (1296)
Prudens prouideas humana nouissima que sunt (837)
Psallite discrete, constanter, cordis amore (1164)
Pugnat et impugnat solito nunc seuius hostis (1065)
Pulsat nec frangit, impellit ne mouet, auget (1245)
Puluis siue cinis Abraham fertur Iob et Adam (180)
Purpura cum clamide rubicunda, candida uestis (1360)

Qua specie Martis cedit uictoria Parthis (1333)
Quadraginta dies pia per ieiunia complens (1134)
Quadrupedes adaquare nequis dum percutis illos (1089)
Quales nos illi, talis nobis Deus extat (247)
Qualis, ubi, quando, quare uel qualiter, unde (3)
Quam sit uitanda derisio quamque nefanda (346)
Quam texit Dominus culpam non detegat ullus (454)
Quamuis perfecti, mortali carne grauati (529)
Quando repugnatur, calcari bis stimulatur. (1101)
Quando temptaris, Christi mala si meditaris (1244)
Quatuor hiis fastus speciebus fit manifestus (1197)
Quatuor in uelo designant ista colores (1307)
Que bona sunt bonus in lingua uel pectore tractat (73)
Que bona sunt oculis cordis colliria si uis (218)
Que bona sunt per se, pactio praua facit. (970)
Que forsan reputo contraria soluere quero (312)
Que secum non ferre potest hominis bona non sunt (74)
Que sors et qualis, quando quibusue datur (1177)
Quem rapit atque leuat fluctus uite trahit huius. (1341)
Quem ter ternus apex diuini numinis index (256)

Querit ut expoliet uenatibus, alite, pisce (543)
Qui cadit in faciem quo decidat aspicit ipse (207)
Qui conuertentur, quando, cur, qualiter, unde. (125)
Qui dat diuitias tibi si Deus adicit ullas (399)
Qui de peccatis confusus penitet, illa (137)
Qui fuerit mendax et amans mendacia fallax (822)
Qui gradiuntur ubi, uel quo duce, quomodo, quando (48)
Qui iustos uexant, merito tandem cruciantur (1057)
Qui mandit non mandentem non spernat inique (594)
Qui numerantur, ubi, quotiens et quando uel ad quid. (833)
Qui proprie carnis dape corda fidelia ditas (410)
Qui sumus addicti pro nostro crimine morti (790)
Qui teneros pueros mergunt merguntur et ipsi (1043)
Qui timet ille sibi cauet et reueretur et horret (1220)
Qui uendunt uel emunt res quaslibet ecclesiales (1199)
Qui uenient, ad quem, quando uel qualiter, unde. (1290)
Qui uitant falsa, ueniunt ad uera scienda (1112)
Qui uitiis mille se tradit, consecrat ille (983)
Qui uoluit uerbum de se sine tempore natum (260)
Quid fueris, quid sis, quid eris, circumspice, si te (794)
Quid fugis ex illo qui claudit cuncta pugillo (495)
Quid lucra terrea uos male ferrea corda gerentes (221)
Quid pariat uentura dies nescis, celer esto (850)
Quid sit agendum, quomodo, quando, curque uideto. (847)
Quid tam curate nutritur inutilis a te (154)
Quid, cui uel quantum, cur, qualiter est operandum (848)
Quid, cui uel quantum, cur, qualiter est operandum (856)
Quis, cui, cur uel ubi, decimas det, qualiter, ad quid. (332)
Quis, cui, quando litet quid, ubi, cur intueamur. (1131)
Quis Domino seruit inductus amore metuue (1135)
Quis Dominum querat, ubi, quando, quomodo, quare (1064)
Quis cursus, quis currat, ubi, quibus auxiliis, quo (205)
Quis dormire facit concentus carmina celi (1059)
Quis labor et quantum uel quomodo quisque laborat (663)
Quis liget aut soluat, ubi, quem, cur, quomodo, quando. (200)
Quis per quem scandat ubi cerne uel unde uel ad quid (16)
Quis, quales et quos, quot, quomodo, quando, uel ad quos (820)
Quis, quid, cui cantet, ubi, quando, quomodo, quare (201)
Quis, quid, ubi, cui precipiat, cur, quomodo, quando (1050)
Quis, quid, ubi, quando serat, ad quid, quomodo, quantum (1150)
Quis, quid, ubi, quando, cur offerat intueamur (859)

Quis, quid, ubi, quando, quo, qualiter, ad quod et unde (603)
Quis, quid, ubi, quibus auxiliis, cur, quomodo, quando (191)
Quis, quid uel quantum, cui, quomodo, quando remittat (1082)
Quis, quo, cur, quando, uideas, et qualiter intret. (606)
Quis, quo, quos, unde, cur, quomodo congregat, ad quid. (212)
Quis quos educat, quo, quando, qualiter, unde. (447)
Quis, quotus ascendat, quare, uel quomodo, quando (11)
Quis sit amandus, quomodo, quantum, curque uideto. (100)
Quis uel ubi surgat, cur, quando, qualiter, unde. (1368)
Quis ueniat uideas, quo, quando, quomodo, quare. (1)
Quis uidet agnoscens quid credendum, quid agendum (216)
Quisque suos, sua, se, pro Christi spernat amore. (30)
Quod dicis facto doctor complere memento (1060)
Quod doceas sane tu multo tempore disce (305)
Quod festum, cuius, que sunt adnexa uideto (484)
Quod fornax auro, quod ferro lima, flagellum (1230)
Quod leo non tetigit dum mordet aranea ledit (117)
Quod noua testa capit, inueterata sapit (165)
Quod plusquam tollat, promittat siue petatur (273)
Quod scio, quod ualeo, totum simul offero Christo (863)
Quomodo, cui, qualis, in quo, cur, quando ministret. (746)
Quomodo, cur, quantum, Dominus sit amandus et a quo. (101)
Quomodo, quo, quando, cur, unde reuersio fiat. (1075)
Quomodo uel de quo, qualis uel qualiter, ad quid (558)
Quos informat amor actus, deuotio condit. (851)
Quot Deus assumat, unde et quo, quomodo, quando. (18)

Radicem prauam, mens leti, falco necabit (225)
Rampnus, apis, Ioab, mulier, pars infima siche. (1194)
Rara fides, simulatus amor, speciosa supellex (493)
Rebus in humanis tria sunt gratissima laude (539)
Recte progrediens, oblitus posteriora (1282)
Recte uiue, feri, flexus propera misereri. (84)
Reddat se populumque fide factisque disertum (907)
Regi paret eques, uerbis munitus et armis (767)
Regis ad aduentum sunt hec uenientis in urbem (4)
Regula fabrilis est hec terrena potestas (589)
Religiosorum sunt hee species uitiorum (1081)
Rem templi, uotum, laudem, grates et honorem (1069)
Rem uariant tempus, locus, etas, causa modusque (1259)
Res modice, magne Domini magnalia monstrant (651)

Res, persona, locus, gestum, tempus, numerusque (1148)
Res pretiosa merum, potu, libamine dignum (1303)
Respiciens retro, collum uelud Orpha reflectens (1104)
Resplendet sole paries pelui mediante (236)
Respondere Deo quid sit si querimus, hoc est (1071)
Rex sacer Oswaldus seuas acies feriturus (841)
Rex sedet in solio, mala dissipat aspiciendo. (1347)
Ridens derisit, flens defleuit mala mundi. (333)
Riuulus et medici puer exto, fistula plumbi (1054)
Roma manus rodit, quos rodere non ualet odit. (1080)
Ros est ipse Deus et copia, gratia, uerbum. (1090)
Ros in scriptura Deus est et gratia, uerbum (1091)
Rosio, ruptio, demptio, pressio, temporis huius (1322)
Ruscus inhorrescens et eisdem rampnus in armis (1100)

Sacre scripture succendunt crimina prune. (1275)
Sal, modus in dandis, et circumstantia queuis (425)
Sal sacrificii cithare discretio plectrum (303)
Sal sacrificii personaque iussio, causa (424)
Saluator cibus et uitis, lux atque leuamen (1366)
Salue crux, hoc est, sis nobis causa salutis. (194)
Sancta Maria, Ioseph, panni, presepeque fenum (823)
Sancti nascuntur cum migrantes moriuntur (800)
Sanctificans alios, sanctus proprie Deus in se (1120)
Sanctorum nos reliquias quasi pignus habemus (1074)
Sanctorum uita nobis est lectio uiua (436)
Sanctorum uita uiuendi sit tibi forma (434)
Sanguine non uesci, mel non offerre iuberis (227)
Sanguinis et fletus, operis quoque cordis et oris (161)
Sanguis, opus, testes dant Christum uera locutum. (1374)
Sanguis, rana, culex, musce, pecus, ulcera, grando (1046)
Scandalon equiuocant obex, impactio, casus (1203)
Scito quod a multis laicis erratur in istis (459)
Scorpius ac dipsas et serpens flatibus urens (339)
Scorpius, eruca, Venus, ignis, uirus, yrudo (687)
Scorpius et laqueus, uestis, stercus, poliandrum (757)
Scriptura teste sunt in legis datione (935)
Scripture uerba, miracula, uita pudica (580)
Sedes firma Dei, lenis subiectaque mollis (281)
Sensus corporei fiant tibi causa merendi (949)
Sepe crumena tumens, emuncta cohercet auarum (1045)

Sepius unius in plures culpa redundat (997)
Septem uocales sunt hore totque reales (570)
Sermo Dei lux est, si diligis hunc tibi dux est (1208)
Sermo Dei sanat, seruat, corroborat, armat. (1209)
Sermo Dei uiuus ueraxque per omnia, castus (1274)
Sermo diuinus acus est dissuta retexens (909)
Sermo diuinus est aduersarius, ignis (1271)
Serpens antiquus a quo uix est homo tutus (368)
Serpens, ceruus, auis, arbor, sol lunaque tellus (1077)
Serpentem innocuum faciunt deserta locorum (815)
Serpentis cibus est fenum puluisque fauilla (235)
Seruat et adiuuat, instruit, expedit angelus, istuc (13)
Serues sollicitus carnis cum sensibus artus (111)
Seruilis bonus est timor ac effectus et usus (1223)
Seruus seruatur ut seruiat inde uocatur. (1138)
Set postremus Adam, natus de uirgine quadam (824)
Si bene membra regis es dignus nomine regis (1084)
Si bona uicinis dentur congratulor illis (171)
Si Christus meruit, cui, quando, qualiter et quid (1361)
Si desit panis est mensa et inops et inanis (240)
Si donas tristis et dona et munera perdis (316)
Si gaudet membrum congaudent omnia membra (747)
Si male iurandi species sit cura notandi (596)
Si mundo moreris moriendo non morieris. (114)
Si probus es tepet hoc, formosus abit, locuplex es (1111)
Si quis ad altare malus accedit celebrare (1128)
Si timor abscedat Domini pastorque recedat (900)
Sic foueam uici, pene, uirtutis, et orti (522)
Siccat et indurat sol presens, lucet et ardet (1180)
Sicut amor Domini cunctorum fons meritorum (24)
Signa futurorum sunt hec presentia queuis (1161)
Signabat labarum clipeorum insignia Christus (667)
Signat, submittit, purgat, conseruat et auget (1235)
Sinapis granum, calidum, siccum, modicumque (1184)
Sint comites Iude pudor et submissio spesque. (131)
Sint funes opus atque fides constantia funda (521)
Sis mundus, firmus, agyos, Dominoque dicatus (1121)
Sis uitulus te sacrificans, homo sis ratione (50)
Sit cita, discreta, conuersio plena, fidelis. (126)
Sit distincta crucis, distincta statera sit oris (1192)
Sit laus discreta, concors et uiuida, leta (653)

Sit mens in Christo, cor defigatur in ipso (1072)
Sit testamenti ueterisque nouique peritus (908)
Sit tibi potus aqua, cibus aridus, aspera uestis (1020)
Sit tibi presagus, presignans, pseudo propheta (933)
Sit tibi presagus, presignans, pseudo propheta (1063)
Sobrietas uires uitiorum comprimit omnes (1117)
Sobrius a mensis, a lecto surge pudicus. (552)
Sol est doctrina, tenebras pellendo chorusca. (308)
Sol trahit ardore nebulas, nos Christus amore (270)
Sol ueluti solus lucens est orbicularis (1178)
Sola reuiuiscunt que quondam uiua fuerunt (849)
Solatur scriptura, Deus pius, actaque pena. (208)
Sollicite scrutans et lustrans lustra ferarum (354)
Sollicitudo cauet culpam, confessio delet (138)
Sollicitudo, uenus, discordia, murmur et ira (737)
Solus prelucens, exsiccans, letificansque (1179)
Sorte nocent equa stultis aduersa, secunda (954)
Sperne deos, non periures, requies celebretur (313)
Spes, amor, exemplum sunt et meditatio mortis (1309)
Spes est pes nobis ad Christum progrediendi (1114)
Spes mola, pes, cedrus, altum crucis, anchora, tectum (1113)
Spes triplex triplexque fides, dilectio triplex. (1263)
Spes uenie, cor contritum, confessio culpe (1019)
Spina facultatis suppungit corda, maresque (326)
Spirituique uiro mulier caro sepe repugnat (155)
Spiritus est ignis precellens atque columba. (1108)
Spiritus et motus ignis, post sibilus aure (33)
Spissus uel rarus, tenuisque leuisque capillus (173)
Splendorem meriti sceleris caligine fuscant (1000)
Spongia, ianua, uiscus et ignis, rete, uorago (224)
Sponsor baptismi uotum dissoluere noli (71a)
Spurcus homo porcus est, mergendus, scabiosus (683)
Sta stabilis, firmus, pugnans et prouidus altus (1126)
Stat Dominus stabilis, prouidus atque uiuans. (280)
Statim post culpam dolet et rubet et pauet Adam (1002)
Stella fides, Christus, sancta exhortatio, sermo est (1182)
Stella Maria maris, uel amarum sit mare dicta (712)
Stella maris, regina poli, miseratio mundi (702)
Stent in mente Dei uerbum Dominique flagellum (773)
Stephanus et Christus mulierque pudica Susanna (!228)
Stramen fedatur, calcatur, et igne crematur. (1188)

Stulte quid egisti, cur non miser extimuisti (976)
Stuppa caro fragilis, cooperta ligataque pixis (21)
Sub specie recti fallit temptatio plures. (363)
Sub tecto nupte sunt plurima, uestis honesta (829)
Subsidium, cautela, Dei clementia, gressus (1285)
Subtrahe consilio dilectum quem petit hostis. (122)
Subtrahe ligna foco si uis extinguere flammam (105)
Subuertunt Sodomam tumor, otia, copia panis (1204)
Suggerit in primis serpens, deliberat Eua (1087)
Sumas exemplum quod tanquam calceus aptus (217)
Summe Pater uerbi, perimentis iura superbi. (259)
Summus ab extremis nebulas leuat opiliones (271)
Sunt adamantina nostri non cerea corda. (1118)
Sunt bustum, domus, infernus, corpus, monumentum. (1206)
Sunt ewangelia paradisi flumina, dragme (419)
Sunt euuangelica nature themata Christi (418)
Sunt extrema crucis contriti quatuor ista (1032)
Sunt fluuius, Pharius, maris unde, sarcina, gibbus (329)
Sunt hec in Pascha: uituli duo, sunt simul agni (864)
Sunt immunda lepus, cirogrillus, susque camelus. (51)
Sunt in deserto serpens, sitis, ardor, harena. (337)
Sunt inopum uitia murmur, detractio, liuor (956)
Sunt legis festa cum iugi sabbata festo (486)
Sunt mala mixta bonis humane conditionis (1232)
Sunt nobis uarie scripture sicut et esce. (1146)
Sunt palee reprobi, sunt purgamenta metalli (1102)
Sunt Pater et Verbum Christi cum Pneumate testes (1372)
Sunt peccata fores inferni, scoria, feces (988)
Sunt persepe simul solaris fulgor et imber (1033)
Sunt pompe mundi tanquam fantasmata noctis. (986)
Sunt porte uite clementia iudiciumque (721)
Sunt preponenda maiora minoribus atque (439)
Sunt primogenita uestis benedictio dupla (958)
Sunt pulcri flores, set fructus utiliores. (853)
Sunt qui cum clauso putrefacta est spina sepulcro (1326)
Sunt septem panes enarrans sermo saluber (939)
Sunt speculum quo conspicitur Deus ista creata (1155)
Sunt sponse Christi uel amice, lumina mundi (736)
Sunt timor et tenebre, uermes, in carcere fetor (158)
Sunt tria grandia: laus, sapientia, gloria rerum (750)
Sus de sorde leuat, saltem dum colligit escam (982)

Suscipiunt ignem sanctum bonus atque beatus (621)
Sustinet atque probat, placet et proponit et optat (1277)

Talpa, canis, Naas, coruus Samsonque Thobias (182)
Tanquam fax ardens de celo decidit ingens (351)
Tardior in nobis set et ictibus apta ferendis (1265)
Te parere docent Bethania, sidera, uenti (867)
Tedia torpentem faciunt, labor atque secunda. (1240)
Telluris loca Tigris obit, qua sorbuit aurum (219)
Tellus purgetur, scindatur, deinde seratur (1249)
Tellus sustentat, induit atque cibat. (1248)
Tempestas, tenebra, seruire, parasceue, limpha (1068)
Tempestas uento, tonitru fit, fulgure, nimbo. (1238)
Tempora cum stellis numerat Deus utile, carum (277)
Tempora cum ueniunt abeunt, sic tempora fiunt (1250)
Tempore uel genere, numero, pretio, minus affert (744)
Temporis ac anime, necnon et uirginitatis (344)
Temporis hec bona sunt non effectu licet usu. (75)
Temptant nos homines, Deus et demon, caro nostra (1243)
Tempus, opes et opus, operam quoque diuide recte. (320)
Tempus sudoris breue, mercedis prope iusto (739)
Ter Dominum Petrus funesta uoce negauit (825)
Terra argillosa, uirgeque Iacob tibi sancti (1122)
Terra, lutum, uestis, uas, fascis, seruus, et hostis (151)
Terra, solum uel humus uirgo est, glis, arida, tellus. (700)
Terre curuatur, amat hanc, finemque minatur (762)
Terreat hos pena quos non inuitat amena (1222)
Terret et illudit per sompnia uana malignus (365)
Terribilis, durus et grandis, semper acutus (546)
Terris uicina mutabilis et uaga luna (670)
Testantur Christum Moyses, Pater atque Iohannes (579)
Timpana, sal, munus, reddit concordia grata. (106)
Tollit opes, animam, sensum cum nomine famam (686)
Tot Dominus nobis et tanta dedit bona quod non (72)
Tramitis amfractus, fraus cordis, fetor et oris (1319)
Transire et capere, simul in coniunge decore (357)
Transit preclara nubes, fecunda, leuata (707)
Tres Herebi furie sunt ira, cupido, libido. (517)
Tristes ac humiles Dominum sancte mulieres (934)
Tristitiam culpa, dampnum, contritio, pena (1239)
Truncus, pons, glacies, bosilac dans, talpa, columba (429)

Tu Deus adiutor, medicus, dux, rex, mihi pastor (254)
Tu fons signatus, tu clausula, clausaque porta (703)
Tu nisi peccatum nil reputes proprium (966)
Tu sapiens, instans, mundus, constans et amans sis (882)
Tu te non alius celis auferre ualebis (110)
Tunc stulti cernit ratio, scelus horret et odit (996)
Turtur, soliuaga uolucris, gemebunda, pudica (1258)
Tutior in terra locus est quam turribus altis (1144)
Tutus uir quis, quoque statu, cur, quomodo, quando. (1205)

Vehementi occurrite morbo (121)
Vel rem uel uerbum tribuas cuicumque petenti (317)
Vellet, si uellent, Deus omnes saluificari. (266)
Vendere cum possis captiuum occidere noli. (1139)
Venimus a Domino per quem redeamus ad ipsum (377)
Ventilabrum dextra gerit et paleas facit extra (289)
Ventris ob ingluuiem mus nulla pericula uitat. (811)
Ventus, caligo, fulmen, tonitrus sonus, imber (374)
Verbi rete, doli, peccati, iudiciique (1098)
Verbum, sputamen, hec egrediuntur ab ore (878)
Vermis corrodens, subtractio gratuitorum (1321)
Vertat pre silo presbiter officio. (892)
Vertitur, opprimit, atterit, eicit ut mola mundus (760)
Verum dixit anus quod piscis olet triduanus (560)
Vesicam loculo preponens stultus habetur (765)
Vespere gallina scandit pro uulpibus alta (1167)
Veste, loco, uase, cultu potuque ciboque (148)
Vestio, poto, cibo, tectum do, uisito, soluo (719)
Vestitur tellus gramine, fronde nemus (1310)
Vilior est humana caro quam pellis ouina (153)
Villa, boues, uxor, cenam clausere uocatis (143)
Vim tu caute caue, retinens moderamina lingue. (1004)
Vinctos educit Dominus de carcere ceco (157)
Vinea culta fuit, cultores premia querunt (1300)
Vinea uallatur, complantatur foditurque (1298)
Vir rationis apex, mulier pars ima uocatur (1088)
Virga Dei rectos regit et contundit iniquos (1292)
Virgo Dei genitrix, rosa, lilia, fons, paradisus (696)
Virgo Deum peperit, set si quis quomodo querit (1350)
Virgo, presepe, crux tumbaque mundus, olimpus (1354)
Virgo tibi sponsus sit is est cui grata iuuentus (1358)

Virtus exornat mentem, contritio mundat (336)
Virtus res simplex, nec crescere nec minui scit (1264)
Virtutes et uerba Dei fletusque precesque (36)
Virtutes, uitia, quid credendum, quid agendum (917)
Vis est in uerbis, gemmis, oculis, et in herbis. (1273)
Visibus intentis scrutatur ab ethere terram (366)
Visio, laus, locus et socii, saluatio iusti (475)
Vita breuis, casusque leuis, nec spes remeandi (1151)
Vita, salus, requies, substantia, doxa, uoluptas (90)
Vitam maiorum disponit uita minorum (890)
Vitam pastoris perdit commissio plebis (889)
Vite labentis et in arto tempore mortis (1289)
Vite presentis si comparo gaudia uentis (534)
Vitet homo culpam ne seruus damnificetur (1008)
Viuens eternum Deus omnia condidit una (262)
Viuere natura dat, gratia, gloria, culpa. (1287)
Viuere natura dat, gratia, gloria, culpa. (1295)
Vix sine sorde potes participare luto. (22)
Vna fides in te faciens subsistere uitam (479)
Vnde et quo, qualis conuersio, quomodo, quare (127)
Vnde Ihesus saluet, quos, quando, quomodo, quare. (1145)
Vnde habeas nemo querit set oportet habere. (324)
Vno rinoceros cornu pugnans, elephantem (1106)
Voce Deum laudes: Vt lingua Deo famuletur (654)
Vrbes munitas uastat bonus aut malus ignis. (1314)
Vsus et ara, liber et gratia, gloria, culpa (177)
Vsus, homo, culpa, cordis contritio, pena (1191)
Vt colatorum locuples, loculusque camelus (330)
Vt Deus alliciat, ut dampnet, premia soluat (382)
Vt dimittaris, aliis peccata remitte (1036)
Vt domet, ut dampnet, ut purget et ut mereatur (291)
Vt dominis plenus honor, obsequiumque fidele (1124)
Vt duo conferret, niue mulcet, fulgure terret (14)
Vt ficte narratur, equi sunt bis duo Phebi (1181)
Vt medicus, rethor, Dominus curare, tueri (405)
Vt naute uigiles, pastores, angelus, ales (1291)
Vt pariat dignos homini contritio fructus (1035)
Vt plus committat culpe memor impius extat (774)
Vt prohibent aliqui bona sunt tantum uia, signum (880)
Vt proruperunt quondam cathaclismus et ignis (285)
Vt reprobi penas uigilanti corde reuoluas (1047)

Vt rota principio uel fine carere uidetur (245)
Vt sambucus eris plebs israelitica, tigris (931)
Vt sit pena rubor tibi uilis ut efficiaris (136)
Vt sompnolentes, sementis, et archa resurgit (1094)
Vt tabulas uectes, sic iustos ista tenebunt (1255)
Vt te ipsum serues, non expergisceris (112)
Vt uox, lux, anima simul hic ibi, sic Deus extat (378)
Vtilis est herba succosaque, lenis, amena (572)
Vtilis ut sermo sit et ut uideatur honestus (1270)
Vulneris ardorem lenit, seditque tumorem (444)
Vxorem quare locupletem ducere nolim (715)

Ydropi languet male luxuriosus, auarus (639)
Ydrops et dipsas, species, bitumen, irudo (60)

Appendix C

Alphabetical list of *themata* of
William de Montibus's sermons

Abiit Iesus trans mare Galilee (36)
Absit mihi gloriari nisi in cruce (80)
Ad uesperum demorabitur fletus et ad matutinum letitia (72)
Adducet Dominus urentem uentum de deserto (133)
Ait angelus de beato Iohanne: Multi in natiuitate eius (86)
Apparuerunt illis lingue dispertite (12)
Ascendens Christus in altum captiuam duxit captiuitatem (84)
Ascendet sicut uirgultum et sicut radix de terra sitienti (40)
Ascendit Deus in iubilo et Dominus in uoce tube (107)
Assumpta est Maria in celum, etc. (147)
Audiui orationem tuam et uidi lacrimam tuam (33)
Aue Maria gratia plena. Eisdem uerbis (103)

Beati misericordes quoniam ipsi misericordiam consequentur (66)
Beati mundo corde. Congrue sollempnitatem (55)
Beati pauperes spiritu quoniam ipsorum est regnum celorum (94)
Beati qui audiunt uerbum Dei et custodiunt illud (124)
Beatus est, et erit, uir qui timet Dominum (23)
Beatus qui habet partem in resurrectione prima (105)
Beatus uir cuius auxilium est abs te, etc. (48)
Benedictus qui uenit in nomine Domini (132)
Bona est oratio cum ieiunio et elemosina. Hiis uerbis (83)
Bona est oratio cum ieiunio et elemosina. Memini (106)

Cananea in oratione perstat et instat (32)
Christus hodie natus est, gaudeamus (74)
Christus humiliauit semetipsum factus obediens (141)
Circumdabo domum meam ex his qui militant mihi (19)
Constituit Dominus populum suum super excelsam terram (1)
Cum appropinquaret Iesus Ierusalem uidens ciuitatem fleuit (79)
Cum complerentur dies Pentecostes (52)
Cum exaltatus fuero a terra, omnia traham ad me ipsum (113)

Cum natus esset Iesus in Bethlehem (118)
Cum optulerit homo sacrificium coctum Domino in clibano (137)
Cum summa deuotione celebranda est beati Michaelis festiuitas (93)
Cum uenerit paraclitus. Quis ueniat uideas, quando (51)

Declina a malo et fac bonum (123)
Descendit sicut pluuia in uellus (117)
Deus ab austro ueniet, de Bethleem scilicet (136)
Dilectissimi emendemus nos ab omni inquinamento carnis (88)
Dilectus meus candidus et rubicundus. Salomon (39)
Dilectus meus candidus et rubicundus. Hiis uerbis (115)
Dilexit Andream Dominus in odorem suauitatis (95)
Dispersit dedit pauperibus (89)
Dixit Iesus phariseis: Homo quidam erat diues (5)
Domine dilexi decorem domus tue. Dei plures sunt (63)
Domine tu omnia scis (110)
Dominus memor fuit nostri et benedixit nobis (8)
Dum implerentur dies Pentecostes erantque pariter in eodem (14)
Duo sunt genera dilectionem proximi conseruanda (120)

Ecce Dominus ueniet et omnes sancti eius cum eo (130)
Ecce quam bonum et quam iocundum. Hac tuba Spiritus sancti (9)
Ecce sacerdos magnus, pater multitudinis gentium (91)
Educens nubes ab extremo terre, fulgura in pluuiam fecit (7)
Ego sum Deus Abraham (2)
Egredere de terra tua. Per hec uerba que Dominus (104)
Erat Iesus eiciens demonium (34)
Erraui sicut ouis que periit (26)
Estote imitatores Dei sicut filii karissimi (35)
Et cantent in uiis Domini, quia magna est gloria Domini (11)
Ex Egipto uocaui filium meum (49)
Exaltare super celos Deus (29)
Expecta me, dicit Dominus, in die resurrectionis mee (142)

Fac tibi archam de lignis leuigatis (21)
Facite uobis amicos de mammona ut cum defeceritis recipiant (25)
Facite uobis amicos de mammona. Mammona lingua Syrorum (24)
Fasciculus mirre dilectus meus mihi (131)
Figura dominice ascensionis fuit ante legem translatio Enoch (50)
Fili si habes benefac tecum (69)
Fulcite me floribus, stipate me malis, quia amore langueo (143)

Gaudeamus omnes in Domino diem festum celebrantes
    sub honore (92)
Gustate et uidete quoniam suauis est Dominus (116)

Hic Iesus qui assumptus est a uobis (45)
Hodie descendit lux magna super terram (98)
Homo quidam diues. Homo iste a quibusdam dictus est Tantalus (3)
Homo quidam erat diues. In diuite isto quattuor (57)
Homo quidam erat diues, quasi ignotus et alienus apud Deum (4)
Homo quidam erat diues [see Dixit Iesus, no. 5]
Honora patrem et matrem. Honora parentes carnales (56)
Honora patrem tuum et matrem tuam ut sis longeuus (67)

Ignem ardentem extinguit aqua et elemosina resistit peccatis (65)
Ignem ueni mittere in terram. Venit autem Dominus (54)
In conspectu angelorum psallam tibi (31)
In hac sacra sollemnitate que sancte Trinitati assignatur (129)
In lapide uno septem oculi sunt (97)
In nouissimis diebus circumcides cor tuum (75)
Inspice et fac secundum exemplar quod tibi in monte (17)
Iustus ut palma florebit (109)

Karitas in dilectione Dei et proximi constat (119)

Lapidem quem reprobauerunt edificantes (62)
Lauamini mundi estote. In hiis uerbis Ysaie (82)
Lauamini mundi estote, auferte malum cogitationum uestrarum (122)

Magnificat anima mea Dominum (111)
Meror in corde iusti humiliabit eum, et sermone bono (38)
Mulier que dampnauit saluauit, et sicut per inobedientiam (37)
Multe filie congregauerunt diuitias (90)
Multi in natiuitate eius [see Ait angelus, no. 86]

Nam et Maria et Ioseph et Symeon et Anna hodie (77)
Nescitis quod hii qui in stadio currunt (15)
Nisi Dominus custodit ciuitatem (71)
Nisi Dominus edificauerit domum (70)
Nisi conuersi fueritis (60)
Nolite thesaurizare uobis thesauros in terra (22)
Non est Deus alius ut Deus rectissimi (6)

Nudus egressus sum de utero matris mee (61)
Nunc dimittis seruum tuum Domine [*see* Nam et Maria, no. 77]

Obtulerunt Magi Domino aurum, thus, et mirram (76)
Offer Domino candelam accensam, benedictam et sanctificatam (135)
Offer filium tuum quem diligis (134)
Omne datum optimum et omne donum perfectum desursum est (73)
Omnia facite sine murmurationibus (59)

Passer, hec auis Christus (47)
Penitentiam agite, appropinquabit enim regnum celorum (102)
Per montem oliueti tendit Dominus Ierusalem (140)
Precepit Dominus Moisi ut faceret tabernaculum (114)

Qui crediderit et baptizatus fuerit, saluus erit (125)
Qui habet mandata mea et seruat ea (127)
Qui sedes super cherubin manifestare (96)
Qui sunt isti qui ut nubes uolant (87)
Quis ueniat, quid agat, in quos, ubi, quomodo, quando (53)

Renouabitur ut aquile iuuentus tua (99)
Respexit humilitatem ancille sue (112)

Sacerdotes qui ad Dominum accedunt sanctificentur (28)
Sacrificium Deo spiritus tribulatus (78)
Sapientia edificauit sibi domum. Maria est domus (148)
Sapientia edificauit sibi domum, excidit columpnas septem (138)
Scrutemur uias nostras. Verba sunt Ieremie (41)
Sedete in ciuitate quoadusque induamini uirtute ex alto (126)
Sex annis seres agrum tuum (16)
Si consurrexistis cum Christo (81)
Si quis diligit me sermonem meum seruabit. Dilectio alia (108)
Si quis diligit me sermonem meum seruabit. Hiis uerbis (85)
Sic Deus dilexit mundum ut Filium suum unigenitum daret (13)
Similis factus sum pellicano solitudinis (144)
Soluite et adducite mihi (139)
Spiritus sanctus detestatur et odit simultatem (146)
Spiritus sanctus discipline effugiet fictum [*see* no. 146]
State succincti lumbos uestros in ueritate (64)
Stelle manentes in ordine suo et cursu (27)
Surge illuminare Ierusalem quia uenit lumen tuum (100)
Surrexit Dominus sicut predixit (42)

Tota religiosorum debet intentio circa hoc uersari (128)
Tria sunt difficilia mihi et quartum penitus ignoro (145)
Tulerunt Iesum in Ierusalem (101)

Vado ad eum qui me misit. Euuangelia que hiis diebus (44)
Vado ad eum qui misit me. Pauperi (10)
Vado parare uobis locum. Verba Domini sunt in cena (43)
Vendite que possidetis et date elemosinam (68)
Venite post me, faciam uos fieri piscatores hominum (18)
Videte quomodo caute ambuletis (30)
Vigili cura, mente sollicita, summo conatu et sollicitudine (121)
Vinea mea coram me est. Ex hodierna euuangelii (20)
Virgo sapiens desponsata est filio regis summi (149)
Vnde Iesus scandat, uel quo, uel ubi uideamus (46)
Vos estis sal terre (58)

Bibliography

Abelard, Peter. *Historia calamitatum*. Ed. Jacques Monfrin. Paris: Vrin, 1959.

Adam of Eynsham. *Magna vita Sancti Hugonis: The Life of St. Hugh of Lincoln*. Ed. Decima L. Douie and David Hugh Farmer. 2 vols. 1961-1962; rept. with corrections Oxford: Clarendon Press, 1985.

Alan of Lille. *Distinctiones dictionum theologicalium*. PL 210: 687-1012.

———. *Liber parabolarum*. PL 210: 581-594.

———. *Regulae caeliestis iuris*. Ed. Nikolaus Häring. "Magister Alanus de Insulis Regulae caelestis iuris." *Archives d'histoire doctrinale et littéraire du moyen âge* 48 (1981) 97-226.

Alexander Neckam. See Neckam, Alexander.

Alexander of Hales. *Summa Theologica: Indices in Tom. I-IV*. Grottaferra: Collegii S. Bonaventurae, 1979.

Analecta hymnica medii aevi. See Dreves, Guido Maria.

Anciaux, Paul. *La théologie du sacrement de pénitence au XIIe siècle*. Louvain: E. Nauwelaerts, 1949.

Annales Monastici, III. Ed. Henry Richard Luard. Rolls Series, 36. London: Longman, 1866.

Auerbach, Erich. *Literatursprache und Publikum in der lateinischen Spätantike und im Mittelalter*. Bern: Francke, 1958.

Avril, Joseph. "La pastorale des malades et des mourants aux XIIe et XIIIe siècles." In *Death in the Middle Ages*, ed. Herman Braet and Werner Verbeke, pp. 88-106. Louvain: Leuven University Press, 1983.

Balbi, John, of Genoa. *Catholicon*. Mainz, 1460.

Baldwin, John W. "A Debate at Paris over Thomas Becket between Master Roger and Master Peter the Chanter." *Studia Gratiana* 11 (1967) 121-132.

———. "Masters at Paris from 1179 to 1215: A Social Perspective." In *Renaissance and Renewal in the Twelfth Century*, ed. Robert L. Benson, Giles Constable, and Carol Lanham, pp. 138-172. Cambridge MA: Harvard University Press, 1982.

———. *Masters, Princes and Merchants: The Social Views of Peter the Chanter and His Circle*. 2 vols. Princeton: Princeton University Press, 1970.

———. *The Scholastic Culture of the Middle Ages 1000-1300*. Lexington MA: Heath, 1971.

Bale, John. *Index Britanniae scriptorum*. Ed. Reginald L. Poole and Mary Bateson. Anecdota oxoniensia, Medieval and Modern Series, 9. Oxford, 1902.

———. *Scriptorum illustrium maioris Brytannie ... Catalogus*. Basel, 1557-1559.

Bartholomew of Exeter. See Morey, Adrian.

Bartlett, Robert. *Gerald of Wales 1146-1223*. Oxford: Clarendon Press, 1982.

Bataillon, Louis-Jacques. "*Similitudines* et *Exempla* dans les sermons du XIIIe siècle." In *The Bible in the Medieval World: Essays in Memory of Beryl Smalley*, ed. Katherine Walsh and Diana Wood, pp. 191-205. Oxford: Blackwell, 1985.

Bazan, Bernardo C., Gérard Fransen, John W. Wippel, and Danielle Jacquart. *Les questions disputées et les questions quodlibétiques dans les facultés de théologie, de droit et de médecine*. Typologie des sources du moyen âge occidental, 44-45. Turnhout: Brepols, 1985.

Beleth, John. *Summa de ecclesiasticis officiis*. Ed. Heribert Douteil. 2 vols. Corpus Christianorum Continuatio Mediaevalis, 41, 41A. Turnhout: Brepols, 1976.

Bennett, H.S. "Medieval Ordination Lists in the English Episcopal Registers." In *Studies Presented to Sir Hilary Jenkinson*, ed. J. Conway Davies, pp. 20-34. London: Oxford University Press, 1957.

Biblioteca apostolica vaticana: Codices reginenses latini. Ed. André Wilmart. 2 vols. Vatican City: Biblioteca Apostolica Vaticana, 1941.

Binkley, Peter. "Unedited Poems from Cotton Titus A.XX with a Note on Chaucer's Sparrowhawk." *Scintilla: A Student Journal for Medievalists* 2-3 (1985-1986) 66-100.

Bischoff, John Paul. "Economic Change in Thirteenth Century Lincoln: Decline of an Urban Cloth Industry." PhD dissertation: Yale University, 1975.

Bloomfield, Morton W. *The Seven Deadly Sins*. [East Lansing MI]: Michigan State College Press, 1952.

Bloomfield, Morton W., B.-G. Guyot, D.R. Howard, and T.B. Kabealo. *Incipits of Latin Works on the Virtues and Vices, 1100-1500 A.D.* Cambridge MA: Mediaeval Academy of America, 1979.

Bonaventure. *Ars concionandi. S. Bonaventurae Sermones de tempore, de sanctis. Opera omnia*, 9. Quaracchi: Collegii S. Bonaventurae, 1901.

Bonaventure, Brother. See Miner, John N.

The Book of St Gilbert. Ed. Raymonde Foreville and Gillian Keir. Oxford: Clarendon Press, 1987.

Bougerol, Jacques Guy. *Les manuscrits franciscains de la Bibliothèque de Troyes*. Rome: Collegii S. Bonaventurae, 1982.

Boyle, Leonard E. "Aspects of Clerical Education in Fourteenth-Century England." In *The Fourteenth Century*, Proceedings of the State University of New York Conferences in Medieval Studies, ed. Paul E. Szarmach and Bernard S. Levy, pp. 19-32. Binghamton NY: Center for Medieval and Early Renaissance Studies, 1977. Rept. in *Pastoral Care, Clerical Education and Canon Law, 1200-1400*.

———. "The Constitution 'Cum ex eo' of Boniface VIII: Education of Parochial Clergy." *Mediaeval Studies* 24 (1962) 263-302. Rept. in *Pastoral Care*.

———. "The Fourth Lateran Council and Manuals of Popular Theology." In *The Popular Literature of Medieval England*, ed. Thomas J. Heffernan, pp. 30-43. Knoxville: University of Tennessee Press, 1985.

———. "The Inter-conciliar Period 1179-1215 and the Beginnings of Pastoral Manuals." In *Miscellanea Rolando Bandinelli Papa Alessandro III*, ed. Filippo Liotta, pp. 45-56. Siena: Accademia Senese degli Intronati, 1986.

———. "The *Oculus sacerdotis* and Some Other Works of William of Pagula." *Transactions of the Royal Historical Society*, 5th series, 5 (1955) 81-110. Rept. in *Pastoral Care*.

———. *Pastoral Care, Clerical Education and Canon Law, 1200-1400*. London: Variorum Reprints, 1981.

———. Review of *Thomae de Chobham Summa Confessorum*, ed. F. Broomfield. Louvain: Nauwelaerts, 1968. In *Catholic Historical Review* 57 (1971) 487-488.

———. "A Study of the Works Attributed to William of Pagula with Special Reference to the *Oculus sacerdotis* and *Summa summarum*." 2 vols. D.Phil. dissertation: Oxford University, 1956.

———. "The *Summa confessorum* of John of Freiburg and the Popularization of the Moral Teaching of St. Thomas and Some of his Contemporaries." In *St. Thomas Aquinas, 1274-1974: Commemorative Studies*, ed. Armand A. Maurer, 2: 245-268. Toronto: Pontifical Institute of Mediaeval Studies, 1974.

———. "The 'Summa summarum' and Some Other English Works of Canon Law." In *Proceedings of the Second International Congress of Medieval Canon Law* ed. Stephan Kuttner and J.J. Ryan, pp. 415-456. Vatican City: Biblioteca Apostolica Vaticana, 1965. Rept. in *Pastoral Care*.

———. "Summae confessorum." In *Les Genres littéraires dans les sources théologiques et philosophiques médiévales: Définition, critique, et exploitation*, Actes du Colloque international de Louvain-la-Neuve, 25-27 mai 1981, pp. 227-237. Louvain: Institut d'études médiévales, 1982.

———. "Three English Pastoral Summae and a 'Magister Galienus.'" *Studia Gratiana* 11 (1967) 135-144

Brady, Ignatius. "Peter Manducator and the Oral Teachings of Peter Lombard." *Antonianum* 41 (1966) 454-490.

Bremond, Claude, Jacques Le Goff, Jean-Claude Schmitt. *L'"exemplum."* Typologie des sources du moyen âge occidental, 40. Turnhout: Brepols, 1982.

Bühler, Curt F. "The Apostles and the Creed." *Speculum* 28 (1953) 335-339.

Burton, Rosemary. *Classical Poets in the "Florilegium Gallicum."* Frankfurt (am Main): Peter Lang, 1983.

Bynum, Carolyn Walker. *Jesus as Mother: Studies in the Spirituality of the High Middle Ages*. Berkeley: University of California Press, 1982.

Caecilius Balba. *Caecilii Balbe De nugis philosophorum*. Ed. Eduard von Wölfflin. Basel, 1885.

Caesarius of Heisterbach. *Caesarii Heisterbacensis monachi Ordinis Cisterciensis Dialogus Miraculorum.* Ed. Joseph Strange. 2 vols. Cologne, 1851.

Canterbury Hymnal. Ed. Gernot R. Wieland. Toronto Medieval Latin Texts, 12. Toronto: Pontifical Institute of Mediaeval Studies, 1982.

Cartulaire général de Paris, 528-1180. Ed. R.C. de Lasteyrie du Saillant. Paris, 1887.

Charland, Thomas. "Les auteurs d''artes predicandi' au XIIIe siècle d'apres les manuscrits." *Etudes d'histoire littéraire et doctrinale du XIIIe siècle* 1 (1932) 41-60.

Chartularium Universitatis Parisiensis, Tomus I: Ab anno MCC usque ad annum MCCLXXXVI. Ed. Heinrich Denifle and E.L.M. Chatelain. Paris, 1889.

Chaucer, Geoffrey. *Canterbury Tales.* In *The Riverside Chaucer*, ed. Larry D. Benson, pp. 3-328. 3rd ed.; Boston MA: Houghton Mifflin, 1987.

Cheney, Christopher Robert. *English Bishops' Chanceries, 1100-1250.* Manchester: Manchester University Press, 1950.

——. *English Synodalia of the Thirteenth Century.* 1941; rept. (with new introduction) London: Oxford University Press, 1968.

——. *From Becket to Langton: English Church Government 1170-1213.* Manchester: Manchester University Press, 1956.

——. "King John and the Papal Interdict." *Bulletin of the John Rylands Library* 31 (1948) 295-317. Rept. in *The Papacy and England 12th-14th Centuries.*

——. *The Papacy and England 12th-14th Centuries.* London: Variorum Reprints, 1982.

——. *Pope Innocent III and England.* Stuttgart: Anton Hiersemann, 1976.

Cheney, Mary. *Roger, Bishop of Worcester 1164-1179.* Oxford: Clarendon Press, 1980.

Chobham, Thomas of. See Thomas of Chobham.

Chronica de Mailros. Ed. Joseph Stevenson. Edinburgh, 1835.

Chronicon de Lanercost. Ed. Joseph Stevenson. Edinburgh, 1839.

Clanchy, M.T. *From Memory to Written Record: England, 1066-1307.* Cambridge MA: Harvard University Press, 1979.

Collon, M. *Catalogue général des manuscrits des bibliothèques publiques des départements de France*, 37. Paris, 1900.

Conciliorum oecumenicorum decreta. Ed. Joseph Alberigo, J.A. Dossetti, P. Joannou, C. Leonardi, and P. Prodi. 3rd ed. Bologna: Istituto per le Scienze Religiose, 1973.

Constable, Giles. "Aelred of Rievaulx and the Nun of Watton: An Episode in the Early History of the Gilbertine Order." In *Medieval Women*, ed. Derek Baker, pp. 205-226. Oxford: Blackwell, 1978.

Constitutiones Concilii quarti Lateranensis una cum Commentariis glossatorum. Ed. Antonius Garcia y Garcia. Monumenta iuris canonici,

Series A: Corpus glossatorum, 2. Vatican City: Biblioteca Apostolica Vaticana, 1981.

Councils & Synods, with Other Documents Relating to the English Church, II: A.D. 1205-1213. Ed. F.M. Powicke and C.R. Cheney. 2 vols. Oxford: Clarendon Press, 1964.

Courtenay, William J. *Schools & Scholars in Fourteenth-Century England.* Princeton: Princeton University Press, 1987.

D'Alverny, Marie-Thérèse. *Alain de Lille: Textes inédits avec une introduction sur sa vie et ses oeuvres.* Paris: Vrin, 1965.

D'Avray, David L. *The Preaching of the Friars: Sermons Diffused from Paris before 1300.* Oxford: Clarendon Press, 1985.

De la Mare, Albinia. *Catalogue of the Collection of Medieval Manuscripts Bequeathed to the Bodleian Library Oxford by James P.R. Lyell.* Oxford: Clarendon Press, 1971.

Delhaye, Philippe. "Deux textes de Senatus de Worcester sur la pénitence." *Recherches de théologie ancienne et médiévale* 19 (1952) 203-224.

——. "Florilèges médiévales d'ethique." In *Dictionnaire de spiritualité* (1962) 5: 460-475.

——. "L'organisation scolaire au XIIe siècle." *Traditio* 5 (1947) 211-268.

Dictionary of Medieval Latin from British Sources. Fasc. II C. London: Oxford University Press, 1981.

Distelbrink, Balduinus. *Bonaventurae scripta: Authentica, dubia, vel spuria critice recensita.* Rome: Istituto Storico Cappuccini, 1975.

Dobson, E.J. *Moralities on the Gospels: A New Source of "Ancrene Wisse."* Oxford: Clarendon Press, 1975.

Dreves, Guido Maria, ed. *Hymnographi Latini: Lateinische Hymnendichter des Mittelalters.* 2nd Series. Analecta Hymnica Medii Aevi, 50 (1907).

Dumoutet, Edouard. *Le désir de voir l'hostie et les origines de la dévotion au saint sacrement.* Paris: Beauchesne, 1926.

——. "La théologie de l'eucharistie: la fin du XIIe siècle: Le témoignage de Pierre le Chantre d'après la 'Summa de sacramentis.'" *Archives d'histoire doctrinale et littéraire du moyen âge* 14 (1943-1945) 181-262.

Dutton, Paul Edward. "The Uncovering of the *Glosae super Platonem* of Bernard of Chartres." *Mediaeval Studies* 46 (1984) 192-195.

Edwards, Kathleen. *The English Secular Cathedrals in the Middle Ages: A Constitutional Study with Special Reference to the Fourteenth Century.* 2nd ed. Manchester: Manchester University Press, 1967.

Egger, Carolus. "De praxi paenitentiali Victorinorum." *Angelicum* 17 (1940) 156-179.

Emden, A.B. *A Biographical Register of the University of Cambridge to 1500.* Cambridge: Cambridge University Press, 1963.

Evans, Gillian R. "A Work of 'Terminist Theology'? Peter the Chanter's *De Tropis Loquendi* and Some *Fallacie.*" *Vivarium* 20 (1982) 40-58.

———. *Alan of Lille: The Frontiers of Theology in the Later Twelfth Century.* Cambridge: Cambridge University Press, 1983.

———. "Alan of Lille's *Distinctiones* and the Problem of Theological Language." *Sacris erudiri* 24 (1980) 67-86.

———. *The Language and Logic of the Bible: The Earlier Middle Ages.* Cambridge: Cambridge University Press, 1984.

———. "The Place of Peter the Chanter's *De Tropis Loquendi*." *Analecta Cisterciensia* 39 (1983) 231-253.

———. "Peter the Chanter's *De Tropis Loquendi*: The Problem of the Text." *New Scholasticism* 55 (1981) 95-103.

Eynde, Damien van den. *Les définitions des sacrements pendant la première période de la théologie scolastique (1050-1240).* Rome: Antonianum, 1950.

Faire croire: Modalités de la diffusion et de la réception des messages religieux du XIIe au XVe siècle. Rome: Ecole Française de Rome, 1981.

Farmer, David Hugh. *Saint Hugh of Lincoln.* Kalamazoo MI: Cistercian Publications, 1985.

Ferruolo, Stephen C. *The Origins of the University: The Schools of Paris and their Critics 1100-1215.* Stanford: Stanford University Press, 1985.

Final Concords of the County of Lincoln. Ed. C.W. Foster. 2 vols. Horncastle: Lincoln Record Society, 1920.

Finkenzeller, Josef. *Die Lehre von den Sakramenten im allgemeinen: Von der Schrift bis zur Scholastik.* Freiburg im Br.: Herder, 1980.

Flint, Valerie I.J. "The 'School of Laon': A Reconsideration." *Recherches de théologie ancienne et médiévale* 43 (1976) 89-110.

Floyer, John Kestell. *Catalogue of Manuscripts Preserved in the Chapter Library of Worcester Cathedral.* Ed. and rev. by S.G. Hamilton. Oxford: J. Parker, 1906.

Foulds, Trevor. "Thurgarton Priory and Its Benefactors with an Edition of the Cartulary." 3 vols. PhD dissertation: University of Nottingham, 1984.

Franz, Adolph. *Die kirchlichen Benediktionen im Mittelalter.* 2 vols. 1909; rept. Graz: Akademische Druck, 1960.

Friedman, Lionel J. *Text and Iconography for Joinville's "Credo."* Cambridge MA: Mediaeval Academy of America, 1958.

Gabriel, Astrik L. *Garlandia: Studies in the History of the Mediaeval University.* Notre Dame IN: Mediaeval Institute, 1969.

Gerald of Wales. *De rebus a se gestis, libri III.* Ed. J.S. Brewer. Rolls Series, 21/1, London: Longman, 1861.

———. *Gemma ecclesiastica.* Ed. J.S. Brewer. Rolls Series 21/2. London: Longman, 1862.

———. *The Life of St. Hugh of Avalon, Bishop of Lincoln 1186-1200.* Ed. and transl. Richard M. Loomis. Garland Library of Medieval Literature, 31. New York: Garland Press, 1985.

——. *Speculum duorum: or, A Mirror of Two Men*. Ed. Yves Lefevre and R.B.C. Huygens. Transl. Brian Dawson. Cardiff: University of Cardiff, 1974.

——. *Speculum ecclesiae*. Ed. J.S. Brewer. Rolls Series 21/4. London: Longman, 1873.

Gesta Regis Henrici Secundi Benedicti Abbatis. Ed. William Stubbs. 2 vols. Rolls Series, 49. London: Longman, 1867.

Ghellinck, Joseph de. *L'essor de la littérature latine au XIIe siècle*. 2nd ed. Brussels: Desclée de Brouwer, 1954.

——. "Medieval Theology in Verse." *Irish Quarterly Review* 9 (1914) 336-354.

——. "'Originale' et 'Originalia.'" *Archivum latinitatis medii aevi* 14 (1939) 95-105.

Gibbs, Marion and Jane Lang. *Bishops and Reform, 1215-1272: With Special Reference to the Lateran Council of 1215*. London: Oxford University Press, 1934.

Gilbert of Poitiers. See Häring, Nikolaus.

Gilbertine Rite. Ed. Reginald Maxwell Wooley. 2 vols. Henry Bradshaw Society, 59. London: Henry Bradshaw Society, 1921-1922.

Gillespie, Vincent. "*Doctrina* and *Predicacio*: The Design and Function of Some Pastoral Manuals." *Leeds Studies in English*, ns 11 (1980) 36-50.

Gilmour, B.J.J. and D.A. Stocker. *St. Mark's Church and Cemetery*. The Archaeology of Lincoln, vol. 13-1. London: Council for British Archaeology, 1986.

Giraldus Cambrensis. See Gerald of Wales.

Giusberti, Franco. *Materials for a Study on Twelfth Century Scholasticism*. Naples: Bibliopolis, 1982.

Glorieux, Palémon. "L'enseignement au moyen âge: Techniques et méthodes en usage: la Faculté de Théologie de Paris, au XIIIe siècle." *Archives d'histoire doctrinale et littéraire du moyen âge* 43 (1968) 65-186.

——. "Sommes théologiques." In *Dictionnaire de théologie catholique* (1941), 14: 2341-2350.

Glossa ordinaria; Glossa interlinearis. *Biblia sacra cum glossa ordinaria et glossa interlineari ... et postilla Nicolai Lyrani*. 7 vols. Lyons, 1545; 1590; Paris, 1590; Venice, 1603.

Goddu, A.A. and Richard H. Rouse. "Gerald of Wales and the *Florilegium Angelicum*." *Speculum* 52 (1977) 488-521.

Goering, Joseph. "The Changing Face of the Village Parish: The Thirteenth Century." In *Pathways to Medieval Peasants*. Ed. J.A. Raftis, pp. 323-333. Toronto: Pontifical Institute of Mediaeval Studies, 1981.

——. "The *Diffinicio eucaristie* Formerly Attributed to Robert Grosseteste." *Journal of Theological Studies*, ns 37 (1986) 91-104.

——. "The Popularization of Scholastic Ideas in Thirteenth Century England and an Anonymous *Speculum iuniorum*." PhD dissertation: University of Toronto, 1977.

——. "The *Summa de penitentia* of Magister Serlo." *Mediaeval Studies* 38 (1976) 1-53.

——. "The *Summa* of Master Serlo and Thirteenth-Century Penitential Literature." *Mediaeval Studies* 40 (1978) 290-311.

Goering, Joseph and F.A.C. Mantello. "The Early Penitential Writings of Robert Grosseteste." *Recherches de théologie ancienne et médiévale* 54 (1987) 52-112.

——. "The *Meditaciones* of Robert Grosseteste." *Journal of Theological Studies*, ns 36 (1985) 118-128.

——. "Notus in Iudea Deus: Robert Grosseteste's Confessional Formula in Lambeth Palace MS 499." *Viator* 18 (1987) 253-273.

——. "The 'Perambulauit Iudas ...' (Speculum confessionis) Attributed to Robert Grosseteste." *Revue bénédictine* 96 (1986) 125-168.

Gordon, James D. "The Articles of the Creed and the Apostles." *Speculum* 40 (1965) 634-640.

Grabmann, Martin. *Die Geschichte der scholastischen Methode.* 2 vols. 1909-1911; rept. Darmstadt: Wissenschaftliche Buchgesellschaft, 1957.

Graham, Rose. *Saint Gilbert of Sempringham and the Gilbertines: A History of the Only English Monastic Order.* London: Elliot Stock, 1901.

Gratian. *Decretum magistri Gratiani.* Ed. E. Friedberg. Corpus iuris canonici, 1. Leipzig: 1881.

Gründel, Johannes. *Die Lehre von den Umständen der menschlichen Handlung im Mittelalter.* Münster: Aschendorffsche Verlag, 1963.

Gsell, Benedict. *Verzeichniss der Handschriften in der Bibliothek des Stiftes Heiligenkreuz.* Vienna, 1891.

Guy of Orchelles. See Kennedy, Vincent L.

Hackett, M.B. *The Original Statutes of Cambridge University: The Text and Its History.* Cambridge: Cambridge University Press, 1970.

Haines, Roy M. "Education in English Ecclesiastical Legislation of the Later Middle Ages." In *Councils and Assemblies,* ed. G.J. Cuming and Derek Baker, pp. 161-175. Studies in Church History, 7. Cambridge: Cambridge University Press, 1971.

Häring, Nikolaus M. "The Augustinian Axiom: *Nulli Sacramento Injuria Facienda Est.*" *Mediaeval Studies* 16 (1954) 87-117.

——. "Character, Signum, und Signaculum: Die Einführung in die sacramentalischen Theologie des 12. Jahrhunderts." *Scholastik* 31 (1956) 182-212.

——. "Commentary and Hermeneutics." In *Renaissance and Renewal in the Twelfth Century,* ed. Robert L. Benson, Giles Constable, and Carol Lanham, pp. 173-200. Cambridge MA: Harvard University Press, 1982.

——. "The Interaction between Canon Law and Sacramental Theology in the 12th Century." *Proceedings of the Fourth International Congress of Medieval Canon Law,* pp. 483-493. Vatican City: Biblioteca Apostolica Vaticana, 1976.

——. "Chartres and Paris Revisited." In *Essays in Honour of Anton Charles Pegis*, ed. J. Reginald O'Donnell, pp. 268-329. Toronto: Pontifical Institute of Mediaeval Studies, 1974.

——. "Die *Sententie magistri Gisleberti Pictavensis Episcopi.*" *Archives d'histoire doctrinale et littéraire du moyen âge* 45 (1978) 83-180.

Hauréau, Barthélmy. *Notices et extraits de quelques manuscrits latins de la Bibliothèque Nationale*, 2 and 3. Paris, 1891.

Helssig, Rudolf. *Katalog der lateinischen und deutschen Handschriften der Universitäts-Bibliothek zu Leipzig*. 2 vols. Leipzig: S. Hirzel, 1926-1935.

Hewlett, Henry G., ed. *Rogeri de Wendover Liber qui dicitur Flores historiarum*. 3 vols. Rolls Series, 84. London: His Majesty's Stationer, 1886-1889.

Hildebert of Le Mans. *De mysterio missae.* PL 171: 1177-1194.

——. *Biblical Epigrams.* See Scott, A.B., et al., ed.

Hill, Francis. *Medieval Lincoln.* Cambridge: Cambridge University Press, 1948.

Hill, Peter and Richard Sharpe. "Peter of Cornwall and Launceston." *Cornish Studies* 13 (1986) 5-53.

Holdsworth, C.J. "John of Ford and English Cistercian Writing 1167-1214." *Transactions of the Royal Historical Society*, 5th series, 11 (1961) 117-136.

Honorius Augustodunensis. *Gemma animae.* PL 172: 541-738.

Hunt, Richard W. "A Manuscript Containing Extracts from the *Distinctiones monasticae.*" *Medium aevum* 44 (1975) 238-241.

——. "English Learning in the Late Twelfth Century." *Transactions of the Royal Historical Society*, 4th series, 19 (1936) 19-35.

——. *The Schools and the Cloister: The Life and Writings of Alexander Nequam (1157-1217).* Ed. and rev. Margaret Gibson. Oxford: Clarendon Press, 1984.

Huygens, R.B.C. "Guillaume de Tyr étudiant." *Latomus* 21 (1962) 811-829.

Innocent III, Pope. *De sacro altaris mysterio.* PL 217: 773-914.

——. *The Letters of Pope Innocent III (1198-1216) concerning England and Wales: A Calendar with an Appendix of Texts.* Ed. Christopher R. Cheney and Mary G. Cheney. Oxford: Clarendon Press, 1967.

——. *Selected Letters of Pope Innocent III concerning England (1198-1216).* Ed. Christopher R. Cheney and W.H. Semple. London: Thomas Nelson and Sons, 1953.

James, Montague Rhodes. *A Descriptive Catalogue of the Manuscripts in the Library of Gonville and Caius College.* 2 vols. Cambridge: Cambridge University Press, 1907.

——. "Lists of Manuscripts Formerly in Peterborough Abbey Library." *Transactions of Bibliographical Society (Supplement)* 5 (1926).

John of Salisbury. *Metalogicon*. Ed. Clement C.J. Webb. Oxford: Clarendon Press, 1929.

———. *Policratici sive De nugis curialium*. Ed. Clement C.J. Webb. 2 vols. Oxford: Clarendon Press, 1909.

Kemmler, Fritz. *"Exempla" in Context: A Historical and Critical Study of Robert Mannyng of Brunne's "Handlyng Synne."* Tübingen: Gunter Narr, 1984.

Kennedy, Vincent L. "The Handbook of Master Peter Chancellor of Chartres." *Mediaeval Studies* 5 (1943) 1-50.

———. "The Moment of Consecration and the Elevation of the Host." *Mediaeval Studies* 6 (1944) 121-150.

———. "The 'Summa de officiis ecclesiae' of Guy d'Orchelles." *Mediaeval Studies* 1 (1939) 23-62.

Ker, Neil R. "From 'Above Top Line' to 'Below Top Line': A Change in Scribal Practice." *Celtica* 5 (1960) 13-16.

———. *Medieval Libraries of Great Britain: A List of Surviving Books*. 2nd ed. London: Royal Historical Society, 1964.

Knapp, Fritz Peter. *Similitudo: Stil- und Erzählfunktion von Vergleich und Example in der lateinischen, französischen und deutschen Grossepik des Hochmittelalters*. Vienna: Wilhelm Braumüller, 1975.

Kristeller, Paul Oskar. *Latin Manuscript Books Before 1600: A List of the Printed Catalogues and Unpublished Inventories of Extant Collections*. 3rd ed. New York: Fordham University Press, 1960.

Kuttner, Stephan. "The Barcelona Edition of St. Raymond's First Treatise on Canon Law." *Seminar* 8 (1950) 52-67.

———. *Repertorium der Kanonistik (1140-1234): Prodromus Corporis Glossarum, I*. Vatican City: Biblioteca Apostolica Vaticana, 1937.

Lacombe, Georges. *La vie et les oeuvres de Prévostin*. Kain: Le Saulchoir, 1927.

Landgraf, Artur. *Dogmengeschichte der Frühscholastik*. 4 vols. Regensburg: F. Pustet, 1952-1956.

———. "Grundlagen für ein Verständnis der Busslehre der Früh- und Hochscholastik." *Zeitschrift für katholische Theologie* 51 (1927) 161-194.

———. "Scholastische Texte zur Liturgie des 12. Jahrhunderts." *Ephemerides liturgicae* 45 (1931) 211-214.

Lawrence, Clifford Hugh. *St. Edmund of Abingdon: A Study in Hagiography and History*. Oxford: Clarendon Press, 1960.

Leland, John. *Commentarii de scriptoribus Britannicis*. Oxford, 1709.

Le Neve, John. *Fasti ecclesiae Anglicanae, 1066-1300: III, Lincoln*. Ed. Diana E. Greenway. London: Institute of Historical Research, University of London, 1977.

Lesne, Emile. *Les écoles de la fin du VIIIe s. à la fin du XIIe s.* Histoire de la propriété ecclésiastique en France, 5. Lille: Giard, 1940.

Longère, Jean. *La prédication médiévale.* Paris: Etudes Augustiniennes, 1983.

Luscombe, David. "Peter Comestor." In *The Bible in the Medieval World: Essays in Memory of Beryl Smalley*, ed. Katherine Walsh and Diana Wood, pp. 109-129. Oxford: Blackwell, 1985.

Maccarrone, Michele. "'Cura animarum' e 'parochialis sacerdos' nelle costituzioni del IV concilio lateranense (1215). Applicazioni in Italia nel sec. XIII." In *Pievi e parrocchie in Italia nel basso medioevo (sec. XIII-XV)*, 1: 81-195. 2 vols. Rome: Herder, 1984.

MacKinnon, Hugh. "The Life and Works of William de Montibus." D.Phil. dissertation: Oxford University, 1959.

——. "William de Montibus: A Medieval Teacher." In *Essays in Medieval History Presented to Bertie Wilkinson*, ed. T.A. Sandquist and Michael R. Powicke, pp. 32-45. Toronto: University of Toronto Press, 1969.

Manuale ad usum percelebris ecclesiae Sarisburiensis. Ed. Arthur J. Collins. Henry Bradshaw Society, 91. London: Henry Bradshaw Society, 1960.

Martin, Janet. "Classicism and Style in Latin Literature." In *Renaissance and Renewal in the Twelfth Century*, ed. Robert L. Benson, Giles Constable, and Carol Lanham, pp. 537-568. Cambridge MA: Harvard University Press, 1982.

Mezey, Ladislaus. *Codices latini Medii Aevi Bibliothecae Universitatis Budapestinensis.* Budapest: Akadémiai Kiado, 1961.

Michaud-Quantin, Pierre. "A propos des prèmieres *Summae confessorum.*" *Recherches de théologie ancienne et médiévale* 26 (1959) 264-306.

——. "Un manuel de confession archaique dans le manuscrit Avranches 136." *Sacris erudiri* 17 (1966) 5-54.

——. *Sommes de casuistique et manuels de confession au moyen âge (XII-XVI siècles).* Louvain: Analecta mediaevalia Namurcensia, 1962.

[Miner, John N.], Br. Bonaventure. "The Teaching of Latin in Later Medieval England." *Mediaeval Studies* 23 (1961) 1-20

Missale Romanum Mediolani, 1474. Ed. Robert Lippe. 2 vols. Henry Bradshaw Society, 17, 33. London: Henry Bradshaw Society, 1899, 1907.

Moore, Philip S. *The Works of Peter of Poitiers, Master in Theology and Chancellor of Paris (1193-1205).* Notre Dame IN: University of Notre Dame Press, 1936.

Morey, Adrian. *Bartholomew of Exeter, Bishop and Canonist: A Study in the Twelfth Century, with the Text of Bartholomew's Penitential from the Cotton MS Vitellius A. XII.* Cambridge: Cambridge University Press, 1937.

Murray, Alexander. *Reason and Society in the Middle Ages.* Oxford: Clarendon Press, 1978.

Mynors, Roger A.B. *Catalogue of the Manuscripts of Balliol College Oxford.* Oxford: Clarendon Press, 1963.

Neckam, Alexander. *Alexandri Neckam De naturis rerum libri duo. With the Poem of the Same Author, De laudibus divinae sapientiae.* Ed. Thomas Wright. Rolls Series, 34. London: Longman, 1863.

Noone, Timothy B. "An Edition and Study of the *Scriptum super Metaphysicam*, bk. 12, dist. 2: A Work Attributed to Richard Rufus of Cornwall." PhD dissertation: University of Toronto, 1988.

Obituaires de la province de Sens. In *Recueil des historiens de la France*, 1. Ed. Auguste Molinier. Paris: Imprimerie nationale, 1902.

O'Conner, Mary C. *The Art of Dying Well, the Development of the "Ars moriendi."* New York: Columbia University Press, 1942.

Olsen, B. Munk. "Les classiques latins dans les florilèges médiévaux antérieurs au xiii siècle." *Revue d'histoire des textes* 9 (1979) 47-121, and 10 (1980) 115-164.

Orme, Nicholas. *English Schools in the Middle Ages.* London: Methuen, 1973.

Os, H.W. van. "Credo." In *Lexikon der christlichen Ikonographie*, ed. Engelbert Kirschbaum, pp. 461-463. Rome: Herder, 1968.

Owen, Dorothy M. *Church and Society in Medieval Lincolnshire.* History of Lincolnshire, 5. Lincoln: History of Lincolnshire Committee, 1971.

Pantin, William A. *The English Church in the Fourteenth Century.* Cambridge: Cambridge University Press, 1955.

——. "The Halls and Schools of Medieval Oxford: An Attempt at Reconstruction." In *Oxford Studies Presented to Daniel Callus*, pp. 31-100. Oxford: Clarendon Press, 1964.

Paré, Gérard M., A. Brunet, and P. Tremblay. *La renaissance du XIIe siècle: Les écoles et l'enseignement.* Ottawa: Institut d'Etudes Médiévales, 1933.

Payer, Pierre. "The Humanism of the Penitentials and the Continuity of the Penitential Tradition." *Mediaeval Studies* 46 (1984) 340-354.

Peter Abelard. See Abelard, Peter.

Peter Comestor. "Pierre le Mangeur *De sacramentis*, Texte inédit." Ed. Raymond M. Martin. In *Maître Simon et son groupe "De sacramentis": Textes inédits*, ed. Henri Weisweiler, appendix. Louvain: Spicilegium sacrum, 1937.

Peter Lombard. *Collectanea in epistolas Pauli.* PL 191: 1297-1696; 192: 9-520.

——. *Commentarium in Psalmos Davidicos.* PL 191: 55-1296.

——. *Sentences. Magistri Petri Lombardi Parisiensis episcopi Sententiae in IV libris distinctae.* 2 vols. 3rd edition. Grottaferrata: Collegium S. Bonaventurae, 1971-1981.

Peter of Blois. *Petri Blesensis...Opera omnia.* Ed. J.A. Giles. 4 vols. Oxford, 1847.

——. *Petri Blesensis...Opera omnia.* Ed. Pierre de Goussainville. Paris, 1667.

Peter of Poitiers. *Sententiae Petri Pictaviensis.* Ed. Philip S. Moore, Marthe Dulong, and Joseph N. Garvin. 2 vols. Notre Dame IN: University of Notre Dame Press, 1943, 1950.

Peter of Poitiers (of St. Victor). *Summa de confessione: Compilatio praesens.* Ed. Jean Longère. Corpus Christianorum Continuatio Mediaevalis, 51. Turnhout: Brepols, 1980.

Peter of Roissy. See Kennedy, Vincent L. "The Handbook of Master Peter Chancellor of Chartres."

Peter Riga. *Aurora Petri Rigae Biblia versificata: A Verse Commentary on the Bible.* Ed. Paul E. Beichner. 2 vols. Notre Dame IN: University of Notre Dame Press, 1965.

Peter the Chanter. *Pierre le Chantre, Summa de sacramentis et animae consiliis.* Ed. Jean-Albert Dugauquier. 5 vols. Louvain: Analecta mediae-valia Namurcensia, 1954-1967.

——. *Verbum abbreviatum.* PL 205: 23-554.

Petrus Alfonsi. *The Scholar's Guide: A Translation of the Twelfth-Century "Disciplina Clericalis" of Pedro Alfonso.* Ed. and trans. Joseph Ramon Jones and John Esteen Keller. Medieval Sources in Translation, 8. Toronto: Pontifical Institute of Mediaeval Studies, 1969.

Pitra, Jean Baptiste. *Spicilegium Solesmense.* 4 vols. Paris, 1882-1858.

Platts, Graham. *Land and People of Lincolnshire.* History of Lincolnshire, 4. Lincoln: History of Lincolnshire Committee, 1985.

Pontal, Odette. *Les statuts synodaux.* Typologie des sources du moyen âge occidental, 11. Turnhout: Brepols, 1975.

Poorter, Alphonse de. "Un catéchisme du XIII siècle." *Revue d'histoire ecclésiastique* 28 (1932) 70-74.

Poschmann, Bernhard. *Penance and the Anointing of the Sick.* Trans. and rev. Francis Courtney. Freiburg i.B.: Herder, 1964.

Post, Gaines. "Alexander III, the 'Licentia docendi' and the Rise of the Universities." In *Anniversary Essays in Mediaeval History by Students of Charles Homer Haskins.* Boston: Houghton Miflin, 1929.

Power, Eileen. *Medieval English Nunneries c. 1275 to 1535.* Cambridge: Cambridge University Press, 1922.

Powicke, F.M. *Stephen Langton.* Oxford: Clarendon Press, 1928.

Praepositinus of Cremona. *Praepositini Cremonensis Tractatus de officiis.* Ed. James A. Corbett. Notre Dame IN: University of Notre Dame Press, 1969.

Prosdocimi, Aldo Luigi. "Chierici e laici nella societ: occidentale del secolo XII: a proposito di Decr. Grat. C. 12 q. 1 c. 7: 'Duo sunt genera Christianorum.'" In *Proceedings of the second International Congress of Medieval Canon Law,* ed. Stephan Kuttner and J. Joseph Ryan, pp. 105-122. Vatican City: S. Congregatio de Seminariis et Studiorum Universitatibus, 1965.

Publilius Syrius. *Publilii Syri sententiae.* Ed. Eduard von Wölfflin. Leipzig, 1869.

Rashdall, Hastings. *The Universities of Europe in the Middle Ages*. Oxford, 1895. New ed. F.M. Powicke and A.B. Emden. 3 vols. Oxford: Clarendon Press, 1936.

Raymund of Peñafort. *Summa sti Raymundi de Peniafort ... De poenitentia, et matrimonio ...*. Rome, 1603; rept. Farnborough, 1967.

Raymund of Peñafort (Ps.). "Libellus pastoralis de cura et officio archidiaconi." In *Catalogue général des manuscrits des bibliothèques publiques des départements de France*. Ed. F. Ravaisson. 1: 592-649. Paris, 1849.

Registrum Antiquissimum of the Cathedral Church of Lincoln. Ed. C.W. Foster and Kathleen Major. 10 vols. Publications of the Lincoln Record Society, 27-29, 32, 34, 41, 42, 46, 51, 62, 67, 68. Hereford: Lincoln Record Society, 1931-1973.

Renaissance and Renewal in the Twelfth Century. Ed. Robert L. Benson, Giles Constable, and Carol D. Lanham. Cambridge MA: Harvard University Press, 1982.

Reynolds, Roger E. *The Ordinals of Christ from their Origins to the Twelfth Century*. New York: W. de Gruyter, 1978.

———. "Patristic 'Presbyterianism' in the Early Medieval Theology of Sacred Orders." *Mediaeval Studies* 45 (1983) 311-342.

Rhodes, W. E. "William de Leicester, or William du Mont." In *Dictionary of National Biography*. Ed. Sidney Lee. 21: 363-364. London: Smith, Elder and Co., 1909.

Richardson, H.G. "The Schools of Northampton in the Twelfth Century." *English Historical Review* 56 (1941) 595-605.

Rigg, A. George, and David Townsend. "Medieval Latin Poetic Anthologies (V): Matthew Paris' Anthology of Henry of Avranches (Cambridge, Univ. Library MS. Dd.11.78)." *Mediaeval Studies* 49 (1987) 352-390.

Rijk, Lambertus Marie de. *Logica modernorum: A Contribution to the History of Early Terminist Logic*. 2 vols. Assen: Van Gorcum, 1962-1967.

Robert of Flamborough. *Liber poenitentialis: A Critical Edition with Introduction and Notes*. Ed. J.J. Francis Firth. Studies and Texts, 18. Toronto: Pontifical Institute of Mediaeval Studies, 1971.

Robert Grosseteste. *Templum Dei*. Ed. Joseph Goering and F.A.C. Mantello. Toronto Medieval Latin Texts, 14. Toronto: Pontifical Institute of Mediaeval Studies, 1984.

Roberts, Phyllis Barzillay. *Stephanus de Lingua-tonante: Studies in the Sermons of Stephen Langton*. Studies and Texts, 16. Toronto: Pontifical Institute of Mediaeval Studies, 1968.

Robson, C.A. *Maurice of Sully and the Medieval Vernacular Homily: With the Text of Maurice's French Homilies from a Sens Cathedral Chapter MS*. Oxford: Blackwell, 1952.

Rochais, H. Marie. "Florilèges spirituels." In *Dictionnaire de spiritualité* (1962), 5: 435-460.

Rotuli Hugonis de Welles, Episcopi Lincolniensis, A.D. MCCIX-MCCXXXV. Ed. W.P.W. Phillimore. 3 vols. London: Canterbury and York Society, 1907-1909.

Rouse, Richard H. "Backgrounds to Print: Aspects of the Manuscript Book in Northern Europe of the Fifteenth Century." In *Proceedings of the PMR Conference*: Annual Publication of the Patristic, Mediaeval, and Renaissance Conference, 6: 37-50. Villanova: Augustinian Historical Institute, 1981.

——. "Florilegia and Latin Classical Authors in Twelfth- and Thirteenth-Century Orleans." *Viator* 10 (1979) 131-160.

Rouse, Richard H. and Mary A. Rouse. "Biblical *Distinctiones* in the Thirteenth Century." *Archives d'histoire doctrinale et littéraire du moyen âge* 41 (1974) 27-37.

——. "Florilegia of Patristic Texts." In *Les genres littéraires dans les sources théologiques et philosophiques médiévales: Définition, critique et exploitation*. Actes du Colloque international de Louvain-la-Neuve, 25-27 mai 1981, pp. 165-180. Louvain-la-Neuve: Institut d'études medievales, 1982.

——. "The *Florilegium Angelicum*: Its Origin, Content, and Influence." In *Medieval Learning and Literature: Essays Presented to R.W. Hunt*, ed. J.J.G. Alexander and M. Gibson, pp. 66-114. Oxford: Clarendon Press, 1976.

——. *Preachers, Florilegia and Sermons: Studies on the "Manipulus florum" of Thomas of Ireland*. Studies and Texts, 47. Toronto: Pontifical Institute of Mediaeval Studies, 1979.

——. "*Statim invenire*: Schools, Preachers, and New Attitudes to the Page." In *Renaissance and Renewal in the Twelfth Century*, ed. Robert L. Benson, Giles Constable, and Carol Lanham, pp. 201-225. Cambridge MA: Harvard University Press, 1982.

——. "The Verbal Concordance to the Scriptures." *Archivum Fratrum Praedicatorum* 44 (1974) 5-30.

Russell, Josiah Cox. *Dictionary of Writers of Thirteenth Century England*. 1936; rpt. New York: Burt Franklin, 1971.

Sarum Missal Edited from Three Early Manuscripts. Ed. John Wickham Legg. Oxford: Clarendon Press, 1916.

Sayers, Jane E. *Papal Judges Delegate in the Province of Canterbury 1198-1254: A Study in Ecclesiastical Jurisdiction and Administration*. Oxford: Oxford University Press, 1971.

Schmidt, Paul Gerhard. *Proverbia sententiaeque Latinitatis medii ac recentioris aevi*. New Series, 7-9. Göttingen: Vandenhoech and Ruprecht, 1982-1986.

Schneyer, Johannes B. *Repertorium der lateinischen Sermones des Mittelalters*. Beiträge zur Geschichte der Philosophie und Theologie des Mittelalters, 43/2. Münster: Aschendorff, 1970.

Scott, A.B., Deirdre F. Baker, and A.G. Rigg. "The *Biblical Epigrams* of

Hildebert of Le Mans: A Critical Edition." *Mediaeval Studies* 47 (1985) 272-316.

Silano, Giulio. "The 'Distinctiones Decretorum' of Ricardus Anglicus: An Edition." 2 vols. PhD dissertation: University of Toronto, 1981.

Smalley, Beryl. "The Gospels in the Paris Schools in the Late 12th and Early 13th Centuries: Peter the Chanter, Hugh of St. Cher, Alexander of Hales, John of la Rochelle." *Franciscan Studies* 39 (1979) 230-254.

———. *The Gospels in the Schools, 1100-1250*. London: Hambledon Press, 1985.

———. "Peter Comestor on the Gospels and His Sources." *Recherches de théologie ancienne et médiévale* 46 (1979) 84-129.

———. *Study of the Bible in the Middle Ages*. 2nd ed. Notre Dame IN: University of Notre Dame Press, 1964.

Smalley, Beryl and G. Lacombe. "The Lombard's Commentary on Isaias and Other Fragments." *New Scholasticism* 5 (1931) 123-162.

Smith, David. "The Rolls of Hugh of Wells, Bishop of Lincoln 1209-35." *Bulletin of the Institute of Historical Research* 45 (1972) 155-195.

Southern, Richard W. "From Schools to University." In *The History of the University of Oxford*, I, *The Early Oxford Schools*, ed. Jeremy I. Catto, pp. 1-36. Oxford: Clarendon Press, 1984.

———. "Master Vacarius and the Beginning of an English Academic Tradition." In *Medieval Learning and Literature: Essays Presented to Richard William Hunt*, ed. J.J.G. Alexander and M.T. Gibson, pp. 257-286. Oxford: Clarendon Press, 1976.

———. *Robert Grosseteste: The Growth of an English Mind in Medieval Europe*. Oxford: Clarendon Press, 1986.

———. "The Schools of Paris and the School of Chartres." In *Renaissance and Renewal in the Twelfth Century*, ed. Robert L. Benson, Giles Constable, and Carol Lanham, pp. 113-137. Cambridge MA: Harvard University Press, 1982.

Spencer, Helen L. "A Fifteenth-Century Translation of a Late Twelfth-Century Sermon Collection." *Review of English Studies*, ns 28 (1977) 257-267.

———. "Vernacular and Latin Versions of a Sermon for Lent: 'A Lost Penitential Homily' Found." *Mediaeval Studies* 44 (1982) 271-305.

Spicq, Ceslaus. *Esquisse d'une histoire de l'exégèse latine au moyen âge*. Paris: Vrin, 1944.

Statuta Antiqua Vniuersitatis Oxoniensis. Ed. Strickland Gibson. Oxford: Clarendon Press, 1931.

Statutes of Lincoln Cathedral. Ed. Henry Bradshaw and Christopher Wordsworth. 2 parts. Cambridge, Cambridge University Press, 1892-1897.

Stohlmann, Jürgen. "Nachträge zu Hans Walther, Initia carminum ac versuum medii aevi." *Mittellateinisches Jahrbuch* 7 (1972) 293-314; 8 (1973) 288-304; 9 (1974) 320-344; 12 (1977) 297-315; 15 (1980) 259-286; 16 (1981) 409-441.

——. "Nachträge zu Hans Walther, Proverbia sententiaeque latinitatis medii aevi." *Mittellateinisches Jahrbuch* 12 (1977) 316-329; 13 (1978) 315-333.

Talbot, C.H. "The *Centum Sententiae* of Walter Daniel." *Sacris erudiri* 11 (1960) 266-383.

Tentler, T.N. *Sin and Confession on the Eve of the Reformation*. Princeton: Princeton University Press, 1977.

Thomas of Chobham. *Thomae de Chobham Summa Confessorum*. Ed. F. Broomfield. Analecta mediaevalis Namurcensia, 25. Louvain: Nauwelaerts, 1968.

Thomson, Samuel Harrison. *The Writings of Robert Grosseteste, Bishop of Lincoln, 1235-1253*. Cambridge, 1940; rept. New York, 1971.

Thorndike, Lynn. "Unde versus." *Traditio* 11 (1955) 163-193.

Thurston, Herbert. *Life of St. Hugh of Lincoln*. London: Burns and Oates, 1898.

Tiele, P.A. *Catalogus codicum manu scriptorum bibliothecae Universitatis Rheno-Trajectinae*. 2 vols. Utrecht, 1887.

Transcripts of Charters relating to the Gilbertine Houses of Sixle, Ormsby, Catley, Bullington and Alvingham. Ed. Frank M. Stenton. Lincoln Record Society, 18. Horncastle: Morton and Sons, 1922.

Van Engen, John H. "Observations on the *De consecratione*." In *Proceedings of the Sixth International Congress of Medieval Canon Law*, pp. 309-320. Vatican City: Biblioteca Apostolica Vaticana, 1985.

Vansteenkiste, C.M. Joris. "'Versus' dans les oeuvres de Saint Thomas." In *St. Thomas Aquinas 1274-1974: Commemorative Studies*, ed. Armand A. Maurer. 2 vols. 1: 77-85. Toronto: Pontifical Institute of Mediaeval Studies, 1974.

Verger, Jacques. "Des Ecoles à l'université: La mutation institutionelle." In *La France de Philippe Auguste: Le temps des mutations*, ed. Robert-Henri Bautier, pp. 817-845. Paris: Centre National de la recherche scientifique, 1982.

Vogel, Cyrille. *Les "Libri paenitentiales."* Typologie des sources du moyen âge occidental, 27. Turnhout: Brepols, 1978.

Walther, Hans. *Initia carminum ac versuum medii aevi posterioris latinorum*. Göttingen: Vandenhoech and Ruprecht, 1959.

——. *Proverbia sententiaeque latinitatis medii aevi*. 6 vols. Göttingen: Vandenhoech and Ruprecht, 1963-1967.

Walz, Angelus. "Des Aage von Dänemark, *Rotulus pugillaris* im Lichte der alten dominikanischen Konventstheologie." *Classica et mediaevalia* 15 (1954) 198-252, and 16 (1955) 136-94.

Warichez, Joseph. *Etienne de Tournai et son temps, 1128-1203*. Tournai: Casterman, 1936.

Weisweiler, Henri. "Das Sakrament der Firmung in den systematischen Werken der ersten Frühscholastik." *Scholastik* 7 (1933) 481-523.

Welter, J.-Th. *L'exemplum dans la littérature religieuse et didactique du moyen âge.* Paris: Guitard, 1927.

Wenzel, Siegfried. "Robert Grosseteste's Treatise on Confession, *Deus est.*" *Franciscan Studies* 30 (1970) 218-293.

——. *Verses in Sermons: "Fasciculus Morum" and Its Middle English Poems.* Cambridge MA: Mediaeval Academy of America, 1978.

——. "Vices, Virtues, and Popular Preaching." *Medieval and Renaissance Studies* 6 (1976) 28-54.

Wieland, Georg. *Ethica — Scientia practica: Die Anfänge der philosophischen Ethik im 13. Jahrhundert.* Münster: Aschendorff, 1981.

Wilmart, André. "Les mélanges de Mathieu Préchantre de Rievaulx au début du XIIIe siècle." *Revue bénédictine* 52 (1940) 15-84.

——. "Un répertoire d'exégèse composé en Angleterre vers le début du XIIIe siècle." *Mémorial Lagrange*, pp. 307-346. Paris, 1940.

Wordsworth, Christopher and Henry Littlehales. *The Old Service-Books of the English Church.* London: Methuen, 1904.

Zink, Michel. *La prédication en langue romane avant 1300.* Paris: Champion, 1976.

Index

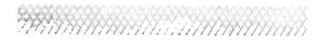